Orbital Tumors

Orbital Tumors

Diagnosis and Treatment

ZEYNEL A. KARCIOGLU, MD
Professor of Ophthalmology and Pathology
Dr. George Haik, Sr./St. Giles Professor of Ocular Oncology
Director, O'Brien Ocular Pathology Laboratory
Consultant, Tulane Cancer Center
Tulane University Health Sciences Center
New Orleans, Lousiana

With 482 Illustrations, 276 in Color

Springer

Zeynel A. Karcıoglu, MD
Professor of Ophthalmology and Pathology
Dr. George Haik, Sr./St. Giles Professor of Ocular Oncology
Director, O'Brien Ocular Pathology Laboratory
Consultant, Tulane Cancer Center
Tulane University Health Sciences Center
New Orleans, LA 70112
USA

Library of Congress Cataloging-in-Publication Data
Orbital tumors : diagnosis and treatment / [edited by] Zeynel A. Karcıoglu.
p. ; cm.
Includes bibliographical references and index.
ISBN 0-387-21321-X (h/c : alk. paper)
1. Eye-sockets—Tumors. I. Karcioglu, Zeynel A.
[DNLM: 1. Orbital Neoplasms—diagnosis. 2. Orbital Neoplasms—therapy. WW 202 O645 2004]
RC280.E9O75 2004
616.99'484—dc22 2004046867

ISBN 0-387-21321-X Printed on acid-free paper.

Printed in China. (MP/EVB)

9 8 7 6 5 4 3 2 1 SPIN 10938430

springeronline.com

Preface

About every 10 years a new book appears on any given medical specialty subject. Naturally, this is not because the entire body of knowledge in that specialty is overhauled every 10 years but because the progress made over a decade usually warrants expressing new perspectives on quite a few diseases. Orbital oncology certainly qualifies as a subspecialty that merits an update every decade. At least two or three excellent textbooks on orbital tumors have been written since the mid-1980s. This book reports advances in knowledge about orbital diseases and their treatment and offers an up-to-date, single-volume reference for orbital tumors with particular emphasis on new improvements in diagnostic and therapeutic measures.

I cannot claim deep personal knowledge on all the topics covered; this work would not have been possible without the expert help of the contributing authors and the work of others who published their findings in the medical literature of the past four decades. The contributors were selected not only from ocular oncologists but also from practitioners in other fields, including radiology, pathology, neurosurgery, medical and radiation oncology, and plastic surgery to expand the input from other clinical disciplines into daily practice. My role as the editor and author was to study others' work, analyze it critically by sifting it through the filter of my own experience in ophthalmology and oncology, and present the whole as an informative package. My contributions as an author in 16 chapters are influenced by my ways of thinking and doing; the reader should be aware of these prejudices; I alone am responsible for any errors of omission and commission.

Part I comprises advances in oncogenesis and its relationship to orbital tumors. Changes in the biological behavior of diseases in the general patient population are much slower than technological advances; nevertheless, those alterations take place as well. One of the major medical issues of our time, for example, is the changes in the immunological status of individuals. This issue influences the entire field of medicine, particularly oncology, including the treatment of orbital tumors. Chapters 2 to 5 summarize these influences.

Medical genetics gained momentum during the past two decades and now affects the clinical practice of almost every discipline of medicine, including ophthalmology and orbitology. Chapters on principles of molecular genetics and immunosurveillance mechanisms of neoplasia and on the occurrence of multiple, malignant neoplasms in retinoblastoma have been included to apply molecular concepts to clinical practice related to orbital tumors.

Advances in one discipline often directly benefit practice in another field. In orbitology, no development has been more influential than the revolution in imaging techniques, including ultrasonography, computerized tomography, and magnetic resonance methods. Four chapters in Part II are devoted to the role of imaging in diagnosis of orbital tumors. Other diagnostic advances entailing immunohistochemistry, flow cytometry, gene microarray, and the polymerase chain reaction are summarized in a separate chapter on orbital biopsy.

A brief section on inflammatory, space-occupying lesions of the orbit is presented in Part VI, including infectious and other inflammatory conditions and thyroid-associated orbitopathy (Graves disease).

Up-to-date information on treatment of orbital tumors is summarized in Part VII. Brief but current staging of malignant orbital tumors is included and advances in surgical, radiation,and chemotherapy are summarized in a practical fashion. Not only is the book intended to help general ophthalmologists, oculoplastic surgeons, and orbitologists in their daily practice, it is also a reference for pediatricians, radiologists, pathologists, neurosurgeons, and otolaryngologists who are dealing with orbital tumors.

ZEYNEL A. KARCIOGLU, MD

Acknowledgments

Many people helped me during the preparation of this book, ranging from friends offering advice on its structure and contents to colleagues generously allowing me to use their case material to skilled archivists and librarians; I am sorry that I will not be able to acknowledge them all. Fellow physicians, residents, and students have read the chapters at various stages and have shared their thoughts and criticisms with me and called my attention to bibliographic items I would otherwise have missed. I am indebted to all who have helped to focus the book on its objectives. My primary goal was to make a single-volume book that would be a practical guide to help general ophthalmologists and other specialists, as well as fellows, residents, and other postgraduate trainees in their daily practice.

The staff of the Medical Library at Tulane Health Sciences Center has been very helpful in search and retrieval of materials; I specifically want to mention the help of Katherine Puglia and Patricia Copeland.

Donald Oliveras and James LeBlanc were of immeasurable assistance in the digital preparation of medical photographs and figure composites. Susanne V. Harbin-Remus, Susan Gilbert, and Anne-Marie H. Williams were also extremely helpful with the figures and illustrations. I also acknowledge the help of my clinical assistant, Tammy Vollmer-Slowey, and the Tulane University Hospital operating room personnel, Denise Indorf, Ann Bonvechio, Sharon Wilson, and Rhonda Lindblom, who patiently tolerated many interruptions of my surgical cases for photographs and helped me immensely to document surgical and pathological material with still photography and videos.

New to me have been the professional support and friendship I have received from Springer-Verlag New York, Inc., particularly Merry Post, the developmental editor of the book, and executive editors Paula Callaghan and Laura Craven. Without the unwavering attention and diligence of Mrs. Post, this book could not have materialized. I greatly acknowledge the assistance of my secretaries Nedra Roper and Judy Marcus, as well as the help of Paula Hildebrand, Sheila Lawshe, Bea Delucca, and Corlis Trepagnier.

I am also thankful to the American Joint Committee on Cancer for allowing the use, in Chapter 30, of parts of the sixth edition of *The Cancer Staging Manual*. I am also indebted to the St. Giles Foundation of New York City and the Turkish American Ophthalmic Society, Inc. of Atlanta for their unrestricted grants, which were in part utilized for this book.

Above all, I thank my wife and son, who have always given their intellectual, practical, and moral support from beginning to end.

Zeynel A. Karcioglu, MD

Contents

Part III Primary Tumors of the Orbit

Part IV Secondary Tumors of the Adult Orbit

Part V Pediatric Orbital Tumors and Pseudotumors

Part VI Tumorlike Conditions in the Orbit

Contributors

MICHAEL D. ABRAMOFF, MD, PHD, MSC
Staff, Department of Ophthalmology, Vrije Universiteit University Hospital, 1081 HV Amsterdam, The Netherlands

GRACE ABOU CHACRA, MD
Staff, Department of Ophthalmology, American University of Beirut, Beirut, Lebanon

J. OSCAR CROXATTO, MD
Chairman, Department of Ophthalmic Pathology, Fundacion Oftalmologica Argentina Jorge Malbran, Azcuenaga 1077 2B, Buenos Aires, Argentina

ANTONIO AUGUSTO V. CRUZ, MD, PHD
Faculdade de Medicina de Ribeirão Preto, Departmento de Oftalmologia e Otorrinolaringologia e Cirurgia de Cabeça e Pescoço, Universidade de São Paulo, Hospital das Clinicas-Campus, Ribeirão Preto, São Paulo, Brazil

PATRICK DE POTTER, MD
Professor and Chair, Department of Ophthalmology, Cliniques Universitaires St-Luc, B 1200 Brussels 1200 Belgium

BITA ESMAELI, MD, FACS
Associate Professor and Chief, Department of Plastic Surgery, Section of Ophthalmology, The University of Texas M. D. Anderson Cancer Center, Houston, TX 77030, USA

MISHA FAUSTINA, MD
Fellow in Oculoplastic Surgery, MD Anderson Cancer Center, The University of Texas MD Anderson Cancer Center, Houston, TX 77030, USA

PAUL T. FINGER, MD, FACS
Clinical Professor of Ophthalmology, New York University School of Medicine, New York, NY 10016, USA; Director, The New York Eye Cancer Center, New York, NY 10021, USA

GUILLERMO A. FRIDRICH, MD
Oculoplastic Surgeon, Clinica de Ojos Dr Nano—Universidad de Buenos Aires, San Miguel, Buenos Aires, Argentina

CARLOS GALINDO-RODRIQUEZ, MD
Department of Hematology-Oncology, University of Tennessee, Memphis, TN 38163, USA

KAAN GÜNDÜZ, MD
Associate Professor of Ophthalmology, Ankara University Medical School, Maltepe 06570, Ankara, Turkey

Doris Hadjistilianou, MD
Associate Professor of Ophthalmology, Chief, Retinoblastoma Referral Center, Department of Ophthalmology, University of Siena, Italy

Barrett G. Haik, MD
Hamilton Professor and Chair, Department of Ophthalmology, University of Tennessee, Memphis, TN 38163, USA

Jeffrey J. Hurwitz, MD
Professor and Chair, Department of Ophthalmology, Mount Sinai Hospital, Toronto, Ontario M5G 1X5, Canada

Zeynel A. Karcioglu, MD
Professor of Ophthalmology and Pathology, Dr. George Haik, Sr./St. Giles Professor of Ocular Oncology, Director, O'Brien Ocular Pathology Laboratory, Consultant, Tulane Cancer Center, Tulane University Health Sciences Center, New Orleans, LA 70112, USA

Yoon-Duck Kim, MD
Professor and Chair, Department of Ophthalmology, Sungkyunkwan University, School of Medicine, Samsung Medical Center, Seoul, Korea 135–230

Georgina Kourt, FANZCO
Consultant, Oculoplastic Unit, Sydney Eye Hospital, Sydney, 2000 Australia

Andrew G. Lee, MD
Professor of Ophthalmology, University of Iowa Hospitals and Clinics, Iowa City, IA 5222, USA

Peter Martin, MBBS, FANZCO
Director, Oculoplastics Department, Sydney Eye Hospital, Lecturer, Save Sight Institute, Sydney University, Sydney 2022, Australia

Christopher R. Mascott, MD
Professor, Department of Neurosurgery, Paul Sabatier University, 3103 Toulouse, France

Domenico Mastrangelo, MD
Staff, Department of Ophthalmology, Ocular Oncology Unit, University of Siena, 53100 Siena, Italy

Alan A. McNab, FRANZCO
Director, Orbital Plastic and Lacrimal Clinic, Royal Victorian Eye and Ear Hospital, Melbourne, Australia

Amin M. Nasr, MD
Professor of Clinical Ophthalmology, American University of Beirut, Beirut, Lebanon

Luis E. Remus III, MD, PhD
Resident in Pathology and Laboratory Medicine, Department of Pathology, Tulane University Health Sciences Center, New Orleans, LA 70112, USA

Paul Rosel, MD
Chief of Neuroradiology, Section of Interventional Neuroradiology, Tulane Hospital and Clinics, Tulane University Health Sciences Center, New Orleans, LA 70112, USA

Marta K. Rozans, MD, PhD
Associate Professor of Clinical Pediatrics, Tulane University Health Sciences Center, New Orleans, LA 70112, USA

Daniel Weil, MD
Centro Andaluz de Oftalmologia. Sevilla, Glorieta Plus Ultra number 1. Av. de la Palmera 10131, Sevilla, Spain

Matthew W. Wilson, MD, FACS
Assistant Professor of Ophthalmology, University of Tennessee Health Science Center, Department of Ophthalmology, Memphis, TN 38163, USA

Johan Zwaan, MD
Clinical Professor of Ophthalmology, The University of Texas Health Science Center of San Antonio, San Antonio, TX 78229, USA

PART ONE

Current Concepts of Oncogenesis

1

Molecular Models of Cancer Development

Domenico Mastrangelo

HISTORICAL OVERVIEW

Cancer is every malignant tumor whose cells have the properties of endless replication, loss of contact inhibition, invasiveness, and the ability to metastasize and whose result, generally, if left untreated, is fatal.[1] Cancer cells typically display three distinct phenotypes that are not associated with normal cells:

1. Immortalization: an indefinite proliferative life span
2. Transformation: the loss of response to normal regulation of cell growth
3. Metastasis: the ability to leave the tumor and invade other tissues at another location in the body

A close relationship between chromosomal alterations and cancer was postulated by Theodor Boveri, who conducted experiments on double-fertilized sea urchin eggs. Boveri demonstrated the following:

- Individual chromosomes carry different information.[2,3]
- The unresticted growth of tumor cells resembles the same abnormal growth of double-fertilized sea urchin eggs carrying the wrong chromosomal complement.[4]

In his last book, on the origin of malignant tumors, Boveri[5] concluded that malignancy is the result of inappropriate balance of instructions (genetic information) in the tumor cells.

The extraordinary relevance of the discoveries made by Boveri in the field of cancer can be fully appreciated only in light of the fact that it took almost 50 years after the publication of his monograph to find out that chronic myeloid leukemia (CML) is associated with a characteristic chromosomal aberration (the Philadelphia chromosome),[6] another decade to identify the chromosomes involved in the translocation producing this aberrant chromosome,[7] a further decade to identify the genes fused and activated as a result of this translocation,[8] and almost two more decades to develop a drug against the fusion protein (BCR-ABL) produced by the gene activated as a result of the chromosomal translocation.[9]

At the time of Boveri's investigations, the concept of the gene was not developed yet. Subsequent research on his observations seemed to demonstrate the following:

- Except for the Philadelphia chromosome in CML, "cancer-specific" aneuploidy is very rare.
- Aneuploidy may not necessarily be associated to cancer development (as shown by the Down Syndrome).
- Cancers can be diploid (in the early stages of cancers of viral origin).[10]

This last observation originated from studies made by Peyton Rous who in 1911 was able to repeatedly induce tumors in a particular breed of chicken by means of tumor-derived cell-free filtrates, probably containing a virus.[11] By the early 1970s, virologist Hidesaburo Hanafusa showed that the *Rous sarcoma virus* (RSV) contains a gene (called *src* for sarcoma) that produces a protein necessary for cancer development.[12] Removing the gene prevented the virus from inducing cancer.[13] These discoveries led researchers to entirely abandon Boveri's idea that aneuploidy was at the basis of the unregulated growth of tumor cells and to shift the focus of cancer research to genes and gene mutations.

At about the same period, Howard Temin,[14–16] together with David Baltimore and Renato Dulbecco, observed that certain viruses were able to synthesize DNA from RNA by using an enzyme called *reverse transcriptase* (RT). The viruses that produce this enzyme were called *retroviruses*, and the RSV was found to belong to this group.

This discovery not only definitively disproved the accepted dogma that protein synthesis within the cell proceeds as a one-way process, from DNA to RNA and to protein, it also had relevant consequences for further investigations in the field of cancer research. In the late 1970s, Michael Bishop and Harold Varmus identified cellular *src* (c-*src*) homologues in organisms as diverse as fruit flies, chicken, fish, mammals, and humans. These cellular genes (c-*onc*) are present in normal cells, where they play an essential role in cell growth regulation (*proto–oncogenes*). When they become overexpressed or mutated (*oncogenes*), they are able to confer to the cells the traits of rapid, uncontrolled growth that are typical of many tumors.[17–19]

ONCOGENES

Oncogenes represent the first identified class of activated human genes responsible for tumor development in humans. A short list of these genes is given in Table 1.1. The distinction between the terms "*proto-oncogene*" and "*oncogene*" relates to the activity of the protein product of the gene. A *proto-oncogene* is a gene whose protein product plays an essential role in cell growth regulation and has the capacity to induce cellular transformation if it sustains a genetic insult. An *oncogene* is a gene that has sustained genetic damage and therefore produces a protein capable of cellular transformation.

Many proto-oncogenes code for proteins that relay growth stimulating signals from outside the cell to deep within its interior. Cell-to-cell signaling begins when one cell secretes a protein called growth factor. The growth factor moves into the intercellular space and binds to the receptors located on the target cell membrane. After that binding, the receptor conveys a proliferative signal to proteins located in the cytoplasm, in a cascade of protein activation that, in turn, brings the signal to the nucleus, where other proteins, known as *transcription factors* (TFs), respond by activating a cohort of genes to usher the cell through its growth cycle (Figure 1.1).

Some oncogenes force cells to overproduce growth factors. Sarcomas and gliomas, of particular interest for this book, overproduce *platelet-derived growth factor* (PDGF). Other cancers overproduce *transforming growth factor* α (TGF-α). These growth factors can drive proliferation in the same cell producing them.

Oncogenic versions of growth factors' receptor genes that induce aberrant receptors to release a flood of proliferative signals within the cell, in the absence of growth factors have been also identified. This is the case, for example, of the Erb-b2 oncogenic protein. In other cases, oncogenes perturb the cytoplasmic signal cascade. This is the case with the RAS *oncogene*, which normally (proto-oncogene) conveys stimulatory signals from growth factor receptors farther down the line, but, when activated, fires continuously even when growth factors are not prompting it.

Still another family of oncogenes, such as those belonging to the *Myc* family, alter the activity of transcription factors within the nucleus. Cells normally produce *Myc transcription factor* when the cell surface is stimulated by growth factors. Myc proteins, in turn, activate genes that stimulate cell growth. However, in many types of cancer, such as blood malignancies, Myc levels are kept high even in the absence of growth factors.[20] Since the discovery and characterization of the first oncogene, a great number of other oncogenes have been added to the list. For detailed information regarding the types, mechanisms of action, and related tumors and proto-oncogenes see the Park reference[21]. For the purposes of this chapter, the list in Table 1.1 is an acceptable synthesis.

From the point of view of Mendelian genetics, oncogenes act in a dominant fashion: that is, a single activated copy (oncogene) of the allelic pair is able to induce cell transformation.

TUMOR SUPPRESSOR GENES

In 1971, while researchers were still identifying new members of the family of oncogenes, Alfred G. Knud-

TABLE 1.1. Oncogenes.[a]

Growth factors or receptors for growth factors	PDGF: platelet-derived growth factor (brain and breast cancer) erb-B receptor for epidermal growth factor (brain and breast cancer) erb-B2 receptor for growth factor (breast, salivary, and ovarian cancers) RET growth factor receptor (thyroid cancer)
Cytoplasmic relays in stimulatory signaling pathways	K*ras* activated by active growth factor receptor proteins (lung, ovarian, colon, and pancreatic cancer) N-*ras* activated by active growth factor receptor proteins (leukemias) c-*src*, a protein kinase that becomes overactive in phosphorylation of target proteins
Transcription factors that activate growth promoting genes	c-*myc* activates transcription of growth stimulation genes (leukemia, breast, stomach, and lung cancer) N-*myc* (nerve and brain cancer) L-*myc* (lung cancer) c-*jun* and c-*fos* function as transcription factors
Molecules of other types	Bcl-2 normal protein blocks cell suicide (lymphoma) Bcl-1 codes for cyclin D1, stimulatory protein of the cell cycle (breast, neck, and head cancers) MDM2 codes for antagonist of p53 (sarcomas)

These genes are associated with the stimulation of cell division. Cancers result from mutation in only one allele of the gene.

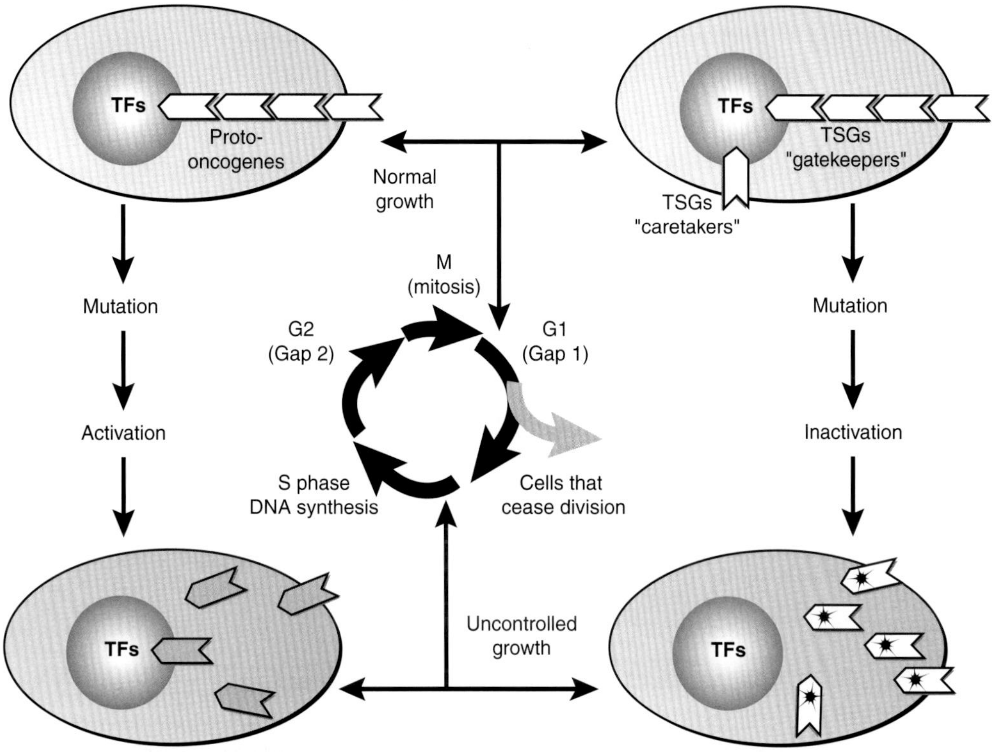

FIGURE 1.1. The relationship between the activation of oncogenes or the inactivation of tumor suppressor genes (TSGs) and the cell cycle. When the normal activity of these cancer genes is lost, cells are pushed toward the S phase of the cell cycle, inevitably leading to increased mitotic activity and uncontrolled proliferation.

son,[22] by studying several cases of retinoblastoma (Rb) demonstrated that this rare eye tumor affecting infants and young children, is likely to depend on two sequential mutations affecting a key gene, still unknown at that time. The hypothesis, formulated by Knudson to explain the different clinical phenotypes of retinoblastoma, was based on the study of the relationships between age at diagnosis, clinical phenotype (unilateral vs bilateral disease), and number of tumor foci per affected eye. When the first mutation is transmitted genetically from one of the parents, all the somatic cells of the individual will carry it. As a consequence, the individual will be likely to develop, at an early age, a tumor affecting both eyes (bilateral Rb), with multiple foci and, given the first mutation in all somatic cells, an increased susceptibility to develop second nonocular tumors. On the other hand, when both the first and second mutations affect the somatic cell (the retinoblast), the individual will develop, later in life, a retinoblastoma affecting, commonly a single eye (unilateral Rb), with a single tumor focus and no susceptibility to second nonocular tumors.

Molecular studies using genetic markers that are heterozygous in the majority of individuals showed that tumor genotypes of affected patients usually differ from the corresponding constitutional genotype (e.g., the genetic makeup of patient's blood cells). In its most simplified expression, this was evidenced as difference in the electrophoretic migration pattern of selected DNA markers. When these markers were found to show a typical two-band model indicating heterozygosity in the patient's constitutional genotype (e.g., nucleated blood cells), it was common to find a single band, indicating homozygosity, when the tumor DNA of the same patient was comparatively analyzed (Figure 1.2). As described by Cavenee et al.,[23] this phenomenon, called *loss of heterozygosity (LOH)*, was considered to be specific to tumors involving the loss or inactivation of a new type of cancer gene and, as shown in Figure 1.2, seemed to represent the physical demonstration of the "two-hit" model hypothesized by Knudson in the genesis of retinoblastoma.

With the introduction of the polymerase chain reaction (PCR), which allows the amplification of large amounts of specific DNA fragments, and the concurrent discovery of a number of new genetic markers from within specific genes, molecular analysis of cancer became available on a larger scale and armed clinical oncologists with a powerful new tool for genetic counseling and prenatal/presymptomatic diagnosis of different types of cancer.[24] Further investigations of a suspect gene for the development of this tumor led to the identification of the gene *Rb1*, located in the long arm of chromosome 13 (13q14), and, most important, opened a completely new line of research on cancer genes. When

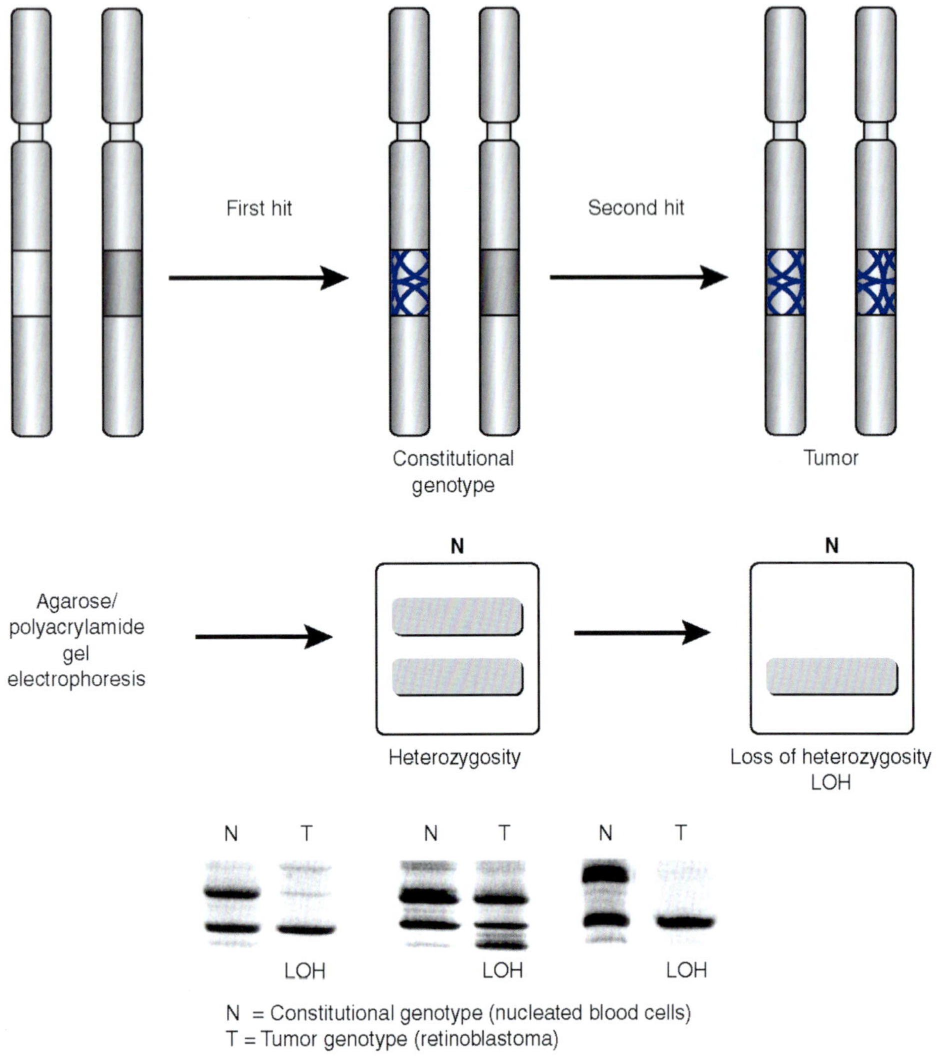

FIGURE 1.2. Schematic illustration of the "two-hit" hypothesis of cancer development. A number of different mechanisms have been postulated to explain how a heterozygous genetic marker is reduced to homozygosity in the tumor cells. Whatever the mechanism involved, the final result is a characteristic band pattern when DNA electrophoresis is performed to compare the constitutional (blood) and the tumor genotypes. The tumor cells are said to show a loss of heterozygosity (LOH). The bonds for the three retinoblastomas at the bottom of the figure show a clear LOH pattern.

considered from the point of view of Mendelian genetics, *Rb1*, as opposed to the known oncogenes, seemed to behave in a "recessive" way. That is, to develop a fully expressed disease, it seemed necessary for *both copies* of the gene to be lost or inactivated, thus implying that even a single functional gene is normally sufficient to inhibit the proliferative activity of the cell.[25] Therefore, it became evident that the cell contains genes of two different types that regulate its proliferative capacity, one with stimulatory (oncogenes) and the other with inhibitory activity. This last category of cancer genes, of which *Rb1* represents the prototype,[26,27] was called *tumor suppressor genes* (TSGs).

TSGs normally function to inhibit, or "put the brakes on," the cycle of cell growth and division; that is, they function to prevent the development of tumors. As for oncogenes, this task is accomplished by a number of heterogeneous proteins in a number of different ways.

- TGF-β can stop the growth of normal cells of various kinds; some colon cancer cells become oblivious to TGF-β by inactivating a gene that encodes a surface receptor for this substance.
- A variety of cancers discard the p15 gene, which normally codes for a protein needed to shut down the machinery guiding the cell through its growth cycle.
- Some TSGs, such as *NF1*, the gene for *neurofibromatosis* type 1, block the flow of signals through the growth stimulatory pathway (RAS *oncogene)*.
- Some other genes, currently considered TSGs, are involved in the repair of DNA mismatches; still others are involved in the apoptotic cascade.

More recently, a simplified classification proposed two different functions for these genes, namely that of *caretakers*, or guardians of the integrity of the genetic material, and that of *gatekeepers*, or regulators of tumor growth by inhibition of cell growth or by promotion of cell death. According to this classification, both *caretakers* and *gatekeepers* share the characteristics of "recessive" genes (i.e., two mutations are necessary for inactivation), whose mutation predisposes to neoplasia. However, the *caretaker* pathway to neoplasia, leading to genetic instability, requires more mutational events than the *gatekeeper* pathway.[28] A short list of TSGs is given in Table 1.2.

The discovery of TSGs seemed to complete the picture of how the cell can be transformed by endogenous influences of opposite sign on its proliferative activity, that is, the activation of the stimulatory pathway (oncogenes) or the disruption of the inhibitory pathway (TSGs). In both cases, the deregulation implies the loss of the normal control these genes exert on the entrance into the cell cycle or the permanence of the cell in a quiescent state (G0) (Figure 1.1).

DNA MUTATIONS AND CANCER

The discovery and characterization of both oncogenes and TSGs represented outstanding achievements in the understanding of the molecular pathogenesis of cancer. An important step in this process has been the elucidation of the mechanisms by which proto-oncogenes are activated to oncogenes and TSGs are inactivated, resulting in the uncontrolled growth that characterizes cancer cells. Further investigations on oncogenes made it clear that their activation in cancer cells can be ascribed to several different mechanisms, as follows:

1. Structural alterations of the genes:
   - Point mutations
   - Chromosomal translocations, such as the t(9;22) in chronic myeloid leukemia
2. Gene amplification (e.g., *NMYC* amplification in neuroblastoma) evidenced as either
   - Small separate chromosomes (double minutes) or
   - Insertions within normal chromosomes (homogeneously staining regions, or HSR)
3. Loss of appropriate control mechanisms, by either
   - Chromosome translocation (translocation of the *MYC* gene on chromosome 8 to one of the immunoglobulin loci on chromosome 14 in Burkitt's lymphoma) or
   - Insertional mutagenesis (insertion of a DNA copy of a retrovirus into the cellular genome close to a proto-oncogene)[29]

Despite the reported variety of the mechanisms involved in the activation of proto-oncogenes, the proposed mechanisms of inactivation of TSGs has remained limited to the structural alteration evolving from a single base (point mutation) to wider portions of the genome. With the increasing interest in TSGs and the potential application of genetic testing to the early diagnosis or identification of predisposition to cancer, the role of mutations in cancer development has become increasingly relevant. Indeed, most researchers worldwide acknowledge no "cause" of cancer other than mutation.

In one of the following paragraphs on gene methylation, we will see that the close relationship between mutations and cancer should be viewed with a more relativistic eye, since gene expression may be altered even in the absence of structural alterations of genes. Moreover, considering the complexity of cell structure and function, and the number of different environmental influences a cell undergoes during its vital cycle, limiting the possible molecular pathogenesis of cancer to one or two mutations within a single gene, as in the case of retinoblastoma, appears to be a very restricted view of the problem.

NEW PERSPECTIVES ON DNA MUTATIONS

Studies on hereditary nonpolyposis colorectal cancer (HNPCC) have shown that affected individuals may inherit an inactive copy of one of the *DNA mismatch repair genes*. The main function of these genes is to produce proteins whose primary function is to iden-

TABLE 1.2. Tumor Suppressor Genes.[a]

Genes for cytoplasmic proteins	*APC* (colon and stomach cancers)
	DPC4 codes for relay molecule in cell division inhibitory pathway (pancreatic cancer)
	NF1 codes for protein that inhibits a stimulatory (Ras) protein (brain, nerve, and leukemia)
	NF2 (brain and nerve cancers)
Genes for nuclear proteins	*MTS1* codes for p16 protein, brake on cell cycle clock (many cancers)
	RB codes for pRB protein, master brake on cell cycle (retinoblastoma, bone, bladder, lung, and breast cancer)
	p53 codes for p53 protein, halts cell cycle in G1, and induces cell suicide (many cancers)
	p16 inhibits cyclin D-dependent kinase activity
	WT1 (Wilms tumor of the kidney)
	BRCA1 functions in repair of damage to DNA (breast and ovarian cancers)
	BRCA2 functions in repair of damage to DNA (breast cancer)
Location not clear	*VHL* (kidney cancer)

These genes are associated with inhibition of cell division. Cancers require both alleles of the gene to be altered.

tify and correct DNA replication errors. Mismatch repair prevents spontaneous mutation; therefore, cells defective in the *DNA mismatch repair enzymes system* may accumulate mutations at rates several hundredfold higher than normal.

Randomly dispersed throughout the human genome are tens of thousands of *microsatellites*, long stretches of reiterated mono- or dinucleotides: for example A_n (A = adenine; *n* = repeated *n* times) or $(C\text{-}A)_n$ (C-A = cytosine–adenine dinucleotide; e.g., $CACACACA_n$). The accurate replication of such repetitive DNA is usually compromised by the tendency of template and daughter DNA strands to misalign during DNA synthesis. In cells with defective DNA mismatch repair enzyme system, the precise control of *microsatellite* length is lost, and therefore, the cells contain many thousands of altered *microsatellites*. This accumulation of mutated repeats is commonly known as *microsatellite instability (MSI)*, which is the defining characteristic of mismatch-repair-deficient tumors.

MSI is a continuing process and is a direct consequence of failure to rectify replication errors. In practice, MSI is defined by differences in the lengths of several microsatellites between DNA from tumor and normal tissue of the same individual.[30] In principle, the two alleles of a given chromosome of an individual contains microsatellite DNA made of repeats (e.g., CA repeats) of unequal length. In "genetic" terms this means that individuals are most frequently heterozygous (they have two different copies of the same DNA portion in the two homologue copies of the same chromosome) for most of the known microsatellite sequences within their genome. This implies that microsatellites are genetic markers of great value in detecting the LOH process, which characterizes cancers that are due to the loss or inactivation of TSGs. In routine laboratory activity, microsatellite DNA can be easily amplified by using the PCR. The amplified DNA is analyzed by resolving it through a polyacrylamide gel, where it can be evidenced as a band pattern that is characteristic of any single microsatellite in each individual.

While microsatellites have long been considered to be genetic markers useful in detecting LOH in the tumor genotype, as opposed to the somatic genotype of the affected individual, their widespread use in the characterization of different tumors has revealed that MSI is another relevant process in carcinogenesis. In simplified terms, the difference between LOH and MSI resides in the qualitative difference of the DNA migration patterns one can find when the constitutional (nucleated blood cells) and the tumor genotypes of an affected individual are compared. LOH is the loss of one or more bands in the tumors with respect to the related constitutional genotype. MSI is not a loss but a band shift, as shown in Figure 1.3, which presents three cases of MSI in embryonal rhabdomyosarcoma of the orbit.

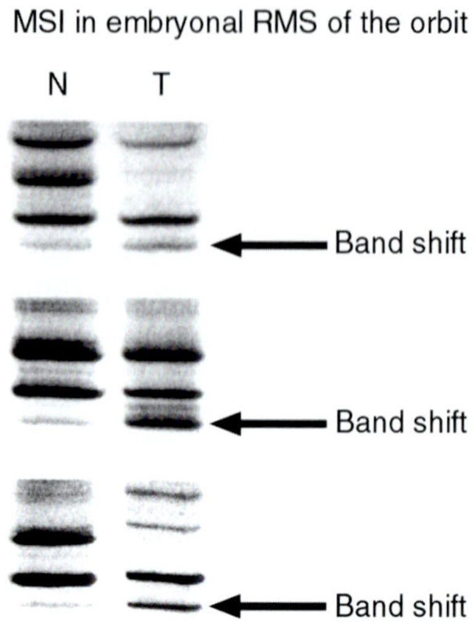

FIGURE 1.3. Three examples of MSI in embryonal rhabdomyosarcoma of the orbit. MSI, like LOH, is a modification, in comparison to the normal constitutional cells (blood) of the affected individual, of the DNA migration pattern of tumor cells as revealed on agarose or polyacrylamide gel. Unlike LOH, which is evidenced as the loss of one or more bands in the tumor DNA, MSI is a qualitative difference that is evidenced as a "band shift."

Cells with a defective mismatch repair system are said to carry a *mutator phenotype*, a phenotype in which many genes carry mutations because of uncorrected errors in DNA replication. These cells are also said to carry *genome instability*, the process leading, through accelerated somatic evolution, to a genomically heterogeneous population of cells naturally selected for their ability to proliferate and invade, while simultaneously evading host defenses.[31] This picture leads to at least two different considerations.

1. It is likely that *several mutations* in different mismatch repair genes, rather than a single mutation in one gene, represent the most relevant early event in carcinogenesis.
2. The genome instability theory brings us back to Boveri's observations, since an unstable genome is more likely to produce unbalanced distribution of chromosomes between the daughter cells during mitosis, as observed by Boveri in his experiments on double-fertilized sea urchin eggs.

RELEVANCE OF MSI TO ORBITAL TUMORS

Several reasons could be suggested for the extreme rarity of reports on molecular analysis of orbital tumors. For example, these tumors are relatively rare and in many countries a consistent gap exists between ophthalmology and molecular biology. Moreover, some of the most recent reports on this subject were neither conclusive nor enthusiastic about the application of molecular biology techniques to the study of orbital tumors.[32] However, studies on orbital rhabdomyosarcoma[33] and metastatic spread to the orbit of intraocular tumors, such as retinoblastoma,[34] have shown the potential for a substantial contribution of molecular biology to an improved understanding and treatment of these tumors. In particular, studies on chromosome 11 in some cases of *embryonal rhabdomyosarcoma* of the orbit have shown that several genes seem to be involved in the pathogenesis of this disease. Moreover, molecular investigations reveal a wide variety of alterations, ranging from allelic losses to LOH and MSI.[35] In light of findings of MSI in embryonal rhabdomyosarcoma of the orbit[36] and the potential implications of this finding for prognosis and treatment, it is likely that more ophthalmic oncologists will be interested in applying molecular biology techniques to the diagnosis of orbital tumors.

EPIGENOMICS: DNA METHYLATION AND HISTONE ACETYLATION

Methylation of DNA of certain control regions in our genome can cause genes to be inappropriately "silenced."[37] DNA methylation is a chemical modification of cytosine, one of DNA's four bases. This modification consists of the addition of a methyl group (CH3−) to the cytosine residues of the DNA double helix. The altered cytosine is called methyl-cytosine, and it represents a critical factor in gene regulation. The enzyme responsible for DNA methylation in humans is known as DNA cytosine methyltransferase (DNA MTase). Abnormal methylation events occur during aging and in the development of many cancers. It is now well known that up to 65% of all cancers originate from inappropriate DNA methylation of some key genes rather than from mutations.

In many instances, hypermethylation of DNA is the suspected cause of the cancer. Hypermethylation inappropriately switches off critical genes, thus allowing cancer to develop. Studies on DNA methylation in cancer have revealed that aberrant methylation of normally unmethylated CpG islands (portions of DNA containing an elevated percentage of cytosine on one side and guanine, the complementary base, on the other) located in the promoter region of genes (the regions promoting or enhancing gene transcription, and hence, expression), is associated with transcriptional inactivation of defined TSGs.[38,39] Other genes, such as those involved in the apoptosis process (e.g., *CSP8*)[40] or DNA mismatch repair,[41] may also be involved, leading to their "silencing" or lack of expression, and hence to cancer initiation and progression.

One relevant aspect of the methylation process, which was already known to operate in the inactivation of the X chromosome[42] and loss of imprinting,[43] is that it can be pharmacologically reversed. If DNA MTase, the enzyme responsible for methylating the DNA, can be inhibited by a methyltransferase inhibitor, the overmethylation can be reversed, thereby switching the tumor suppressor gene back on. This approach will provide a powerful platform for the development of anticancer drugs (Figure 1.4).

In summary, four different features of DNA methylation make this process relevant to understanding the molecular bases of tumor development and potential new approaches in cancer treatment:

1. DNA methylation is a functional and hence "epigenetic" process (no mutation is involved).
2. It, therefore, affects the function of genes, but not their structure, as mutation does.
3. It explains functional phenomena involved in tumor development, such as loss of imprinting or "silencing" of TSGs.
4. It can be reversed with drugs such as 5-azacytidine.

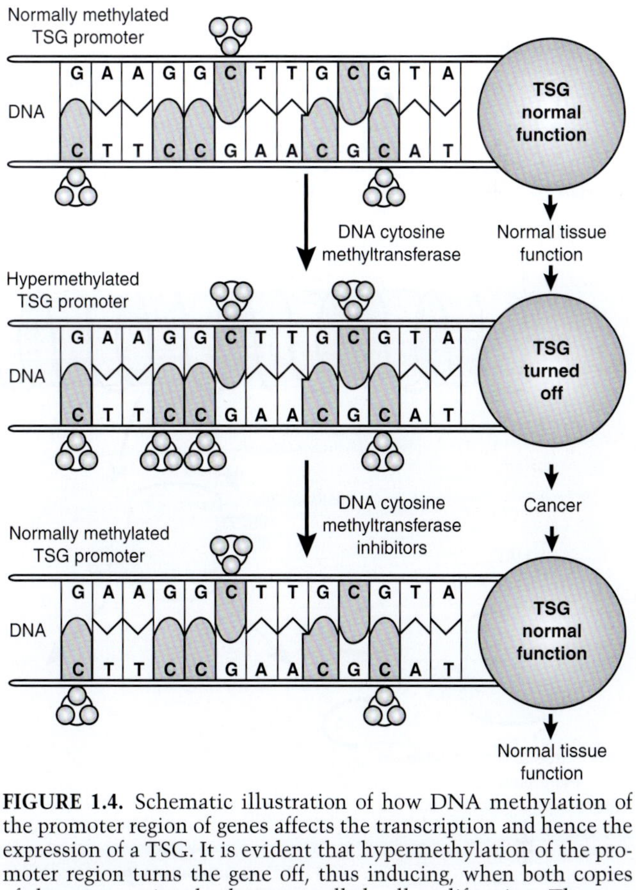

FIGURE 1.4. Schematic illustration of how DNA methylation of the promoter region of genes affects the transcription and hence the expression of a TSG. It is evident that hypermethylation of the promoter region turns the gene off, thus inducing, when both copies of the gene are involved, uncontrolled cell proliferation. The normal gene expression can be restored by inhibiting the enzyme responsible for DNA methylation (DNA methyltransferase).

In eukaryotic cells, genes are complexed with core histones and other chromosomal proteins to form chromatin. The basic repeating unit of chromatin is called a nucleosome. Each nucleosome is made of two copies of each of the four core histones (H2A, H2B, H3, and H4) wrapped by 146 base pairs (bp) of DNA (Figure 1.5). With the aid of additional proteins, including histone H1, the nucleosomes are further packaged into 30 nm fibers. When these fibers unfold, DNA becomes accessible for transcription; on the contrary, when they are packaged together, DNA becomes inaccessible. The unfolding involves posttranslational modifications of the core histone amino-terminal tails. Each core histone is composed of a structured, three-helix domain and two unstructured tails. These tails are susceptible to a variety of covalent modifications, such as acetylation, phosphorylation, and methylation, whose roles are now beginning to be unveiled.[44]

At present, both genetic and biochemical studies support an important role for histone tail acetylation in transcriptional regulation. The acetylation status of histones, in turn, depends on the activity of two enzymes with opposite actions: histone acetylase (HAT) and histone deacetylase (HDAC). Both these enzymatic activities are required for the activation or repression of transcription. Because of their important roles in the regulation of such events, enzymes that affect histone acetylation status are increasingly being associated with tumors.[45] Histone deacetylation, as operated by HDAC, involves the removal, through hydrolysis, of the acetyl groups (COO^-) from the ε-amino group of the histone's lysine side chain, with an overall increase of histone's positive charge and affinity for the negatively charged DNA, thus making the DNA itself relatively inaccessible to transcription factors (reduced gene expression). When HDAC is inhibited, the amount of counterenzyme, HAT, becomes excessive, and hyperacetylation occurs. Hyperacetylation, in turn, leads to an increase in the negative charge of histones, disrupting the structure of the histone and allowing its DNA to unfold. The unfolded state of histone then permits transcription factors to reach previously hidden genetic information, with a consequent increase in gene expression.[46]

The anticancer potential of HDAC inhibitors stems from their ability to affect several cellular processes that are unregulated in cancer cells. For example, assuming that one or more TSGs are silenced in cancer cells, the theoretical role of HDAC inhibitors

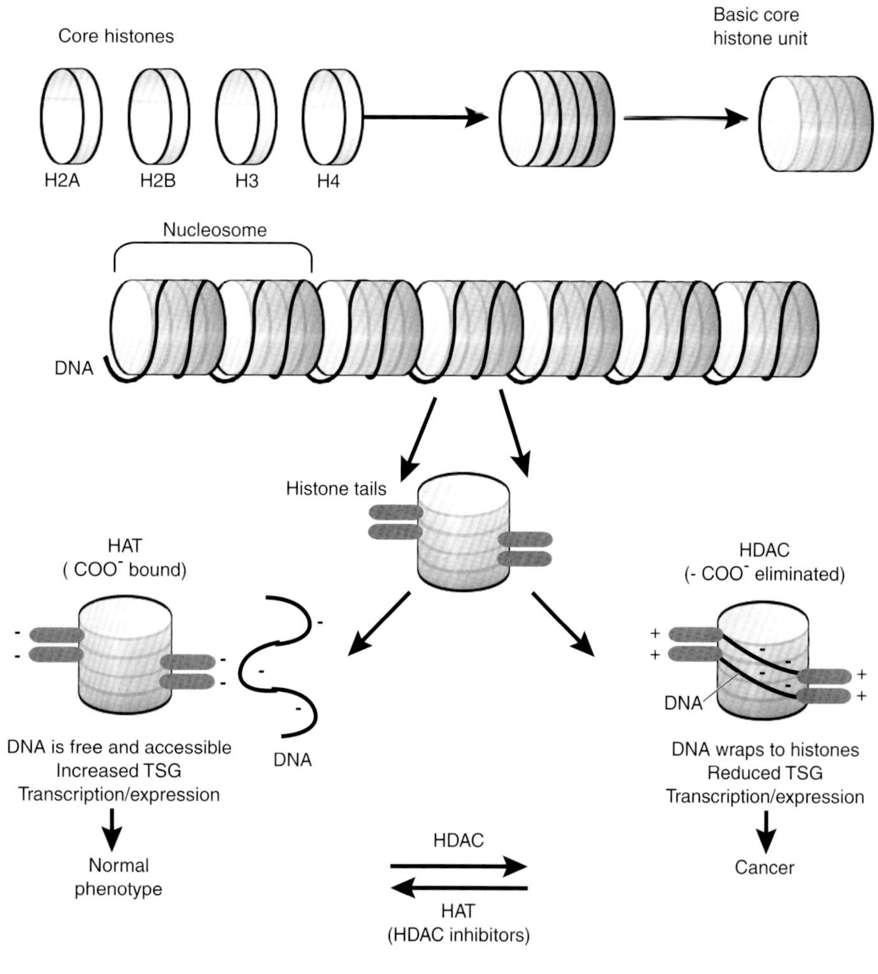

FIGURE 1.5. Schematic illustration of how the degree of acetylation of histones modulates gene expression, based on a hypothetical TSG. In the normally acetylated histone, the acetyl groups add a negative charge to histone proteins, thus allowing the negatively charged DNA to unfold to become accessible to transcription factors for regular gene expression. When histone deacetylase (HDAC) removes acetyl groups from histone proteins, the global charge of histones becomes positive, thus attracting the negatively charged DNA, which wraps around histone proteins, thus becoming inaccessible to transcription factors. This process will silence the normal expression of TSGs, thus pushing the cell toward an uncontrolled condition of proliferation. This condition can be reversed and a normal TSG expression restored by using HDAC inhibitors.

consists of promoting the transcription of the silenced gene or genes, thus reversing the cancer phenotype. Preliminary reports indicate that HDAC inhibitors activate differentiation programs, inhibit the cell cycle, and induce apoptosis; but they also seem to activate the host immune response and play a role in inhibition of angiogenesis. Hence the mechanisms whereby HDAC inhibitors induce tumor cell growth arrest, differentiation, and/or apoptosis are presumably more complex than those suggested by this short review. Intensive research in phase I and II clinical trials using several HDAC inhibitors has been initiated. HDAC inhibitors seem to possess minimal toxicity and are well tolerated at the doses needed to hyperacetylate histones and achieve clinical outcomes.[47,48] It is worthwhile, when mentioning the potentialities of histone acetylation status in regulating gene expression, to note that histone methyltranferases have been found to contain a potential methyl-CpG-binding domain, raising the important possibility that histone methylation, in a manner similar to histone deacetylation, might function in concert with DNA methylation to switch off tumor suppressor or DNA mismatch repair genes in cancer.

DO MUTATIONS MATTER IN CANCER?

For nearly a century cancer has been blamed on somatic mutation. As we have seen, one of the fundamental distinctions between oncogenes and TSGs is based on the assumption that a single mutation involving one allelic copy of an oncogene (cancer "dominant" gene) or two sequential mutations involving both copies of a TSG (cancer "recessive" gene), are sufficient to determine cancer. However, it has been shown that many, if not all of the predictions made by the somatic mutation model, as applied to cancer, are difficult to meet.[10] As shown in Table 1.3, the arguments against the somatic mutation model in cancer are numerous and consistent. For example, the somatic mutation model predicts that carcinogens induce cancer by causing mutations within the DNA. This prediction, however, is largely disproved by the existence of a growing list of carcinogens (such as asbestos, Ni^{2+}, hormones, butter yellow, arsenic, acrylamide, urethan) that do not cause DNA mutations. For decades, the search for "cancer genes" and mutations affecting them has been considered to be the most relevant target of cancer research, and arguments that disprove such consolidated knowledge sound like heresy. However, if we look without prejudice at the evidence emerging in the past few years, we can easily convince ourselves that mutation represents only one aspect of cancer pathogenesis and probably not the most relevant one. The study of the genes involved in the DNA mismatch repair system teaches us the following:

1. DNA mutations are still compatible with a normal cell life if the mismatch repair system is working properly.
2. Mutations affecting both oncogenes and TSGs can be the result of uncorrected errors in the mismatches occurring during DNA replication. Therefore these mutations (or their permanence within the genome) can be due to defects in the DNA mismatch repair system, thus configuring the so-called mutator phenotype in cancer.
3. The genome of cells showing microsatellite instability is, in turn, unstable.[49]

Studies on DNA methylation have clearly shown that the degree of methylation of CpG islands within the DNA is a key factor in the regulation of gene expression. These studies have yielded the following insights:

1. DNA hypermethylation (with no structural alteration like mutation) of CpG islands within the promoter regions of genes is the main mechanism of gene silencing of TSGs.
2. DNA hypermethylation is also responsible for the silencing of genes of the DNA mismatch repair system that are considered to belong to the "caretaker" category of TSGs. It is therefore reasonable to infer that the hypermethylation of the promoter regions of these genes is responsible for the permanence and accumulation of mutations in cancer genes such as oncogenes and TSGs.

TABLE 1.3. Predictions Based on the Somatic Mutation Model as Applied to Cancer.

Predictions	*Arguments countering these predictions*
Carcinogens cause mutations.	There is a large list of carcinogens that do not cause mutations.
Mutations are cancer-specific.	No cancer-specific mutations have been found yet.
Cancer-specific genes can transform normal human cells into cancer cells.	No genes isolated from cancer are able to transform normal human cells into cancer cells.
Transformation is coincident with mutation.	The latent period between carcinogen treatment and cancer ranges from many months to decades.
Cancer phenotypes are as stable as conventional mutations.	The phenotypes of cancer cells are notoriously unstable.
Cancer cells are diploid, since mutations do not depend on karyotype alterations for expression.	Virtually all cancers are aneuploid.

3. DNA hypermethylation can be reversed with drugs.[50]

It has become evident that both histone acetylation and methylation represent still another key factor in the regulation of gene expression. From the studies of these processes, and chromatin dynamics, we have learned the following:

1. Acetylation of histone tails correlates with the "opening" of chromation structure to allow transcription (i.e., increased gene expression).
2. The reverse happens when histone tails are deacetylated.
3. Histone acetylation is an enzymatic process that can be modulated with specific drugs (e.g., HDAC inhibitors).
4. Histone methylation, similar to histone deacetylation, may function in concert with DNA methylation in gene silencing.
5. The complex system of interactions of histone proteins with DNA and the known consequences on gene transcription and expression considerably extend the information potential of the genetic code, thus configuring the existence of the so-called histone code.[44,51,52]

Recent investigations have aimed at characterizing and defining the role of "epigenetic" factors in cancer development, with special reference to the DNA mismatch repair system, DNA methylation, and histone acetylation. Concurrently, researchers have published new hypotheses on the genesis of cancer that, while discarding the somatic mutation model, exalted the role of aneuploidy. These authors point out that cancer encompasses an extremely complex cell phenotype. Cancer cells are often undifferentiated, invasive, and metastatic, showing abnormal morphology and metabolism, genetic instability, and progression to malignancy.

All this extraordinary complexity and perturbation of normal cell function and morphology can be better explained and understood by assuming that aneuploidy, rather than gene mutation, is responsible for cell transformation and, consequently, tumor development. Aneuploidy is the gain or loss of individual chromosomes from the normal diploid set of 46. Since it is known that each chromosome contains thousands of genes, the imbalance of chromosome distribution between the daughter cells, represented by aneuploidy, implies an imbalanced expression of all these genes and consequently the great perturbation of cell functions and morphology known to be at work in cancer. Aneuploidy destabilizes a cell in much the same way that a dent disrupts the symmetry of a wheel. It leads to ever greater distortions with each revolution.

Accordingly, two phases can be hypothesized in the development of cancer. In the first phase, carcinogens induce aneuploidy by chemically or physically altering one or more of the many proteins of the spindle apparatus of the chromosomes. In the second phase, aneuploidy destabilizes the karyotype and thus initiates an autocatalytic karyotype evolution that generates lethal preneoplastic or neoplastic karyotypes.[10,53,54] In Chapter 2, the possible causes of aneuploidy will be discussed briefly. However, for the purposes of this chapter it is worth noting that the hypothesized first phase of cancer development, with specific reference to the "physically altered proteins of chromosomes," recalls the process of histone acetylation, whereas the second phase, involving aneuploidy, brings us back a century to Boveri's observations on double-fertilized sea urchin eggs. All this knowledge from Boveri's observations leading back to almost the same conclusions a hundred years later, should stimulate some philosophical considerations about the reductionistic attitude of modern science and the value of direct observation of phenomena in science. In more pragmatic terms, the evolution of knowledge seems to teach us that the time of the somatic mutation theory is over and that fundamental role of "epigenetic" events in cancer development must be acknowledged.[55]

References

1. http://www.harcourt.com/dictionary
2. Boveri T. Über morphologie Mitosen als Mittel zur Analyse des Zellkerns. *Verh D Phys Med Ges Wurzberg N F* 1902;35:67–90.
3. Boveri T. *Ergebnisse über die Konstitution der chromatischen Substanz des Zellkerns*. Jena: Fischer; 1904.
4. Balmain A. Cancer genetics: from Boveri and Mendel to microarray. *Nat Rev Cancer* 2001;1:77–82.
5. Boveri T. In *Zur Frage der Entstehung maligner Tumoren* 1914. Jena: Fischer; 1–64.
6. Nowell P, Hungerford D. Chromosomes of normal and leukemic human leukocytes. *J Natl Cancer Inst* 1960;25:85.
7. Rowley JD. A new consistent chromosomal abnormality in chronic myelogenous leukaemia. *Nature* 1973;243:290–293.
8. Heisterkamp N, Stephenson JR, Groffen J, et al. Localization of the c-*abl* oncogene adjacent to a translocation break point in chronic myelocytic leukaemia. *Nature* 1983;306:239–242.
9. Druker BJ, Sawyers CL, Kantarjian H, et al. Activity of a specific inhibitor of the BCR-ABL tyrosine kinase in the blast crisis of chronic myeloid leukemia and acute lymphoblastic leukemia with the Philadelphia chromosome. *N Engl J Med* 2001;344:1038–1342.
10. Li R, Sonik A, Rasnik D, Duesberg P. Aneuploidy vs gene mutation hypothesis of cancer: recent studies claims mutation but is found to support aneuploidy. *Proc Natl Acad Sci USA* 2000;97:3236–3241.
11. Rous P. A sarcoma of the fowl transmissible by an agent separable from the tumor cells. *J Exp Med* 1911;13:397–411.
12. Chen JH, Hayward WS, Hanafusa H. Avian tumor virus proteins and RNA in uninfected chicken embryo cells. *J Virol* 1974;14:1419–1429.
13. Hanafusa H, Halpern CC, Buchhagen DL, Kawai S. Recovery of avian sarcoma virus from tumors induced by transformation-defective mutants. *J Exp Med* 1977;146:1735–1747.
14. Temin HM. On the origin of RNA tumor viruses. Harvey Lect 1973–1974:173–196.

15. Temin HM. On the origin of the genes for neoplasia: G.H.A. Clowes Memorial Lecture. *Cancer Res* 1974;34:2835–2841.
16. Temin HM. On the origin of RNA tumor viruses. *Annu Rev Genet* 1974;8:155–177.
17. Stehelin D, Varmus HE, Bishop JM, Vogt PK. DNA related to the transforming gene(s) of avian sarcoma viruses is present in normal avian DNA. *Nature* 1976;260:170–173.
18. Bishop J.M. Enemies within: the genesis of retroviral oncogenes. *Cell* 1981;23:5–6.
19. http://www.nobel.se/medicine/laureates/1989/bishop-lecture.pdf
20. Weinberg RA. How cancer arises. *Sci Am* 1996;275:62–70. Review.
21. Park M. Oncogenes. In: Scriver CR, Beaudet AL, Sly WS, Valle D, eds. *The Metabolic and Molecular Bases of Inherited Disease.* 8th ed. New York: McGraw-Hill Medical Publishing; 2001:645–664.
22. Knudson AG Jr. Mutation and cancer: statistical study of retinoblastoma. *Proc Natl Acad Sci U S A* 1971;68:820–823.
23. Cavenee WK, Dryja TP, Phillips RA, et al. Expression of recessive alleles by chromosomal mechanisms in retinoblastoma. *Nature* 1983;305:779–784.
24. Perucho M. PCR and cancer diagnostics: detection and characterization of single point mutations in oncogenes and antioncogenes. In: Mullis K.B, Ferré F., Gibbs RA, eds. *PCR: The Polymerase Chain Reaction.* Basel: Birkhauser; 1994:369–394.
25. Knudson AG. Two genetic hits (more or less) to cancer. *Nature Rev Cancer* 2001;1:157–162.
26. Friend SH, Bernards R, Rogelj S, et al. A human DNA segment with properties of the gene that predisposes to retinoblastoma and osteosarcoma. *Nature* 1986;323:643–646.
27. Friend SH, Dryja TP, Weinberg RA. Oncogenes and tumor-suppressing genes. *N Engl J Med* 1988;318:618–622.
28. Kinzler KW, Vogelstein B. Familial cancer syndromes: the role of caretakers and gatekeepers. In: Scriver CR, Beaudet AL, Sly WS, Valle D, eds. *The Metabolic and Molecular Bases of Inherited Disease.* Vol. 1. 8th ed. New York: McGraw-Hill Medical Publishing Division; 2001:675–676.
29. http://www.ich.ucl.ac.uk/cmgs/onc99.htm
30. Karran P. Human mismatch repair: defects and predisposition to cancer. *Encyclopedia of Life Sciences. www.els.net*
31. Anderson GR. Genomic instability in cancer. *Curr Sci* 2001; 81:501–507.
32. Johnson TE, Tse DT, Byrne GE Jr, et al. Ocular-adnexal lymphoid tumors: a clinicopathologic and molecular genetic study of 77 patients. *Ophthalmol Plast Reconstr Surg* 1999;15:171–179.
33. Brinkschmidt C, Poremba C, Schafer KL, et al. Evidence of genetic alterations in chromosome 11 in embryonal and alveolar rhabdomyosarcoma. *Verh Dtsch Ges Pathol* 1998;82:210–214.
34. Finger PT, Harbour JW, Karcioglu ZA. Risk factors for metastasis in retinoblastoma. *Surv Ophthalmol* 2002;47:1–16.
35. Mastrangelo D, Sappia F, Bruni S, et al. Loss of heterozygosity of chromosome 11 in orbital embryonal rhabdomyosarcoma (OERMS): a microsatellite study of seven cases. *Orbit* 1998;17: 89–95.
36. Mastrangelo D, Hadjistilianou T, Mazzotta C, Loré C. Microsatellite instability in three cases of embryonal rhabdomyosarcoma of the orbit. *Med Pediatr Oncol* 2002;39:132–133.
37. Brown R, Strathdee G.: Epigenomics and epigenetic therapy of cancer. *Trends Mol Med* 2002;8:S43–S48.
38. Baylin SB, Herman JG, Graff JR, et al. Alterations in DNA methylation: a fundamental aspect of neoplasia. *Adv Cancer Res* 1998;72:141–196.
39. Esteller M, Corn PG, Baylin SB, Herman JG. A gene hypermethylation profile of human cancer. *Cancer Res* 2001;61: 3225–3229.
40. Teitz T, Wei T, Valentine MB, et al. Caspase 8 is deleted or silenced preferentially in childhood neuroblastomas with amplification of *MYCN*. *Nat Med* 2000;6:529–535.
41. Deng G, Peng E, Gum J, Terdiman J, Sleisenger M, Kim YS. Methylation of hMLH1 promoter correlates with the gene silencing with a region-specific manner in colorectal cancer. *Br J Cancer* 2002;86:574–579.
42. Goto T, Monk M: Regulation of X-chromosome inactivation in development in mice and humans. *Microbiol Mol Biol Rev.* 1998;62:362–378.
43. Plass C, Soloway PD. DNA methylation, imprinting and cancer. *Eur J Hum Genet* 2002;10:6–16.
44. Zhang Y, Reinberg D. Transcription regulation by histone methylation: interplay between different covalent modifications of the core histone tails. *Genes Dev* 2001;15: 2343–2360.
45. Gray SG, The BT. Histone acetylation/deacetylation and cancer: an "open" and "shut" case? *Curr Mol Med* 2001;4:401–429.
46. http://www.acdlabs.com/download/publ/scholar/jstockdill.pdf
47. Johnstone RW. Histone deacetylase inhibitors: novel drugs for the treatment of cancer. *Nat Rev Drug Discovery* 2002;4:287–299.
48. Vigushin DM, Coombes RC. Histone deacetylase inhibitors in cancer treatment. *Anticancer Drugs* 2002;13:1–13.
49. Atkin NB. Microsatellite instability. *Cytogenet Cell Genet* 2001;92:177–181.
50. Esteller M, Herman JG. Cancer as an epigenetic disease: DNA methylation and chromatin alterations in human tumors. *J Pathol* 2002;196:1–7.
51. Nakayama J, Rice JC, Stahl BD, et al. Role of histone H3 lysine 9 methylation in epigenetic control of heterochromatin assembly. *Science* 2000;292:110–113.
52. Jenuwein T, Allis CD. Translating the histone code. *Science* 2001;293:1074–1080.
53. Rasnick D, and Duesberg HP. How aneuploidy affects metabolic control and causes cancer. *Biochem J* 1999;340:621–630.
54. Duesberg P, Li R, Rasnick D, et al. Aneuploidy precedes, and segregates with chemical carcinogenesis *Cancer Genet Cytogenet* 2000;119:83–93.
55. Jones PA, Baylin SB. The fundamental role of epigenetic events in cancer. *Nature Rev Genet* 2002;1:415–428.

2

Immune Surveillance and Cancer Pathogenesis

Domenico Mastrangelo

Scientists have debated the existence of a surveillance role for the normal immune system (NIS) in regulating the growth and spread of human cancer since the first observation of spontaneous tumor regression in experimental animals.[1] This observation led to the concept that through surveillance, the NIS could detect and destroy newly formed cancer cells. This concept persists even though 90% of the most common cancers occur in a host with a fully functioning NIS,[2] and no good evidence has been reported of an increase of common carcinomas in the presence of severely decreased immune function.[3] However, some degree of immunological response against cancer exists both in animals and humans, as shown by the following observations:

1. Components of the immune system that are capable of recognizing cancer cells have been identified in cancer patients.
2. Laboratory investigations have shown that cells of the immune system can kill cancer cells.
3. The stimulation of the immune system with bacterial products or components of the immune system itself can lead to tumor regression.
4. Patients with an impaired immune system (as in HIV/AIDS) are more likely to develop certain types of cancer, and cancer may display a more aggressive behavior in these individuals.[4]

A detailed description of the mechanisms and biological components involved in the immune response against cancer is far beyond the scope of this chapter; therefore we summarize only the most relevant and practical aspects concerning the interaction between the immune system and cancer.

IMMUNOLOGICAL RESPONSE TO CANCER

For the immune system to react against a tumor, tumor cells must express antigens that are recognized to be foreign by the individual's immune system. As outlined in Chapter 1, structural alterations of chromosomes (i.e., aneuploidy) typical of cancerous transformation lead to complex cancer-specific phenotypes, including abnormal cellular and nuclear morphology, metabolism, growth, DNA indices, invasiveness, metastasis, and neoantigens.[5,6] Neoantigens are usually subdivided into two major classes:

1. *Tumor-specific antigens (TSAs):* These substances are unique to cancer cells and cannot be found in their normal counterparts. Shared TSAs found on related tumors from separate individuals include oncoviral antigens expressed on the surfaces of infected cells. Oncogenic viruses found in humans include Epstein–Barr virus (EBV) in Burkitt's lymphoma and nasopharyngeal carcinoma, human T-cell lymphotrophic virus 1 (HTLV-I) in adult T-cell leukemia, human papilloma virus in cervical cancer, hepatitis B virus (HBV) in primary hepatoma, and human herpes virus 8 in Kaposi sarcoma.

2. *Tumor-associated antigens (TAAs):* The TAAs can be found in both normal and cancer cells, but their expression is greatly increased in tumors. They include the so-called oncofetal antigens, usually present during embryonic and fetal development, but either absent or present at very low levels in normal adult tissue. The two most important antigens of this group are represented by the carcinoembryonic antigen (CEA) (colon, pancreas, lung, breast, and prostate cancers, cirrhosis of the liver, chronic lung disease, and serum of heavy smokers), and α-fetoprotein (AFP) (liver and testicular cancer).[7]

The immune system is a complex network of specialized cells and organs that has evolved to defend the body against attacks by foreign invaders. When functioning properly, it fights off infections; when its function is compromised, a number of diseases, ranging from allergy to cancer, may arise.

Two major types of immune response can be distinguished in humans:

1. The humoral immune (HI) response is essentially operated by B lymphocytes through the produc-

tion of antibodies. Antibodies can kill tumor cells by different mechanisms:

- IgG or IgM antibodies that fix the complement and can destroy soft tumors.
- Antibodies directed against antigens expressed on tumor cell surfaces, which may interfere with the adhesion molecules some tumor cells need to survive
- IgG antibodies, which may mediate tumor cell lysis through antibody dependent cell–mediated cytotoxicity (ADCC), involving effector cells such as macrophages, natural killer (NK) cells, cytotoxic T lymphocytes (CTLs), and perhaps blood neutrophils

2. The cell-mediated immune (CMI) response is operated essentially by macrophages, NK cells, and T lymphocytes. The mechanisms of cancer cell killing vary, in this case, according to the cell type involved, as follows:
   - Macrophages, activated by T-cell γ-interferon, which kill tumor cells by the same mechanisms they use to kill microorganisms (tumor necrosis factor α, lysozyme, oxygen radicals)
   - NK cells, which kill tumors by the same mechanisms they use to kill virus-infected cells (perforin, granzymes, interferon gamma (IFN-γ), FasL-mediated apoptosis)
   - Cytotoxic T lymphocytes (CTLs), which kill tumors in an antigen-specific and MHC-restricted manner (perforin, granzymes, IFN-γ, FasL-mediated apoptosis)[7]

As our discussion of the mechanisms of the immune response to cancer will illustrate, CMI, with the intervention of both CTLs (also defined as "killer" cells) and NKs, represents the most efficient mechanism of immune surveillance and immune response to cancer. NK and killer CTL cells represent, therefore, the key players in tumor immunity, being ultimately responsible for the destruction of malignant cells. NKs participate early as the effectors of the innate immune system, and CTLs provide long-lasting effects.[8]

At the heart of the immune system is its ability to distinguish between antigens that belong to the individual ("self") and those that do not ("non-self"). Virtually every cell of the body carries distinctive molecules that identify it as a self. Molecules that mark a cell as self are encoded by a group of genes that is contained in a section of a specific chromosome and is known as the major histocompatibility complex (MHC). MHC is essential to immune defense because it determines which antigens an individual can respond to and how strongly. Two different classes of MHC are usually recognized:

1. Class I molecules, which alert killer T cells to the presence of body cells that have been changed for the worse (infected with a virus or transformed by cancer) and need to be eliminated
2. Class II molecules, which are found on B cells, macrophages, and other cells responsible for presenting foreign antigen to helper T cells

Regarding the distinction between "self" and "non-self," it must be noted that the innate immune system uses three strategies, which can be described in terms of recognition of "microbial non-self" or "infectious non-self," recognition of "missing self," and recognition of "induced or altered self." The basis of microbial non-self recognition is the ability of the host to recognize products (antigens) that are unique to microorganisms and are not produced by the host. The second strategy relies on the detection of "markers of the normal self." The third strategy, the one of interest for cancer immunology, is based on the detection of "markers of abnormal self" that are induced upon infection (i.e., viral infection) and cellular transformation (cancer). Markers of abnormal self tag the affected cells for elimination by the immune system.[9] The concept of self/non-self discrimination has recently evolved toward a model of immunity based on the idea that the immune system is more concerned with entities that do damage than with those that are foreign.[10]

The first line in the immune response to cancer is represented by the natural killer cells, which account for approximately 10 to 20% of peripheral blood lymphocytes and do not express surface antigens typical of both T and B lymphocytes. Unlike CTLs, they do not need to be activated to exert their cytotoxic action. They are primarily restricted to peripheral blood, bone marrow, spleen, and liver and are not found in lymph nodes. NK cells are thought to represent an important defense mechanism against various intracellular pathogens, such as herpesvirus, and against certain tumors.

Through specific membrane receptors, NK cells are able to recognize MHC class I molecules [human leukocyte antigen (HLA) class I in humans] on normal cells, leading to the delivery of signals that inhibit their function. As a consequence, NK cells destroy only the target cells that have lost or express insufficient amounts of MHC class I molecules, a frequent event following cancer transformation or viral infection.[11]

Traditionally, the effectors of the more specific and long-lasting anticancer responses are CTLs. Like NK cells, the CTLs kill tumor cells, but they do it more efficiently and specifically. Also, their intervention requires a network of specific interactions between different cells and molecules. The first element in this network is represented by the so-called antigen presenting cells (APCs), such as macrophages and dendritic cells. APCs are not a single category but rather a group of cells that share the same function, that is, the processing of an antigen and presenting it to the immune system in a form recognizable by T lymphocytes. The processing of an antigen by an APC involves several steps:

1. The APC engulfs the antigen.
2. Enzymes in the APC break down the antigen into smaller fragments.
3. These fragments are transported on the APC's surface and bound to MHC class I molecules.
4. A CTL is now able to recognize the antigen and bind it.

A simplified scheme of the processes involved in the activation of CTLs, which is valid for both virally infected and transformed (cancer) cells, encompasses the following phases:

1. The APC engulfs the antigen.
2. The antigen is processed and associated with MHC class I antigen for recognition.
3. The MHC-associated antigen is recognized by CD8+ lymphocytes.
4. The presence of costimulatory molecules, such as B7-1 and B7-2 on APC and the secretion of interleukin 2 (IL-2), promote the differentiation of CD8+ lymphocytes (T cytotoxic) into CTLs;
5. CTLs lyse tumor cells.[12]
6. The same processing is simultaneously operating within the MHC class II antigens for recognition by CD4+ lymphocytes (T-helper cells). As a consequence, CD4+ lymphocytes produce lymphokines that stimulate B lymphocytes to enter the cell cycle and start producing antibodies. No major emphasis, however, is placed on this pathway, given its secondary role in the immune response to tumor (Figure 2.1).

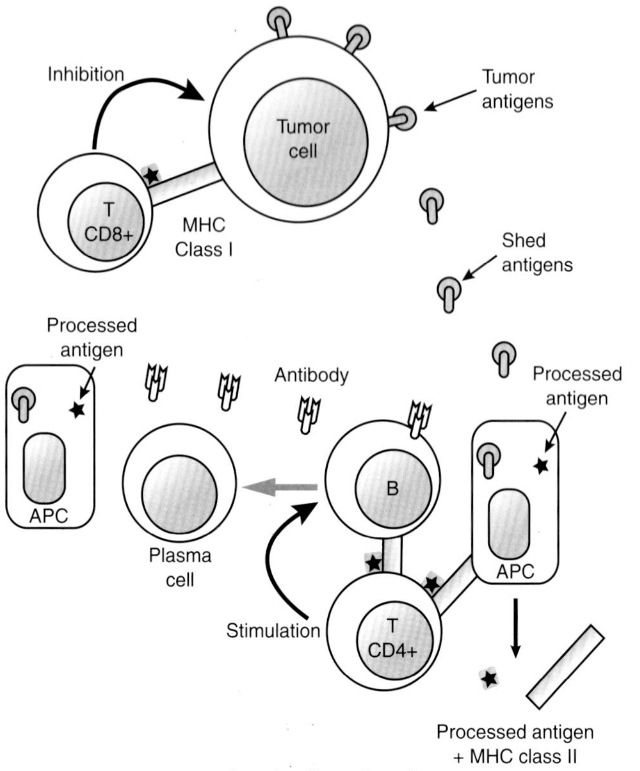

FIGURE 2.1. Humoral and cell-mediated immunity to cancer.

If the proposed mechanisms of immunological response to tumor worked as effectively as described, cancer probably would not exist; unfortunately, this is not the reality. It must therefore be assumed that, for various reasons, the killing of tumor cells by an immunological route is not as effective as described. Among explanations that have been suggested are the following:

1. Most tumor cells are poor APCs because they lack costimulatory molecules (such as B7), and this may determine anergy (lack of response) of T cells to cancer cells.
2. Tumor cells may also lack other molecules (LFA-3 and ICAM-1) required for adhesion of lymphocytes.
3. Some tumor cells show a reduction or complete loss of MHC class I molecules. As reported, this may help recognition by NK cells but, at the same time, it may compromise recognition by CTLs.
4. Molecular complexes made of tumor antigens and specific antibodies (blocking antibodies) can saturate Fc receptors on macrophages, NK cells, neutrophils, and CTLs, thus preventing the interaction of these cells with the tumor.
5. Tumor surface antigens may be internalized by endocytosis and degraded (antigenic modulation), thus reducing the stimulatory effects of new antigens on the immune system.
6. Some tumors secrete factors (e.g., prostaglandin E_2, tumor growth factor β) that inhibit the development and proliferation of T lymphocytes.
7. Tumors may secrete factors that induce apoptosis in T cells.

More recently, major emphasis has been put on the role of chemokines in both cancer immunotherapy and development. Chemokines are a family of 40 to 50 proteins that regulate leukocyte transport by mediating the adhesion of leukocytes to endothelial cells and the initiation of transendothelial migration and tissue invasion. It has been found that tumors divert chemokines' function to favor tumor development through several mechanisms, including direct growth activity, stimulation of angiogensis, control of spreading and metastatization, and interference with the recruitment of different leukocyte populations. At the same time, it is becoming increasingly evident that through the manipulations of these factors, robust anti-tumor responses can be induced.[13,14] Still much remains to be understood on the manipulation of the immune response.[15] This is the ultimate scope of research in the field of cancer immunology, and it is therefore worthwhile to mention some of the major achievements of immunology as applied to the field of clinical cancer research. Immunology can be applied for the detection of tumor antigens (CEA, AFP, etc.) shed in the blood or urine, both in vitro and in vivo, by antibody-based techniques such as ELISA (enzyme-linked immunosorbent assay), radio immune detection (RAID), and immunoscintigraphy. Also, laboratory techniques, such as the mixed lymphocyte–tumor culture (MLTC), test allow the study of the efficiency of cytotoxicity of different cell populations to cancer cells. Finally, immunology has shown a great potential in the field of cancer treatment, allowing the application, with variable but promising results, of new treatment modalities. In this regard, the following are worth mentioning:

1. ***Anticancer vaccines.*** The expression of neoantigens on cancer cell surfaces raises the possibility of using them exactly as bacterial or viral antigens have been used to induce either active or passive immunity to cancer.

2. ***Therapy with lymphokine-activated killer (LAK) cells.*** When human peripheral blood mononuclear cells are cultured in vitro with IL-2, they become highly cytotoxic to a wide variety of tumor targets, many of which are resistant to freshly isolated NK cells.

3. ***Therapy with tumor-infiltrating lymphocytes (TILs).*** This is a variant type of LAK therapy in which the population of killer cells is directly isolated from the tumor. The population of lymphocytes isolated from the tumor and expanded under the influence of IL-2 possesses receptors with high specificity for the tumor, and the final result is a great improvement in the specificity of treatment and reduction of side effects compared with LAK.

4. ***In vivo cytokine therapy.*** Some cytokines, such as α-interferon, γ-interferon, IL-2, and TGF-α, have been used with some success in cancer treatment.

5. ***Monoclonal antibodies.*** A number of treatment modalities exploiting the principle of antigen–antibody reaction have been used with some success in the treatment of cancer and still show great potential. The following three applications deserve mention:
   - Chimeric monoclonal antibodies (murine or human antibodies). These substances are much less likely to elicit production of human antimouse antibodies than a standard murine monoclonal antibody
   - Monoclonal antibodies conjugated with radioisotopes, toxins, or enzymes. In this case, the specificity of the antibody for its particular antigen on the cancer cell surface is exploited to bring drugs or toxins directly into contact with the cancer cell; the result is an overall decrease of the drug dosage and the side effects of treatment;
   - Monoclonal heteroconjugates (bispecific monoclonal antibodies). Monoclonal antibodies have been engineered to bind simultaneously to a specific antigen expressed on cancer cell surface and to a specific receptor on either CTLs or NK cells.

AGING AND ONCOGENESIS

Advancing age has been described as the most potent of all carcinogens.[16] In humans, the incidence of cancer rises exponentially in the final decades of life, culminating in a lifetime risk of 1 in 2 for men and 1 in 3 for women.[17] This dramatic escalation in the incidence of cancer among the aged is largely due to epithelial carcinomas that develop between ages 40 and 80.

Until recently, the most common explanation for the increased incidence of cancer among older people has been the accumulation of somatic mutations due to cumulative exposure to both endogenous and exogenous DNA damaging agents[18,19] and failure to repair mismatches occurring during DNA replication.[20] In Chapter 1 it was shown that failure to repair mismatches occurring during DNA replication represents an early event in carcinogenesis[21,22] and configures the so-called "mutator phenotype," in which many genes carry mutations because of uncorrected errors in DNA replication.[23] The inability of the cell to correct mismatches that "normally" occur during DNA replication leads to an abnormal accumulation of "spontaneous mutations" and a consequent increase in DNA damage and genome instability.

The demonstration of the "mutator phenotype"[24,25] resolved one of the most important issues linked to the theory of the accumulation of somatic mutation with age: the insufficiency of the observed spontaneous mutation rate to account for the extensive tumor-associated genomic changes. In fact, in the new scenario of the "mutator phenotype," the age-dependent increase in the incidence of cancer stems from mutations affecting the genes governing the correction of mismatches occurring during DNA replication and the genome's stability, with a consequent accelerated pace of mutation overall.

Within this fundamental issue concerning the age-related increase in the incidence of cancer, it must be noted that several groups have provided experimental evidence in support of the suggestion that DNA repair activity declines with age. We showed in Chapter 1 that microsatellite instability (MSI) represents the "signature" associated with DNA repair defects,[26] and can be found in several cancer types. However, MSI is not always associated with cancer in the aged. Therefore, although the failing DNA mismatch repair system surely accounts for a consistent explanation of many age-associated cancer types, it does not explain them all. Other mechanisms must be at work, including those described in Chapter 1 as "epigenetic" which entail both DNA methylation and modifications of chromatin structure. Age-progressive CpG island methylation (and consequent gene silencing) has been observed to take place in subsets of cells residing in normal tissues. One example may be represented by the age-progressive methylation of the genes for estrogen receptors, with consequent silencing of these genes and increased cancer incidence in older women.

It has been outlined that the root source of genomic instability, which, in turn, represents the hallmark of nearly all solid tumors and adult-onset leukemia, is represented by the imbalance between DNA damage and repair, with damage prevailing because of either an increased rate of mutation or a decreased ability of the system to repair the damage incurred. Also, epigenetic events, such as gene methylation or histone acetylation, play a fundamental role in the process of genomic destabilization leading to cancer. Inherent in the concept of damage accumulation is the concept of time; it seems logical to assume that to allow for damage to accumulate and produce the irreversible alterations typical of cancer, a close relationship between increased age and cancer incidence must exist at the systemic level.

When aging and its relationship to cancer are considered at the cellular level, new and very interesting aspects are discovered. Investigations on the physiology of cell senescence and proliferative aging have led to the discovery of the telomere–telomerase system, which seems to be of extreme relevance to both aging and cancer. It is known that with each cell division, the genetic code is transferred as chromosomes are replicated and distributed into daughter cells. To ensure that the transfer is carried out in an accurate and efficient manner, different cellular mechanisms are in place, including the semiconservative replication of DNA and cell senescence.

The semiconservative replication of DNA is the process of replicating the original DNA in such a way that the finished products are two double DNA strands, each with one original and one new strand, to be distributed to the daughter cells. The mechanism of DNA replication in linear chromosomes is different for the so-called leading and the lagging strands. DNA synthesis proceeds from the 5′ to the 3′ DNA ends, but native (double-stranded) DNA is a polar molecule; that is, the leading strand has a 5′–3′ orientation, whereas the lagging strand has a 3′–5′ orientation. Therefore, although in the leading strand the synthesis of new DNA is straightforward, the process becomes more complicated in the lagging strand. Semiconservative DNA replication requires a labile short RNA primer to begin DNA polymerization in the 5′-to-3′ direction, in the lagging strand. After DNA polymerization, the RNA primers are degraded and replaced by DNA synthesized from an upstream primer. Because there is no DNA beyond the end of the chromosome to serve as a template for an RNA priming event, the gap between the final lagging strand segment (Okazaki fragment) and the end of the chromosome cannot be filled in (the "end replication problem"). Thus the 5′ end of the lagging strand will lose some nucleotides each time a cell replicates its DNA (Figure 2.2). Thus, the extreme end of a chromosome is not replicated and progressively shortens. This end, called the telomere (telos = end, meros = part), is made of repeats of 6 base pairs: $(TTAGGG)_n$ on one strand and $(AATCCC)_n$ on the complementary DNA strand. Human telomeres vary in length with age and cell type, with a range of 6 to 12 kilobase pairs (kbp: 6000–12,000 bp) in somatic cells. With the mechanism of Okazaki fragment replication, 50 to 100 bp are usually lost with each cell cycle. More important, loss of telomeric DNA continues with successive cell divisions until the telomeres reach such a critically short length that replication is halted. This happens, on average, after 60 to 70 divisions in human cells, and at this point the cell stops growing and enters senescence.

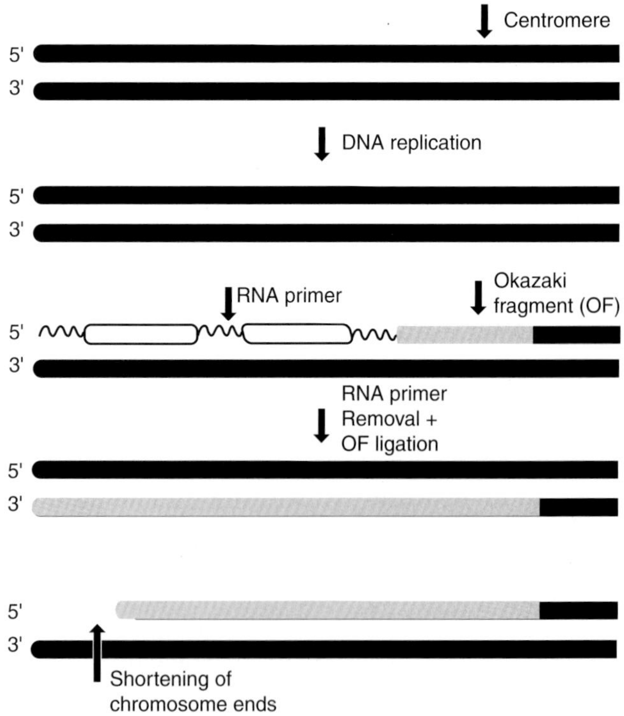

FIGURE 2.2. Mechanism of telomere shortening with advancing replicative age of the cell (the "end replication problem").

The fundamental issue concerning telomeres and their relationship with aging is the idea that progressive telomere shortening represents a biologic or mitotic clock of the cell keeping track of the number of replications a cell has used and indicating the time for permanent growth arrest when telomeres are sufficiently short. Telomere function is strictly associated with the function of the related enzyme, telomerase. Telomerase is a reverse transcriptase (i.e., an enzyme capable of synthesizing DNA starting from a template made of RNA) that can add TTAGGG examers to chromosome ends, thus extending and maintaining the length of telomeres and, as a consequence, the number of divisions a cell may undergo.

The most outstanding discovery concerning the telomere–telomerase system is that nearly the complete spectrum of human tumors has been shown to be telomerase positive, thus implying that tumor cells use telomerase to gain the capacity for unlimited proliferation and thus immortality. An exhaustive list of telomerase-positive human cancers has been reported by Granger et al.[27] The discovery of the appearance of telomerase activity as a distinctive feature of cancer in comparison to normally growing cells has opened new horizons in both diagnosis and treatment of cancer, since cancer cells can be identified for their distinctive expression of the enzyme telomerase, which in not expressed by normal cells and can be treated with telomerase inhibitors to "induce" cell senescence. This model assumes that because many divisions are needed to accumulate all the changes needed to transform a normal cell into a cancerous one,[28,29] cell senescence acts as an initial "cancer brake."

At this point it must be emphasized that telomerase is not the only tool a cell can use to lengthen its proliferative capacity; other mechanisms, which effect alternative lengthening of telomeres (ALT), have been identified.[30] Increasing the proliferative potential by either telomerase or ALT pathway is only one aspect of the process of malignant transformation.[31] As reported by Granger et al.,[27] there are at least six essential alterations necessary for malignancy shared by virtually all types of cancer. These are the generation of self-stimulatory growth signals, insensitivity to inhibitory growth signals, resistance to apoptosis, unlimited potential for proliferation (telomere lengthening), capacity for angiogenesis, and tissue invasion and metastasis. Whatever the implications of these arguments, the role of telomere shortening in proliferative aging remains unquestionable, as does the role of telomere lengthening in increasing the proliferative potential of the cell.

The final picture that can be inferred from major investigations concerning telomere physiology and pathology sounds rather paradoxical with respect to the introductory statement of this section. As a matter of fact, it is assumed from these investigations that the progressive shortening of telomeres is indicative of progressive cell senescence, and cell senescence, in turn, acts as a "cancer brake," theoretically allocating cancer and aging at the two opposite ends of the same spectrum. This seems to imply that, at the cellular level, the notion that advancing age is the most potent of all carcinogens is absolute nonsense.

Once again, the research on the role of chromosomal ploidy and genome stability in cancer and speciation gives us insight into a possible unifying theory to solve the apparent paradox concerning the role of aging in cancer in the light of telomere dynamics. In summary, it has been found that telomere shortening (and thus cell aging), plays an important role in genetic instability, including chromosomal loss, reciprocal translocations, and cancer development.[32] These observations have led authors to propose that the following sequence of events in cancer transformation is related to telomere dynamics. In ordinary somatic cells, certain chromosomes may lose or have reduced amounts of telomeric DNA (aging) and, therefore, may undergo translocations or other structural alterations. Because of this DNA rearrangement, cells get arrested in the G2/M phase of their life cycle. Their chromosomes replicate, but the cytoplasm does not, thus resulting in tetraploidy (four copies of the normal euploid number of chromosomes) and, if this continues in the absence of telomerase, the cell undergoes apoptosis. On the other hand, it may happen that telomeres are stabilized because of activation or upregulation of telomerase or other pathways (ALT), in which case the cell will survive and push to undergo mitosis. The high number of chromosomes within this cell, and the presence of only two centrosomes will trigger the amplification of other centrosomes to allow the cell to divide. (Centrosomes are the structures joining the two chromosomes of a couple within the cell. Their function is to help organize the mitotic spindle, which is the collection of microtubules that pull the duplicated chromosomes apart during cell division, ensuring that each of the two daughter cells has received the same number of chromosomes.) At this point, the cell will show a number of structural anomalies, including telomere erosion, double chromosome number, and amplification of centrosomes. This will give rise to multipolar mitosis, aneuploidy, and subsequent cancer formation.[33] In light of this view, telomere erosion due to cell senescence is the key factor in inducing the genome instability that represents the hallmark of malignant transformation, and the telomerase- or ALT-dependent lengthening of telomeres intervenes in a second phase of malignant transformation to confer on the cell the capacity to overcome the apoptotic pathway and push toward mitosis and consequent expansion of the structural abnormalities to future generations. This view seems to perfectly reconcile telomere dynamics with both aging and cancer and to validate the assumption that aging is the most potent of all carcinogens.

VIRUSES AND ONCOGENESIS

In Chapter 1, we pointed out the role that viruses have historically played in our understanding of the molecular bases of cancer. Viruses have been defined as the Rosetta Stone for unlocking the mysteries of cell growth control. They have also revealed the functional foundations of the genetic bases of cancer and provided a conceptual framework applicable to all cancers.[34] The concept that viruses cause cancer dates back to the first decade of the twentieth century, when Francis Peyton Rous demonstrated that tumors can be induced in particular breeds of chickens by inoculating tumor derived cell-free filtrates, containing a transmissible agent, most probably a virus.[35]

Viruses are a type of infectious agent that must invade living cells in order to reproduce. According to the type of nucleic acid that represents the virus genome, a distinction is usually made between DNA and RNA oncogenic viruses, the latter also being referred to as retroviruses. This basic distinction is not only qualitative; it also reflects a substantial difference in the way viruses attack and are assumed to transform a normal cell into a cancerous one. All RNA oncogenic viruses (or retroviruses) show the unusual characteristics of reverse transcription. After infecting the host cell, the viral RNA genome is transcribed into double-stranded DNA by the viral enzyme reverse transcriptase—typical of this kind of viruses. The double-stranded DNA is then integrated into the chromosomal DNA of the host cell with the help of the enzyme integrase. The integrated copy, termed a *provirus*, is similar to a cellular gene, but its expression is regulated by the virus rather than by the cell. Also, cellular genes, particularly cellular oncogenes, are usually copied together with the integrated proviral DNA in such a way that the viral genome carries cellular oncogenes after infection. Once incorporated into the viral genome, an oncogene is freed from normal cellular constraints and is expressed constitutively in infected cells under the direct control of the virus, leading to cell transformation and cancer development. Alternatively, a retrovirus containing a cellular oncogene may infect a cell type that does not express that oncogene and thus lacks controls to regulate it. Therefore, in the case of retroviruses, a combination of *overexpression* or *inappropriate expression* of a modified oncogene leads to malignant transformation of the target cell.

Unlike retroviruses, the oncogenes of small DNA tumor viruses are of viral, not cellular origin, and are essential for both viral replication and cell transformation. Small DNA tumor viruses are dependent on the host cell machinery to replicate the viral DNA. Viral DNA encodes nonstructural proteins that stimulate resting cells to enter the S phase of the cell cycle, to provide an environment that enhances DNA replication. One such protein, the large-T antigen of the simian virus 40 (SV-40), is required both for initiation of viral DNA synthesis and for stimulation of cell entry into the S phase. The large-T antigen of SV-40 was found to form a complex with a host cell protein (p53) in SV-40 transformed cells,[36] and this led to the conclusion that the gene synthesizing this protein (the *p53* gene) could be included in the growing list of oncogenes. However, a decade later it was definitely demonstrated that the *p53* gene is in fact a tumor suppressor gene,[37] that is, a gene that inhibits instead of stimulating cell growth. A second tumor suppressor protein, the retinoblastoma gene product (pRb) was also identified as one of several host cell proteins complexed with the E1A oncoprotein in adenovirus transformed cells.[38] The SV-40 T antigen also forms complexes with pRb and, by binding to and abolishing the normal function of both p53 and pRb inhibitory proteins, disrupts cell growth control mechanisms (Figure 2.3).[39] Once again it is clear from the previous outline that the study of both RNA and DNA oncogenic viruses and their close relationship with oncogenes and tumor suppressor genes, respectively, has played an outstanding role in the elucidation of the mechanisms of control of cell proliferation in normal cells and cancer. It may therefore sound rather paradoxical to question whether there is a role for viruses in cancer development, and the great majority of scientists working with tumor viruses would have no doubt at all. However, it is clear that even in cancers with proven viral etiology, the virus appears to be necessary but not sufficient, for tumor development. The interpretation is that viruses do not behave as complete carcinogens, but rather act as initiating or promoting factors. Additional changes must necessarily accumulate to complement those produced by the virus, to disable the multiple regulatory pathways and checkpoints that control proliferation in normal cells. Different data support this interpretation:

1. It is well known that the majority of individuals infected with a tumor virus do not develop cancer. As demonstrated by epidemiologic data, more than 90% of humans are infected with Epstein–Barr virus, but cancer due to EBV is rare, unless an individual becomes immunocompromised.
2. The latent period between the initial virus infection and tumor appearance is often too long to establish a clear-cut relationship between infection and tumor development. This is clearly illustrated by epidemiological evidence showing that, for example, Chinese with chronic HBV infections ac-

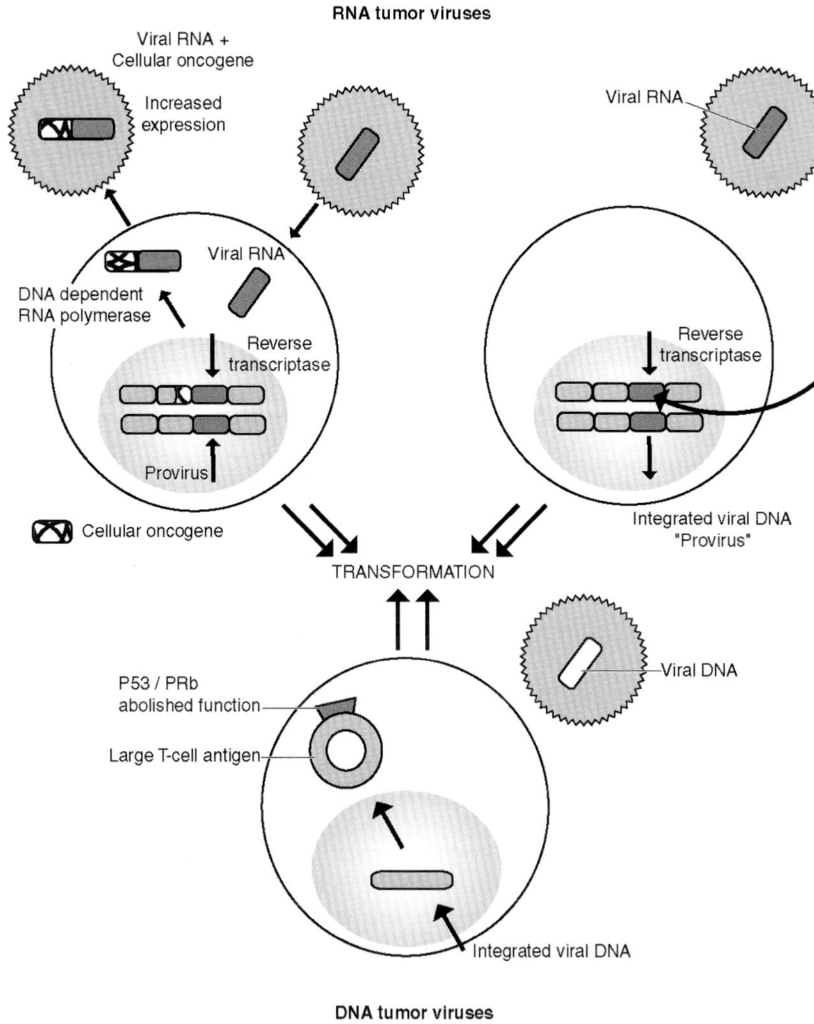

FIGURE 2.3. Mechanisms of cell transformation by RNA and DNA viruses.

quired as newborns usually develop hepatocellular carcinoma (HCC) beyond 50 years of age.

3. Finally, although it could be assumed that the host immune response may play a major role in explaining outcome, evidence from in vitro experiments conducted on isolated cell systems still confirms that additional changes must accumulate within a virus-infected cell for it to be fully transformed and that the transformation potential of a virus, given the necessity of these additional changes, is not instantaneous but requires a long latency period. Note that SV 40 or its cloned antigen alone has been known since 1962 to be a particularly efficient aneuploidogen in human cells. This effect would be produced, particularly by the T antigen, by displacing histone proteins from chromosomal DNA, thus inducing unwinding of nucleosomally organized DNA, with the block of the normal chromosomal binding sites for tubulin fibers.[5]

A list of some of the major viruses and related human cancers is presented in Table 2.1. The recognition of the viral etiology of human cancer provides the rationale to develop preventive strategies to inhibit viral infection, thus reducing cancer risk. Prophylactic vaccines can induce antibodies that can neutralize the virus before it infects the cell. The HBV vaccine has been used for more than 15 years to prevent transmission of the virus to newborns and to prevent the establishment of a lifelong persistent infection. Large-scale immunization programs have been undertaken in some countries to clarify the efficacy of the vaccine in reducing the incidence of HCC.[40] Given the worldwide burden of HPV-related diseases, papillomavirus vaccines are under development, recombinant virus–like particles (VLPs) are also under investigation.

Viruses can be also harnessed for novel approaches to cancer treatment. A number of gene-based therapies use viral vectors to deliver tumor suppressor genes (e.g., *p53*): immune response genes (cytokines), drug resistance genes, drug sensitivity genes, and genes to inhibit activated oncogenes. A further application of viruses to cancer therapy is represented by the so-called viral oncolysis. A prototype of this approach is represented by a mutant form of adenovirus

TABLE 2.1. Major Viruses Implicated in Human Cancer.

Name of virus	*Type of cancer*	*Cofactors*
Epstein–Barr virus (EBV)	Burkitt's lymphoma	Malaria
	Nasopharyngeal carcinoma	Nitrosamines
	B-cell lymphoma	Immunodeficiency
	Hodgkin's disease	Unknown
Hepatitis B virus (HBV)	Liver cancer	Aflatoxin, alcohol
Human immune deficiency virus (HIV)	Severe immune deficiency predisposing to Kaposi sarcoma, lymphoma, and cervical cancer	EBV, HPV, herpes virus
Human papilloma virus (HPV)	Cervical cancer	Smoking
	Skin cancer (*epidermodysplasia verruciformis*, a rare hereditary condition) and conjunctival cancer	Sunlight
Human T-cell lymphotropic virus type I (HTLV-1)	Adult T-cell leukemia/lymphoma	Unknown
Human T-cell lymphotropic virus type 2 (HTLV-2)	Hairy cell leukemia	Unknown
Kaposi sarcoma-associated herpesvirus (KSHV)	Kaposi sarcoma	Unknown
	Body-cavity-based lymphoma	EBV and HIV

that fails to express E1B that can replicate and destroy cancer cells that lack *p53*.[41] For updated information on this kind of therapy, see Reference 42.

IONIZING RADIATION, CHEMICALS, AND CANCER

The carcinogenic potential of ionizing radiation was soon recognized after Roentgen's discovery of x-rays in December 1895. The first report of leukemia in five radiation workers dates back to 1911.[43] (Marie Curie and her daughter, Irene, are both thought to have died from complications of radiation-induced leukemia.) Follow-up studies on atomic bomb survivors in Hiroshima and Nagasaki have confirmed that ionizing radiation is a "universal carcinogen" in that it induces tumors in most tissues of most species at all ages, including the fetus. The universal nature of radiation as a carcinogen is based on its ability to penetrate cells and deposit energy within them in a random manner, unaffected by the usual cellular barriers presented to chemical agents. As a consequence, all cells of the body are susceptible to ionizing radiation, and the amount of damage will depend on the physical parameters that determine the radiation dose received by a particular cell or tissue. Radiation can induce DNA lesions including damage to nucleotide bases, cross-linking, and DNA single- and double-strand breaks (DSBs). It is now accepted that misrepaired DSBs are the main lesions of importance in the induction of both chromosomal abnormalities and gene mutations.[44,45]

DSBs in DNA are produced when the two complementary DNA strands are simultaneously broken at sites close enough to one another and cannot be kept juxtaposed. The two fragments generated by this process are liable to become physically dissociated, making repair difficult and providing an opportunity for inappropriate recombination with other sites of the genome. However, despite posing major threats to genomic integrity, DSBs can be deliberately produced for "physiologic" purposes in the cells of the immune response. Moreover, DSBs are potent inducers of mutations and cell death.

There are two main pathways for DNA DSBs repair: homologous recombination (HR) and nonhomologous end joining (NHEJ). HR requires that the damaged chromosome enter into synapsis with, and retrieve genetic information from, an undamaged DNA molecule with which it shares extensive sequence homology; NHEJ does not have these requirements. As a consequence, NHEJ is more prone to error than HR and may facilitate the production of chromosomal rearrangements and other large-scale changes frequently occurring in irradiated cells.[46,47] As a consequence of DSBs, large-scale mutational events, such as deletions, chromosomal rearrangements, and recombinational processes, are associated with ionizing radiation. However, the search for genetic changes specifically associated with radiation has been disappointing, and there is no evidence of site specificity for mutations induced by radiation. Studies of oncogene activation or tumor suppressor gene inactivation in radiation transformation in vitro have been also disappointing. As we have seen in Chapter 1, however, there is increasing evidence that genomic instability may represent the earliest and most important event in both radiation and chemical carcinogenesis and may represent, as well, the best explanation for the reported lack of specificity of genomic lesions induced by both radiation and chemical carcinogens.

As outlined, genomic instability is a hallmark feature of nearly all solid tumors and adult-onset leukemia. Genomic instability is the process by which the entire cellular genome becomes more prone than a normal (stable) genome to make mistakes in the arrangement of chromsomes and fragments of chromosomes within the cell itself and, during mitosis, within the daughter cells. As already mentioned, the root source of genomic instability has to be researched in the processes of DNA damage and repair. As a matter of fact, intrachromosomal genomic instability in cancer reflects an increased rate of appearance of DNA alterations in tumor cells, which arises from either an increased rate of damage overwhelming the ability of a normal repair system to restore genetic integrity or a defective repair system unable to cope with a normal rate of damage. It is clear that preserving genomic integrity is of immense relevance for cells and organisms. That is evident when we consider that our genome contains around 250 genes for the purpose of DNA repair, 230 for high-fidelity DNA replication, and 500 for chromosome segregation, cell cycle checkpoints, telomeres, centromeres, and so on.

When the cell becomes unable to repair DNA damage for either of the reported conditions, genomic instability will follow and will propagate to daughter cells for a number of generations, thus amplifying both the number of damaged cells and the amount of damage per cell until, eventually, transformation occurs and cancer develops.[48]

Evidence has been presented that an unstable genome persists for at least 12 and perhaps 25 population doublings after radiation exposure. This transmissible instability may enhance the rate at which spontaneous mutations arise in the descendants of the irradiated cells. The widespread and apparently random nature of genomic instability may account for the reported lack of specificity of genomic lesions induced by both radiation and chemicals; also, genomic instability tells us that ionizing radiation may produce nontargeted effects, or, in other words, important genetic consequences of radiation may arise in cells born from the irradiated ones that in themselves received no direct nuclear exposure.

At this point, it will be of interest to notice that early investigations have shown that cytoplasmic irradiation with low fluences of α particles can induce a significant frequency of mutations in mammalian cells,[49] thus indicating that nuclear irradiation is not required for the production of important genetic effects. The production of gene mutations after cytoplasmic irradiation has been hypothesized to involve an enhanced production of reactive oxygen species (ROS) within the process globally indicated as oxidative stress. As demonstrated, DNA can be damaged in a sequence-specific manner by oxidative stress.[50] Oxidative stress results when the balance between the production of ROS overrides the antioxidant capabilities of the target cells; the interaction between reactive oxygen and critical cellular macromolecules may then occur,[51] with subsequent modification of cellular proteins, lipids, and DNA, which results in altered target cell function.

One further step in the mechanism of oxidative stress within radiation-induced carcinogenesis is represented by the so-called bystander effect, that is, the production of biologically relevant effects in cells that receive no direct radiation exposure. Evidence has been presented that cells irradiated with α particles secrete cytokines and other factors that lead to enhanced production of oxygen species in cells not directly irradiated, with subsequent damage of their proteins, lipids, and DNA[52] and have increased potential for genomic instability and cancer transformation (Figure 2.4). The International Agency for Research in Cancer (IARC) has defined chemical carcinogenesis as "the induction by chemicals of cancers that are not usually observed, the earlier induction by chemicals of cancers that are usually observed, and the induction by chemicals of more cancers than are usually found."[53] Although operationally useful, this definition does not address the fundamental distinction between direct-acting carcinogens and those acting indirectly through complex interactions with the test organism.[54] In 1973 the term "genotoxicity" was introduced to denote toxic, lethal, and heritable effects to karyotic and extrakaryotic material in germinal and somatic cells[55] and was assumed to be the basis of carcinogenicity of all chemicals. Subsequently, this paradigm was largely questioned, and the distinction between DNA-reactive (genotoxic) and epigenetic (nongenotoxic) carcinogens was well established.[56] DNA-reactive carcinogens are those that act in the target cell of tissue(s) to form DNA adducts that are the basis for neoplastic transformation. Epigenetic carcinogens lack chemical reactivity and hence do not form DNA adducts, but produce their effects indi-

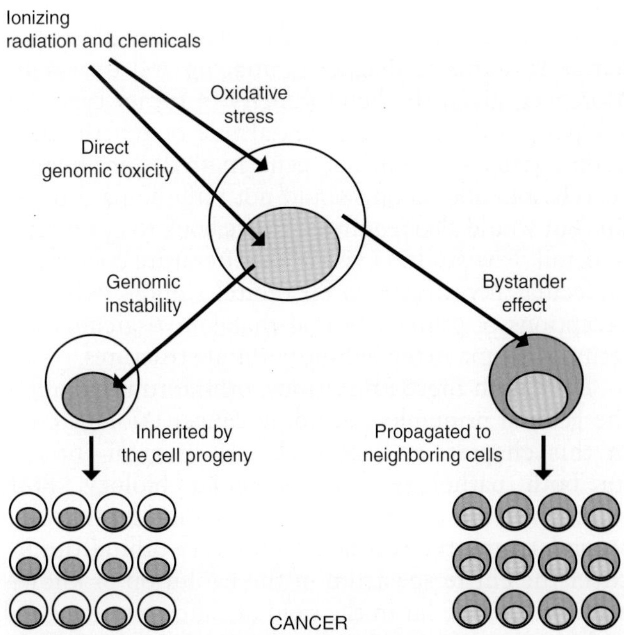

FIGURE 2.4. Proposed mechanisms of radiation and chemical carcinogenesis.

rectly (Figure 2.4). A comprehensive list of chemical carcinogens classified according to this distinction is reported by Williams.[56] The past two decades have witnessed an extraordinary impulse of the genetics, particularly under the influence of the Human Genome Project, and cancer has been increasingly viewed as a genetic disease. This radical and partial view of the pathogenesis of human cancer has been tempered by the discovery that gene expression can be modulated in the absence of structural damage of the genes themselves. Therefore, cancer should be more appropriately defined as a "disease of genes," implying that while an altered gene expression is almost invariably found in cancer, it does not necessarily derive from spontaneous gene changes but from either a direct or indirect insult on the DNA structure.

The paradigm of chemical carcinogenesis represents a milestone in the understanding of the real complexity inherent the processes of cell transformation and cancer development. As we have seen, together with "direct" DNA-reactive chemicals, a number of chemicals must be taken into account whose action, through the intermediary of oxidative stress, can modify intercellular communication, protein–kinase activity, membrane structure and function, and gene expression, to finally lead to deregulation of cell growth.[57]

RELEVANCE OF IMMUNOLOGICAL RESPONSE TO ORBITAL TUMORS

Orbital tumors constitute a heterogeneous array of lesions that may originate from tissues of the orbit itself (primary tumors), extend from neighboring structures (secondary tumors), or come from distant sites (metastatic tumors),[58] and, as such, they pose numerous challenges in terms of diagnosis, imaging and treatment. Moreover, given the heterogeneity of tumor types developing in the orbit, the causal role of genetic alterations, viruses, chemicals, gene methylation, histone acetylation, and so on, would not only be hard to define but would also require an entire book to be reported in detail. Few studies exist in the literature concerning molecular investigations on orbital tumors, with the exceptions of primary orbital rhabdomyosarcoma and retinoblastoma extended into orbital structures.

Even with these limitations, orbital tumors follow the general principles regarding cancer etiology cited in this chapter, and, as such, are of great interest for both pathology and molecular biology. Both retinoblastoma and rhabdomyosarcoma, the first as a secondary and the second as a primary orbital tumor, cover the entire spectrum of the evolution of knowledge reported so far in the field of cancer etiology and pathogenesis. Retinoblastoma has represented the prototype of cancer due to the loss or inactivation of a tumor suppressor gene, and for a long time has remained the most significant example of cancer determined by small structural modifications of a gene.[59] Rhabdomyosarcoma of the orbit, to the contrary, while occurring at an average age quite close to that reported for retinoblastoma, has always shown a more complex pathogenesis. In particular, gross chromosomal alterations, such as the translocation t(2;13) (q35-q14) or t(1;13) (q36-q14), involving the *PAX3* and *PAX7* genes, have been detected in alveolar rhabdomyosarcoma,[60] while a number of different genes (either oncogenes or tumor suppressor genes) have been reported to be involved in the genesis of the embryonal form of the disease.[61] More recently, the investigation of the methylation profile of retinoblastoma has shown that *RASSF1A* and *CASP8* (a tumor suppressor gene and a gene involved in the apoptotic process, respectively) are frequently methylated and "silenced" in retinoblastoma, thus showing that other genes may play a role in the genesis of retinoblastoma and that reducing its pathogenesis to the alteration of a single gene represents an oversimplification.[62,63] Moreover, the recent observation that microsatellite instability often occurs in embryonal rhabdomyosarcoma of the orbit represents an important clue into the pathogenesis of this disease, possibly implying a role for genomic instability and the related events in the process of cancer development.[64]

The same reasoning can be applied to orbital malignant tumors arising later in life. A recent review[65] has shown that malignant lymphoma is the most common malignant tumor of the orbit in the population over the age of 60 years, accounting for 24% of cases.[65] Malignant lymphoma, particularly the diffuse large-cell lymphoma (DLCL) has been shown to depend from an aberrant hypermutation state whose nature and consequences appear to be very similar to those described elsewhere under the generic term of genomic instability, which can be in part, considered "physiologic" for lymphocytes belonging to the B-cell lineage.[66] Finally, human papilloma virus has been reported in neoplastic and nonneoplastic conditions of the external eye,[67] as well as its possible relationship with an increased expression of the p53 protein, with consequent prognostic implications, particularly in conjunctival squamous cell carcinoma (CSCC),[68] thus demonstrating the potential of the application of molecular techniques in the study of orbital tumors.[68]

In summary, although the application of the principles and procedures of the molecular biology to cancer arising in the orbit is not very common, it can be of great potential value for both diagnostic and therapeutic purposes. Therefore, it is highly desirable for the ophthalmologist to become acquainted with the basic principles in the perspective of a modern and more effective approach to patients with tumors involving the orbit.

References

1. Burnet FM. The concept of immunological surveillance. *Prog Exp Tumor Res* 1970;13:1–23.
2. Wick M, et al. Antigenic cancer cells grow progressively in immune competent hosts without evidence of T-cell exhaustion or systemic anergy. *J Exp Med* 1997;186:229–238.
3. Joklik WK, Willett HP, Amos DB. Immunity to tumors and pregnancy. In: *Zinsser Microbiology*. 18th ed. Norwalk, CT: Appleton-Century-Crofts; 1984.
4. http://www.cancerresearch.org/immincid.html
5. Li R, Sonik A, Stindl R, et al. Aneuploidy vs gene mutation hypothesis of cancer: recent study claims mutation but is found to support aneuploidy. *Proc Natl Acad Sci U S A* 2000; 97:7, 3236–3241.
6. http://www.annieappleseedproject.org/antheorofcan.html
7. http://www.kcom.edu/faculty/chamberlain/Website/MSTUART/Lect14.htm
8. Djeu JY, Jiang K, Wei S. A view to a kill: signals triggering cytotoxicity. *Clin Cancer Res* 2002;8:636–640.
9. Medzhitov R, Janeway CA Jr. Decoding the patterns of self and non-self by the innate immune system. *Science* 2002;296: 298–300.
10. Metzinger P. The danger model: a renewed sense of self. *Science* 2002;296:301–305.
11. Moretta L, Biassoni R, Bottino C, et al. Natural killer cells: a mystery no more. *Scand J Immunol* 2002;55:229–232.
12. Foss FM. Immunologic mechanisms of antitumor activity. *Semin Oncol* 2002;29(suppl 7):5–11.
13. Vicari AP, Caux C. Chemokines in cancer. *Cytokines Growth Factors Rev* 2002;13:143–154.
14. Homey B, Muller A, Zlotnik A. Chemokines: agents for the immunotherapy of cancer? *Nat Rev Immunol* 2002;2:175–184.
15. Finn OJ, Lotze MT. A decade in the life of tumor immunology. *Clin Cancer Res* 2001(suppl);7:759–760.
16. De Pinho RA. The age of cancer. *Nature* 2000;408:248–254.
17. American Cancer Society. *Cancer Facts and Figures, 2000*. Atlanta: American Cancer Society; 2000:1–7.
18. Harman D. Aging: a theory based on free radical and radiation chemistry. *J Gerontol* 1956;6:298–300.
19. Ames BN, Shigenega MK, Hagen TM. Oxidants, antioxidants, and the degenerative diseases of aging. *Proc Natl Acad Sci U S A* 1993;90:7915–7922.
20. Minnik DT, Kunkel DA. DNA synthesis errors, mutations and cancer. *Cancer Surv* 1996;28:3–20.
21. Kinzler KW, Vogelstein B. Familial cancer syndromes: the role of caretakers and gatekeepers. In: Scriver CR, Beaudet AL, Sly WS, Valle D, eds. *The Metabolic and Molecular Bases of Inherited Disease*. Vol 1. 8th ed. New York: McGraw-Hill Medical Publishing; 2001:675–676.
22. Karran P. Human mismatch repair: defects and predisposition to cancer. *Encyclopedia of Life Sciences*. www.els.net
23. Anderson GR. Genomic instability in cancer. *Curr Sci* 2001;81: 501–507.
24. Loeb LA. Mutator phenotype may be required for multistage carcinogenesis. *Cancer Res* 1991;51:3075–3079.
25. Kinzler KW, Vogelstein B. Lessons from hereditary colorectal cancer. *Cell* 1996;87:159–170.
26. Atkin NB. Microsatellite instability. *Cytogenet Cell Genet* 2001;92:177–181.
27. Granger MP, Wright WE, Shay JW. Telomerase in cancer and aging. *Crit Rev Oncol/Hematol* 2002;41:29–40.
28. Wright WE, Shay JW. Telomere dynamics in cancer progression and prevention: fundamental differences in human and mouse telomere biology. *Nat Med* 2000;6:849–851.
29. Mathon NF, Lloyd AC. Cell senescence and cancer. *Nat Rev Cancer* 2001;1:203–213.
30. Sheel C, Poremba C. Telomere lengthening in telomerase negative cells: the ends are coming together. *Virchows Arch* 2002; 440:573–582.
31. Shay JW, Wright WE. Telomeres and telomerase: implications for cancer and aging. *Radiat Res* 2001;155:188–193.
32. Artandi S, Chang S, Lee S-L, et al. Telomere dysfunction promotes non-reciprocal translocations in epithelial cancer in mice. *Nature* 2000;406:641–645.
33. Pathak S, Multani AS, Furlong CL, Sohn SH. Telomere dynamics, aneuploidy, stem cells, and cancer [review]. *Int J Oncol* 2002;20:637–641.
34. Butel JS. Viral oncogenesis: revelation of molecular mechanisms and etiology of human disease. *Carcinogenesis* 2000;21: 405–426.
35. Rous P. A sarcoma of the fowl transmissible by an agent separable from the tumor cells. *J Exp Med* 1911;13:397–411.
36. Lane TP, Crawford LV. T antigen is bound to a host protein in SV-40 transformed cells. *Nature* 1979;278:261–263.
37. Finlay CA, Hinds PW, Levine AJ. The p53 proto-oncogene can act as a suppressor of transformation. *Cell* 1989;57:1083–1093.
38. Whyte P, Buchowich KJ, Horowitz JM, et al. Association between an oncogene and an anti-oncogene. The adenovirus E1A protein binds to the retinoblastoma gene product. *Nature* 1988;334:124–129.
39. Butel JS, Ledniky JA. Cell and molecular biology of simian virus 40: implications for human infections and disease. *J Natl Cancer Inst* 1999;91:119–134.
40. Chang MH, Chen CJ, Lai MS, et al. for the Taiwan Childhood Hepatoma Study Group (1997). Universal hepatitis B vaccination in Taiwan and the incidence of hepatocellular carcinoma in children. *N Engl J Med* 1997;336:1855–1859.
41. Bischoff JH, Kim DH, Williams A, et al. An adenovirus mutant that replicates selectively in p53-deficient human tumor cells. *Science* 1996;274:373–376.
42. Mullen JT, Tanabe KK. Viral oncolysis. *Oncologist* 2002;7: 106–119.
43. Upton AC. Historical perspectives in radiation carcinogenesis. In: Upton AC, Albert RE, Burns FJ, Shore RE, eds. *Radiation Carcinogenesis*. New York: Elsevier; 1986:1–10.
44. Goodhead DT. Initial events in the cellular effects of ionising radiations: clustered damage in DNA. *Int J Radiat Biol* 1994;142:362–368.
45. Ward JF. Radiation mutagenesis: the initial DNA lesions responsible. *Radiat Res* 1995;79:7763–7767.
46. Jackson SP. Sensing and repairing DNA double-strand breaks. *Carcinogenesis* 2002;23:687–696.
47. Little JB. Radiation carcinogenesis. *Carcinogenesis* 2000;21: 397–404.
48. Anderson AG. Genomic instability in cancer. *Curr Sci* 2001;81: 501–507.
49. Wu L, Randers-Perhson G, Xu A, et al. Targeted cytoplasmic irradiation with alpha particles induces mutations in mammalian cells. *Proc Natl Acad Sci U S A* 1999;96:4959–4964.
50. Kawanishi S, Hiraka Y, Oikawa S. Mechanism of guanine-specific DNA damage by oxidative stress and its role in carcinogenesis and aging. *Mutat Res* 2001;488:65–76.
51. http://lowdose.org/pubs/ehp/members/klaunigfull.html
52. Prise KM, Belyakov OV, Folkhard M, Michael BD. Studies of bystander effects in human fibroblasts using a charged particle microbeam. *Int J Radiat Biol* 1998;74:793–798.
53. International Agency for Research on Cancer. IARC Monographs on the Evaluation of the Carcinogenic Risk of Chemicals in Humans. No 29. Lyons, France: IARC, 1982:16.
54. Weisburger J, Williams G. Chemical carcinogens. In: Klaasen CD, Amdur MO, eds. *Toxicology: The Basic Science of Poisons*. 2nd ed. New York: Macmillan; 1980:84–138.
55. Ehremberg L, Brookes P, Druckrey H, et al. The relation of cancer induction and genetic damage. In: Ramel C, ed. *Evaluation of Genetic Risks of Environmental Chemicals*. Stock-

holm: University of Stockholm; 1973. AMBIO Special Report No 3, pp. 15–16.
56. Williams GM. Mechanisms of chemical carcinogenesis and application to human cancer risk assessment. *Toxicology* 2001; 166:3–10.
57. Klaunig JE, Xu SI, Isenberg JS, Bachowski S, et al. The role of oxidative stress in chemical carcinogenesis. *Environ Health Perspect* 1998;106(suppl 1):289–295.
58. Darsaut TE, Lanzino G, Lopes MB, Newman S. An introductory overview of orbital tumors. *Neurosurg Focus* 2001;10:1–9.
59. Newsham IF, Hadjistilianou T, Cavenee WK. Retinoblastoma. In: Vogelstein B, Kinzler KW, eds: *The Genetic Basis of Human Cancer*. 2nd ed. New York: McGraw-Hill; 2002:357–386.
60. Meltzer PS, Kallioniemi A, Trent JM. Chromosome alterations in human solid tumors. In: Vogelstein B, Kinzler KW, eds. *The Genetic Basis of Human Cancer*. 2nd ed. New York: McGraw-Hill; 2002:93–113.
61. Mastrangelo D, Sappia F, Bruni S, et al. Loss of heterozygosity on the long arm of chromosome 11 in orbital embryonal rhabdomyosarcoma (OERMS): a microsatellite study of seven cases. *Orbit* 1998;17:89–95.
62. Harada K, Toyooka S, Maitra A, et al. Aberrant promoter methylation and silencing of the *RASSF1A* gene in pediatric tumors and cell lines. *Oncogene* 2002;21:4345–4349.
63. Harada K, Toyooka S, Shivapurkar N, et al. Deregulation of Caspase 8 and 10 expression in pediatric tumors and cell lines. *Cancer Res*. 2002;62:5897–5901.
64. Mastrangelo D, Hadjistilianou T, Mazzotta C, Loré C. Microsatellite instability in three cases of embryonal rhabdomyosarcoma of the orbit. *Med Pediatr Oncol* 2002;39:132–133.
65. Demirci H, Shields CL, Shields JA, et al. Orbital tumors in the older adult population. *Ophthalmology* 2002;109:243–248.
66. Pasqualucci L, Neumeister P, Goossens T, et al. Hypermutation of multiple proto-oncogenes in B-cell diffuse large-cell lymphoma. *Nature* 2001;412:341–346.
67. Karcioglu ZA, Tawfik MI. Human papilloma virus in neoplastic and nonneoplastic conditions of the external eye. *Br J Ophthalmol* 1997;81:595–598.
68. Karcioglu ZA, Toth J. Relation between p53 overexpression and clinical behavior of ocular/orbital invasion of conjunctival squamous cell carcinoma. *Ophthalmol Plast Reconstr Surg* 2000;16:443–449.

3

The Changing Nature and Behavior of Orbital and Periorbital Tumors

Alan A. McNab

This chapter discusses the changes over time in the nature and behavior of orbital tumors and related diseases, looking in particular at the influence of certain forms of viral and iatrogenic immunosuppression.

CHANGES IN THE INCIDENCE OF ORBITAL DISEASES OVER TIME

A glance through older textbooks of ophthalmology reveals a number of orbital disorders almost unknown to the modern ophthalmologist. Duke-Elder, in his seminal *System of Ophthalmology*,[1] describes such conditions as orbital syphilis (syphilitic periostitis, orbital gummas, etc.), orbital tuberculosis (which may return to the West with the emergence of resistant strains of *Mycobacteria* and the increase in immunosuppression), and echinococcus (hydatid disease) of the orbit (still common in some parts of the world). The most significant change, however, has been in the classification and nomenclature of disorders that have probably always existed but are now better understood. These include the idiopathic inflammatory disorders ("pseudotumors"), lymphoproliferative disorders, and the vascular lesions of the orbit.

Some orbital tumors have increased in incidence over time. One of the commonest tumors of the orbit in current clinical practice is non-Hodgkin's lymphoma (NHL). Although the classification of NHL has changed, making comparison of older reports with current reports difficult, good epidemiological data confirm the clinical impression of many specialists that NHL is increasing in incidence over time, including NHL of the orbit. Margo and Mulla examined the Florida Cancer Registry from 1981 through 1993 and showed a large increase in orbital NHL over this time, with a steady but smaller increase in primary orbital malignancy in general.[2] A study from Singapore failed to show any significant change over the period 1968 to 1995,[3] but given the widely reported increase in NHL, it is likely the increase noted in Florida is real. In Australia, there was a steady increase in the incidence of NHL (whole body) between 1982 and 1989 among both males and females,[4] but between 1993 and 1998 the increase was confined to females, with an increase of 1.8% per year.[5] There is no adequate explanation for this observed increase. A study from Denmark, where a national orbital tumor registry was established in 1974, has also shown a steady increase in the incidence of both benign and malignant orbital tumors over the period 1974 to 1997.[6] All tissue specimens derived from the orbit were registered during this time, making the increased incidence observed very likely to be a real increase rather than an artifact. Data are limited on changes in incidence of secondary orbital tumors, but one study from Japan has shown a small but steady increase in orbital metastasis from primary tumors in the lung, liver, and adrenal gland since 1980.[7] As the incidence of primary tumors changes over time, it is likely the pattern of orbital metastases will change also.

IMMUNOSUPPRESSION AND CANCER

Perhaps the greatest change in the nature and frequency of some orbital disorders has been in those that occur more frequently in the immunosuppressed patient. The treatment of many disorders, especially for those of an autoimmune type and for the immunosuppression required for solid organ transplants, has involved general suppression of the immune system at the expense of an increased risk and incidence of formerly rare disorders.

Immunodeficiency may be congenital, therapeutic, or infectious [human immunodeficiency viruses (HIV)]. We have seen increases in the latter two, and in some parts of the world, HIV is the most prevalent and serious infectious disease in the community. Immunodeficiency increases the risk of some but not all cancers. The common feature of these cancers is that specific infectious agents may be important in their etiology; this may extend to a lesser extent beyond the immunodeficient population to the normal population. People with acquired immune deficiency syndrome (HIV/AIDS) are more susceptible to a variety of malignant neoplasms (see Table 3.1). These include

TABLE 3.1. Malignant Neoplasms of the Orbit and Ocular Adnexa Associated with AIDS.

Lymphoma	Small, non-cleaved cell (Burkitt) lymphoma
	Large non-cleaved-cell immunoblastic lymphoma
	Hodgkin's lymphoma (rare)
Kaposi's sarcoma	Eyelid
	Conjunctiva
	Orbit (rare)
Squamous cell carcinoma	Eyelid
	Conjunctiva (common especially in Africa)

Kaposi sarcoma (which is associated with human herpes virus type 8 (HHV-8)), non-Hodgkin's lymphoma of the Burkitt type (associated with another herpesvirus, the Epstein–Barr virus (EBV)), and conjunctival squamous cell carcinoma (associated with human papilloma virus (HPV)). In some studies, however, HIV/AIDS has not been shown to lead to an increase in cervical cancer, which has a known association with HPV infection. This requires further study, as does the apparent lack of certain other cancers that might be expected to be increased in HIV/AIDS.[8]

Despite the worldwide epidemic of HIV/AIDS and the increased incidence of these cancers, there has been a relative paucity of cases of orbital non-Hodgkin's lymphoma. NHL in AIDS is typically higher grade, is extranodal, and has a poorer outcome. The first case of orbital involvement was reported in 1982[9] and the second as late as 1990.[10] Since that time, a handful of other cases has been reported.[11–13]

Here then is a paradox. We have a worldwide epidemic of HIV/AIDS. There has been a documented increase in the incidence of NHL and, in particular, NHL of the orbit; but there have been very few cases of NHL of the orbit reported to be associated with AIDS. Our own experience has mirrored this. In a survey of 73 cases of orbital and ocular adnexal lymphoma from our institution, not one was known to be associated with HIV/AIDS.[14] Other large series also show no cases of HIV/AIDS-associated NHL. NHL of the ocular adnexa typically occurs in the older population (median age 65 in our series),[14] whereas NHL in association with HIV/AIDS occurs most commonly in the third decade, coinciding with the median decade in which AIDS is found.[15] From a practical perspective, a younger patient with a higher grade lymphoma of the orbit probably should be tested for HIV, although the likelihood of a positive result is fairly low, and most cases reported have been in patients already known to have HIV/AIDS. Another large group of immunodeficient patients are those receiving solid organ transplants. It is well recognized that this group is also more susceptible to a range of cancers and infections. Many of these are associated with particular viruses and may occur in the orbit or ocular adnexa.

Infection by HPV is well documented to increase after organ transplantation and the concomitant immunosuppression. The incidence of warts increases after transplantation, and at a later date, the incidence of squamous cell cancers of the skin also increases. Within these tumors can be found evidence of HPV of various types, often more than one type in each tumor.[16]

Within the first 5 years of immunosuppression, 40% of transplant recipients experience premalignant skin tumors such as actinic keratoses and Bowen's disease, as well as squamous cell carcinoma (SCC) and basal cell carcinoma (BCC).[17] These tumors often have a more aggressive pattern of growth and atypical morphology.[18] Sun exposure is a clear risk factor, and the presence of skin cancers or premalignant skin lesions may be a contraindication to organ transplantation because of the increased mortality associated with organ transplantation from cancer, including skin cancer. In addition to the association between immune suppression and HPV infection and the development of nonmelanoma skin cancer, there is evidence of a link with herpes-like virus infection and skin cancers other than Kaposi sarcoma in transplant patients.[19] In a group of non-AIDS immunocompromised patients, 82% of 33 skin lesions (BCC, SCC, actinic keratoses, etc.) demonstrated herpes virus-like sequences of DNA.

The incidence of skin cancers (other than Kaposi sarcoma) is also increased in patients whose immune system is compromised by the HIV/AIDS virus. A study from Italy found a threefold increase in nonmelanoma skin cancer (mostly BCC) in AIDS patients.[20] This increase in nonmelanoma skin cancer was noted to be less than that occurring in transplant patients. Cutaneous SCC is often more aggressive when it occurs in patients with HIV/AIDS,[21] and such lesions should be managed aggressively rather than palliatively because they may be fatal, particularly with antiretroviral therapies now prolonging survival in HIV-infected patients for many years.[22] Basal cell carcinoma may behave more aggressively in AIDS patients also. Although metastasis from BCC is extremely rare, it is documented to occur when cellular immunity is compromised, as occurs in AIDS.[23] The commonest mucocutaneous malignancy associated with AIDS is Kaposi sarcoma, which is associated with infection with HHV-8. The condition may occur in the eyelids or conjunctiva but rarely affects the orbit.[24] Conjunctival Kaposi sarcoma may be the presenting feature of AIDS, but by far the commonest conjunctival tumor associated with AIDS is SCC. This is particularly true for AIDS occurring in Africa, where conjunctival SCC is one of the commonest AIDS-associated cancers. In African HIV patients, non-Hodgkin's lymphoma may be less frequent than in the West.[25] It is unclear whether this represents differences in prevalence of other associated viral infections. Because of the dramatic rise in incidence of AIDS, Kaposi sarcoma has emerged as the most common cancer in parts of Africa.[26] Conjunctival SCC has dramatically increased in incidence in areas of Africa where AIDS is prevalent, and it behaves in a particularly aggressive manner.[27] This dramatic rise in SCC of the conjunctiva has not been mirrored in the West, although SCC of the conjunctiva has certainly been seen[28] and may be the presenting sign in AIDS.[29]

IMMUNOSUPPRESSION AND INFECTION

The hallmark of the acquired immunosuppression appearing after infection with HIV is the occurrence of life-threatening infections by organisms that are usually opportunistic or nonpathogenic. A range of orbital infections has been seen, which may be bacterial, fungal, parasitic, or protozoan. These are listed in Table 3.2.

Invasive Aspergillosis

The commonest orbital infection seen in association with HIV/AIDS is invasive aspergillosis.[30] Risk factors for invasive aspergillosis apart from HIV/AIDS include other causes of decreased cellular immunity, neutropenia below 1000/mm^3, defects of phagocytosis, hematological malignancy, steroids or other immunosuppressive agents, and diabetes mellitus.[31] *Aspergillus* is a ubiquitous fungus found especially in soil and in decaying vegetable matter. *A. fumigatus* and *A. flavus* are the species most commonly seen in orbital and paranasal sinus disease. A range of patterns of disease may be associated with this organism, broadly divided into noninvasive and invasive forms. In nonimmunocompromised patients, two forms, both less aggressive, may occur. *Aspergillus* sinusitis may cause a chronic form of sinusitis in patients with atopy whose immune systems are otherwise normal. The sinuses may expand dramatically, with resultant telecanthus and structural changes in the facial skeleton. A fungus ball (aspergilloma) may occur in poorly aerated sinuses. Both these types of infection are characterized by a lack of tissue reaction, invasion, or necrosis. By contrast, in immunocompromised individuals, infection with *Aspergillus* may take the form of an invasive granulomatous inflammation with concomitant fibrosis, or a more fulminant necrotizing form characterized by vascular invasion and associated tissue necrosis.

When invading the orbit, aspergillosis usually spreads from the adjacent paranasal sinuses but may spread hematogenously from distant sites of infection, most commonly, the lung. The posterior orbit is commonly involved, presenting as an orbital apex syndrome, with loss of vision, ophthalmoplegia, loss of sensation in the first division of the trigeminal nerve and proptosis, often with pain.[32] In the early phases of the process, single nerves may be affected before progression to a full orbital apex syndrome. The cavernous sinus is usually also involved by the process. All too often, spread occurs to the cranial cavity and brain, with cerebral infarction or subarachnoid hemorrhage being terminal events. The diagnosis of invasive aspergillosis is aided by clinical imaging. Computed tomography (CT) images often show opacification of adjacent paranasal sinuses, with enhancing soft tissue masses usually invading the posterior orbit, with or without bone destruction. Intraluminal calcification visible on CT images is said to be characteristic but is present in less than 50% of cases.[33] Magnetic resonance imaging often shows more widespread enhancement than is seen on CT, showing involvement of adjacent dura or optic nerve, for example.[34] The definitive diagnosis of invasive aspergillosis is made by examination of affected tissue, both for histopathology and microbiology. If the condition is suspected, tissue should be obtained as soon as possible. It is important to alert the laboratory to the suspicion of fungal infection. Tissue may be obtained by fine needle aspirate,[35] or biopsy via an endoscopic or open approach. Frozen sections should be requested, since the establishment of an immediate diagnosis may allow the surgeon to proceed to appropriate debridement.

Treatment of invasive aspergillosis is difficult. Reversal of any immunosuppression, if possible, is important. In AIDS patients, in whom invasive aspergillosis is often fatal, treatment with antiretroviral drugs, including protease inhibitors, may prolong survival for extensive periods, even in the presence of invasive aspergillosis.[36] The role of wide surgical debridement is unclear.[37] Systemic and local antifungal therapy is the mainstay of treatment, with the less toxic liposomal form of amphotericin B most widely used.[38]

TABLE 3.2. Infectious Diseases of the Orbit Occurring in HIV/AIDS Patients.

Bacterial	Orbital cellulitis/abscess Syphilitic periostitis
Fungal	Invasive aspergillosis Mucormycosis (uncommon)
Parasitic/protozoan	Infection with *Pneumocystis carinii* Toxoplasmosis

Mucormycosis

Mucormycosis is usually a fulminant form of fungal infection occurring in a group of patients somewhat different from those who are susceptible to invasive aspergillosis (see also Chapter 27). Often referred to as phycomycosis or zygomycosis, mucormycosis is a disease caused by a variety of fungi from the order *Mucorales* in the class *Zygomycetes*. These organisms are widespread molds that we are exposed to regularly in daily life, but disease is rare because of their low virulence and because of host defenses. The people most susceptible are the debilitated, injured, and diabetic (especially ketoacidotic, poorly controlled diabetics), and those who are immunocompromised, most commonly by corticosteroids. Renal dialysis patients have also been commonly affected possibly because of the previous widespread use of deferoxamine in these patients to treat aluminum or iron overload.[39] Iron overload of itself may be a risk factor also,[40] with some evidence that the acidosis found in diabetics alters iron metabolism and enhances the ability of the *Mucor* organisms to grow in tissues.[41] AIDS patients do not appear to have an increased susceptibility to mucormycosis. This is probably because of the vital role of polymorphonuclear neutrophils (PMNs) in the prevention of the disease and the relatively normal function of PMNs in AIDS.[42]

Spores enter the airways, and for rhino-orbital-cerebral mucormycosis, the infection begins in the paranasal sinuses, or nasal airway, then spreading to the orbit and cranial cavity. The organism causes ischemic necrosis and invades blood vessels, including major arteries. The disease process is usually more fulminant than in invasive aspergillosis, with time from onset of symptoms to death often measured in days. The predisposed patient presents with pain, headache, swelling of the lids, ophthalmoplegia, and visual loss, occasionally with a central retinal artery occlusion. The classic black eschar due to tissue necrosis, which may be seen in the skin, nasal mucosa, or palate, is a late sign. Signs of intracranial involvement usually occur within a short period, with death resulting from cerebral infarction or subarachnoid and intracerebral hemorrhage. Early diagnosis is essential in mucormycosis. The tissue required for diagnostic purposes can be obtained from the sinuses or the orbit and processed both for histopathology (frozen section) and microbiology. Reversal of any immunosuppression and reversal of acidosis improves survival significantly. Widespread surgical debridement has a clearer role in mucormycosis than in aspergillosis and often involves orbital exenteration and widespread removal of affected paranasal sinuses.[43] Antifungal therapy, both local and systemic, is critical. There may be a role for adjunctive hyperbaric oxygen therapy.[44] Despite these measures, mortality rates remain high in mucormycosis.

Other Infections and Orbital Inflammation in AIDS Patients

Fulminant bacterial infections of the orbit have been reported in AIDS patients. Francis et al. reported a case of orbital streptococcal gangrene (necrotizing fasciitis) in an AIDS patient with extensive tissue necrosis and visual loss secondary to infection with group A β-hemolytic *Streptococcus*.[45] Kronish et al. also documented a variety of bacterial infections in AIDS patients, including cases caused by low virulence organisms such as *Propionibacterium acnes*.[30] Parasitic orbital infections have also been reported, including cases of *Toxoplasma* orbital cellulitis.[46] Orbital infection from *Pneumocystis carinii* is rare,[47] but *Pseudomonas* orbital cellulitis has been reported by several authors.[30,48]

Noninfectious Orbital Inflammation in AIDS

A small number of cases of apparently noninfectious inflammation of the orbit have been described in AIDS patients. This includes a case of "pseudotumor"[49] and one of "ocular myositis" that responded to high doses of corticosteroids.[50] Extreme caution needs to be exercised in accepting such a diagnosis and then treating with further immunosuppression. If the diagnosis is erroneous and the condition is, for example, a fungal infection, the addition of the steroids may accelerate the process.

OTHER VIRUS-ASSOCIATED NEOPLASMS OF THE ORBIT AND OCULAR ADNEXA

A variety of neoplasms has been shown to be associated with viruses (in the absence of infection with HIV); many of these may affect the orbit and ocular adnexa. The best-recognized ones are listed in Table 3.3.

Epstein–Barr Virus

EBV is a herpes-type virus, well recognized to be associated with some types of lymphoma, particularly Burkitt's lymphoma (small non-cleaved-cell lymphoma). Burkitt's lymphoma may also be linked to a heritable or familial predisposition, which in turn is associated with a chromosomal abnormality (translocation from chromosome 8 to chromosome 14). It is

TABLE 3.3. Neoplasms and Diseases of the Orbit and Ocular Adnexa Linked to Specific Viruses.

Virus	*Neoplasm or disease*
Epstein–Barr virus	Burkitt's lymphoma Nasal T/natural killer cell lymphoma (lethal midline granuloma) Nasopharyngeal carcinoma
Human papilloma virus	Squamous cell carcinoma (eyelid, conjunctiva, lacrimal excretory system)
Human T-cell lymphotropic/leukemia virus 1	Orbital T-cell leukemia/lymphoma Graves disease

endemic in some parts of Africa and had been well before the onset of the HIV/AIDS epidemic. It also is common in New Guinea, and its incidence parallels that of malaria in its distribution. Sporadic cases do occur outside these areas but are relatively uncommon; in these cases, EBV is not often found to be expressed in the tumor cells. Burkitt's lymphoma also occurs more frequently in patients infected with HIV. Burkitt's lymphoma is often rapidly progressive and in the endemic form occurs usually in childhood with a mean age of 8 years. In Uganda it is the commonest orbital tumor.[51] The mandible is most commonly affected, but the orbit and meninges are affected in about 10 to 20% of patients. Bone defects are common. The sporadic form tends to affect older children (mean age 12 years), and the orbit may also be affected but with less bony involvement. EBV has also been shown to be associated with the nasal condition formerly called lethal midline granuloma, now designated as a lymphoma characterized by T and natural killer cells.[52] This disease is commonest in Asian, Native American, and Hispanic peoples, and in Hong Kong Chinese, it represents a third of nasal lymphomas.[53] Because it usually arises in the nose and paranasal sinuses, secondary involvement of the orbit may occur, with orbital infiltration or uveitis being the commonest.[54] Another tumor linked to EBV is nasopharyngeal carcinoma, which also has an interesting epidemiology; this tumor represents up to 18% of all cancers in the south of China.[55] Orbital signs are frequently due to skull base invasion with cranial neuropathies or, less commonly, direct orbital invasion.

Human Papilloma Virus

HPV is linked to squamous cell neoplasia of skin and conjunctiva, particularly in immunosuppressed patients, and SCC of the conjunctiva is a major health issue in parts of Africa where AIDS is endemic. In nonimmunosuppressed patients, the role of HPV in the development of SCC of the conjunctiva has been debated. Some researchers have failed to link HPV with conjunctival SCC,[56–58] but others have shown a strong link.[57] A similar link has been shown for epithelial neoplasms of the lacrimal sac.[60,61]

Human T-Cell Leukemia Virus 1

HTLV-1 was the first oncogenic retrovirus to be identified. HTLV-1 infection is endemic to the Caribbean, Central and South America, southern Africa, and Japan. It is linked to an adult form of T-cell leukemia characterized by a malignant proliferation of T lymphocytes and a neuromyelopathy, usually causing a progressive paraplegia. Ocular lesions may occur, including uveitis in 15%, keratoconjunctivitis sicca in 37% with a lymphoplasmacytoid infiltrate of salivary and lacrimal glands, interstitial keratitis in 10%, and occasionally optic neuritis.[62] A case of orbital T-cell lymphoma has been reported in this infection,[63] as well as cases of optic nerve infiltration[64] and orbital and intracranial spread from nasal disease.[65] Another fascinating association noted with HTLV-1 is with Graves disease.[66] A number of reports have noted an increased incidence of Graves disease in patients with HTLV-1 infection, often associated with uveitis. It is postulated that the HTLV-1 infection induces an autoimmune process manifesting as uveitis and/or Graves disease. Up to 17% of patients with uveitis associated with HTLV-1 had a history of Graves disease in one report.[66]

Mucosa-Associated Lymphoid Tissue Lymphoma and Microbial Infection

A fascinating insight into tumor biology has arisen with the observation of an association between mucosa-associated lymphoid tissue lymphoma (MALT lymphoma, or marginal cell lymphoma) of the gastric mucosa and infection with the bacterium *Helicobacter pylori*. An association between *H. pylori* infection and adenocarcinoma of the stomach has also been noted.[67,68] Additionally, a role for chronic infection with hepatitis C virus has been suggested in MALT lymphoma of the stomach.[69] Inasmuch as MALT lymphoma is common in the orbit and ocular adnexa, future research may detect an association with other infective agents.

CONCLUSIONS

The incidence of disease processes of the orbit and ocular adnexa, both infective and neoplastic, has changed over time and varies enormously in geographic distribution. These trends have been largely due to changes in the incidence of infections with some bacteria and viruses. In addition, our understanding of the role of infectious agents in the development of neoplasms has increased, and it is likely that their role is greater than had been recognized in a large number of orbital and ocular adnexal neoplasms.

References

1. Duke-Elder S. Inflammations of the orbit. In: *System of Ophthalmology*. Vol 13. Pt 2. London: Henry Kimpton; 1974:859–931.
2. Margo CE, Mulla ZD. Malignant tumors of the orbit. Analysis of the Florida Cancer Registry. *Ophthalmology* 1998;105:185–190.
3. Lee SB, Au Eong KG, Saw SM, et al. Eye cancer incidence in Singapore. *Br J Ophthalmol* 2000;84:767–770.
4. Anti-Cancer Council or Victoria Epidemiology Centre. Can-

Stat—Cancer in Victoria 1999–2001. Melbourne: Anti-Cancer Council of Victoria; 2002.
5. Cancer incidence in Australia. www.aihw.gov.au/dataonline/index/.
6. Johansen S, Heegaard S, Bogeskov L, et al. Orbital space-occupying lesions in Denmark 1974–1997. *Acta Ophthalmol Scand* 2000;78:547–552.
7. Amemiya T, Hayashida H, Dake Y. Metastatic orbital tumors in Japan: a review of the literature. *Ophthalmic Epidemiol* 2002;9:35–47.
8. Beral V, Newton R. Overview of the epidemiology of immunodeficiency-associated cancers. *J Natl Cancer Inst Monogr* 1998; 23:1–6.
9. Ziegler JL, Drew WL, Miner RC, et al. Outbreak of Burkitt's-like lymphoma in homosexual men. *Lancet* 1982;2:631–633.
10. Antle CM, White VA, Horsman DE, et al. Large cell orbital lymphoma in a patient with acquired immunodeficiency syndrome. Case report and review. *Ophthalmology* 1990;97:1494–1498.
11. Shapiro AL, Shectman FG, Guida RA, et al. Head and neck lymphoma in patients with the acquired immune deficiency syndrome. *Otolaryngol Head Neck Surg* 1992;106:258–260.
12. Font RL, Laucirica R, Patrinely JR. Immuno-blastic B-cell lymphoma involving the orbit and maxillary sinus in a patient with acquired immune deficiency syndrome. *Ophthalmology* 1993;100:966–970.
13. Reifler DM, Warzynski MJ, Blount WR, et al. Orbital lymphoma associated with acquired immune deficiency syndrome. *Surv Ophthalmol* 1994;38:371–380.
14. McKelvie P, McNab AA, Francis IC, et al. Ocular adnexal lymphoproliferative disease. A series of 73 cases. *Clin Exp Ophthalmol* 2001;29:387–393.
15. Ziegler JL, Beckstead JA, Volberding PA, et al. Non-Hodgkin's lymphoma in 90 homosexual men; relation to generalized lymphadenopathy and the acquired immunodeficiency syndrome. *N Engl J Med* 1984;311:565–570.
16. Bouwes Bavinck JN, Feltkarmp M, Struijk L, et al. Human papillomavirus infection and skin cancer risk in organ transplant recipients. *J Invest Dermatol Symp Proc* 2001;6:207–211.
17. Stockfleth E, Ulrich C, Meyer T, et al. Epithelial malignancies in organ transplant patients: clinical presentation and new methods of treatment. *Recent Results Cancer Res* 2002;160: 251–258.
18. Berg D, Otley LL. Skin cancer in organ transplant recipients: epidemiology, pathogenesis and management. *J Am Acad Dermatol* 2002;47:1–17.
19. Rady PL, Yen A, Rollefson JL, et al. Herpesvirus-like DNA sequences in non-Kaposi's sarcoma skin lesions of transplant patients. *Lancet* 1995;345:1339–1340.
20. Franceschi S, Dal Maso L, Arniani S, et al. Risk of cancer other than Kaposi's sarcoma and non-Hodgkins's lymphoma in persons with AIDS in Italy. Cancer and AIDS registry linkage study. *Br J Cancer* 1998;78:966–970.
21. Wang CY, Brodland DG, Su WP. Skin cancers associated with the acquired immunodeficiency syndrome. *Mayo Clin Proc* 1995:70:766–772.
22. Nguyen P, Vin-Christian K, Ming ME, et al. Aggressive squamous cell carcinomas in persons infected with the human immunodeficiency virus. *Arch Dermatol* 2002;138:758–763.
23. Sitz KV, Keppen M, Johnson DF. Metastatic basal cell carcinoma in acquired immunodeficiency syndrome-related complex. *JAMA* 1987;257:340–343.
24. Collaco L, Gonçalves M, Gomes L, et al. Orbital Kaposi's sarcoma in acquired immunodeficiency syndrome. *Eur J Ophthalmol* 2000;10:88–90.
25. Thomas JO. Acquired immunodeficiency syndrome-associated cancers in sub-Saharan Africa. *Semin Oncol* 2001;28:198–206.
26. Wabinga HR, Parkin DM, Wabwire-Mangen F, et al. Trends in cancer incidence in Kyadondo County, Uganda, 1960–1997. *Br J Cancer* 2000;82:1585–1592.
27. Chokunga E, Levy LM, Bassett MT, et al. AIDS and cancer in Africa: the evolving epidemic in Zimbabwe. *AIDS* 1999;13: 2583–2588.
28. Muccioli C, Belfort R Jr, Burnier M, et al. Squamous cell carcinoma of the conjunctiva in a patient with the acquired immunodeficiency syndrome. *Am J Ophthalmol* 1996;121:94–96.
29. Fogla R, Biswas J, Kumar SK, et al. Squamous cell carcinoma of the conjunctiva as initial presenting sign in a patient with acquired immunodeficiency syndrome (AIDS) due to human immunodeficiency virus type-2. *Eye* 2000;14:246–247.
30. Kronish JW, Johnson TE, Gilberg SM, et al. Orbital infections in patients with human immunodeficiency virus infection. *Ophthalmology* 1996;103:1483–1492.
31. Levin LA, Avery R, Shore JW, et al. The spectrum of orbital aspergillosis: a clinicopathological review. *Surv Ophthalmol* 1996;41:142–154.
32. Case records of the Massachusetts General Hospital: case 33–1991. *N Engl J Med* 1991;325:494–504.
33. Kopp W, Fotter R, Steiner H, et al. Aspergillosis of the paranasal sinuses. *Radiology* 1985;156:715–716.
34. Ashdown BC, Tien RD, Felsberg GJ. Aspergillosis of the brain and paranasal sinuses in immunocompromised patients: CT and MR imaging findings. *AJR Am J Roentgenol* 1994;162: 155–159.
35. Austin P, Dekker A, Kennerdell JS. Orbital aspergillosis. Report of a case diagnosed by fine needle aspiration biopsy. *Acta Cytol* 1983;27:166–169.
36. Jihnson TE, Casiano RR, Kronish JW, et al. Sino-orbital aspergillosis in acquired immunodeficiency syndrome. *Arch Ophthalmol* 1999;117:57–64.
37. Denning DW, Stevens DA. Antifungal and surgical treatment of invasive aspergillosis: review of 2,121 published cases. *Rev Infect Dis* 1990;12:1147–1201.
38. Lopez-Berestein G, Bodey GP, Fainstein V, et al. Treatment of systemic fungal infections with liposomal amphotericin B. *Arch Intern Med* 1989;149:2533–2536.
39. Slade MP, McNab AA. Fatal mucormycosis associated with deferoxamine therapy. *Am J Ophthalmol* 1991;112:594–595.
40. McNab AA, McKelvie P. Iron overload is a risk factor for zygomycosis. *Arch Ophthalmol* 1997;115:919–921.
41. Artis WM, Fountain JA, Delcher AK, et al. A mechanism of susceptibility to mucormycosis in diabetic ketoacidosis: transferrin and iron availability. *Diabetes* 1982;31:109–114.
42. Diamond RD, Haudenschild CC, Erickson NF III. Monocyte mediated damage to *Rhizopus oryzae* hyphae in vitro. *Infect Immunol* 1982;38:292–297.
43. Yohai RA, Bullock JD, Aziz AA, et al. Survival factors in rhino-orbital-cerebral mucormycosis. *Surv Ophthalmol* 1994;39: 3–22.
44. De La Paz MA, Patrinely JR, Marines HM, et al. Adjunctive hyperbaric oxygen therapy in the treatment of bilateral cerebro-rhino-orbital mucormycosis. *Am J Ophthalmol* 1992;114: 208–211.
45. Francis BA, Mui AL, Calonje D. Orbital streptococcal gangrene and AIDS. *Orbit* 2000;20:243–248.
46. Moorthy RS, Smith RE, Rao NA. Progressive ocular toxoplasmosis in patients with acquired immunodeficiency syndrome. *Am J Ophthalmol* 1993;115:742–747.
47. Friedberg DN, Warren FA, Lee MH, et al. Pneumocystis carinii of the orbit. *Am J Ophthamol* 1992;113:595–596.
48. Cano-Parra J, Espana E, Esteban M, et al. *Pseudomonas* conjunctival ulcer and secondary orbital cellulitis in a patient with AIDS. *Br J Ophthalmol* 1994;78:72–73.
49. Benson WH, Linberg JV, Weinstein GW. Orbital pseudotumor in a patient with AIDS. *Am J Ophthalmol* 1988;105:697–698.
50. Fabricius EM, Hoegl I, Pfaeffl W. Ocular myositis as first pre-

senting symptom of human immunodeficiency virus (HIV-1) infection and its response to high-dose cortisone treatment. *Br J Ophthalmol* 1991;75:696–697.
51. Templeton AC. Tumors of the eye and adnexa in Africans of Uganda. *Cancer* 1967;20:1689–1698.
52. Kwong YL, Chan AC, Liang RH. Natural killer cell lymphoma/leukemia: pathology and treatment. *Hematol Oncol* 1997;15:71–79.
53. Cheung MM, Chan JK, Lau WH, et al. Primary non-Hodgkin's lymphoma of the nose and nasopharynx: clinical features, tumor immunophenotype, and treatment outcome in 113 patients. *J Clin Oncol* 1998;16:70–77.
54. Hon C, Kwok AKH, Shek TWH, et al. Vision-threatening complications of nasal T/NK lymphoma. *Am J Ophthalmol* 2002; 134:406–410.
55. Neel HB. Nasopharyngeal carcinoma: clinical presentation, diagnosis, treatment and prognosis. *Otolaryngol Clin North Am* 1985;18:463–470.
56. Eng Hl, Lin TM, Chen SY, et al. Failure to detect human papillomavirus DNA in malignant epithelial neoplasms of conjunctiva by polymerase chain reaction. *Am J Clin Pathol* 2002;117:429–436.
57. Karcioglu ZA, Tawfik MI. Human papilloma virus in neoplastic and non neoplastic conditions of the external eye. *Br. J. Ophthalmol.* 1997;81:595–598.
58. Karcioglu ZA, Toth J. Relation between p53 overexpression and clinical behavior of ocular/orbital invasion of conjuctival squamous cell carcinoma. *Ophthal. Plast. Reconstr. Surg.* 2000; 16:443–449.
59. Scott IU, Karp CL, Nuovo GJ. Human papillomavirus 16 and 18 expression in conjunctival intraepithelial neoplasis. *Ophthalmology* 2002;109:542–547.
60 Madreperla SA, Green WR, Daniel R, et al. Human papillomavirus in primary epithelial tumors of the lacrimal sac. *Ophthalmology* 1993;100:569–573.
61. Nakamura Y, Mashima Y, Kameyama K, et al. Detection of human papillomavirus in squamous cell tumours of the conjunctiva and lacrimal sac by immunohistochemistry, in situ hybridisation, and polymerase chain reaction. *Br J Ophthalmol* 1997;81:308–313.
62. Merle H, Cabre P, Olindo S, et al. Ocular lesions in 200 patients infected by the human T-cell lymphotropic virus type 1 in Martinique (French West Indies). *Am J Ophthalmol* 2002; 134:190–195.
63. Lauer SA, Fischer J, Jones J, et al. Orbital T-cell lymphoma in human T-cell leukemia virus-1 infection. *Ophthalmology* 1988;95:110–115.
64. Yamamoto N, Kiyosawa M, Kawasaki T, et al. Successfully treated optic nerve infiltration with adult T-cell lymphoma. *J Neuro-Ophthalmol* 1994;14:81–83.
65. Hayashi K, Anda T, Yasanuga A. et al. Intracranial and orbital extension of nasal cavity adult T-cell leukemia: a case report. *No Shinkei Geka* 1999;27:55–59.
66. Yamaguchi K, Mochizuki M, Watanabe T. et al. Human T lymphotropic virus type 1 uveitis after Graves' disease. *Br J Ophthalmol* 1994;78:163–166.
67. Du MQ. Molecular biology of gastric MALT lymphoma: application in clinical management. *Hematology* 2002;7:339–344.
68. Sanders MK, Peura DA. *Helicobacter pylori*-associated diseases. *Curr Gastroenterol Rep* 2002;4:448–454.
69. Vallisa D, Berte R, Rocca A, et al. Association between hepatitis C virus and non-Hodgkin's lymphoma, and effects of viral infection on histologic subtype and clinical course. *Am J Med* 1999;106:556–560.

4

Mechanisms of Tumor Metastasis in the Orbit

J. Oscar Croxatto

CONCEPT OF METASTASIS

The most dreadful point in the progression of neoplasia is invasion and dissemination beyond the original limits of tumor, since most deaths from cancer are due to metastases.[1,2] Metastasis refers to the spread of neoplastic cells from the primary cancer site to other areas of the body. Metastases develop after malignant cells gain phenotypic characteristics that facilitate access to lymphatic channels and blood vessels. Once they outgrow local defense mechanisms in the distant organs, they establish a new phase of independent neoplastic proliferation.[3] The survival of a patient with metastatic disease depends on the extent and size of the dissemination and which vital organs are affected. This chapter provides a brief review of the basic mechanisms associated with invasion and metastasis.

INVASION AND METASTASIS

The basic condition of cancer is invasion. Cancers may either express their invasive behavior initially or progress into malignancy from preexisting benign tumors, premalignant conditions, or neoplasias in situ. Invasion may compromise the function of any organ (e.g., the eye) by compression, by local destruction, or by inhibition of normal function. Invasion and local extension in the head region beyond the orbit may result in the destruction of vital structures and death. Invasion, dissemination, and metastasis may also develop early in the process of the disease when the tumor is relatively small and has not been detected.[2]

DISSEMINATION AND METASTASES

Growing tumors may disseminate throughout the body in several ways including through the cerebrospinal fluid, serous cavities, virtual spaces, lymphatic channels, and blood vessels. Tumor cells enter blood circulation, resist hemodynamic shear stress of the blood circulation, eventually extravasate, and migrate through tissue stroma to a site favorable for tumor growth. Dissemination, however, does not necessarily end in metastatic spread. Some tumor cells must therefore be endowed with exceptional abilities to successfully metastasize, since others, although capable of forming tumors in specific organs, do not metastasize. Therefore, the cells that have access to the routes of spread require the incorporation or development of a metastatic molecular phenotype and imbalance of cytoskeletal regulation.[4] On the other hand, the local microenvironment, the development of angiogenesis, stroma–tumor interactions, and the elaboration of cytokines all influence metastatic potential.[5] Thus, the malignant phenotype is a culmination of a series of genetic changes in the primary tumor and its disseminated cells.[6]

THE METASTASIC EVENT IN THE TEMPORAL PROGRESSION OF CANCER

Tumorigenesis is a multistep process associated with accumulated genetic alterations in somatic cells.[3] The progression of a tumor through preneoplasia to frank neoplasia and then invasion and metastasis is the result of successive rounds of clonal expansion of somatic cells that acquire a selective growth advantage as a result of mutations in genes that control cellular proliferation and death (Table 4.1).[7,8] Figure 4.1 is a schematic representation of tumor progression including multiple sequential steps involving host–tumor interactions. Although modern medical technology permits early detection of neoplasias, most tumors manifest or are detected relatively late in the progression after the tumor has acquired cell heterogeneity as result of spontaneous mutations and chromosomal abnormalities. This heterogeneity, detected at clinical presentation of tumors, indicates higher growth rates and greater metastatic potential.

TABLE 4.1. Carcinogenic Steps During the Metastatic Cascade.

Step	*Characterized by*
I. Tumor initiation	Carcinogenic insult; gene and chromosomal disarrangements
II. Promotion and progression	Gene amplification; inactivation of suppressor genes
III. Uncontrolled proliferation	Growth factors and hormones
IV. Angiogenesis	Multiple stimulating and promoting factors
V. Invasion of tissues, blood vessels, and lymphatic channels	Metalloproteinases; loss of MTP inhibitors, receptors, and adhesion molecules
VI. Vascular endothelial cell tumor arrest and extravasation	Adhesion molecules and receptors; MTP; chemotaxis factors
VII. Tumor growth at secondary sites	Homing factors, angiogenesis, growth factors
VIII. Evasion of host defenses and resistance to therapy	Surpass macrophages; natural killer cells and blocking of T-cell response; expression of drug-resistant genes

Source: Modified from Liotta LA, Kohn EC. Invasion and metastasis. In: Bast RC, Kufe DW, Pollock RE, et al, eds. *Cancer Medicine.* 5th ed. New York: BC Decker; 2000:121–131.

TUMOR CELLS AND STROMAL INTERACTIONS

Angiogenesis

Angiogenesis, the growth of new capillary blood vessels, is a prerequisite for cellular growth beyond the size restriction dictated by oxygen and nutrient diffusion. Angiogenesis is regulated by growth factors and properties of the extracellular matrix.[9,10] Promoters of angiogenesis include basic fibroblast growth factor (bFGF), acidic fibroblast growth factor (aFGF), vascular endothelial growth factor (VEGF), and angiopoietin 1. In contrast, endogenous proteins such as angiostatin, endostatin, pigment epithelium derived factor (PEDF), and angiopoietin 2, prevent vascular cells from responding to a wide spectrum of angiogenic factors. The structure of newly formed blood vessels differs from that of normal vessels. The main differences include the cellular components, the properties and integrity of the basement membrane, and permeability. These elements facilitate the leakage and passage of cancer cells into the circulation. Microvessel density and histological arrangement of blood vessels in the tissue are an independent prognostic indicator of the risk for future development of metastasis. Additionally, angiogenesis is necessary for the growth of cells in the new metastatic foci. To survive, tumor cells must gain access to the vasculature within the primary tumor, survive transit, dwell for a time in the microvasculature of the target organ, exit from this vasculature, grow in the target organ, and induce angiogenesis (Figures 4.2 and 4.3).

Cellular Factors

Cell-to-cell interactions and cell-to-stroma interactions are very important during the invasive stages. The homeostasis of surface receptors and the adhesion molecules, integrins and cadherins, favors tissue stability and integrity, whereas the loss or alteration of these cell surface proteins has been associated with increased metastatic potential.[11] Downregulation of gene expression of E-cadherin has been correlated with increased invasiveness and metastatic potential. Another mechanism that facilitates invasion is degradation of surface protein complexes by mutated gene products.

Tumor cell migration is necessary for the initiation of the metastatic cascade. The interaction of surface receptor proteins and components of the extracellular matrix such as laminin, collagens, fibronectin, and vitronectin regulates the shape, polarity, and migration of cells.[12] Some members of the integrin family of adhesion molecules play a fundamental role in the angiogenesis and invasion.[13] Overexpression of integrin $\alpha_V\beta_3$ mediates cellular adhesion with the ex-

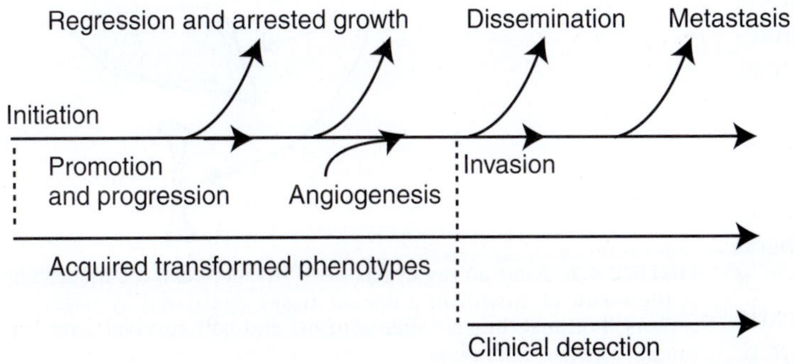

FIGURE 4.1. Tumor progression. The diagram shows that the events of progression, invasion, dissemination, and metastasis are associated with acquired transformed phenotypes.

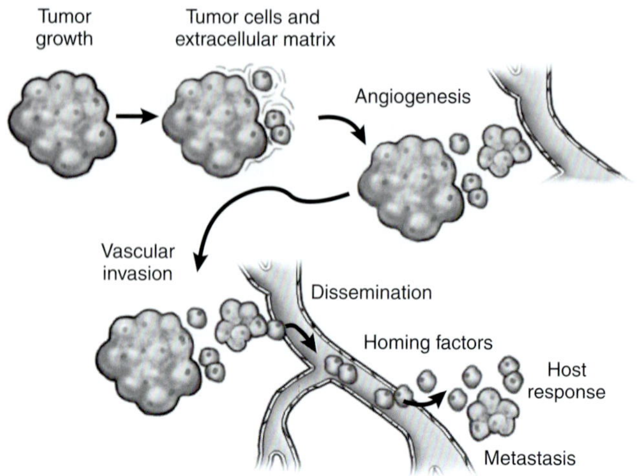

FIGURE 4.2. Angiogenesis is a required step for survival of the tumor, invasion, and dissemination.

tracellular matrix proteins leading to changes in cell shape and increased cell motility. Growth factors that stimulate tumor cell motility include insulin growth factor (IGF), hepatic growth factor (HGF), fibroblast growth factor (FGF), and transforming growth factor β (TGF-β). These factors may play a role in the "homing" of the tumor cell to secondary sites. Cell–matrix interaction also leads to transcription and expression of genes with increased amounts of proteases and disruption of the balance between activated matrix metalloproteinases (MMPs) and free endogenous tissue inhibitors of metalloproteinases (TIMPs) that facilitate invasion and metastasis.[14–16]

GENE OVEREXPRESSION AND DOWNREGULATION

Invasiveness and metastatic ability of the neoplastic cells appear as a result of accumulation of newly acquired genetic alterations beyond those that initiate oncogenesis.[7] Some of these alterations may include more than a few genes.[8] Mutations occur at a higher rate in cancer cells because their genetic material (chromosomes or DNA) is intrinsically unstable.[17] This genetic instability seems to be a "property" of cancer cells. Abnormalities (i.e., loss or gain of chromosomal material) are rather frequent in solid tumors and have been associated with high-grade malignancies.[17,18] During the stepwise progression of cancer, oncogenes are either activated or inactivated, mutation or deletions occur in normal suppressor genes, and there is gene amplification of promotion associated genes and growth factors. Thus, the association between oncogene alterations and prognosis has been extensively investigated, and the demonstration of oncogene amplification is a valuable prognostic marker in certain tumors. Certain genes, such as *p53*, *RB* and *p16*, are altered in diverse tumor types, and others are selectively modified in particular tumors such as those of the von Hippel–Lindau (VHL gene) syndrome.[19] Because of heterogeneity of gene silencing and expression, most primary tumors contain subpopulations of metastastic and nonmetastatic cells. Genes differently expressed in cancer cells that reach the bloodstream have the effect of inducing or suppressing metastasis.

ORBITAL METASTASIS

The development of metastasis in a particular organ depends on vascular architecture and blood flow. In addition, the pattern of spread is influenced by the type and site of the primary tumor. Surface receptors in the cells of the receptor organ and in the disseminated cells together with release hormones, growth factors, and cytokines constitute homing factors for the development of metastasis in specific organs and tissues.

Local Orbital Environment

Orbital Vascular Bed

The cells responsible for metastases must traverse the lungs before reaching the orbit through hematogenous spread, although a few orbital metastases may arrive by retrograde venous flow through the vertebral–basilar plexus. The arterial supply to the orbit arises from the internal carotid artery with some anasto-

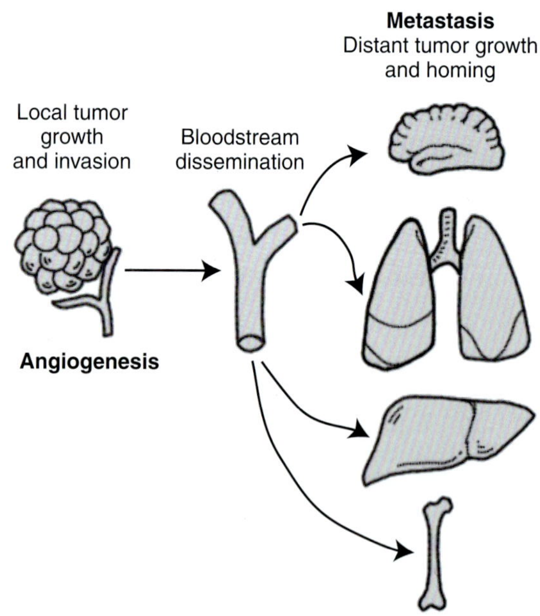

FIGURE 4.3. After an organ has been invaded, distant metastasis is the result of growth in a distant tissue facilitated by tissue receptors (homing), on-site angiogenesis, and cell survival after immune response of the host.

motic connections to the external carotid circulation.[20] The right carotid originates together with the subclavia from the brachiocephalic trunk, whereas the left carotid system originates directly from the aorta.[21] Within the orbit, the ophthalmic artery gives off posterior ciliary vessels and multiple muscular branches, which give rise to the anterior ciliary vessels.[22] These arteries lead into the marginal and peripheral arterial arcades of the eyelid, with anastomoses from the maxillary branch of the external carotid artery. Blood vessels and connective tissue form an integrated system. The microvascular system is predominantly confined to the adipose tissue compartments. The interrelationships of the vascular system and the connective tissue system are likely to be important factors in controlling and regulating orbital blood flow.

Early studies suggested that orbital metastases were more frequent on the left side. This suggestion was supported by the direct origin of the left common carotid artery from the aorta. However, recent reviews of reported series and case reports revealed that unilateral involvement was very similar in both sides, and both sides are simultaneously affected in 7% of cases.[23]

The presence of orbital lymphatics in a primate model was demonstrated by using light and electron microscopic enzyme histochemistry.[24] Lymphatic vessels were identified in the lacrimal gland and in the dura mater of the optic nerve. In addition, structures demonstrating positive staining markers at the orbital apex were highly suggestive of lymphatics but did not meet the morphologic criteria established.[25] Lymphatic vessels were not identified in the extraocular muscles or orbital fat in other studies.[26] Traditionally, lymph node dissemination from ocular and orbital tumors requires prior invasion of the conjunctiva and eyelid, where lymphatic channels are constitutively present.

Orbital Tissue Homing

Based on the presence of different tissue components within the orbit (i.e., bone, striated muscle, fat and connective tissue, lacrimal gland), some tumors appear to disclose specific homing tissue patterns. "Homing" refers to cell trafficking to specific tissues and organs that appears to be regulated by tissue- or cell-specific adhesion molecules and receptors critical to the extravasations process. This may reflect some degree of organ tropism or the production of tumor cells and host cells of some sort of products that specifically bind to or favor the survival and growth of the mestastatic cells. In addition, circulating tumor cells may adhere specifically to the endothelial cells only in the target organ. The expression of particular genes has been recently shown to be associated with the development of metastasis of certain tumors in a particular organ. In addition, preferential growth may be induced by the local microenvironment.

Adhesion of circulating cells to endothelial cells is mediated by a variety of cell adhesion molecules. The first steps in the cell adhesion cascade (rolling and tethering) are regulated by selectins (P, E, and L selectin). The following steps of stable adhesion and transmural migration predominantly involve integrins (LFA-1).[27]

Although homing patterns are relatively well known for normal and neoplastic lymphocytes, the mechanisms for tissue- or organ-specific homing in solid tumors are not fully understood. CD44 is a family of transmembrane glycoproteins encoded by a single gene containing 20 exons, 10 of which (v1–v10) are variant exons inserted by alternative splicing.[28] Some variant isoforms, especially those containing sequences encoded by v6 to v10, might be related to capillary–lymphatic space invasion and metastasis and are overexpressed in both human and animal neoplasms.[29] In a rat pancreatic adenocarcinoma model, one of the variant CD44 isoforms was proven to be determinant in the metastatic process. For some human neoplasms (e.g., carcinomas of the digestive tract, thyroid carcinomas, poorly differentiated endometrioid adenocarcinomas) correlations have been made between the particular pattern of CD44 variants (CD44v6) produced by neoplastic cells and clinicopathological parameters of tumors, such as grade, stage, presence of metastases, and survival. CD44 in normal cells acts mainly as a receptor for hyaluronan and has an affinity for other extracellular matrix ligands such as fibronectin, serglycin, and osteopontin. In orbital diseases, CD44 receptors have been observed in patients with Graves ophthalmopathy, characterized by increased amounts of hyaluronic acid in the extracellular matrix and infiltration by lymphocytes.[30]

Chemoattraction is another mechanism to direct the migration of tumor cells from their primary site via the circulation to preferential targets of metastases.[31] The findings indicate that certain chemokine receptors are found on breast cancer cells, and their ligands are highly expressed at sites associated with breast cancer metastases.[32]

As mentioned, tumor cells express adhesion molecules in the integrin family, and these receptors play a pivotal role in the development of a metastatic colony. Several integrin subunits (α_2, α_4, β_3) were found to have increased expression in orbital metastatic lesions from prostate carcinoma, malignant melanoma, and lobular breast carcinoma in comparison to normal prostate tissue and normal melanocytes.[33] The increased expression of these integrins may be responsible for the tendency of these tumors to metastasize to the orbit, as well as for the tendency of prostate tumors to metastasize preferentially to orbital bones.

METASTATIC DISEASE IN THE ORBIT

Metastatic tumors constitute approximately 3% of all orbital diseases and 10% of orbital neoplasms in most series.[23,34–36] The prevalence of ocular and orbital metastasis in patients with cancer varies from 0.7 to 12%, depending on whether the analysis was clinical or performed in autopsy series.[37–39] The frequency of the site of origin parallels the general incidence of tumors.[40] The most frequent primary organs are breast in women, and lung and prostate in men, and cutaneous melanoma. However, metastases from a large variety of tumors have been reported to occur in the orbit (Table 4.2).[23]

Ocular and adnexal metastasis in children occurs almost exclusively in the orbit.[41] Metastastic tumors of the orbit in children include neuroblastoma, mainly from an abdominal intra-adrenal primary lesion; Ewing sarcoma originating in long bones; and Wilms tumor, an embryonal growth of the kidney.[42,43] In half of the cases, metastastic neuroblastoma affects both orbits, with compromise of the temporal orbit and adjacent bone and periosteum, resulting in bilateral periorbital hematomas.[39]

The spatial and tissue location of metastasis within the orbit is variable. Frequency analysis suggests that tumors from different primary sites tend to metastasize predominantly within certain tissues of the orbit. The orbit is bordered by bone and contains fat and muscle tissues. Melanoma has a strong tendency to metastasize muscle (41–76% of the cases), whereas thyroid and prostate carcinomas metastasize bone.[23] Breast carcinoma usually metastasizes fat and muscle.[44,45] Some tumors are discrete like metastasis of melanoma, breast carcinoma, and renal carcinoma (Box 4.1), whereas others are diffuse like lobular carcinoma of the breast and carcinomas with a scirrhous fibroblastic response.[46] Regarding location, a recent study combining the data from published series and case reports suggests that the lateral and the superior orbit are the most commonly affected quadrants for metastatic tumors.[23,35]

TABLE 4.2. Primary Sites of Orbital Metastasis.

Site	*Cell type*
Breast	Lobular carcinoma, ductal carcinoma
Lung	Bronchiogenic carcinoma, adenocarcinoma, small-cell carcinoma, carcinoid tumor, malignant bronchial adenoma
Prostate	Carcinoma
Skin	Melanoma, squamous cell carcinoma
Kidney	Renal cell carcinoma, Wilms' tumor
Urinary bladder	Transitional carcinoma
Gastrointestinal tract	Adenocarcinoma, carcinoid tumor, gastric carcinoma
Liver	Hepatocellular carcinoma
Pancreas	Adenocarcinoma, islet cell carcinoma
Parotid gland	Malignant mixed tumor
Thyroid	Follicular carcinoma, papillary carcinoma
Adrenal gland	Sympathoblastoma, neuroblastoma, adrenocortical carcinoma
Testis	Seminoma
Choroid	Melanoma
Miscellanea	Bile ducts, gall bladder, ovary, cervix, vagina, peritoneum (mesothelioma), chordoma, pheochromocytoma, sarcomas [Ewing's sarcoma, fibrosarcoma, malignant fibrous histiocytoma, leiomyosarcoma (uterus), liposarcoma, angiosarcoma, osteosarcoma, rhabdomyosarcoma, malignant schwannoma].

BOX 4.1. Extraocular Muscle Involvement in Orbital Metastasis and Dissemination

Breast carcinoma
Cutaneous melanoma
Neuroblastoma
Lung carcinoma
Carcinoid tumor
Seminoma
Pancreatic carcinoma
Lymphoma
Leukemia

Temporal Relationship Between Metastasis and Time of Diagnosis of Primary Tumor

Metastatic carcinomas of the orbit frequently pose a diagnostic challenge because they may occur long after a primary tumor has apparently been successfully treated; they may even occur as the first manifestation of an undetected primary neoplasm (Box 4.2). In approximately 15 to 42% of the cases, the orbital manifestations precede the diagnosis of the primary tumor.[23,35] This group of early-metastasizing tumors includes lung, stomach, colon, pancreas, thyroid, and

BOX 4.2. Clinical Presentations of Orbital Metastases

I. The primary tumor is removed, but within a few months metastases develop.
II. Metastases are already present when the primary tumor is first detected.
III. Metastases appear first, and the primary lesion remains occult.
IV. The primary tumor is removed, and metastases develop several years later.
V. Metastases regress after removal of the primary tumor.

ovary. The evaluation of these patients is facilitated by higher resolution image analysis and available serological tests. The diagnostic procedure when a metastatic orbital tumor is suspected is fine-needle aspiration or incisional biopsy.[47] The use of immunohistochemical techniques is required for confirmation or identification of the primary tumor in case of an unknown or occult primary lesion.

The mean interval from the diagnosis of the primary tumor to the development of the ophthalmic sign or symptom is highly variable and is related to the biology of the primary tumors and the development and application of diagnostic methods and therapy.[23] An interval of more than 3 to 5 years is expected in breast, thyroid, and prostate carcinoma, and carcinoids. Lung, renal, and gastrointestinal tumors are more frequently diagnosed after the appearance of orbital metastatic signs and symptoms and usually follow a fulminant course with short survival.

It is important to note that tumors with isolated orbital metastasis carry the best prognosis for survival. Approximately 2% of the body metastases occur in the setting of cancer of unknown primary site. The initial pathology study usually identifies four light-microscopic diagnoses including poorly differentiated neoplasm, adenocarcinoma, squamous cell carcinoma, and poorly differentiated carcinoma. The optimal management of these patients requires appropriate clinical and pathology evaluation to identify treatable subgroups, followed by the administration of specific therapy.

Metastatic melanoma to the orbit constitutes a unique situation because of the long delay from onset and treatment of the primary tumor and the first appearance of metastasis. It may manifest in one of four clinical settings: from an excised cutaneous lesion, in association with an active skin melanoma, with history or evidence of a spontaneously regressed melanoma, or from an occult primary site. Most patients present with widespread metastatic disease at the time of ocular manifestions.[48] The survival after the diagnosis of metastastic disease is poor: the average time from diagnosis to death is 4 months (range 2–6 months).[23] In addition, a patient with a metastastic melanoma may have had a spontaneously regressed cutaneous melanoma that was unnoticed, or an occult primary melanoma.[49] This scenario most likely explains findings of metastatic melanoma without an apparent primary lesion or in an unknown primary. The long delay between the origin of the primary tumor and the first manifestation of metastatic disease may indicate a superior or more effective host–tumor immunologic response. However, when metastatic disease develops, the survival rate of the patient does not differ among those with a concurrent growing primary tumor, spontaneously regressed melanoma, or occult primary site.[50]

METASTASTIC DISEASE FROM PRIMARY ORBITAL TUMORS

The vascular circulation of the orbit has the peculiar feature that lymphatic vessels are not usually present within the deep orbital tissues. Therefore, dissemination of primary malignant tumors of the orbit occurs through the venous system (Figure 4.4). Lymphatic vessels are seen only in the anterior orbital septum and are related to eyelid and conjunctival lymphatics (see earlier subsection entitled Orbital Vascular Bed). The superior lymphatics drain mainly to the preauricular lymph nodes, and the inferior lymphatics drain into the submandibular nodes (Figure 4.4).

CONCLUSIONS

Invasion and metastasis are currently recognized as early events in cancer progression. Trends in the management of advanced metastatic disease include the use of molecular techniques for the early diagnosis of disseminated disease and the clinical application of serum markers that may indicate a more precise indication of immunomodulation. The knowledge gained by means of sophisticated molecular techniques involving cell adhesion, proteolysis of the extracellular matrix, migration, and angiogenesis signaling has opened a wide field of novel therapies. The use of agents against growth factor receptors and integrin receptors, matrix metalloproteinase inhibitors, and products inhibiting the signaling pathways underlying metastasis, including oncoprotein signaling cascades and calcium mobilization, may lead to the interruption of the metastatic process in selected patients.

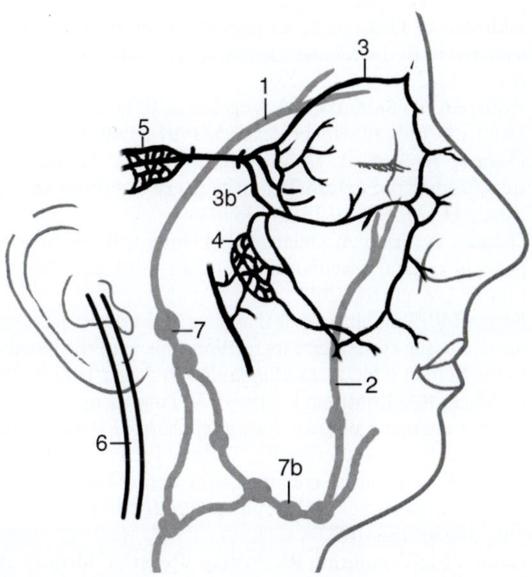

FIGURE 4.4. Orbital venous drainage and the periorbital lymphatic system.

References

1. Liotta LA, Stetler-Stevenson WG. Tumor invasion and metastasis: an imbalance of positive and negative regulation. *Cancer Res* 1991;51:5054–5059.
2. Kohn EC, Liotta LA. Molecular insights into cancer invasion: strategies for prevention and intervention. *Cancer Res* 1995;51:1862–1865.
3. Yokota J. Tumor progression and metastasis. *Carcinogenesis* 2000;21:497–503.
4. Woodhouse EC, Chuaqui RF, Liotta LA. General mechanisms of metastasis. *Cancer* 1997;80:1529–1537.
5. Fidler IJ. Critical factors in the biology of human cancer metastasis: 28th G H A Clowes Memorial Award Lecture. *Cancer Res* 1990;50:6130–6138.
6. Fidler IJ, Hart IR. Biologic diversity in metastastic neoplasms: origins and implications. *Science* 1982;217:998–1003.
7. Nicolson GL. Gene expression, cellular diversification and tumor progression to the metastatic phenotype. *BioEssays* 1991;13:337–342.
8. Yokota J, Sugimura T. Multiple steps in carcinogenesis involving alterations of multiple tumor suppressor genes. *FASEB J* 1993;7:920–925.
9. Pluda JM. Tumor-associated angiogenesis: mechanisms, clinical implications, and therapeutic strategies. *Semin Oncol* 1997;15:61–75.
10. Kerbel RS. Tumor angiogenesis: past, present and the near future. *Carcinogenesis* 2000;21:505–515.
11. Ohene-Abuakwa Y, Pignatelli M. Adhesion molecules in cancer biology. *Adv Exp Med Biol* 2000;465:115–126.
12. Liotta LA. Tumor invasion: role of extracellular matrix. *Cancer Res* 1986;46:1–7.
13. Seftor REB. Role of the $\beta 3$ integrin subunit in human primary melanoma progression. *Am J Pathol* 1998;153:1347–1351.
14. Coussens LM, Werb Z. Matrix metalloproteinases and the development of cancer. *Chem Biol* 1996;3:895–904.
15. Chambers AF, Matisian LM. Changing views of the role of matrix metalloproteinases in metastasis. *J Natl Cancer Inst* 1997;89:1260–1270.
16. Kawamata H, Kawai K, Kameyama S, et al. Over-expression of tissue inhibitor of matrix metalloproteinases (TIMP1 and TIMP2) suppresses extravasation of pulmonary metastasis of a rat bladder carcinoma. *Int J Cancer* 1995;63:680–687.
17. Lengauer C, Kinzler KW, Vogelstein B. Genetic instability in colorectal cancers. *Nature* 1997;386:623–627.
18. Ishimaru G, Ookawa K, Yamaguchi N, et al. Allelic losses associated with the metastatic potential of colorectal carcinoma. *Int J Oncol* 1994;5:267–273.
19. Hollstein M, Sidransky D, Vogelstein B, Harris CC. *p53* mutations in human cancer. *Science* 1991;53:49–53.
20. Ducasse A, Segal A, Delattre JF, Burette A, Flament JB. Participation of the external carotid artery in orbital vascularization. *J Fr Ophtalmol* 1985;8:333–339.
21. Ducasse A, Segal A, Delattre JF, Flament JB. Macroscopic aspects of arterial vascularization of the orbit. *Bull Soc Ophtalmol Fr* 1989;89:989–993.
22. Bergen MP. Some histological aspects of the structure of the connective tissue system and its relationships with the blood vessels in the human orbit. *Acta Morphol Neerl Scand* 1982;20:293–308.
23. Goldberg RA, Rootman J, Cline RA: Tumors metastatic to the orbit: a changing picture. *Surv Ophthalmol* 1990;35:1–24.
24. Sherman DD, Gonnering RS, Wallow IH, et al. Identification of orbital lymphatics: enzyme histochemical light microscopic and electron microscopic studies. *Ophthalmic Plast Reconstr Surg* 1993;9:153–169.
25. Gausas RE, Gonnering RS, Lemke BN, et al. Identification of human orbital lymphatics. *Ophthalmic Plast Reconstr Surg* 1999;15:252–259.
26. McGetrick JJ, Wilson DG, Dortzbach RK, et al. A search for lymphatic drainage of the monkey orbit. *Arch Ophthalmol* 1989;107:255–260.
27. Sanding M, Negrou E, Rogers KA. Changes in the distribution of LFA-1, catenins, and F-actin during transendothelial migration of monocytes in cultures. *J Cell Sci* 1997;110:2807–2818.
28. Naot D, Sionov RV, Ish-Shalom D. CD44: structure, function, and association with the malignant process. *Adv Cancer Res* 1997;71:241–319.
29. Hoffmann M, Rudy W, Zoller M, et al. CD44 splice variants confer metastatic behavior in rats: homologous sequences are expressed in human tumor cell lines. *Cancer Res* 1991;51:5292–5297.
30. Heufelder AE, Bahn RS, Boergen KP, Scriba PC. Detection, localization and modulation of hyaluronic acid/CD44 receptor expression in patients with endocrine orbitopathy. *Med Klin* 1993;88:181–184.
31. Kohn EC, Francis A. Liotta LA, Schiffmann E. Heterogeneity of the motility responses in malignant tumor cells: a biological basis for the diversity and homing of metastatic cells. *Int J Cancer* 1990;46:287–292.
32. Moore MA. The role of chemoattraction in cancer metastases. *BioEssays* 2001;23:674–676.
33. Hartstein ME, Grove AS Jr, Woog JJ. The role of the integrin family of adhesion molecules in the development of tumors metastatic to the orbit. *Ophthalmic Plast Reconstr Surg* 1997;13:227–238.
34. Shields JA, Shields CL, Brotman HK, et al. Cancer metastatic to the orbit: The 2000 Robert M Curts Lecture. *Ophthalmic Plast Reconstr Surg* 2001;17:346–354.
35. Demirci H, Shields CL, Shields JA, et al. Orbital tumors in the older adult population. *Ophthalmology* 2002;109:243–248.
36. Font RL, Ferry AP. Carcinoma metastatic to the eye and orbit III. A clinicopathologic study of 28 cases metastatic to the orbit. *Cancer* 1976;38:1326–1335.
37. Godtfredsen E. On the frequency of secondary carcinomas in the choroid. *Acta Ophthalmol* 1944;22:394–400.
38. Albert DM, Rubenstein RA, Scheie HG. Tumor metastasis to the eye. I. Incidence in 213 adult patients with generalized malignancy. *Am J Ophthalmol* 1967;63:723–726.
39. Bloch MS, Gartner S. The incidence of ocular metastatic carcinoma. *Arch Ophthalmol* 1971;85:673–675.
40. Amemiya T, Hayashida H, Dake Y. Metastatic orbital tumors in Japan: a review of the literature. *Ophthalmic Epidemiol* 2002;9:35–47.
41. Albert DM, Rubenstein RA, Scheie HG: Tumor metastases to the eye. II. Clinical study in infants and children. *Am J Ophthalmol* 1967;63:727–732.
42. Musarella MA, Chen HS, DeBoer G, Gallie BL. Ocular involvement in neuroblastoma: prognostic implications. *Ophthalmology* 1984;91:936–940.
43. Fatkin JD, Purcell JJ, Krachmer JH, Taylor JC. Wilms' tumor metastatic to the orbit. *JAMA* 1977;238:1841–1842.
44. Capone A, Slamovits TL. Discrete metastasis of solid tumors to extraocular muscles. *Arch Ophthalmol* 1990;108:237–243.
45. Bullock JD, Yanes B. Ophthalmic manifestations of metastatic breast cancer. *Ophthalmology* 1980;87:961–973.
46. Char DH, Miller T, Kroll S. Orbital metastases: diagnosis and course. *Br J Ophthalmol* 1997;81:386–390.
47. Dresner SK, Kennerdell JS, Dekker A. Fine needle aspiration biopsy of metastatic orbital tumors. *Surv Ophthalmol* 1983;27:397–398.
48. Orcutt JC, Char DH. Melanoma metastatic to the orbit. *Ophthalmology* 1988;95:1033–1037.
49. Avril MF, Charpentier P, Margulis A, Guillaume JC. Regression of primary melanoma with metastases. *Cancer* 1992;69:1377–1381.
50. Vijuk G, Coates AS. Survival of patients with visceral metastatic melanoma from an occult primary lesion: a retrospective matched cohort study. *Ann Oncol* 1998;9:419–422.

5

Multiple Malignancies in Retinoblastoma

Zeynel A. Karcıoglu

Retinoblastoma (Rb) is considered to be the prototype for hereditary neoplasms in humans.[1,2] Current thinking in tumor pathogenesis is that the regulatory mechanisms of cell division are impaired and control over cell proliferation is lost. In Rb and other tumors, this may be a result of mutations in genes of two types: tumor suppressor genes and oncogenes. One of the first tumor suppressor genes to be isolated was from Rb (*Rb-I*).[3,4] The function of these genes is to act on normal cells to limit their proliferation. In other words, the tumor suppressor gene applies a continuous growth restriction. Therefore, whenever it is genetically absent or otherwise rendered nonfunctional, cell growth is uncontrolled. On the other hand, oncogenes produce proteins that stimulate cell division and proliferation.

Molecular identification of *Rb-I* led to the confirmation of the hypothesis that all retinoblastomas carry two mutations, one in each allele of the gene.[5,6] In hereditary Rb, one mutant allele is inherited and the other develops within the retina. In sporadic cases, both mutations take place during retinal development. The hereditary form of Rb is estimated to constitute approximately 40% of all cases of the disease.[7–9] More than 90% of hereditary cases present with multiple tumors bilaterally at a mean age of I5 months. On the other hand, nonhereditary Rb is typically unilateral and presents with a single focus of tumor at a mean age of 27 months. However, it has been reported that approximately 15% of unilateral cases have inherited mutations.[10]

STUDIES OF THE GENE FOR Rb

After the cloning of *Rb-I* for Rb, which is now considered to be a member of a family of genes including *p107* and *p130*, it became evident that mutations of the Rb tumor suppressor gene were also present in a wide variety of other human neoplasms.[11–18] As is the case in retinoblastomatoma, all *Rb-I* mutations in other neoplasms lead either to loss of expression of Rb protein (pRB) or the production of malfunctioning protein.[19–22] The understanding of the Rb suppressor gene in tumors led to other practical insights. Patients with the hereditary form of Rb were recognized to be at a greater risk than the general population to develop a second malignant neoplasm (SMN) later in life. Today, with early detection and improved treatment modalities, second, third, and even fourth malignant neoplasms are increasingly becoming the leading cause of mortality among Rb survivors. Since second malignant tumor is the most commonly encountered presentation of these multiple tumor-harboring patients in this chapter the term "second malignant neoplasms" designates these lesions.

Prior to the advent of genetic experimentation and examination of the molecular basis of susceptibility to multiple malignancies, the development of second tumors had been reported sporadically as the result of clinical observations. The most startling report was by Abramson and coworkers indicating that the incidence of SMNs in the hereditary form of Rb was 20% after 10 years, 50% after 20 years, and 90% after 30 years.[23] Although the SMN incidences were exaggerated, this paper was significant in attracting attention to the second malignancy issue in Rb, and more reports were published throughout the 1980s.[22–30] Draper and coworkers conducted a population-based study using records from cancer registries and hospitals in England, Scotland, and Wales.[26] All cases listed with the National Cancer Registration Scheme between 1962 and 1977 were included. Their base was 882 patients with Rb, 2% of whom developed an SMN at 12 years' follow-up, and 4.2% at 18 years' follow-up. Three hundred eighty-four of these instances of Rb were determined to be hereditary, and the incidence of SMN in the hereditary group was 8.4% at 18 years.[16]

Abramson's group adjusted their figures to an SMN incidence of 16% at 35 years. The same group later published a more conclusive retrospective cohort study examining the second malignancy mortality rate among long-term survivors of Rb.[31] In the new study, 1603 patients were enrolled at one year after the diagnosis of Rb. A total of 305 deaths was recorded: 167 from Rb, 96 from SMNs, and 42 from other causes. The great majority of Rb deaths (143 of 167 patients) occurred between the first and ninth year after initial diagnosis, agreeing with other studies and indicating the rarity of late mortality due to Rb.[31] Nine hundred nineteen (57%) of the 1603 patients had unilateral disease. The most common second primary malignancies were bone and soft tissue sarcomas, followed by cutaneous melanoma and brain tumors. When the relative risk of mortality was calculated, it was found to exceed the expected rates 300-fold for malignant tumors of bone and soft tissues,[32–34] 100-fold for melanoma, and 24-fold for brain tumors. At 40 years of follow-up, the cumulative mortality for all SMNs was 26 ± 3.5% (expected 1.3%) for bilateral Rb and 1.5 ± 0.7% (expected 1.1%) for unilateral Rb. In the bilateral Rb patients, external beam radiotherapy (EBRT) further increased the risk of mortality (Figure 5.1). The cumulative mortality from SMNs among patients who received radiotherapy was 30.3 ± 4.8% as opposed to 6.4 ± 3.8% for those who did not receive EBRT. Acute leukemias have also been reported among the patients who survive Rb.[35,36] Several investigators have restricted their studies of Rb, some focusing on the bilateral form[37–38] and others on the hereditary.[25,28] Desjardins and coworkers reported nine SMNs in 80 bilateral Rb patients who had been followed for more than 30 years. Six of these SMNs may have been radiation induced.[37] Roarty and coworkers reported cumulative SNN incidence in bilateral disease ranging from 4.4% (10 years postdiagnosis) to 26.1% (30 years postdiagnosis).[38]

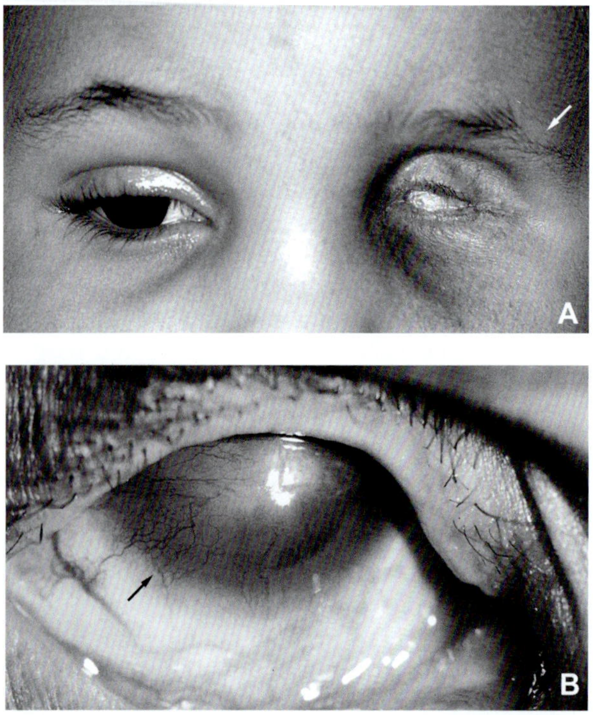

FIGURE 5.1. (A) Socket atrophy, scarring, and contraction of the eyelid tissues, and charring of the skin with loss of eyelashes and eyebrow hair (white arrow) following EBRT for Rb. (B) Extensive scarring and neovascularization (black arrow) of the external eye, secondary to EBRT for Rb.

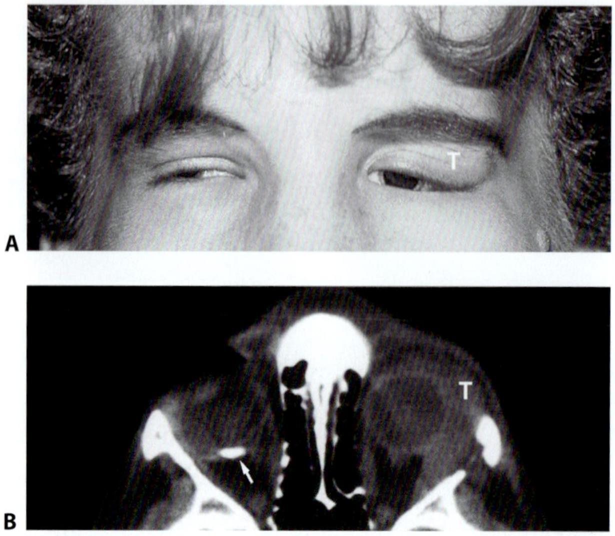

FIGURE 5.2. A 13-year-old girl with osteogenic sarcoma (T) originating from the superior lateral rim of the orbit. The patient had been treated with EBRT for bilateral Rb at the age of 2.

Among studies based exclusively on nonhereditary (unilateral and bilateral) cases, Minoda reported a cumulative SMN incidence of 4.8 and 15.7%, respectively, at 10 and 20 years after diagnosis.[39] In another study that included only hereditary Rb patients, Lueder and coworkers reported cumulative SMN incidences of 6, 14, and 14 at 10, 20, and 30 years after diagnosis, respectively.[28] In another group that included only hereditary disease patients, DerKinderen and coworkers reported a cumulative SMN incidence of 19% in Rb patients at the age of 35 years.[25]

Other studies include both unilateral and bilateral, and hereditary and nonhereditary patients as mixed groups. In a joint study conducted in Europe, DeSutter and coworkers reported a cumulative SMN incidence ranging from 10 to 30% in the Rb population with 40% bilateral disease.[40] In another European study that included approximately 35% hereditary Rb patients, Winther et al. reported a relative risk for SMN development as 15.4% for hereditary and 1.7% for nonhereditary Rb patients.[29] Smith and coworkers in the United States studied 53 Rb patients, 79% of whom were reported as hereditary; their actuarial SMN incidence was 6, 19, and 38% after 10, 20, and 30 years, respectively.[41]

TYPES OF SECOND MALIGNANCY

The most common SMN, osteogenic sarcoma (Figures 5.2 and Figure 5.3), occurs at about the same age as in the normal population, around the second decade.[42–44] The frequency of bone and soft tissue sarcomas is not surprising, since many of these tumors seem to harbor *Rb-1* mutations.[45,46] The osteogenic sarcoma incidence in the literature varies from 19 to 54% of all

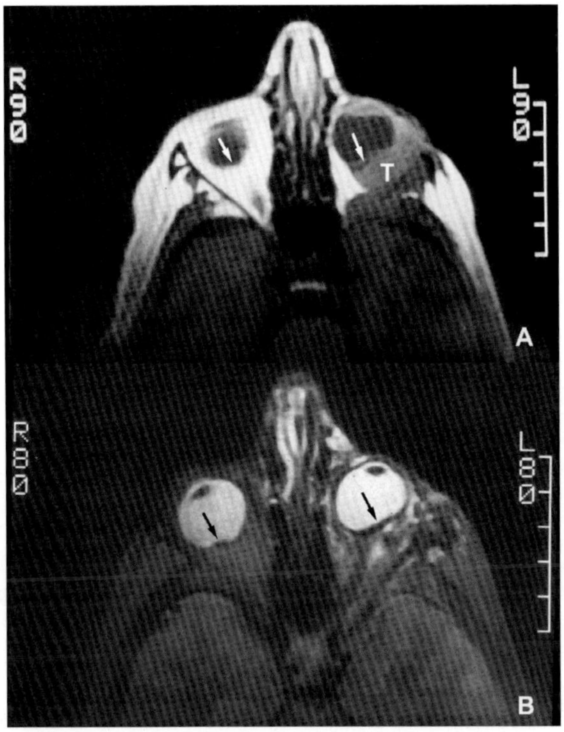

FIGURE 5.3. Axial magnetic resonance images from the same patient depicting the osteogenic sarcoma (T) compressing onto the left globe; arrows indicate remnants of calcified Rb. (A) T1-weighted image. (B) T2-weighted image.

SMNs.[23,26] Hawkins et al., whose survey included at least 90% of children with cancer in the United Kingdom, estimated that the relative risk of bone tumors increased 415 times in patients with Rb.[47] Soft tissue tumors (Figures 5.4 and 5.5) are ranked as the second most common SMN, with an estimated increased relative risk of 130 times.[47]

Mortality from cutaneous melanoma as an SMN seen in Rb survivors is also far above the age-matched expected levels.[47,48] The increased incidence of melanoma is a rather unexpected finding, since melanoma has not been shown to harbor *Rb-1* mutations and more often develops outside the radiotherapy site.[49] Many SMNs, including osteogenic and soft tissue sarcomas and carcinomas of breast and other sites, have proven to have somatic mutations of *Rb-1*; this is thought to be the common pathway of oncogenesis in the development of SMNs in children with Rb.[50] The carriers of *Rb-1* may have a dramatic increase in susceptibility to other common cancers when the usual age of onset of these neoplasms is approached.

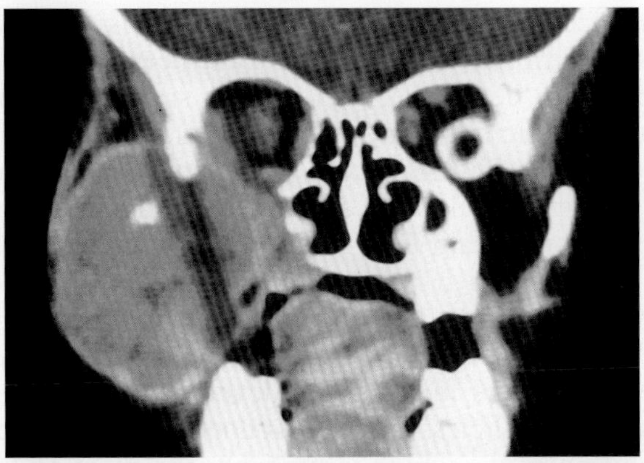

FIGURE 5.4. Large rhabdomyosarcoma originating from the inferior orbital rim and mandible, following EBRT for bilateral Rb. (Courtesy of Dr. Barrett Haik, Memphis, Tennessee.)

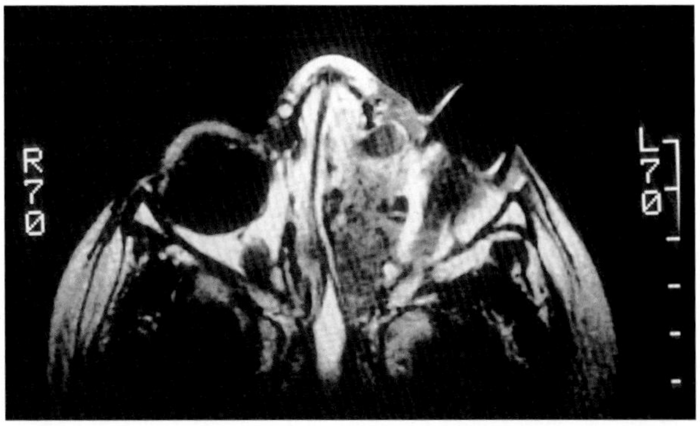

FIGURE 5.5. Extensive esthesioneuroblastoma developed in the left orbit and nasal cavity following enucleation and postoperative irradiation of the left socket for recurrent bilateral Rb.

At present few reliable data are available on patients older than 40 years of age. Two studies of family members of patients with bilateral Rb, however, revealed more deaths due to stomach, bronchial, bladder, and breast carcinoma than expected in the normal population, particularly in first-degree relatives.[51,52] Data indicate that the observed excess mortality due to SMNs is far above the incidence of that expected to occur in the same age group of the normal population. What is not clear, however, is what happens as these patients proceed through life. Is the risk lifelong? If it is, the risk represents a unique situation for Rb patients, since more than 90% of these patients are cured of their primary neoplasm.

The SMN issue is rapidly becoming a significant public health concern, claiming a large segment of the population living with a history of a "cured" malignancy after exposure to chemotherapy, radiation, or both. In the early 1990s it was projected that at the end of the year 2000, one of every 900 individuals in the United States between the ages of 16 and 44 years would be a survivor of a childhood malignancy.[53] In general, it is estimated that 70% of children with a diagnosis of malignancy survive 5 years. In Rb, however, the percentage of survivors and the length of the survival period are greater than for other malignancies. Recent data suggest that 95% of these patients do not develop metastatic disease and are cured of Rb for life.[54] Although the rate of metastasis varies from one series to another, Shields and Shields seem to be correct in their estimate that the mortality rate in Rb today due to the primary disease is less than 5%.[54–56]

Even the small percentage of patients who develop metastatic disease survive longer with aggressive chemotherapy.[57]

The increased risk of developing additional malignancies in the survivors of childhood cancer may well be lifelong. However, from the standpoint of implications for public health, the age range to concentrate on is between I5 and 45 years. After the fourth decade, the overall incidence of malignancies rises sharply in the general population. Whether survivors of Rb are at a higher risk to develop malignancies than the general population over 50 years of age is not yet known; accumulation of data for another 20 to 25 years is needed to provide the answer.

The occurrence of third and additional nonocular malignancies in Rb survivors is another interesting aspect of this problem. Abramson reported that approximately 1% of hereditary Rb patients develop second nonocular neoplasm each year. Approximately 50% of these patients die as a result of these tumors.[58] It is becoming more and more apparent that the survivors of SNMs are at risk for the development of third, fourth, and even fifth nonocular malignancies.[59,60] Abramson and coworkers reported a series of 211 (19 unilateral,192 bilateral) Rb patients who had developed second malignant neoplasms. One hundred forty-two of these patients died within approximately 2 years as a result of their cancers. In 28 patients, a third nonocular tumor developed; all but one had received EBRT for the initial treatment of Rb. A fourth and a fifth tumor developed in 6 and 2 patients, respectively, out of the total of 211 Rb patients.

Another interesting finding is the higher mortality from SMNs in females. In the study of Eng and coworkers, death from second malignancies in females, was reported to be significantly higher than in males.[23] Although there are biological differences between genders, the increased mortality in females is quite striking and difficult to explain. Again, more studies are needed to qualify the gender issue.

ROLE OF EBRT IN SECOND MALIGNANCIES

There is general agreement that radiotherapy increases the incidence of SMNs in patients with Rb.[24,61–64] The only large study reporting that the SMN incidence was independent of radiation therapy was that of DeSutter and coworkers.[40] Radiation-induced tumors of the eye are classified as those that arise within the "field of radiation" (i.e., eyelids, orbit, periorbital sinuses, skin, and subcutaneous tissues overlying the periorbital area). In the study of Roarty and coworkers, the 30-year incidence of SMN following radiation therapy for Rb was reported to be 35.1%; in the same series, only 5.8% of Rb patients who did not receive radiotherapy developed SMNs; 29.3% of these malignancies developed within the field of radiation, 8.1% were outside the radiation field (i.e., elsewhere in the body).[38] Similarly, Draper and Abramson and their colleagues report an increased risk in radiation-treated patients, primarily within the field of radiation.[24,26]

If one considers conceptual and technological advances in radiation therapy over the past 50 years, the risk today may very well be less than what has been stated in the above-mentioned series. The case cited by Roarty et al., for example, dates back to 1922.[38] Similarly, Abramson's series included patients from 60 years ago who received 3500 to 26,000 cGy of radiation with orthovoltage equipment. Others received up to 12,000 cGy of radiation on a betatron, probably in multiple courses. Draper's series dates back to the 1950s, and patients were reported to have received radiation of 1200 to 7500 cGy, although the majority were within the range of 3500 to 4000 cGy, comparable to today's treatments.[26] Modern supervoltage radiation therapy equipment has less effect on normal bone than older orthovoltage equipment, is much more precise, and delivers a lower dose to a smaller area than older methods. It is not yet known, however, whether the use of this modified equipment will reduce the incidence of SMNs in the future.

Whatever improvements have been taking place, the fact remains that radiation treatment in Rb increases the risk of SMNs within the radiation field by a factor of 5 to 6; there is not enough evidence to indicate that it has the same effect on the incidence of SMNs elsewhere in the body. Attempts to determine a dose–response effect have been unsuccessful because radiation doses have decreased over the years and patients who received the highest doses have the longest follow-up periods. Since there is no determined "tumor-forming radiation dose," the only way to minimize the risk of SMNs due to EBRT is to use carefully fractionated treatment with shielding of normal tissues as much as possible. For example, brachytherapy applications with ^{125}I or ^{106}Ru plaques are ideal in that they deliver curative doses to the tumor but minimize radiation toxicity to adjacent tissues. Individuals with hereditary Rb also have been reported to be prone to develop benign tumors such as lipomas and dysplastic nevi that may progress into cutaneous melanoma.[65] Thirty percent of patients with hereditary Rb who had lipomas also developed an SMN, suggesting that certain *Rb-I* mutations may increase the risk of both benign and malignant tumors.

Another issue is the contribution of chemotherapy to SMN development. It is known that treatment with cytotoxic agents may lead to development of subsequent malignancies. This is best documented with cyclophosphamide, which is probably the most widely used alkylating agent.[66] Although there are anecdotal reports of SMNs developing in Rb patients following cyclophosphamide treatment, most of these patients have also received radiotherapy. The real risk of chemotherapy is difficult to determine. Hawkins and coworkers estimate a 26-fold risk of SMN development in Rb patients treated with radiation but no chemotherapy, and a 78-fold risk in patients who receive both radiation and chemotherapy.[47] For bone sarcomas, the relative risks are significantly higher: 174 times for Rb patients who receive no chemotherapy or radiotherapy, and 340 times and 771 times, respectively, in patients who receive radiation but no chemotherapy, and radiation with chemotherapy. The alkylating cytotoxic agents and ionizing radiation are known carcinogens. It is quite conceivable that these agents alone, or in combination, increase the frequency of somatic mutations needed to produce SMNs in Rb patients.[50,67]

The high frequency of SMNs, radiation retinopathy, and orbital growth retardation in Rb patients who are treated with EBRT forced many investigators to look into alternative treatments.[68,69] Neutralization of chemotherapy as a primary treatment for intraocular Rb seems particularly promising. Historically, combination chemotherapy has been utilized only when Rb is accompanied by extraocular extension and metastasis. The preliminary results of the new approach suggest that combination chemotherapy can markedly reduce the tumor bulk so that more conservative, local modalities (cryotherapy, photocoagulation, etc.) can be employed to eradicate the tumor. This approach is particularly useful as a means of avoiding enucleation or EBRT.[70–72] Most chemoreduction regimens consist of vincristine sulfate, etoposide, and carboplatin and achieve tumor shrinkage approximately 70% of the time. Gallie et al. reported better response when cyclosporin was added to the regimen, which may reverse the chemoresistance of the tumor that is due to the expression of phosphoglycoproteins.[70,73]

Although the promising results of the primary application of the chemotherapy in treating intraocular Rb should be celebrated, it should not be forgotten that the possibility of SMN development deterred widespread use of chemotherapy in Rb in the first place. There is evidence that alkylating agents increase the risk of leukemia when used in patients with childhood cancers and that cyclophosphamide may induce SMNs in patients with Rb.[26,66] Therefore, enough follow-up time should be allowed before the use of primary chemotherapy is fully endorsed; after all, it took more than three decades to unveil the role of radiation in the induction of SMNs in Rb patients. It should also be kept in mind that the rapid improvement of the overall survival rate of Rb within the last century is primarily due to timely decision on enucleation. There is no doubt that efforts should be made to maximize the benefits of new chemicals and technologies; however, it is also important to be conscious of the potential danger of tumor dissemination when trying to preserve vision.

MANAGEMENT OF SECOND MALIGNANCIES

Management of SMNs is difficult, and the prognosis is not rewarding. Robinson et al. studied 344 cases of postirradiation sarcomas.[74] Cumulative disease-free survival of patients with these sarcomas was 17% at 5 years with a median survival of 1 year. The mean time from diagnosis of the primary tumor to the diagnosis of SMN was 11 years, and most of these postirradiation sarcomas were high-grade malignancies, detected at advanced stages. Most of the tumors were located in areas where radical surgery could not be performed, and the response rate to chemotherapy was poor. Robinson and coinvestigators comment that the prognosis for sarcomas that develop outside the field of radiation is also very poor in patients with Rb. Smith and coworkers report their experience with a 28.9% "cure" in 162 patients with SMNs; the average time from diagnosis of the primary to development of the second malignancy was 10.8 years.[75] Another series reports eight hereditary Rb patients with 11 SMNs (10 sarcomas) with better results.[41] In this series, an aggressive approach with combined radiation and chemotherapy led to four patients having no evidence of disease for 22 to 72 months following treatment.

CONCLUSIONS

Today it is widely accepted that there is a significantly increased incidence of second malignant neoplasms in Rb survivors, particularly in bilateral and hereditary cases. Most SMNs develop between the ages of 10 and 30, and the cumulative probability of death from SMN is approximately 25% at 40 years after bilateral Rb diagnosis. There is evidence that death from SMNs is more frequent among females than males. There is also general agreement that radiation therapy increases the likelihood of SMN development within the field of radiation and elsewhere. The effect of chemotherapy on the development of SMNs is suspected but not proven, since most of the patients with metastases do not survive long enough to develop other malignancies, and there simply are not enough follow-up data to permit the evaluation of primary chemotherapy patients. Most common SMNs are bone and soft tissue sarcomas, central nervous system malignancies, and cutaneous melanoma. In general, it is believed that hereditary factors, such as oncogenic mutations in specific sites of the *Rb-I* gene, could predispose individuals to develop Rb as well as SMNs. Furthermore, treatment modalities involving cytotoxic drugs and ionizing radiation may raise the incidence by inducing an increased number of somatic mutations.

References

1. Hethcote HW, Knudson AG Jr. Model for the incidence of embryonal cancers: application to retinoblastoma. *Proc Natl Acad Sci U S A* 1978;75:2453–2457.
2. Knudson AG Jr. Retinoblastoma: a prototypic hereditary neoplasm. *Semin Oncol* 1978;5:57–60.
3. Yunis JJ,Ramsay N. Retinoblastoma and subband deletion of chromosome 13. *Am J Dis Child* 1978;132:161–163.
4. Friend SH, Bernards R, Rogelj S, et al. A human DNA segment with properties of the gene that predisposes to retinoblastoma and osteosarcoma. *Nature* 1986;323:643–646.
5. Fung YK, Murphree AL, T'Ang A, et al. Structural evidence for the authenticity of the human retinoblastoma gene. *Science* 1987;36:1657–1667.
6. Lee WH, Bookstein R, Hong F, et al. Human retinoblastoma susceptibility gene: cloning, identification, and sequence. *Science* 1987;235:1394–1399.
7. Mullaney PB, Karcioglu ZA, Al-Mesfer S, Dowaidi M. Retinoblastoma referral patterns in Saudi Arabia. *Ophthalmic Epidemiol* 1996;3:35–46.
8. Vogel F. Genetics of retinoblastoma. *Hum Genet* 1979;52:1–54.
9. Zhang K, Wang MX, Munier F, et al. Molecular genetics of retinoblastoma. *Int Ophthalmol Clin* 1993;33:53–65.
10. Lee EY, To H, Shew JY, et al. Inactivation of the retinoblastoma susceptibility gene in human breast cancers. *Science* 1988;241:218–221.
11. Scotil U, O'Brien JM, Murray TG. Retinoblastoma: A review emphasizing genetics and management strategies. *Semin Ophthalmol* 1997;12:59–71.
12. Dunn JM, Phillips RA, Zhu X, et al. Mutations in the *RBI* gene and their effects on transcription. *Mol Cell Biol* 1989;9:4596–4604.
13. Friend SH, Horowitz JM, Gerber MR, et al. Deletions of a DNA sequence in retinoblastomas and mesenchymal tumors: organization of the sequence and its encoded protein. *Proc Natl Acad Sci U S A* 1987;84:9059–9063.
14. Scholz RB, Kabisch H, Delling G, Winkler K. Homozygous deletion within the retinoblastoma gene in a native osteosarcoma specimen of a patient cured of a retinoblastoma of both eyes. *Pediatr Hematol Oncol* 1990;7:265–273.
15. Shew JY, Lin BT, Chen PL, et al. C-terminal truncation of the retinoblastoma gene product leads to functional inactivation. *Proc Natl Acad Sci U S A* 1990;87:6–10.
16. T'Ang A, Varley JM, Chakraborty S, et al. Structural rearrangement of the retinoblastoma gene in human breast carcinoma. *Science* 1988;242:263–266.
17. Varley JM, Armour J, Swallow JE, et al. The retinoblastoma gene is frequently altered leading to loss of expression in primary breast turnouts. *Oncogene* 1989;4:725–729.
18. Moll AC, Imhof SM, Bouter LM, Tan KE. Second primary tumors in patients with retinoblastoma. *Ophthalmic Genet* 1997;18:27–34.
19. Fearon ER, Cho KR, Nigro JM, et al. Identification of a chromosome 18q gene that is altered in colorectal cancers. *Science* 1990;247:49–56.
20. Finlay CA, Hinds PW, Levine AJ. The p53 proto-oncogene can act as a suppressor of transformation. *Cell* 1989;57:1083–1093.
21. Nishisho I, Nakamura Y, Miyoshi Y, et al. Mutations of chromosome 5q2l genes in FAP and colorectal cancer patients. *Science* 1991;253:665–669.
22. White E. Tumour biology. p53, guardian of Rb. *Nature* 1994;371:21–22.
23. Eng C, Li FP, Abramson DH, et al. Mortality from second tumors among long-term survivors of retinoblastoma. *J Natl Cancer lnst* 1993;85:1121–1128.
24. Abramson DH, Ellsworth RM, Kitchin FD, Tung G. Second monocular tumors in retinoblastoma survivors. Are they radiation-induced? *Ophthalmology* 1984;91:1351–1355.
25. Der Kinderen DJ, Koten JW, Nagelkerke NJ, et al. Non-ocular cancer in patients with hereditary retinoblastoma and their relatives. *Int J Cancer* 1988;41:499–504.
26. Draper GJ, Sanders BM, Kingston JE. Second primary neoplasms in patients with retinoblastoma. *Br J Cancer* 1986;53:661–671.
27. François J, de Sutter E, Coppieters R, de Bie S. Late extraocular tumours in retinoblastoma survivors. *Ophthalmologica* 1980;181:93–99.
28. Lueder GT, Judisch F, O'Gorman TW. Second monocular tumors in survivors of heritable retinoblastoma. *Arch Ophthalmol* 1986;104:372–373.
29. Winther J, Olsen JH, de Nuily-Brown P. Risk of monocular cancer among retinoblastoma patients and their parents. A population-based study in Denmark, 1943–1984. *Cancer* 1988;62:1458–1462.
30. Eng C, Abramson DH, Ellsworth RM, Boice JD, Seddon J, Goldman M, et al. Causes of late mortality in retinoblastoma patients [abstract]. *Proc Am Assoc Cancer Res* 1991;32:221.
31. Abramson DH. Retinoblastoma 1990: diagnosis, treatment, and implications. *Pediatr Ann* 1990;19:387–395.
32. Cope JU, Tsokos M, Miller RW. Ewing sarcoma and sinonasal neuroectodermal tumors as second malignant tumors after retinoblastoma and other neoplasms. *Med Pediatr Oncol* 2001;36:290–294.
33. Wenzel CT, Halperin EC, Fisher SR. Second malignant neoplasms of the head and neck in survivors of retinoblastoma. *Ear Nose Throat J* 2001;80:106–109, 112; Klippenstein KA, Wesley RE, Glick AD: Orbital leiomyosarcoma after retinoblastoma. *Ophthalmic Surg Lasers* 1999;20:579–583.
34. Hasegawa T, Matsuno Y, Niki T, et al. Second primary rhabdomyosarcomas in patients with bilateral retinoblastoma: a clinicopathologic and immunohistochemical study. *Am J Surg Pathol* 1998;22:1351–1360.
35. Gallegos-Castorena S, Medina-Sanson A, Gonzalez-Montalvo P. Acute myeloid leukemia in a patient surviving retinoblastoma [letter]. *Med Pediatr Oncol* 2002;38:450.
36. Nishimura S, Sato T, Ueda K. Acute myeloblastic leukemia as a second malignancy in a patient with hereditary retinoblastoma. *J Clin Oncol* 2001;19:4182–4183.
37. Desjardins L, Haye C, Schlienger P, et al. Second nonocular tumours in survivors of bilateral retinoblastoma. A 30-year follow-up. *Ophthalmic Paediatr Getiet* 1991;12:145–148.
38. Roarty JD, McLean IW, Zimmerman LE. Incidence of second neoplasms in patients with bilateral retinoblastoma. *Ophthalmology* 1988;95:1583–1587.
39. Minoda H. Survival rate and risk factors for patients with retinoblastoma in Japan. The committee for the National Registry of Retinoblastoma. *Jpn J Ophthalmol* 1992;36:121–131.
40. DeSutter E, Messmer E, Hoepping W. Retinoblastoma: importance of time interval in onset of second tumors. *Bull Soc Belge Opthalmol* 1986;213:27–40.
41. Smith LM, Donaldson SS, Egbert PR, et al. Aggressive management of second primary tumors in survivors of hereditary retinoblastoma. *Int J Radiat Oncol* 1989;17:499–505.
42. Aung L,Gorlick RG, Shi W, et al: Second malignant neoplasms in long-term survivors of osteosarcoma: Memorial Sloan-Kettering Cancer Center Experience. *Cancer* 2002;95:1728–1734.
43. Chauveinc I, Mosseri V, Quintana E. Osteosarcoma following retinoblastoma: age at onset and latency period. *Ophthalmic Genet* 2001:77–88.
44. Pratt CB, Michalkiewicz EN, Rao BN, et al. Multifocal osteo-

sarcoma following retinoblastoma. *Ophthalmic Genet* 1999; 20:23–29.

45. Benedict WF, Fung YK, Murphree AL. The gene responsible for the development of retinoblastoma and osteosarcoma. *Cancer* 1988;62:1691–1694.
46. Weichselbaum RR, Beckett M, Diamond A. Some retinoblastomas, osteosarcomas, and soft tissue sarcomas may share a common etiology. *Proc Natl Acad Sci U S A* 1988;85:2106–2109.
47. Hawkins MM, Draper GJ, Kingston JE. Incidence of second primary tumors among childhood cancer survivors. *Br J Cancer* 1987;56:339–347.
48. DerKinderen DJ, Koten JW, Den Otter W, et al. Retinoblastoma, melanoma, and pancreatic cancer [letter]. *Lancet* 1986; 2(8519):1335–1336.
49. Friend SH, Bernards R, Rogelj S, et al. A human DNA segment with properties of the gene that predisposes to retinoblastoma and osteosarcoma. *Nature* 1986;323:643–646.
50. Brachman DG, Hallahan DE, Beckett MA, et al. *p53* gene mutations and abnormal retinoblastoma protein in radiation-induced human sarcomas. *Cancer Res* 1991;51:6393–6396.
51. Strong LC, Stine M, Norsted TL. Cancer in survivors of childhood soft tissue sarcoma and their relatives. *J Natl Cancer Inst* 1987;79:1213–1220.
52. Tarkkanen A, Karjalainen K. Excess of cancer deaths in close relatives of patients with bilateral retinoblastoma. *Ophthalmologica* 1984;189:143–146.
53. Robinson LL. Survivors of childhood cancer and risk of a second tumor. *J Natl Cancer Inst* 1993;85:1102–1103.
54. Shields AJ, Shields CL. *Intraocular Tumors*. Philadelphia: WB Saunders; 1992:390–391.
55. Karcioglu ZA, Al-Mesfer SA, Abboud E, et al. Workup for metastatic retinoblastoma: a review of 261 patients. *Ophthalmology* 1997;104:307–312.
56. Kopelman JE, McLean IW, Rosenberg SU. Multivariate analysis of risk factors for metastasis in retinoblastoma treated by enucleation. *Ophthalmology* 1987;94:371–377.
57. Judisch GF, Apple DJ, Fratkin JD. Retinoblastoma. A survivor 12 years after treatment for metastatic disease. *Arch Ophthalmol* 1980; 98:711–713.
58. Abramson DH. Second non-ocular cancers in retinoblastoma: a unified hypothesis. *Ophthalmic Genet* 1999;20:193–204.
59. Ceha HM, Balm AJM, deJong D, Van Veer LJ. Multiple malignancies in a patient with bilateral retinoblastoma. *J Laryngol Otol* 1998;112:189–192.
60. Abramson DH, Melson MR, Dunkel IJ, Frank CM: Third (fourth and fifth) nonocular tumors in survivors of retinoblastoma. *Ophthalmology* 2001;108:1868–1876.
61. Sagerman RH, Cassady JR, Tretter P, Ellsworth RM. Radiation-induced neoplasia following external beam therapy for children with retinoblastoma. *Am J Roentgenol Radiat Ther Nucl Med* 1969;105:529–535.
62. Soloway HB. Radiation-induced neoplasms following curative therapy for retinoblastoma. *Cancer* 1966;19:1984–1988.
63. Moll AC, Imhof SM, Schouten-Van Meeteren AY, et al. Second primary tumors in hereditary retinoblastoma: a register-based study 1945–1997: is there an age effect on radiation-related risk? *Ophthalmology* 2001;108:1109–1114.
64. Murray T. Cancer incidence after retinoblastoma: radiation dose and sarcoma risk. *Surv Ophthalmol* 1998;43:288–289.
65. Li FP, Abramson DH, Tarone RE, et al. Hereditary retinoblastoma, lipoma, and second primary cancers. *J Natl Cancer Inst* 1997;89:83–84.
66. Tucker MA, Meadows AT, Boice JD, Jr, et al. Leukemia after therapy with alkylating agents for childhood cancer. *J Natl Cancer Inst* 1987;78:459–464.
67. Tucker MA, D'Angio GJ, Boice JD Jr, et al. Bone sarcomas linked to radiotherapy and chemotherapy in children. *N Engl J Med* 1987;317:588–593.
68. Imhof SM, Hofman P, Tan KE. Quantification of lacrimal function after D-shaped field irradiation for retinoblastoma. *Br J Ophthalmol* 1993;77:482–484.
69. MacFaul PA, Badford MA. Ocular complications after therapeutic irradiation. *Br J Ophthalmol* 1970;54:237–247.
70. Gailie BL, Budning A, DeBoer G, et al. Chemotherapy with focal therapy can cure intraocular retinoblastoma without radiotherapy. *Arch Ophthalmol* 1996;114:1321–1328.
71. Murphree AL, Villablanca JG, Deegan WF 3rd, et al. Chemotherapy plus local treatment in the management of intraocular retinoblastoma. *Arch Ophthalmol* 1996;114:1348–1356.
72. Shields CL, DePotter P, Himelstein BP, et al. Chemoreduction in the initial management of intraocular retinoblastoma. *Arch Ophthalmol* 1996;114:1330–1338.
73. Chan HSL, DeBoer G, Thiessen JJ, et al. Combining cyclosporine with chemotherapy controls, intraocular retinoblastoma without radiation. *Clin Cancer Res* 1996;2:1499–1508.
74. Robinson E, Neugut AI, Wylie P. Clinical aspects of postirradiation sarcomas. *J Natl Cancer Inst* 1988;80:233–240.
75. Smith MB, Xue H, Strong L, et al. Forty-year experience with second malignancies after treatment of childhood cancer: analysis of outcome following the development of the second malignancy. *J Pediatr Surg* 1993;28:1342–1349.

PART TWO

Diagnosis of Orbital Tumors

6

Clinical Evaluation of the Orbit

Zeynel A. Karcıoglu

A complete ocular history and a physical examination are mandatory for every orbit patient. In an emergency, some parts of the eye examination can be postponed, unless the results are pertinent for the patient's differential diagnosis.

HISTORY

History taking should begin with the most important issue: the chief complaint of the patient. The answer may be "pain around my eye," "protrusion of my left eye," "double vision," or simply "When I went to my ophthalmologist to renew my glasses, the doctor noticed such and such and advised me to come and see you."

The physician's inquiry should include general questions about the onset and the duration of the chief complaint. The patient's systemic health should be investigated, and inquiries of past and present illnesses, injuries, surgeries, and drug treatment should be made.[1,2] Particular attention should be paid to history of cancer, thyroid disorders, and past episodes of infectious diseases.[2,3] The allergy history of the patient should also be questioned.

If the patient is complaining of "bulging of the eye," it may be beneficial to ask for an old photograph or a driver's license to verify the presence or absence of orbital changes. The onset of proptosis should be questioned in detail. Did it begin with an acute episode of redness and swollen eyelids and/or conjunctiva? Did it begin as a painful episode? Did the pain ease afterward? Did the pain increase or decrease during the course of the disease? Is the pain intermittent, and does it radiate to a particular spot on the patient's face? Does the patient feel a dull pain behind the eye when moving the eyes from right to left and up and down? Was the proptosis totally painless? Does the proptosis get worse when the patient sneezes or coughs? Was the proptosis intermittent, getting worse during certain times of the day, and did this intermittency stabilize later in the course of the disease? Does the patient feel irritated and gritty in the eyes; is the protruding eye worse in this regard? Does or did the patient hear a bruit (running-water sound) after the development of the proptosis? Does the patient have double vision?

Sensory problems, including numbness and tingling, as well as cold/heat sensation, should also be inquired about. Visual history related to clarity and color vision should be questioned. Awareness of a positive or negative scotoma should be checked.

OCULAR EXAMINATION

The ocular examination should include the best corrected visual acuity and intraocular pressure applanation in the primary position and in different vertical and horizontal gazes. A neuro-ophthalmologic examination, including motor and sensory functions, pupillary examination, contrast sensitivity, color vision assessment, confrontation visual fields, and central visual acuity with an Amsler grid should also be done (see Chapter 7).

During biomicroscopy, the integrity of the corneal and conjunctival epithelium should be checked as well as the conjunctival and subconjunctival blood vessels for dilatation, fusiform distension, tortuosity, and congestion. Chemosis of varying degrees is also a common finding in orbital tumor patients (Figure 6.1).

Fully dilated indirect ophthalmoscopy should be performed on every patient because many orbital diseases cause a wide variety of funduscopic changes, which may provide clues regarding the location, size, and the nature of the orbital pathology.[4] The major fundal manifestations of a space-occupying mass in the orbit include chorioretinal folds, retinal vascular changes, and optic disk edema and/or atrophy (Table 6.1).

Chorioretinal folds appear as a series of delicate striae, which are most often present in the posterior pole (Figure 6.2). Lines are usually parallel, but rarely they may radiate haphazardly to all directions.[5] Although chorioretinal folds are most commonly seen with orbital tumors, they are also seen with mucoceles and other types of cysts and also in cases of orbital injury.[6–9] Most chorioretinal folds are without symptoms and do not affect visual acuity.

The etiopathogenesis of chorioretinal folds is not known, but they are most likely due to the compression of the globe by a space-occupying lesion in the orbit.[10] However, the compression theory fails to explain the process fully, since in some cases folds are

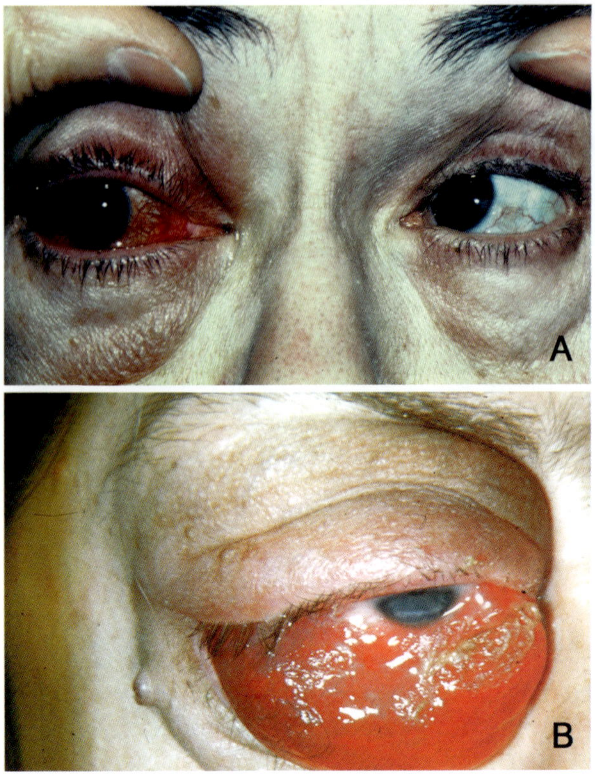

FIGURE 6.1. (A) Congestion of the conjunctiva with tortuous vessels in an orbital tumor. (B) Marked chronic chemosis in a proptotic orbit with long-standing optic nerve meningioma.

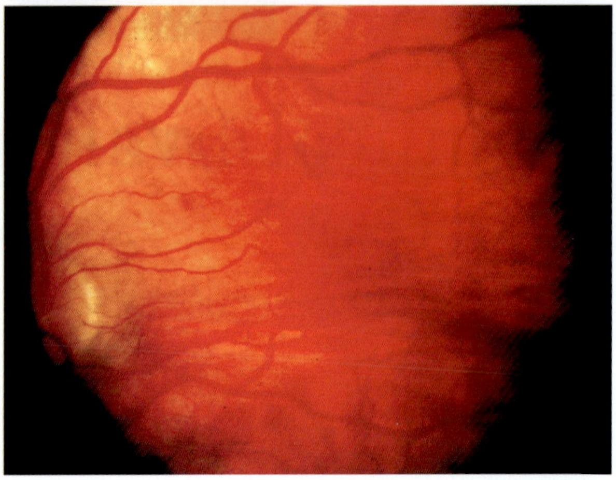

FIGURE 6.2. Fundus photograph showing horizontally aligned choroidal striae in a patient with intraconal cavernous hemangioma.

present without scleral indentation, and in other patients, rapidly expanding orbital tumors lead to scleral indentation without chorioretinal folds.[11] There is no clear relationship between the size of the space-occupying lesion and the extent or direction of the chorioretinal folds. Furthermore, the position of the chorioretinal striae is not a very dependable finding on which to localize the compressing orbital lesion.[5] Although choroidal folds have a typical appearance on fluorescein angiography, appearing as alternating light and dark lines, this test is not helpful in adding anything to the clinical workup of a patient in the presence of chorioretinal folds. The folds usually regress after treatment of the associated orbital pathology.[12] However, they may persist many months or even years after the exclusion of the primary orbital disease.

Congestion and increased tortuosity of retinal veins is another significant finding secondary to space-occupying mass lesions of the orbit, which occur more commonly with masses located in midorbit, causing stasis through the vortex veins. The diameters of engorged retinal veins are best measured and compared with the fellow eye by means of fluorescein angiography.

Disk edema, optic nerve atrophy, and, occasionally, optociliary shunt vessels[13–15] are other findings that should be noted during the funduscopic examination of the orbit harboring a space-occupying lesion (Figures 6.3, 6.4, and 6.5). Optociliary vessels are venous shunts that develop to carry blood from the retinal vasculature to the juxtapapillary choroidal circulation when the retinal venous return at the optic nerve head is blocked secondary to optic nerve tumors and other pathology.[16] Therefore, "retinochoroidal venous shunt" is a better name for these collateral vessels, which usually develop in meningioma, and, rarely, in optic nerve glioma, central retinal vein oc-

TABLE 6.1. Funduscopic Changes That May Be Seen Secondary to Orbital Disease.

Chorioretinal folds	*Retinal detachment*	*Retinal vascular abnormalities*	*Optic disk edema and atrophy*	*Optociliary shunts*
Primary and secondary tumors	Primary and secondary tumors	Primary and secondary tumors	Optic nerve meningioma	Optic nerve meningioma
			Optic nerve glioma	Optic nerve glioma
Metastatic tumors	Metastatic tumors	Metastatic tumors	Intraconal hemangiomas	Cavernous hemangioma
Choroidal tumors	Choroidal tumors	Choroidal tumors	nerve tumors	Orbital vascular
Specific inflammation	Trauma	Trauma	Dermoid cyst	Hamartomas
Pseudotumor		Cavernous sinus thrombosis	Mucocele	Glaucoma
Mucocele and cysts			Fibrous dysplasia	High myopia
Hyperopia		Wegener's granulomatosis, sarcoidosis		
Hypotony		Phycomycoses		
Scleritis, uveitis		Postradiation treatment		
Retinal detachment				
Scleral buckle				

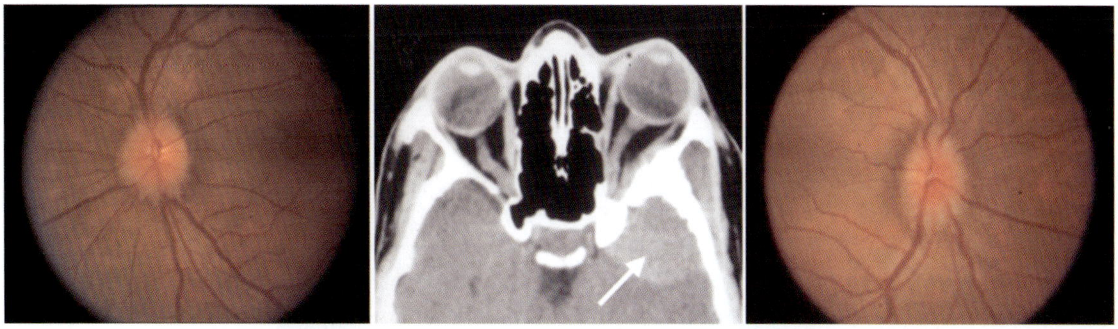

FIGURE 6.3. Papilledema in a patient with sphenoid ridge meningioma.

clusion, juxtapapillary tumors, or cysts. As opposed to choroidal folds and vascular changes, optic disk changes are better seen by means of direct ophthalmoscope or a contact lens. Optic nerve changes and other neuro-ophthalmologic features are detailed in Chapter 7.

The funduscopic examination of the orbit patient is also important to detect posttreatment changes secondary to surgical complications, radiation therapy, chemotherapy, and second primary malignancies.[4,17,18]

ORBITAL EXAMINATION

The external examination of the patient should assess the facial features and critically evaluate the symmetry of the ocular, eyelid, and orbital structures. Physical examination of the periorbital structures, including eyelids and conjunctiva, should include inspection of appearance and function, which are commonly altered by a space-occupying lesion in the orbit. The horizontal distance between interpalpebral fissures and the width of the palpebral fissures should be measured and recorded. Additionally, the distance between the margin of the upper eyelid and the upper eyelid crease, as well as the amount of inferior scleral exposure, should be measured (Figure 6.6). The comparison of these values to those of the fellow eye is usually helpful because most orbital tumors present with unilateral structural abnormalities.

Levator function should be determined on both sides and carefully recorded. Although there are many methods to assess the levator function, it is usually sufficient to measure the margin reflux (MRD: dis-

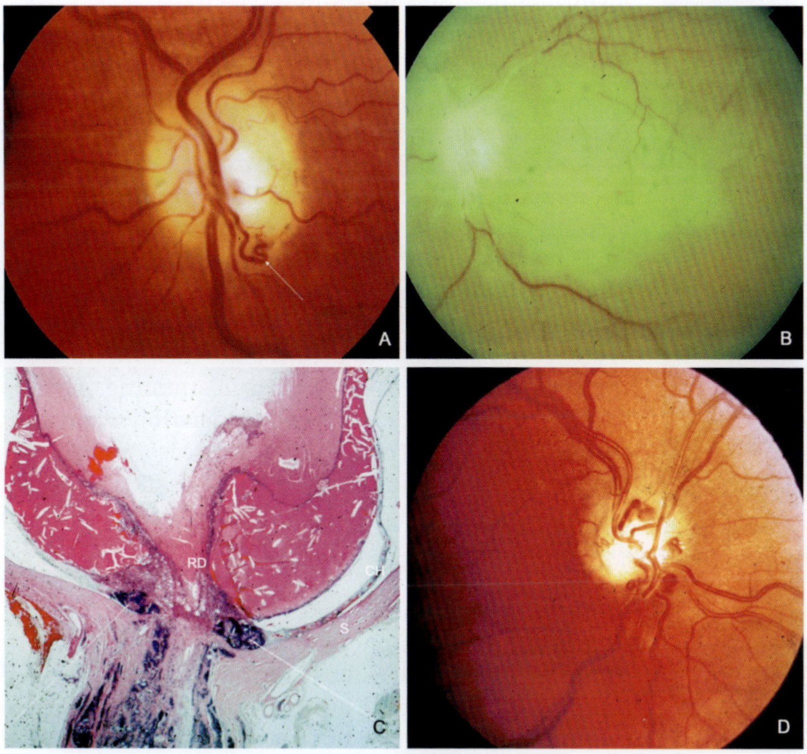

FIGURE 6.4. Optic disk changes in orbital disease: optociliary shunts (arrows) in (A) and (D) and optic nerve atrophy with retinal infarction (B) in optic nerve meningioma (C). (S, sclera; RD, retinal detachment; CH, choroid.)

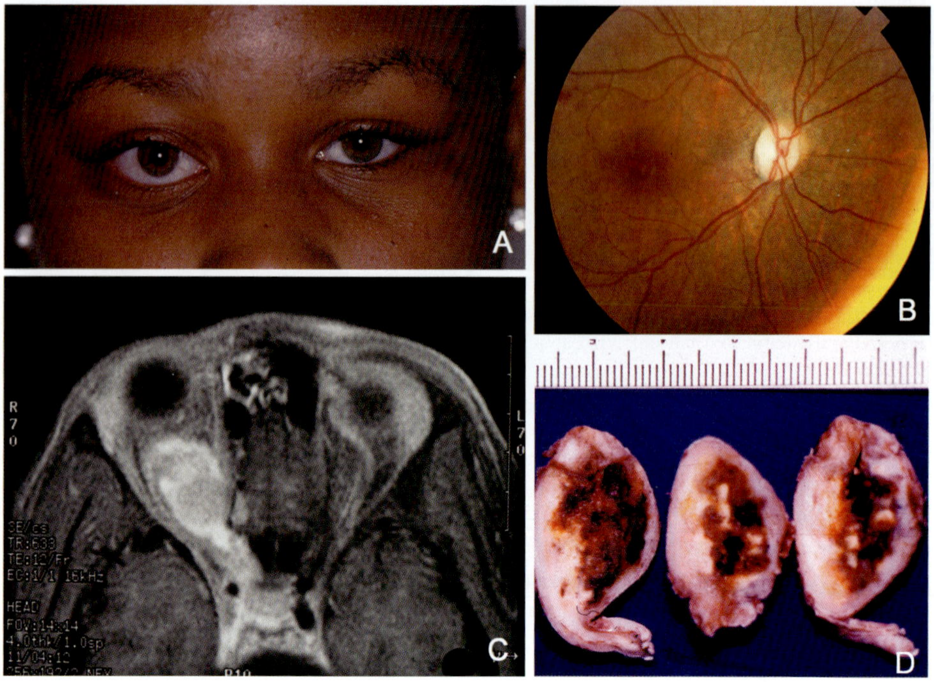

FIGURE 6.5. (A) Minimal proptosis of the right side with (B) severe optic disk atrophy secondary to optic nerve glioma (C, D).

tance between the margin of the upper eyelid and the corneal light reflex) and to obtain the full range of vertical motion [Burke levator function (BLF)] of the upper lid. Normal values for MRD and BLF are 3–5 and 15–18 mm, respectively.[19]

The appearance of the eyelids in relation to the globe should be observed individually by alternate coverage of the eyes while the physician is facing the patient; then the eyes should be viewed simultaneously from the same distance. Slowly growing masses of the orbit usually do not alter the anatomic relationship of the eyelids to the globe, and extraocular motility is affected only at extreme gazes; therefore, when observed one side at a time, these patients may look normal or close to normal. When both eyes are observed simultaneously, however, the proptosis of one eye and/or lid distortion becomes much more obvious.

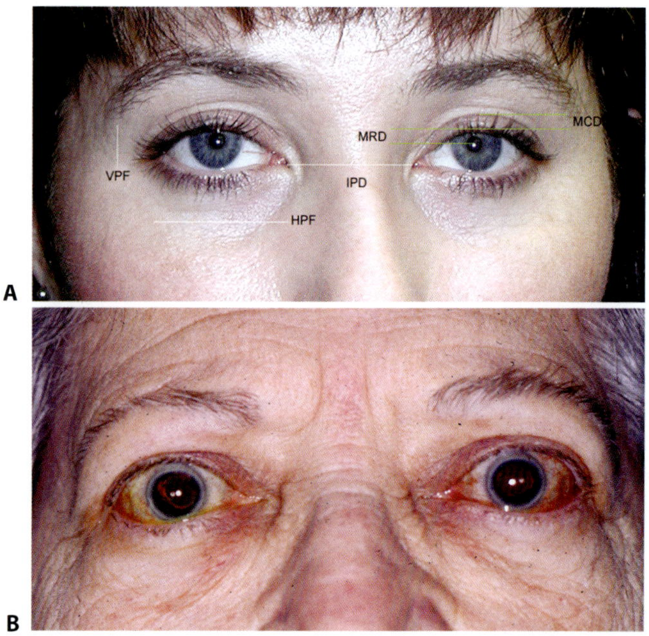

FIGURE 6.6. Normal eyelid and periorbital distances in a young adult (A) versus an elderly patient with bilateral proptosis (B). (VPF, vertical palpebral fissure; HPF, horizontal palpebral fissure; MRD, margin reflex distance; MCD, margin crease distance; IPD, interpalpebral distance.)

The most important structural feature to rate in the examination of an orbit with a space-occupying lesion is proptosis, which is also known as exophthalmos, protrusion, or the displacement of the globe beyond the orbital rim.[20] *Proptosis* is an old term having its roots in Galenic terminology, meaning "falling forward" or "falling out." In its original context, however, it was used for traumatic prolapse of the uvea, particularly of the iris.[21] *Exophthalmos*, on the other hand, is a rather new term, initially appearing in the seventeenth century, to describe the forward thrust of the eyes resulting from a systemic straining, such as hanging. After Robert Graves's association of the protrusion of the eyes with thyroid disease, exophthalmos came to be commonly referred to as a manifestation of thyroid-associated orbitopathy or Graves disease.

The term "proptosis" is commonly used to describe a forward displacement of the eye, secondary to a space-occupying lesion in one orbit, in most cases a tumor or a cyst. The displacement of the eye is determined based on the distance in an anterior–posterior plane between the front surface of the cornea and the anterior margin of the zygomatic arch. This distance normally varies from 16.5 to 21.5 mm in white men and 15.5 to 20 mm in white women. In black adults the measurements are increased by approximately 2 mm.[22] The degree of global displacement is determined with a device called an exophthalmometer.

Many exophthalmometers have been designed, but only a few have gained popularity for practical use in the clinic. One of the earlier exophthalmometers was a simple and a very useful device, designed by Luedde, that consisted of a piece of transparent plastic ruler with a groove to fit onto the lateral orbital rim. Millimetric scales were engraved on both sides of the plastic bar. When the corresponding measurements on both sides of the ruler are aligned, one can superimpose the apex of the cornea on the ruler and read that as the degree of displacement in millimeters.[23] Although dependable measurements can be obtained with this device, it measures the displacement of one eye at a time, and the accuracy of the measurement is dependent on the integrity of the orbital rim anatomy. If there is asymmetry between the two sides, the comparison of measurements would not be accurate.[24,25]

Another device, the Hertel exophthalmometer, is commonly used in today's orbit clinic.[26–29] This instrument with binocular measurements allows the observer to view the images of the cornea profiles and superimpose them on the measuring scale (Figure 6.7). The Hertel exophthalmometer offers accurate and reproducible measurements and the advantage of comparing one eye with the other during the same examination. In Hertel exophthalmometry, the distance between the two lateral orbital rims is engraved on the horizontal bar, which carries the sliding mirrors. This baseline measurement should be kept at a constant in repeat examinations to ensure dependable comparisons between measurements; ideally the same person should perform the exophthalmometry at each evaluation.

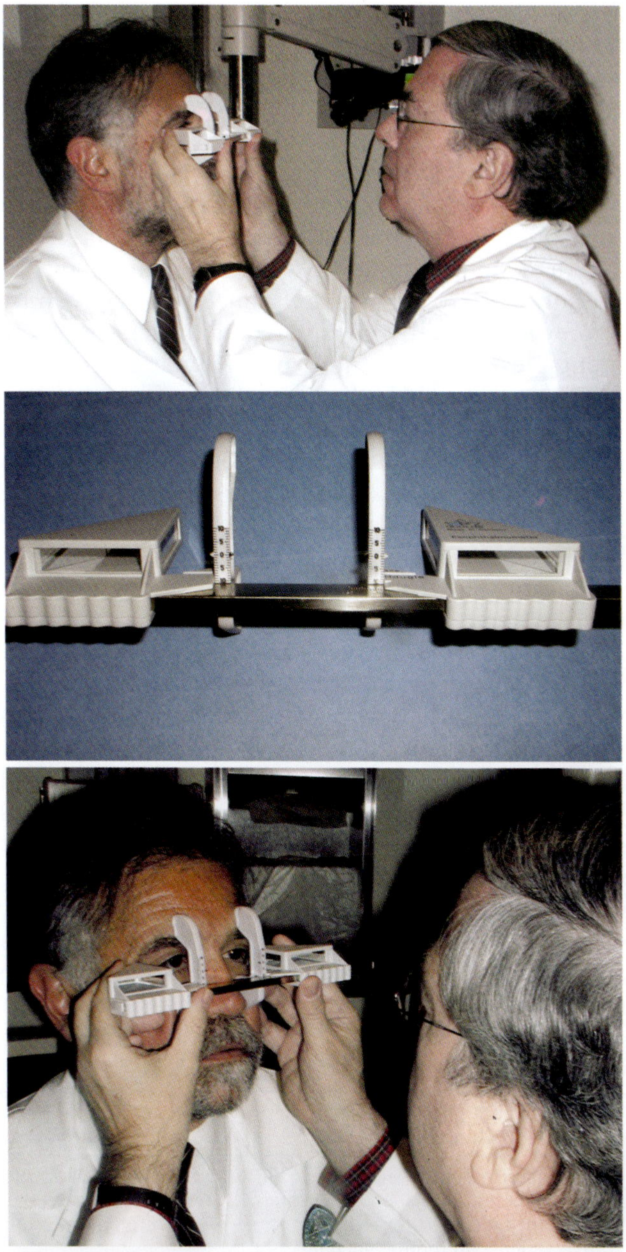

FIGURE 6.8. Evaluation with Naugle exophthalmometer. Dr. Naugle demonstrates the proper application of the instrument. (Courtesy of Dr. Thomas Naugle Jr, New Orleans.)

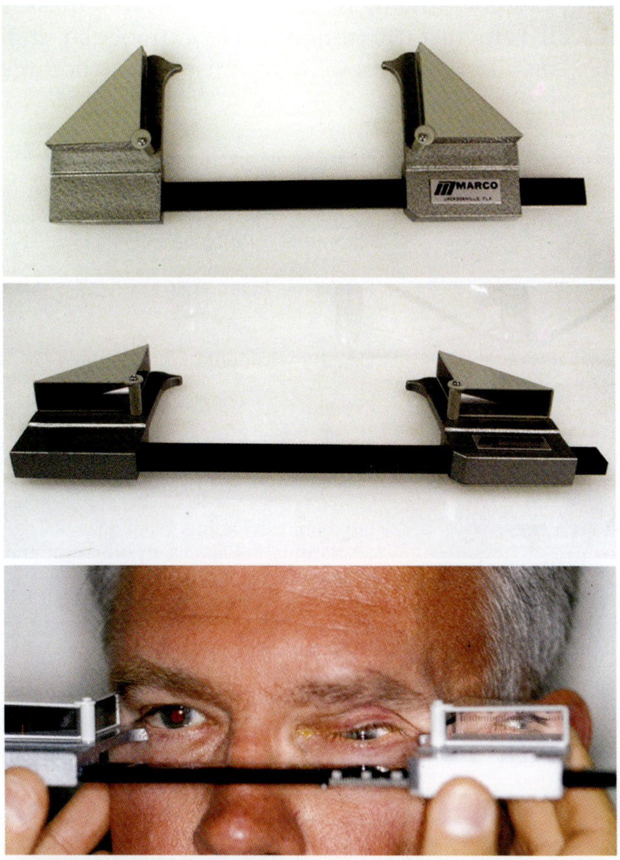

FIGURE 6.7. Evaluation with Hertel exophthalmometer.

The Naugle exophthalmometer (orbitometer) is another instrument used to measure globe displacement (Figure 6.8). This device is designed to sit on vertical fixation bars that rest on superior and inferior periorbital rims, rather than the lateral canthi. Therefore, it measures not only enophthalmos and exophthalmos, but hypo- and hyperophthalmos as well. The main advantage of this instrument is that it renders accurate measurements even when the lateral rim is irregular or missing.[30,31] This instrument is particularly useful in evaluating patients with maxillofacial trauma.[32]

An exophthalmometry measurement above 21 mm or a difference of more than 2 mm between the two eyes is usually considered abnormal. Measurements less than 14 mm are considered to be an enophthalmos.[33,34]

The direction of the globe displacement may carry diagnostic significance; if the globe is pushed down and out, natural location for the space-occupying lesion is superiotemporal (i.e., a lacrimal gland tumor) (Table 6.2).[35] The degree of asymmetry may also be important. Slowly growing, benign lesions may produce extreme asymmetrical proptosis. On the other hand, the thyroid disease usually produces less symmetrical displacement of the globes. The proptosis direction is usually downward because the majority of the primary orbital tumors develop in the upper half of the orbit. Lateral displacement, on the other hand, is usually seen as a result of secondary orbital lesions, such as a mucocele or squamous cell carcinoma, originating from the ethmoidal sinuses. Squamous cell carcinoma may displace the globe upward when it originates from the maxillary sinus. In some instances, simple transillumination with a muscle light reveals the cystic nature of an orbital lesion; this is particularly true for anterior orbital masses (Figure 6.9). Displacement of the globe toward the nose is quite rare because very few space-occupying lesions develop on the lateral aspect of the orbit.

The proptotic eye should also be examined from the standpoint of ocular motility in cardinal positions and compared with the normal eye. Recordings of deviations should be made whenever applicable. Although accurate recordings of prism values may be useful for the posttreatment follow-up of the patient, detailed diplopia measurements in prism diopters are not always possible or necessary. The amount of deviation can be quickly approximated by a red glass test in the clinic.[36] The author's preference is to use a modified Maddox cross engraved on transparent plastic that has a white fixation light in the center (Figure 6.10). When the patient is seated with straight head position at 50 cm, the numbers on the cross indicate the amount of deviation in degrees. A red glass is positioned in front of the fixating eye, and the patient is asked to point at the "white light" and the "red light" on the surface of the device (Figure 6.11).

The position of the visual axis in a proptotic eye may provide useful information. In some patients with slowly growing orbital masses, the proptotic eye adapts to the fellow normal eye and may have parallel visual axis. This is commonly seen in dermoid cysts, benign mixed tumors of the lacrimal gland, and slowly growing neural tumors. In contrast, rapidly growing or posteriorly located masses, as well as metastatic tumors to the extraocular muscles, invade the nearest neuromuscular structures,

TABLE 6.2. Differential Diagnosis of Proptosis.

Location/Pathology	*Type of displacement*	*Associated findings (may or may not be present)*
Benign lacrimal fossa lesions (e.g., pleomorphic adenoma, cysts)	Inferonasal proptosis	Choroidal folds; good EOM
Malignant lacrimal fossa lesions (e.g., adenocarcinoma, adenoid cystic carcinoma)	Inferonasal proptosis	Pain; poor EOM; enlarged lymph nodes
Benign superionasal lesions (e.g., dermoid)	Inferotemporal proptosis	Usually without choroidal folds
Anterior lesions (e.g., lymphoma, dermoid)	Mild proptosis away from the site of lesion	Conjunctival and/or lid involvement
Benign muscle cone lesions (e.g., cavernous hemangioma, schwannoma)	Axial proptosis	Posterior choroidal folds; venous congestion; early disk edema
Extraconal and intraconal lesions (e.g., vascular tumors; rhabdomyosarcoma)	Massive proptosis without a rule	Lid, conjunctiva involvement; choroidal folds; ON dysfunction and disk edema; amblyopia
Diffusely infiltrating lesions (e.g., metastatic carcinoma, diffuse pseudotumor)	Axial with or without "frozen" proptosis or enophthalmos	EOM is abnormal at all gazes; ON dysfunction with/without disk edema, enlarged lymph nodes
Inferior lesions (e.g., SCC of maxillary sinus)	Superior proptosis	Pain; sensory deficit in lower periorbital area
Medial lesions (mucocele; secondary SCC from ethmoid sinus)	Lateral and superiolateral proptosis	Pain; horizontal EOM limitation or diffuse
Posterior orbit, apical lesions (e.g., meningioma, glioma, paraganglioma)	Minimal, late proptosis	ON dysfunction with normal disk; diffuse EOM abnormality

EOM, extraocular motility; ON, optic nerve; SCC, squamous cell carcinoma.

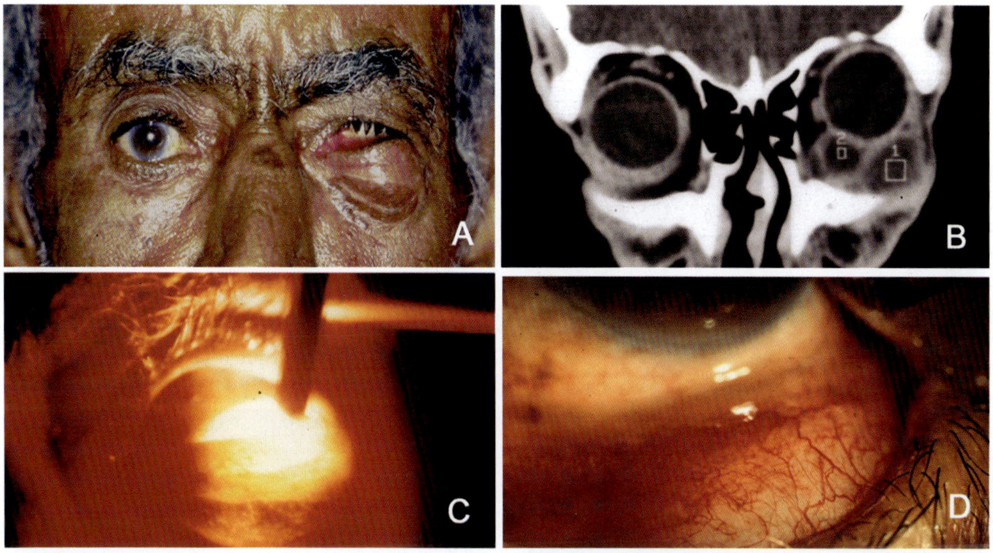

FIGURE 6.9. (A, B, D) A recurrent cystic basal cell carcinoma pushes the left globe up significantly. (C) Transillumination reveals the cystic nature of the anterior–inferior orbital tumor.

resulting in malfunction of the motility with consequent strabismus.

The rotation of the proptotic eye should be assessed. The rotation disturbance caused by proptosis can be grouped into one of two categories: (1) abnormal rotation of the eye turning toward the affected quadrant, usually seen with slowly growing masses, or (2) abnormal rotation resulting from secondary neuromuscular invasion. In the latter situation, the abnormal rotation of the eye is not limited toward the direction of the affected sector. Infiltrating orbital lesions, on the other hand, produce the most severe impairment of ocular rotation, whether they are neoplastic or inflammatory in origin. Orbital cellulitis, diffuse pseudotumor, secondary squamous carcinoma from the ethmoid sinus involving the posterior orbit, and metastatic scirrhous breast carcinoma are good examples of this pathology (see Chapter 24).

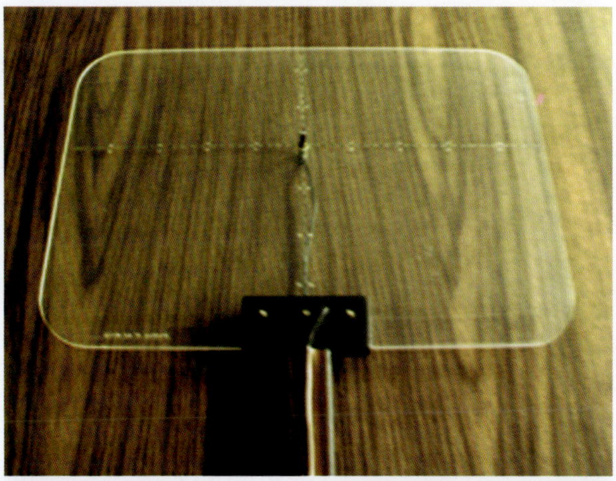

FIGURE 6.10. Maddox cross with a fixation light in the center. The scale of the cross is adjusted so that when the patient is at 50 cm, the engraved numbers on the plastic panel indicate the amount of deviation in degrees.

Generally, extraocular motility disturbance accompanying acute inflammatory disorders develops rapidly and may be painful. The ophthalmoplegia of Graves disease, on the other hand, develops gradually without pain and may, in some instances, appear prior to exophthalmos. In patients with known hyperthyroidism, ophthalmoplegia is usually noted in upward gaze secondary to slow infiltration of the superior rectus muscle by glycoproteins and chronic inflammatory cells. As the disease progresses, the extraocular motility disturbance becomes generalized, and finally, the eye may come to a standstill in the abnormal position of upward or downward gaze owing to extensive scarring of the extraocular muscle, in the direction of the deviation. The infiltrating tumors, on the other hand, have a tendency to "freeze" the eye in the primary position of gaze because of their haphazard infiltration into the muscles and the soft tissues of the orbit.

External examination must include the changes of the soft tissues of the eyelids, conjunctiva, and periorbital skin. Edema, hyperemia, and tenderness of these tissues may be a part of the clinical picture in orbital tumors; however, anteriorly located tumors such as lymphomas may cause a certain degree of lower lid edema and conjunctival chemosis. Edema of the lids, greater in the lower than in the upper eyelid, is occasionally associated with hemangioma and neurogenic tumors, presumably secondary to long-standing venous stasis. Soft tissue involvement with the resulting edema and/or retraction is more commonly associated with Graves disease and pseudotumor (Figure 6.6B). Hyperemia is also more often encountered with inflammatory lesions, particularly in acute pre-

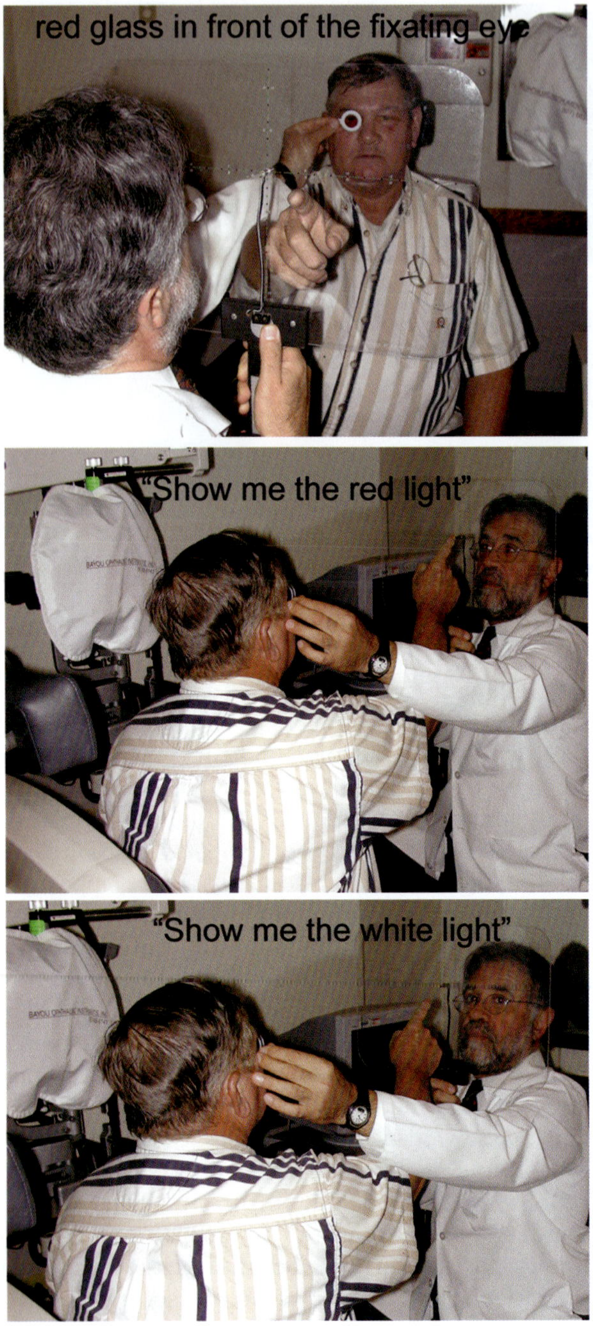

FIGURE 6.11. Evaluation of diplopia with a red glass positioned in front of the fixating eye of the patient. The patient points to white and red lights on the Plexiglas surface of the Maddox cross.

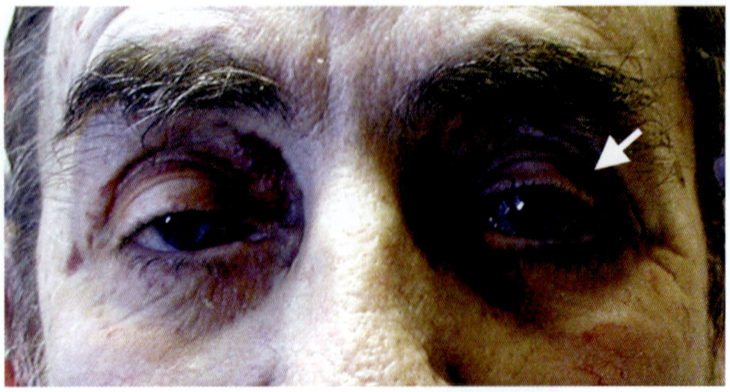

FIGURE 6.12. Bilateral ecchymosis of eyelid and periorbital skin in a patient with multiple myeloma and amyloidosis. Note the dark bruised lesion in the left upper lid; this area corresponds to a thumb imprint, which was made during indirect ophthalmoscopy. (Courtesy of Dr. David Hinkle, New Orleans.)

sentations.[37] However, redness of the eyelids may be seen in any rapidly growing malignant tumor that is located anteriorly, such as more malignant types of lymphoma, leukemia, rhabdomyosarcoma, and metastatic tumors.[38,39] Ecchymosis should not be confused with hyperemia. The former is most often seen in metastatic neuroblastoma but may also be encountered with amyloid and leukemic infiltrates (Figure 6.12). A typical feature of ecchymosis, secondary to neuroblastoma, is its changing appearance from day to day.[40] Xanthelasmas on the eyelids and periorbital skin should also be observed, since they may be a part of orbital xanthogranuloma or systemic disease (see Chapter 15).[41]

The value of palpation of the orbit is limited except for a few specific findings. First, because of the close proximity of tissues, orbital structures are difficult to palpate and may cause a considerable amount of discomfort to the patient unless done under general anesthesia (Figure 6.13). The degree of ballottement is usually measured subjectively and gives an idea about the compressibility or firmness of the underlying mass lesions. Anteriorly located tumors, including lymphomas, lacrimal gland tumors, and mucocele and dermoid cysts, can be palpated. The examiner may get a feel of the nature of their anterior surface; however, in this age of advanced imaging, feeling the tumor to determine its nature is rarely rewarding. On the other hand, palpation of a mass to guide a biopsy needle accurately may be a useful adjunct. Palpation of the orbital rim to feel an irregular edge indicative of tumor infiltrate or an old trauma site may add to the usefulness of the examination. Furthermore, crepitation within the orbit and, in some instances, arteriovenous

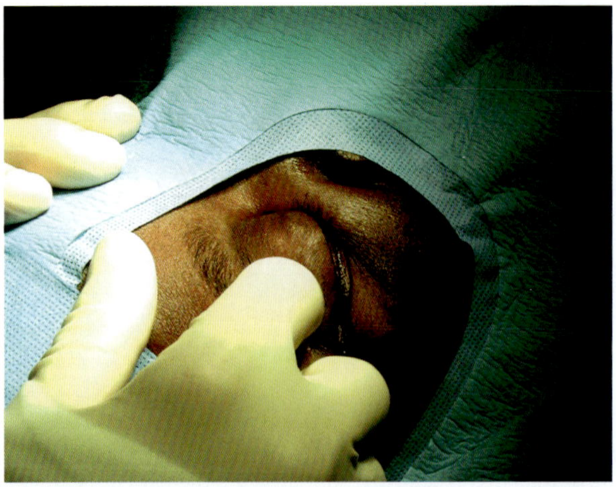

FIGURE 6.13. Palpation of the orbit under general anesthesia prior to surgery.

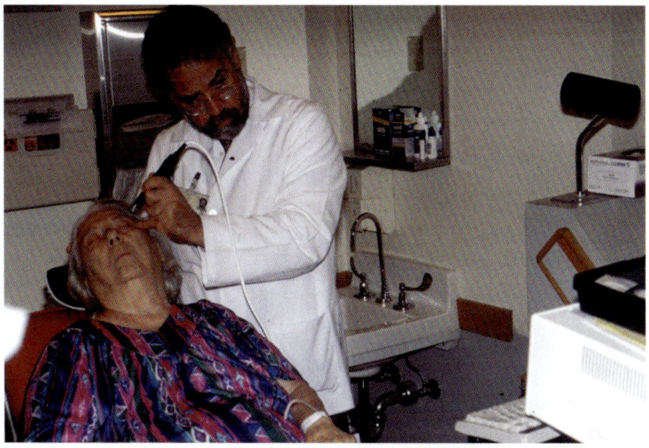

FIGURE 6.14. Examination of the orbit with Doppler instrument.

shunts, can be felt and may be useful findings in the differential diagnosis.[42] Auscultation with a stethoscope or Doppler testing is a much more dependable approach to detect bruit in the orbit (Figure 6.14). The use of a color Doppler instrument with conventional B-scan ultrasonography may be useful to study vascular tumors of the orbit as well as the blood flow characteristics of other tumors (see Chapter 8).[43,44]

During the clinical evaluation, one should keep in mind that the orbit is a small chamber, occupied by tissues of many types, located in a very compact fashion. Because of the close relationship of different tissue types, certain disease entities of different etiology and different tissue origin may clinically present with remarkably similar signs and symptoms. For example, a vascular tumor, a cholesteatoma, and a sarcoidosis granuloma may develop very similar clinical and radiological features. Another example of this dilemma may be experienced in the early stages of a subperiosteal abscess, secondary to ethmoiditis, which may mimic a secondary squamous cell carcinoma originating from the same sinus. Furthermore, there is surprising variability in the clinical manifestations of individual disorders; good examples of this are metastatic tumor to the orbit, idiopathic orbital inflammation, and Graves disease. Similar confusion may occur in the evaluation of ultrasonography, computed tomography scans, and magnetic resonance images. Although many diseases tend to be confidently interpreted on the basis of imaging, others may be very confusing. For instance, although the enlargement of extraocular muscles is quite typical of Graves disease, it may be seen in other conditions, including metastatic carcinoma, hematoma, rhabdomyosarcoma, inflammatory orbital pseudotumor, and parasitic infections.

The ophthalmologist should have a systematic approach to the workup of orbital tumor patients and keep in mind that one aspect of evaluation will not necessarily offer the final diagnosis. Therefore, a systemic history and physical examination, ocular/orbital examination, laboratory, imaging, and consultation findings should be evaluated as a whole to ensure proper assessment of the patient.

References

1. Grove AS. Orbital disease: examination and diagnostic evaluation, *Ophthalmology* 1979;86:854.
2. Kennedy RE. An evaluation of 820 orbital cases. *Trans Am Ophthalmol Soc* 1984;82:134–157.
3. Krohel GB, Stewart WB, Chavis RM. *Orbital Disease: A Practical Approach*. New York: Grune & Stratton; 1981.
4. De La Paz MA, Boniuk M. Fundus manifestations of orbital disease and treatment of orbital disease. *Surv Ophthalmol* 1995;40:3–21.
5. Newell FW. Choroidal folds. *Am J Ophthalmol* 1973;75:930–942.
6. Leatherbarrow B, Noble JL, Lloyd IC. Cavernous hemangioma of the orbit. *Eye* 1989;3:90–99.
7. Bullock JD, Egbert PR. The origin of choroidal folds: A clinical, histopathological, and experimental study. *Doc Ophthalmol* 1974;37:261–293.
8. Cangemi FE, Trempe CL, Walsh JB. Choroidal folds. *Am J Ophthalmol* 1978;86:3880–3887.
9. Newell FW. Fundus changes in persistent and recurrent choroidal folds. *Fr J Ophthalmol* 1984;62:32–35.
10. Friberg TR. The etiology of choroidal folds. A biomechanical explanation. *Graefes Arch Clin Exp Ophthalmol* 1989;227: 459–464.
11. Hampton GR. Scleral foldings: a manifestation of orbital lymphoma. *Ann Ophthalmol* 1982;14:561–562.
12. Kroll AJ, Norton EWD. Regression of choroidal folds. *Trans Am Acad Ophthalmol Otolaryngol* 1970;74:515–526.
13. Karcioglu ZA, Yulug A, Haik BG. Tumors of the optic nerve. In: Margo C, ed. *Clinical Problems in Ophthalmology*. Philadelphia: WB Saunders; 1994:105–114.
14. Sarkies NJ. Optic nerve sheath meningioma: diagnostic features and therapeutic alternatives. *Eye* 1987;1:597–602.
15. Tyson SL, Lesell S. Resolution of optociliary shunt vessels. *J Clin Neuro-Ophthalmol* 1986;6:205–208.
16. Imes RK, Schatz H, Hoyt WF, et al. Evolution of optociliary veins in optic nerve sheath meningioma. *Arch Ophthalmol* 1985;103:59–60.
17. Chacko DC. Considerations in the diagnosis of radiation injury. *JAMA* 1981;245:1255–1258.
18. Alberti WE, Sagerman RH. *Radiotherapy of Intraocular and Orbital Tumors*. Berlin: Springer-Verlag; 1993.
19. Gladstone GJ, Black EH, Myint S, et al. *Oculoplastic Surgery Atlas, Eyelid Disorders*. New York: Springer-Verlag; 2002.
20. Burde RM, Savino PJ, Trobe JD. Proptosis and adnexal masses. In: *Clinical Decisions in Neuro-Ophthalmology*. 2nd ed. St. Louis: CV Mosby; 1992:379–416.
21. Henderson JW. *Orbital Tumors*. New York: Raven Press; 1994.
22. Migliori ME, Gladstone GJ. Determination of the normal range of exophthalmometric values for black and white adults. *Am J Ophthalmol* 1984;98:438.
23. Luedde WH. An improved transparent exophthalmometer. *Am J Ophthalmol* 1938;21:426.
24. Chang AA, Bank A, Francis IC, Kappagoda MB. Clinical exophthalmometry: a comparative study of the Luedde and Hertel exophthalmometers. *Aust N Z J Ophthalmol* 1995;23: 315–318.
25. Nasr AM, Ayyash I, Karcioglu, ZA. Unilateral enophthalmos secondary to acquired hemilipodystrophy. *Am J Ophthalmol* 1997;124:572–575.
26. Hertel E. Ein einfaches Exophthalmometer. *Albrecht von Graefes Arch Ophthalmol* 1905;60:171–174.

27. Tengroth B, Bogren H, Zackrisson U. Human exophthalmometry, *Acta Ophthalmol* 1964;42:864.
28. Knudtzon K. On exophthalmometry: the results of 724 measurements with Hertel's exophthalmometer on normal adult individuals. *Acta Psychiatr Neurol Scand* 1949;24:523–537.
29. Yeats, RP, van Rens E, Taylor CL. Measurement of globe position in complex orbital fractures. I. A modification of Hertel's exophthalmometer, using the external auditory canal as a reference point. *Ophthalmic Plast Reconstr Surg* 1992;8:114–118.
30. Cole HP, Couvillion JT, Fink AJ, et al. Exophthalmometry: a comparative study of the Naugle and Hertel instruments. *Ophthalmic Plast Reconstr Surg* 1997;13:189–194.
31. Naugle TC Jr, Couvillion JT. A superior and inferior orbital rim-based exophthalmometer (orbitometer). *Ophthalmic Surg* 1992;23:836–837.
32. Schmitz JP, Parks W, Wilson IF, Schubert W. The use of the Naugle orbitometer in maxillofacial trauma. *J Craniomaxillofac Trauma* 1999;5:13–18.
33. Iliff NT. The ophthalmic implications of the correction of late enophthalmos following severe midfacial trauma. *Trans Am Ophthalmol Soc* 1991;89:455–548.
34. Cline RA, Rootman J. Enophthalmos: a clinical review. *Ophthalmology* 1984;91:229.
35. Reese AB. Expanding lesions of the orbit. Bowman lecture. *Trans Ophthalmol Soc UK* 1971;91:85.
36. von Noorden GK. Binocular vision and ocular motility therapy and management of strabismus. St Louis: CV Mosby; 1980:175–212.
37. Noel LP, Clarke WN, Peacocke TA. Periorbital and orbital cellulitis in childhood. *Can J Ophthalmol* 1981;16:178.
38. Ridgeway EW, Jaffe N, Walton DS. Leukemic ophthalmopathy in children. *Cancer* 1976;38:1744–1749.
39. Zimmerman LE, Font FL. Ophthalmologic manifestations of granulocytic sarcoma (myeloid sarcoma or chloroma). *Am J Ophthalmol* 1975;80:975–990.
40. Musarella MA, Chan HSL, DeBoer G, et al. Ocular involvement in neuroblastoma: prognostic implications. *Ophthalmology* 1984;91:936–940.
41. Karcioglu ZA, Sharrara N, Boles T, Nasr AM. Orbital xanthogranuloma clinical and morphologic review of eight cases. *Ophthalmolic Plast Reconst Surg* 2003;19:372–381.
42. Hedges TR. Carotid cavernous fistula—a re-evaluation of orbital signs. *Ophthalmic Surg* 1973;4:75.
43. Erickson SJ, Hendrix LE, Massaro BM, et al. Color Doppler flow imaging of the normal and abnormal orbit. *Radiology* 1989; 173:511.
44. Lieb WE, Muller-Forell WS, Wichmann W. Ophthalmologic imaging methods. In: Muller-Forell WS, ed. *Imaging of Orbital and Visual Pathway Pathology*. Berlin: Springer-Verlag; 2002:9–10.

7

Neuro-Ophthalmologic Evaluation of the Orbit

Andrew G. Lee

Diseases of the orbit present with typical localizing findings including proptosis, lid findings (e.g., edema, retraction, ptosis), visual loss (e.g., optic neuropathy), external signs (e.g., palpable mass), or ophthalmoplegia. The clinician dealing with orbital disease should be aware, however, that neuro-ophthalmic disease can coexist with orbital disorders, that orbital findings may be the presenting signs of systemic or neurological conditions, and that certain key portions of the neuro-ophthalmic exam should be performed in selected cases of orbital disease. This chapter discusses the major neuro-ophthalmologic features of orbital disease and the common neuro-ophthalmic pathology of the orbit that may mimic tumors. The orbital tumors are not discussed in detail; instead a review of the tumors of the optic nerve with special emphasis on optic nerve glioma and meningioma is included.

HISTORY

The history is critical in the evaluation of patients with orbital disease and should include the typical assessment of any patient-related risk factors (age, gender, race, past medical history, surgical history, medications, allergies, social and occupational history). The history of present illness should include the tempo, duration, timing, severity, frequency, and quality of the ocular complaint. Associated signs or symptoms, palliating and precipitating factors, and current treatments should be recorded.

Age

The age of the patient may be helpful in the differential diagnosis of orbital disease. Most orbital lesions of childhood are benign (e.g., dermoid, epidermoid, capillary hemangioma, lymphangioma, optic nerve glioma). The most common malignant orbital lesion of childhood is rhabdomyosarcoma, which should be considered in every case of acute proptosis in a child. Leukemic infiltration, metastatic neuroblastoma, or Ewing's sarcoma may also occur in the orbit of children. Conversely, orbital cellulitis is common in children but less common in adults. Thyroid ophthalmopathy and orbital pseudotumor (idiopathic orbital inflammation) may present with findings that can mimic orbital neoplasms. These two conditions are common in adults but less common in children. In addition, younger children with orbital lesions should be evaluated and treated for amblyopia.

Past Medical History

The past medical history should include any prior ocular or sinus disease (e.g., mucocele, malignancy, infection) systemic medical problems (e.g., thyroid disease, diabetes, tuberculosis, sarcoid), prior radiation therapy (e.g., radiation necrosis or secondary neoplasms), immunosuppressive history (e.g., risk for secondary infections or neoplasms), or previous malignancy. Social history (e.g., smoking, alcohol, occupational exposure), family history (e.g., neurofibromatosis), past surgical history (e.g., orbital or sinus surgery), medications (e.g., steroids, antibiotics), and allergies may provide important information in the evaluation of the orbital process.

Time Course of Orbital Process

In general, an acute onset (e.g., hours to days) or a rapidly progressive course suggests infectious or inflammatory disease in the orbit. In the setting of trauma, an orbital retrobulbar hemorrhage or carotid cavernous fistula may produce rapid orbital findings within hours. On the other hand, neoplastic disorders typically produce a painless and progressive course (e.g., proptosis, visual loss, ophthalmoplegia). Some neoplastic disorders may present relatively acutely, however, including metastatic lesions, rhabdomyosarcoma, adenoid cystic carcinoma, and paranasal sinus with orbital extension. Other tumors may masquerade as inflammatory disease by producing rapid inflammatory signs.

Patients with orbital lesions may complain of transient monocular visual loss precipitated by gaze position (gaze-evoked amaurosis). The optic nerve, the ocular blood supply, or the globe itself may be distorted by an underlying mass lesion (e.g., orbital tumor, orbital pseudotumor, thyroid ophthalmopathy) in certain fields of gaze.[1]

Symptoms

Patients with orbital disease may complain of diplopia, visual loss, ptosis, lid retraction, pain, proptosis, or visual loss. A careful history is required to document the onset, course, and progression of these symptoms. Any history of trauma should be noted.

EXAMINATION

The assessment of the patient should include a general workup as well as a complete ocular examination. Table 7.1 lists the major signs in the ocular examination of importance in orbital disease.

General Physical Examination

Patients with systemic thyroid disease may have a goiter. Orbital lesions (e.g., lymphoma or metastatic disease) may be associated with lymphadenopathy. Skin rash may suggest inflammatory etiology (e.g., systemic lupus erythematosus, sarcoid).

External Examination

The external examination of the ocular adenexa and eyelids can provide important information about underlying neuro-ophthalmic or systemic disorders. Lacrimal gland enlargement may be seen in sarcoidosis or underlying malignancy. Lid erythema or edema should be noted. Significant lid swelling, infiltration, or superior orbital mass can produce mechanical ptosis. Any deformity in the eyelid configuration (e.g., S-shaped eyelid in plexiform neurofibroma) should be documented. The lid position should be recorded and any lid retraction (e.g., thyroid ophthalmopathy) or lid lag (lid retraction in downgaze) should be noted specifically.

Palpation for any underlying mass, lymphadenopathy, or point tenderness may be helpful. Auscultation for orbital or cranial areas might reveal a bruit [e.g., carotid cavernous fistula, arteriovenous malformation (AVM)]. The globe position should also be noted (e.g., hypoglobus). The presence of enophthalmos (e.g., orbital floor fracture, metastatic scirrhous breast cancer) should also be recorded.[2] Testing of trigeminal function including corneal sensation may help localize an orbital process with cavernous sinus extension.[3,4] Orbicularis weakness may be seen in patients with seventh nerve weakness or myasthenia gravis.

Proptosis or enophthalmos can be assessed in the primary position or from a "worm's-eye" view, with the examiner looking up at the patient. Formal measurement of proptosis (e.g., by Hertel exophthalmometer) is important in documenting exophthalmos and following progression or regression of this sign. Although thyroid ophthalmopathy is the most common cause of adult proptosis, other etiologies including neoplasms should be considered. In addition, patients with thyroid eye disease may also have an underlying orbital or intracranial tumor. Thyroid ophthalmopathy usually produces symmetric proptosis, lid retraction, and lid lag. Asymmetric proptosis (e.g., greater than 4–5 mm difference between eyes), ptosis rather than lid retraction, severe pain, or pupil involvement should suggest alternative etiologies for the proptosis.[5,6] Other entities may produce proptosis and extraocular muscle enlargement; these are listed in Table 7.2.[7–19]

TABLE 7.1. Signs and Symptoms of Orbital Disease.

Proptosis or enophthalmos	
Conjunctival chemosis and injection	
Lid findings	Lid retraction
	Lid lag
	Lid edema
	Ptosis
Visual loss	Exposure keratopathy
	Optic neuropathy
Ophthalmoplegia and diplopia	

TABLE 7.2. Etiologies for Enlargement of Extraocular Muscles.

Endocrinopathy	Thyroid ophthalmopathy
	Acromegaly
Inflammatory	Orbital inflammatory pseudotumor
	Sarcoidosis
	Wegener's granulomatosis
	Giant cell arteritis
	Myositis
Neoplastic	Lymphoproliferative disorders
	Metastatic tumors
	Primary muscle tumors (e.g., rhabdomyosarcoma)
	Histiocytic
Infiltrative	Amyloidosis
Infectious	Trichinosis
Vascular	Carotid cavernous fistula
	Arteriovenous malformation

Slit Lamp Examination

The anterior segment exam may show conjunctival chemosis or injection in thyroid disease or orbital inflammatory disease. Arterialization of the conjunctival vessels might suggest an underlying carotid cavernous fistula. Orbital AVMs may present with findings similar to cavernous sinus AVMs and may require superselective angiography for diagnosis. Anterior uveitis can be seen in patients with systemic inflammatory disorders including sarcoid.[14–18]

Measurement of Intraocular Pressure

Elevated intraocular pressure may occur in thyroid ophthalmopathy and carotid cavernous fistula. Increased pulse pressure (e.g., pulsatile mires on applanation) may suggest an underlying carotid cavernous fistula. Orbital tumors or hemorrhage may produce elevated intraocular pressure from increased intraorbital pressure.

Testing Afferent Visual Function

Testing of the afferent system, including visual acuity, visual field (e.g., automated perimetry, Goldmann perimetry), and color vision testing (e.g., Ishihara color plates), should be performed on any patient suspected of having an orbital process that is causing an optic neuropathy. Changes in refractive error (e.g., induced hyperopia) may occur from orbital lesions compressing the posterior globe. Orbital lesions may produce severe proptosis with secondary exposure keratopathy that may diminish the visual acuity.

Subjective tests comparing the afferent responses in each eye can provide additional evidence for an optic neuropathy. A red test object (e.g., a red top bottle) can be used to subjectively compare color saturation between hemifields in one eye or between the two eyes. Subjective desaturation of the color suggests an optic neuropathy. The subjective comparison of the brightness of light between eyes can also suggest an underlying optic nerve disturbance. The patient is asked to quantify or compare the brightness of a handlight shone in one and then the fellow eye. The difference can be quantified between the eyes. The clinician arbitrarily assigns the brightness of the better eye as 100% and asks the patient to rate by relative percentage the brightness of the involved eye. Contrast sensitivity tests using various spatial frequencies and contrast levels can also detect small or subtle differences in afferent function. These tests are highly sensitive but not as specific as the others just described.

Visual Field Testing

Visual field testing can help to localize a lesion affecting the anterior visual pathway. Optic nerve related defects may be central, cecocentral, arcuate, or altitudinal (Figure 7.1). Most lesions causing an optic neuropathy in the orbit will produce ipsilateral visual field loss consistent with optic nerve related field loss. Some orbital lesions, however, involve the intracranial optic nerve and chiasm, and combination visual field defects may occur. Lesions that involve the anterior chiasm may cause optic nerve related field loss in one eye and temporal field loss in the fellow eye from compression of the junction of the optic nerve

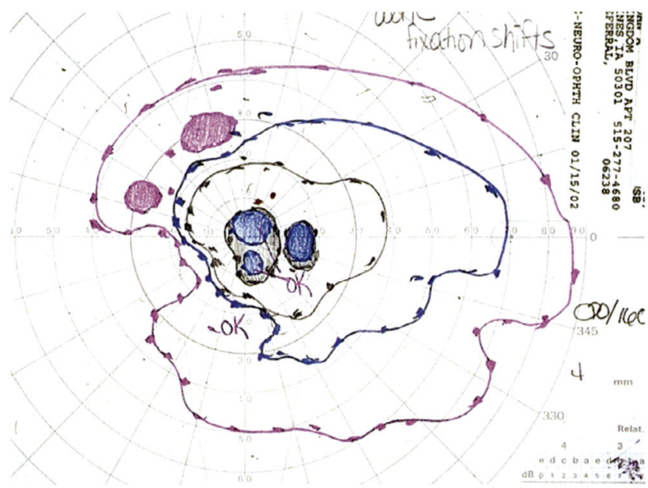

FIGURE 7.1. Goldmann visual field of the right eye shows a central scotoma and inferior arcuate visual field loss due to an optic neuropathy.

and chiasm. Lesions of the body of the optic chiasm produce a bitemporal hemianopsia. Lesions of the optic tract and other retrochiasmal diseases produce a contralateral homonymous hemianopsia.

Confrontation visual testing can easily be performed in the clinic. The clinician sits facing the patient and tests each eye separately, using his or her own eye as a control. The field can be tested with static or kinetic targets of various sizes or with the examiner's fingers or hand as the target. Formal visual field testing provides more information than confrontation field testing. Kinetic manual perimetry (e.g., Goldmann perimetry) offers the ability to vary the test object size and brightness and the ability to test the peripheral visual field; another advantage is that the technician can monitor the testing. Goldmann perimetry also provides excellent information about the shape of visual field defects. The disadvantages of Goldmann perimetry are that the test is time-consuming, requires a trained technician, and is not universally available. Automated computed perimetry (e.g., Humphrey visual field) has the advantage of reproducibility, and the depth of field loss can be quantified in decibels. The disadvantages of automated perimetry are the need for a reliable patient, who is able to follow instructions and pay attention to the testing stimuli. Elderly, very young, inattentive, or acutely ill patients may perform better on the Goldmann perimetry than automated testing. The Humphrey automated perimetry strategies can test the central 10 (e.g., 10-2 strategy), 24, 30, or 60 degrees. Patients with poor visual acuity (e.g., 20/200 or worse) may not be able to perform automated perimetry using the default stimulus size (e.g., Goldmann III test object size in Humphrey perimetry). The size of the stimulus can be increased (i.e., to Goldmann V) to improve reliability in patients with impaired central acuity.

Pupil Testing

Testing the pupillary light and near reaction is important in the assessment of afferent and efferent pupillary problems. Patients with visual loss should undergo careful assessment for a relative afferent pupillary defect because orbital lesions may produce an optic neuropathy. Patients with bilateral and symmetric visual loss may not exhibit a relative afferent pupillary defect. The absence of a relative afferent pupillary defect in a patient with a unilateral orbital lesion is strong evidence against an optic neuropathy.

Anisocoria may result from damage to the efferent sympathetic or parasympathetic pupil pathway. The oculosympathetic pathway is a three-neuron arc that begins in the hypothalamus, descends in the brain stem to the spinal cord (C8-T2 level), then arches over the apex of the lung, up the cervical sympathetic chain, and enters the cranial cavity with the internal carotid artery. The third-order neuron travels on the carotid artery into the cavernous sinus and enters the orbit through the superior orbital fissure. This third order neuron of the sympathetic pathway may be affected by orbital disease (postganglionic Horner syndrome). The ciliary ganglion resides within the posterior orbit between the optic nerve and the lateral rectus muscle. A tonic pupil may result from damage to the ciliary ganglion (including orbital surgery) or from orbital lesions.

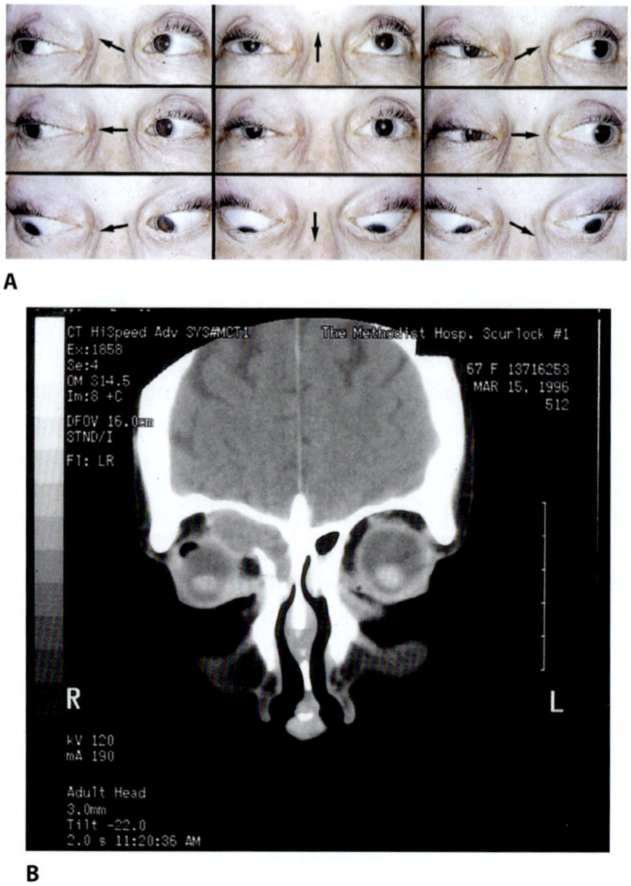

FIGURE 7.2. Ocular motility photos show an elevation deficit and ptosis (A) due to a frontal sinus mucocoele (B).

Ocular Motility Measurements

Patients with orbital disease may present with diplopia and ophthalmoplegia. The ocular motility may be impaired by restrictive disease (e.g., orbital floor fracture, mucocele, orbital tumor) or paretic disease. Figure 7.2 shows a patient with an elevation deficit and ptosis due to a frontal sinus mucocele. A rapid saccade that abruptly terminates ("hits the wall") suggests restrictive disease, whereas a slowed saccade suggests paretic disease. Forced duction and forced generation testing may be positive in restrictive etiologies.

Ophthalmoscopy

Compressive optic neuropathy may occur in patients with orbital disease. The typical features of an optic neuropathy may be present, including visual acuity loss, visual field loss, and a relative afferent pupillary defect. The optic disk in these cases may be normal (i.e., retrobulbar optic neuropathy), swollen, or pale (Figure 7.3). In most cases, if the compressive lesion is producing optic disk edema, it will be located more anteriorly in the eye, orbit, or the optic canal. Intracranial lesions are less likely to produce compressive optic disk edema, although if large enough may produce papilledema (disk edema due to increased intracranial pressure). Optic disk edema that is longstanding may compress the central retinal venous circulation, and collaterals between the retinal and choroidal circulations may form to bypass this obstruction. These new blood vessels are referred to as optociliary shunt vessels (although technically they are collateral vessels and not shunts). Optic nerve collaterals in the setting of compressive optic neuropathy (e.g., progressive visual loss and optic atrophy) are a sign of orbital tumor, usually optic nerve sheath meningioma, or, less likely, optic nerve glioma.

Retinal Findings

Orbital disease may produce retinal and retinal vasculature changes in the fundus.[4] Venous engorgement and tortuousity may be seen in carotid cavernous fistulas or less commonly in compressive orbital disorders. Secondary retinal vein occlusion with intraretinal hemorrhages and macular edema may be seen. Choroidal folds may result from orbital lesions compressing the globe. Fluorescein angiography might demonstrate the folds more dramatically (Figure 7.4).

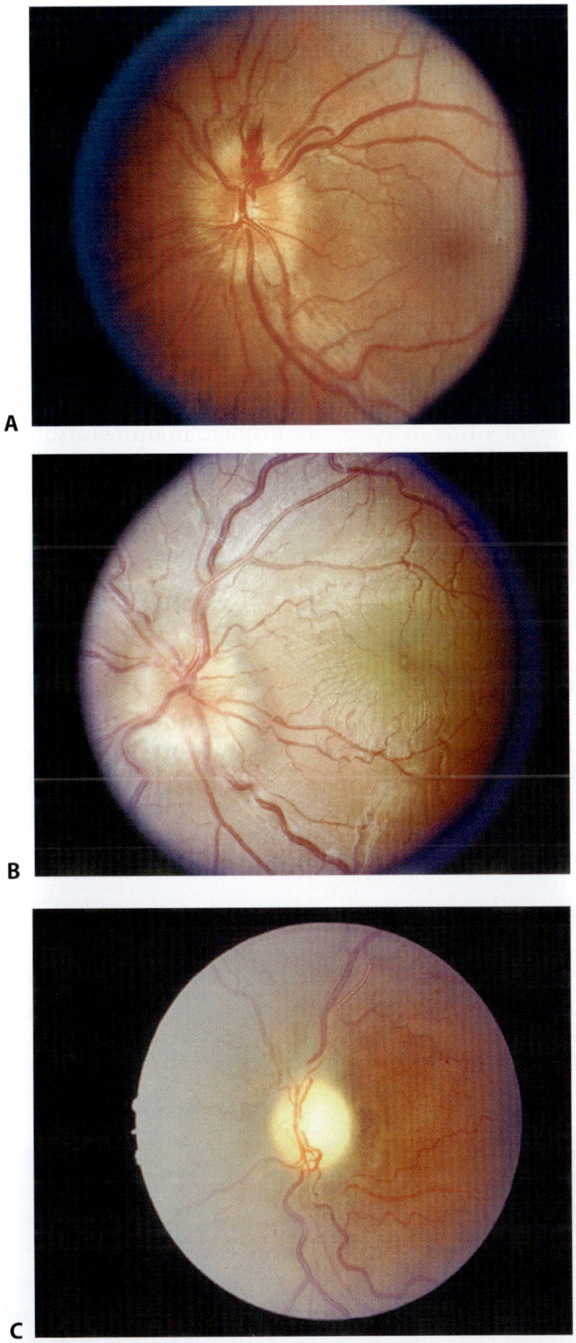

FIGURE 7.3. Optic disk photographs show (A) mild optic nerve swelling, (B) more severe optic disk edema, and (C) optic atrophy.

The evaluation of orbital lesions should include orbital imaging [e.g., orbital ultrasonography, computed tomography (CT), or magnetic resonance imaging (MRI)].

Retinal artery occlusions may result from orbital infections (e.g., angioinvasive aspergillosis or mucormycosis) or in acute orbital trauma (e.g., retroorbital hemorrhage with elevated intraorbital and intraocular pressure). Intraocular inflammation (e.g., exudative retinal detachment, vitreous cells, retinal infiltrates, retinal vasculitis, optic disk edema) may occur in patients with intraorbital inflammatory (e.g., scleritis, systemic lupus erythematosus, Wegener's granulomatosis), infectious (e.g., endophthalmitis with extrascleral extension), or neoplastic (e.g., orbital lymphoma) conditions.

ORBITAL IMAGING

In general, MR is superior to CT scanning for demonstrating intracranial involvement of orbital lesions.

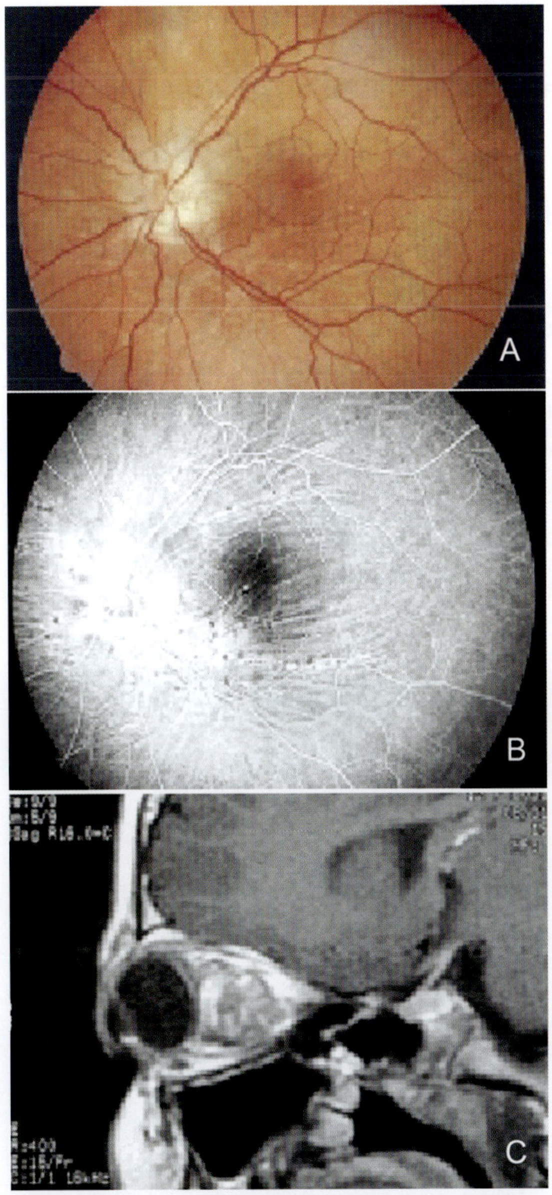

FIGURE 7.4. Optic disk photographs (A) show optic disk edema and choroidal folds that are seen better on the fluorescein angiogram (B) as alternating light (hyperfluorescent) and dark (hypofluorescent) lines. (C) Sagittal T1-weighted MR imaging shows an orbital mass compressing the posterior globe.

CT scans show bony anatomy (e.g., hyperostosis, bone destruction, bone remodeling) and calcifications better than MR scans (Figure 7.5). Fat on T1-weighted MR studies is hyperintense. Gadolinium contrast is also hyperintense on T1-weighted images. Fat suppression is necessary for orbital studies in order to visualize any pathologic enhancement. Thus, MR studies of the orbit should be performed with fat suppression techniques and gadolinium contrast material (Figure 7.6). In addition, specific signal characteristics on MRI may help in distinguishing certain tumor types (Figure 7.7).

SYSTEMIC DISORDERS THAT MAY AFFECT THE ORBIT

Although the focus of this chapter is on orbital tumors and neuro-ophthalmology, the clinician should be aware that other conditions can mimic an orbital tumor. Complete evaluation (including imaging and medical consultation) for these underlying disorders may be necessary.

Sarcoidosis

Sarcoidosis is a multisystem, granulomatous disorder of uncertain etiology. Sarcoid has a predilection for the lungs (e.g., hilar adenopathy) and may produce anterior or posterior uveitis (e.g., choroiditis, retinal vascular disease, optic neuritis, optic nerve granuloma). Although lacrimal gland and extraocular muscle involvement may occur in sarcoid, orbital involvement is uncommon.[14,15] Neurologic manifestations include optic neuropathy, papilledema, intracranial granuloma, vasculitis, and meningitis.[16–18]

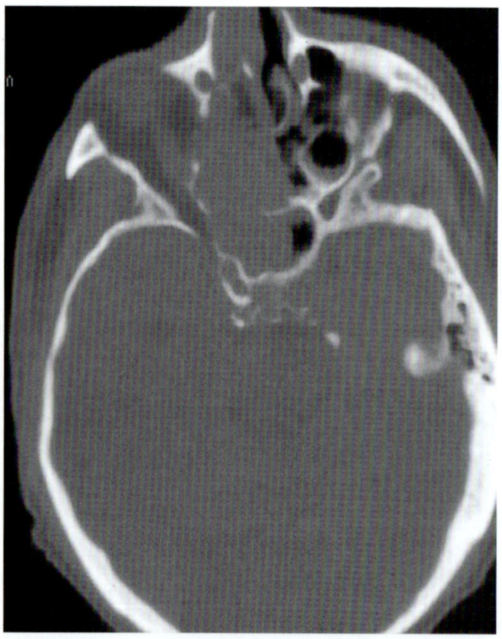

FIGURE 7.5. Axial CT scan with bone windows shows right sinus lesion with orbital extension due to renal cell carcinoma metastasis.

Wegener's Granulomatosis

Wegener's granulomatosis is a systemic inflammatory disorder characterized by necrotizing granulomatous vasculitis of the upper and lower respiratory tract and kidney involvement. The orbit may be involved in 20 to 40% of cases including conjunctivitis, episcleritis, scleritis, keratitis, uveitis, optic neuropathy, and orbital extension (e.g., proptosis, chemosis, ophthalmoplegia) of sinus disease. Neurologic manifestations include peripheral and cranial neuropathy, seizure, cerebritis, and focal neurologic deficit.[10]

Polyarteritis Nodosa

Polyarteritis nodosa is a multisystem small to medium-sized vessel vasculitis that may affect the heart, kidney, liver, and gastrointestinal tract. Orbital inflammatory disease is an uncommon finding, but choroidal and retinal ischemia related to vasculitis may occur.

Giant Cell Arteritis

Giant cell arteritis is a vasculitis of the elderly that typically presents with headache, scalp tenderness, jaw claudication, and visual loss. Orbital involvement is rare but may mimic orbital inflammatory pseudotumor.[15]

ORBITAL EXTENSION OF INTRACRANIAL DISEASE

Intracranial tumors may rarely extend into the orbit. Table 7.3 lists several systemic or intracranial processes that may involve the orbit from direct extension.[11–90] Orbital extension may produce ophthalmoplegia, optic neuropathy, and proptosis. Appropriate head and orbital imaging may be needed in these circumstances.

The two most commonly encountered tumors of the optic nerve that involve the orbit are optic nerve glioma and optic nerve meningioma.

Optic Pathway Glioma

Optic nerve glioma is a tumor of childhood,[20–34] and presentation in adulthood might suggest a more malignant glioma.[21] Although the tumor can present at any age, most patients are less than 10 years old with a mean age of 8.8 years. There is no gender predilec-

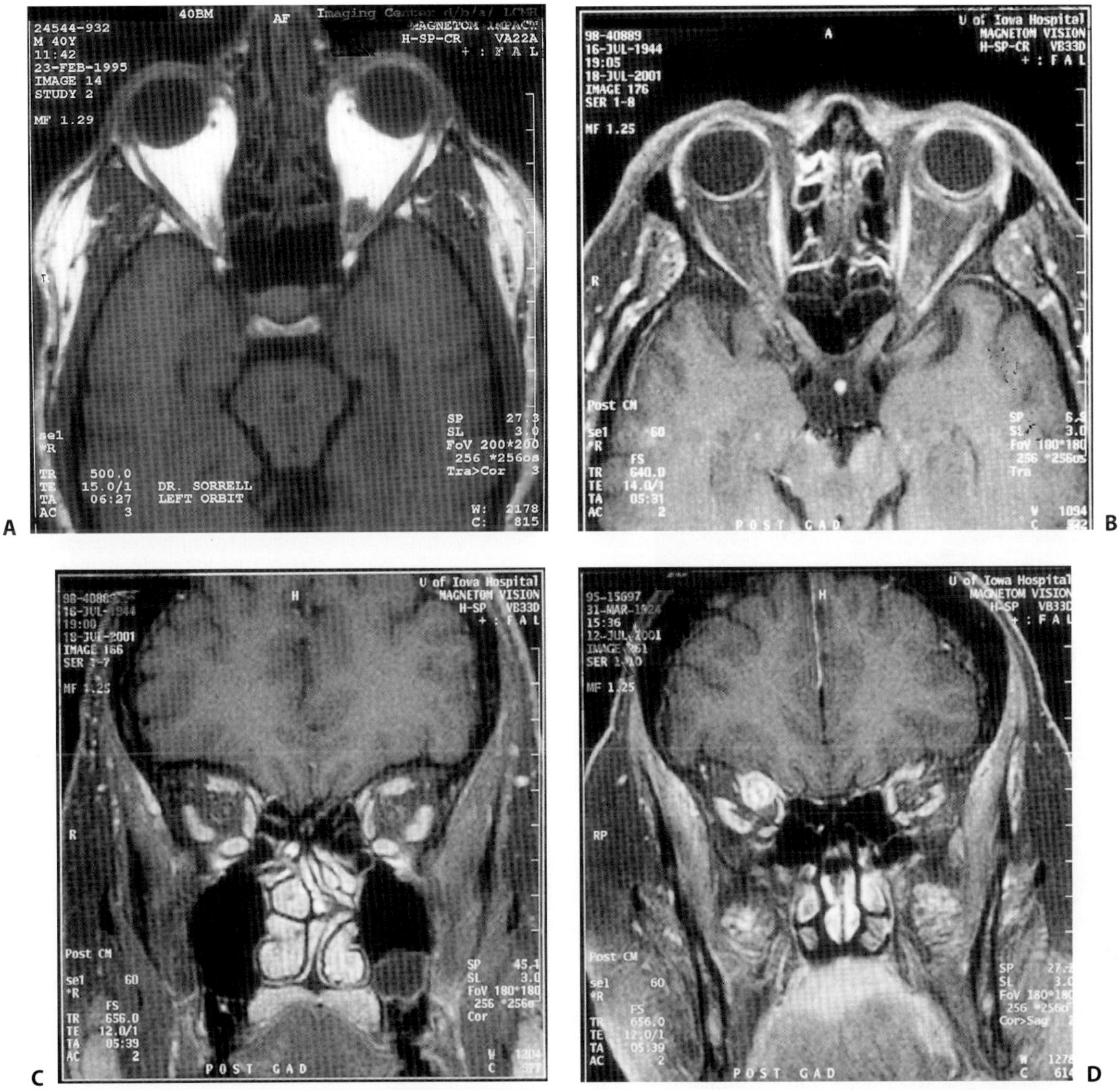

FIGURE 7.6. (A) Axial non-fat-suppressed MR images show the hyperintense fat on T1-weighted imaging (B). Axial and (C) coronal MR studies show fat-suppressed postcontrast T1-weighted images. Note the previously hyperintense fat signal on these T1-weighted images. (D) Metastatic lesion to the right superior rectus muscle.

tion.[34] Optic pathway gliomas are associated with neurofibromatosis type 1 (NF1) (see Chapter 17); the tumor may be asymptomatic in these patients, or appear later in life after initially normal imaging.[22,24,25] Some studies have suggested that patients with NF1 may have borderline favorable prognosis, but other studies have shown little or no difference prognosis.[26,29,31,33,35]

Any part of the optic pathway may be involved with a glioma, and prognosis depends in part upon the extent and location of the tumor. One or both optic nerves alone are involved in 24%, the optic disk is involved in 1.6%, and the optic chiasm or tract is involved in 75%. In general, the more anterior the lesion, the better the prognosis.

Optic pathway gliomas involving the orbit produce proptosis, ophthalmoplegia, and painless progressive visual loss.[32] Visual loss is present at presentation in 87.5%. Hypothalamic symptoms (26%) or endocrinologic manifestations (e.g., diabetes insipidus, diencephalic wasting, precocious puberty, somnolence, growth failure) may occur in chiasmal-hypothalamic tumors.[36] Optic disc swelling (35%) or atrophy (59%) is generally present, and rarely optociliary shunt vessels may occur.[23]

Neuroimaging with an MR scan with gadolinium is superior to CT scan for demonstrating intracranial extension. The imaging typically shows intrinsic enlargement of the optic nerve with variable contrast enhancement.[30,37] Figure 7.8 shows a left optic nerve glioma on an axial fat suppressed MR of the orbit. The treatment of optic pathway gliomas is controversial.[38] Most authors recommend a period of observation for progression prior to initiation of therapy as gliomas are often static lesions (after an initial but variable pe-

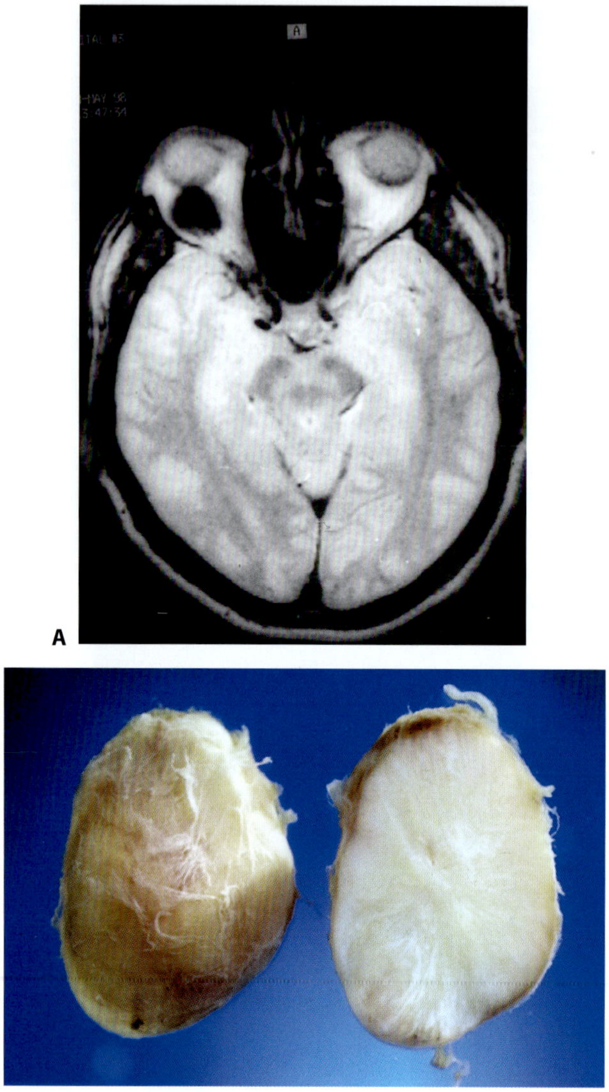

A

B

FIGURE 7.7. T2-weighted MR image of the orbit shows a markedly hypointense lesion (A) consistent with a hypercellular fibrous tumor, in this case solitary fibrous tumor of the right orbit (B).

TABLE 7.3. Systemic or Intracranial Lesions That May Extend into the Orbit.

Neoplastic	Optic pathway glioma
	Secondary intracranial meningioma or sheath meningioma
	Pituitary adenoma
	Lymphoproliferative disorders (e.g., lymphoma and leukemia)
	Germinoma
	Sinus histiocytosis with lymphadenopathy
	Sinus tumors (e.g., nasopharyngeal cancer, metastasis, adenoid cystic carcinoma)
	Metastasis
Extramedullary hematopoiesis	
Trauma	Orbital, facial, and skull base fractures
Inflammatory	Sarcoidosis
	Wegener's granulomatosis
	Collagen vascular disorders
	Giant cell arteritis
	Orbital inflammatory pseudotumor
	Hypertrophic pachymeningitis
Infectious diseases	Mucoceles
	Sarcoidosis
	Aspergillosis
	Mucormycosis
	Cysticercosis
Primary bone diseases	Osteopetrosis
	Fibrous dysplasia
	Craniometaphyseal
	Dysplasia
	Fibrosclerosis
	Paget's disease
	Aneurysmal bone cyst
	Pneumosinus dilatans
Vascular etiologies	Orbital hemorrhage
	Hematic cyst
	Subperiosteal hemorrhage
	Orbital venous and vascular anomalies
	Arteriovenous malformations
Iatrogenic	Intracranial oxidized cellulose hemostat
	Postoperative (e.g., postoptic canal decompression, sinus surgery)

riod of growth). Radiation therapy is generally reserved for patients over age 5 years with progressive radiographic findings or worsening clinical signs and symptoms.[32] The risks of radiation are considerable and include cerebrovascular disease, moya moya disease, cerebral atrophy, subnormal intelligence or learning disabilities, secondary malignancies (e.g., astrocytomas), cataracts, radiation retinopathy or optic neuropathy, endocrinopathy, and hypothalmic dysfunction.[39–41] These risks are generally higher the younger the age of the patient. Chemotherapy is emerging as a possibly safer alternative to radiation therapy particularly in younger children.[32] Various agents and combinations of agents have been used with some anecdotal success including: actinomycin D, vincristine, CCNV, 6-thioguanine, procarbazine, dibromodulatol, topotecan, carboplatin, and etoposide.[32]

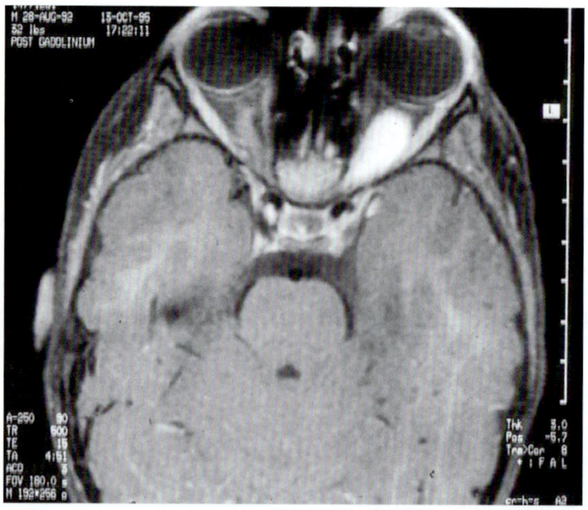

FIGURE 7.8. Axial fat-suppressed T1-weighted postcontrast MR scan of the orbit shows a left fusiform enhancing optic nerve mass consistent with an optic nerve glioma.

Surgical therapy is generally limited. A strictly optic nerve glioma with no useful vision or progression may be resected. Chiasmal, hypothalamic, or optic tract gliomas, cannot be completely resected because of unacceptable visual and surgical morbidity. Any exophytic and symptomatic component of these tumors, however, may be debulked. Secondary hydrocephalus may require shunting procedure.[32]

The prognosis of optic pathway gliomas is quite variable and is in part based upon location.[42] Most (80%) have stable vision after an initial period of visual loss. The 10-year overall survival rate is between 85% to 100% in various series, and spontaneous regression may occur.[27,28]

Adult Malignant Glioma

As opposed to optic pathway gliomas in childhood, gliomas in adults tend to be more malignant. The patients tend to be older males. The clinical signs and symptoms include rapidly progressive loss of vision unilaterally or bilaterally. The visual acuity usually progresses to complete blindness over an average of 11 weeks. Optic nerve related visual field defects occur. The optic disk may be normal or show swelling or atrophy. Proptosis or ophthalmoplegia may occur if the lesion involves the orbital optic nerve. Retro-orbital pain is quite common. Macular edema, a cherry-red spot, and flame hemorrhages or hemorrhagic papillopathy may occur and simulate a central retinal vein occlusion. Unlike childhood optic gliomas, adult malignant gliomas are not associated with NF-1. The treatment options are limited and include radiation therapy or chemotherapy. The pathology is consistent with a malignant astrocytoma. The prognosis is generally poor with an overall mortality of 97% and a mean survival of 8.7 months (range 3 to 24 months).[21,34]

Meningiomas

Meningiomas may occur primarily in the optic nerve sheath or extend into the orbit secondarily from the intracranial cavity.[43–58] Meningiomas typically affect middle-aged patients. There is a female to male ratio of 3 to 1, and Caucasians are more affected than African-American patients.[43,44] There is an increased frequency of meningioma in neurofibromatosis I and II, and multiple meningiomas (e.g., bilateral optic nerve sheath meningiomas in NF-2) may occur in these patients.[45] The symptoms of a meningioma affecting the anterior visual pathway include painless and gradually progressive loss of vision or visual field. Frontal or olfactory meningiomas may have mental status changes. There may be diplopia from extraocular muscle, orbital, or cavernous sinus involvement. The signs of anterior visual pathway meningioma include loss of visual acuity and field and an ipsilateral RAPD. There may be optic disk edema, optic atrophy, or the disk may be normal (retrobulbar optic neuropathy). Optociliary collateral ("shunt") vessels may be present on the optic nerve head.[55]

Neuroimaging typically shows characteristic but not necessarily diagnostic features of meningioma.[58] Some patients may have meningocoele that might mimic a sheath meningioma.[47] MR imaging is superior to computed tomography (CT) scans in the evaluation of meningioma, but a CT scan may show hyperostosis of adjacent bone or calcification within the lesion. Magnetic resonance imaging typically shows an isointense lesion on T1-weighted images with homogenous gadolinium enhancement. There may or may not be a classic but not pathognomonic dural tail of enhancement. Optic nerve sheath meningiomas have a more diagnostic radiographic appearance and may display a classic "tram track" appearance of enhancement of the optic nerve sheath.

The management of symptomatic intracranial meningiomas must be individualized. The tumor is usually histopathologically benign but may compress vital structures. A gross total resection is generally attempted if the patient is a good surgical candidate, is symptomatic with good expectation for improvement with decompression, and if the surgery is technically feasible. If the meningioma is encasing or surrounding vital structures (e.g. cavernous sinus, internal carotid artery), a subtotal excision may have to be performed. Sequential neuro-ophthalmic evaluations and neuroimaging studies are recommended to detect postoperative recurrence or progression. Postoperative radiation may be employed for malignant or aggressive pathology or for residual, recurrent, or non-resectable tumors if signs or symptoms progress.[48–52,56]

Optic Nerve Sheath Meningiomas

Optic nerve sheath meningiomas usually do not require biopsy for diagnosis if the typical clinical and radiographic features are present.[53,58] Figure 7.9 shows a typical sheath meningioma on T1-weighted post-contrast fat suppressed MR scan of the orbit. Observation for progression is a reasonable first step in management. Complete surgical excision usually produces irreversible visual loss and is generally reserved for eyes without visual potential and vision-threatening or cosmetically unacceptable proptosis. Observation is an acceptable protocol to evaluate progression with serial neuroimaging (e.g., MRI head and orbits with gadolinium and fat suppression) every 6 months for 2 years, then yearly if there is no growth. Most authors would consider radiation therapy to be the treatment of choice for optic nerve sheath meningioma if preservation of visual function is the goal.[48] Improved techniques of delivery of radiotherapy (e.g., conformal,

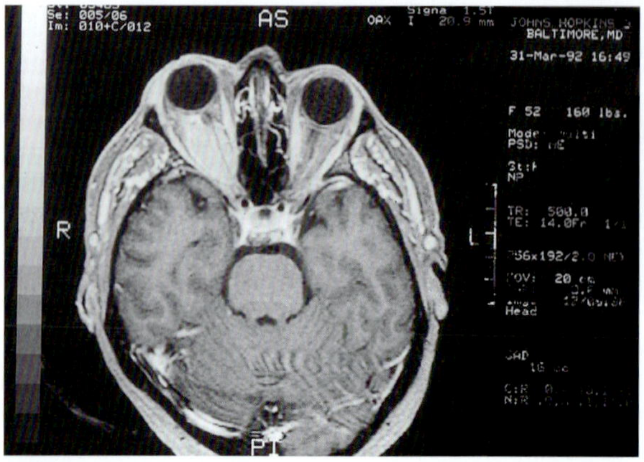

FIGURE 7.9. Axial fat-suppressed T1-weighted postgadolinium MR scan of the orbit shows a left enhancing optic nerve sheath meningioma.

three dimensional, intensity-modulated, radiotherapy) may decrease the risks of radiation side effects.[52,54]

CONCLUSIONS

Orbital disorders may present with neuro-ophthalmologic findings (e.g., optic neuropathy). In addition, neurologic and systemic diseases may present in the orbit. The clinician should understand the neuro-ophthalmic considerations in orbital disease and perform appropriate evaluation and imaging.

References

1. Bradbury PG, Levy IS, McDonald WI. Transient uniocular visual loss on deviation of the eye in association with intraorbital tumors. *J Neurol Neurosurg Psychiatry* 1987;50:615–619.
2. Cline RA, Rootman J. Enophthalmos: a clinical review. *Ophthalmology* 1984;91:229–237.
3. Huna-Baron R, Setton A, Kupersmith MJ, Berenstein A. Orbital arteriovenous malformation mimicking cavernous sinus dural arteriovenous malformation. *Br J Ophthalmol* 2000;84: 771–774.
4. De La Paz MA, Boniuk M. Fundus manifestations of orbital disease and treatment of orbital disease. *Surv Ophthalmol* 1995;40:3–21.
5. Trobe JD, Glaser JS, LaFlamme P. Dysthyroid optic neuropathy: clinical profile and rationale for management. *Arch Ophthalmol* 1978;96:1199–1209.
6. Feldon SE, Muramatsu S, Weiner JM. Clinical classification of Graves' ophthalmopathy. Identification of risk factors for optic neuropathy. *Arch Ophthalmol* 1984;102:1469–1472.
7. Patrinely JR, Osborn AG, Anderson RL, et al. Computed tomographic features of non-thyroid extraocular muscle enlargement. *Ophthalmology* 1989;96:1038–1047.
8. Dal Pozzo G, Boschi MC. Extraocular muscle enlargement in acromegaly. *J Comput Assist Tomogr* 1982;6:796–707.
9. Katz B, Leja S, Melles RB, et al. Amyloid ophthalmoplegia. Ophthalmoparesis secondary to primary systemic amyloidosis. *J Clin Neuro-Ophthalmol* 1989;9:39–42.
10. Nishino H, Rubino FA, DeRemee RA, et al. Neurologic involvement in Wegener's granulomatosis: an analysis of 324 consecutive cases at the Mayo Clinic. *Ann Neurol* 1993;33:4–9.
11. Capone A, Jr., Slamovits TL. Discrete metastasis of solid tumors to extraocular muscles. *Arch Ophthalmol* 1990;108: 237–243.
12. Hornblass A, Jakobiec FA, Reifler DM, et al. Orbital lymphoid tumors located predominantly within extraocular muscles. *Ophthalmology* 1984;94:688–697.
13. Goldberg S, Mahadevia P, Lipton M, Rosenbaum PS. Sinus histiocytosis with massive lymphadenopathy involving orbit: reversal of compressive optic neuropathy after chemotherapy. *J Neuro-Ophthalmol* 1998;18:270–275.
14. Cornblath WT, Elner V, Rolfe M. Extraocular muscle involvement in sarcoidosis. *Ophthalmology* 1993;100:501–505.
15. Simon EM, Zoarski GH, Rothman ML, et al. Systemic sarcoidosis with bilateral orbital involvement. MR findings. *AJNR Am J Neuroradiol* 1998;19:336–337.
16. Ing EB, Garrity JA, Cross SA, Ebersold MJ. Sarcoid masquerading as optic nerve sheath meningioma. *Mayo Clin Proc* 1997;72:38–43.
17. Achiron L, Strominger M, Witkin N, Prime S. Sarcoid optic neuropathy: a case report. *J Am Optom Assoc* 1995;66:646–651.
18. Carmody, RF, Mafee, MF, Goodwin, JA, et al. Orbital and optic pathway sarcoidosis: MR findings. *AJNR Am J Neuroradiology* 1994;15:775–783.
19. Lee AG, Tang RA, Feldon SE, et al. Orbital presentations of giant cell arteritis. *Graefes Arch Ophthalmol* 2001;239:509–513.
20. Alvord EJ, Lofton S. Gliomas of the optic nerve or chiasm. Outcome by patient's age, tumor site, and treatment. *J Neurosurg* 1988;68:85–98.
21. Brodovsky S, ten Hove MW, Pinkerton RM, et al. An enhancing optic nerve lesion: malignant glioma of adulthood. *Can J Ophthalmol* 1997;32:409–413.
22. Chateil JF, Soussotte C, Pedespan JM, et al. MRI and clinical differences between optic pathway tumours in children with and without neurofibromatosis. *Br J Radiol* 2001;74:24–31.
23. Levin LA, Jakobiec FA. Optic nerve tumors of childhood: a decision-analytical approach to their diagnosis. *Int Ophthalmol Clin* 1992;32:223–240.
24. Listernick R, Charrow J, Greenwald M. Emergence of optic pathway gliomas in children with neurofibromatosis type I after normal neuroimaging results. *J Pediatr* 1992;121:584–587.
25. Listernick R, Charrow J, Greenwald M, et al. Optic gliomas in children with neurofibromatosis type I. *J Pediatr* 1994;125: 63–66.
26. Listernick R, Louis DN, Packer RJ, Gutmann DH. Optic pathway gliomas in children with neurofibromatosis 1: consensus statement from the NF1 Optic Pathway Glioma Task Force. *Ann Neurol* 1997;41:143–149.
27. Liu GT, Lessell S. Spontaneous visual improvement in chiasmal gliomas. *Am J Ophthalmol* 1992;114:193–201.
28. Parsa CF, Hoyt CS, Lesser RL, et al. Spontaneous regression of optic gliomas. Thirteen cases documented by serial neuroimaging. *Arch Ophthalmol* 2001;119:516–529.
29. Créange A, Zeller J, Rostaing-Rigattieri S, et al. Neurological complications of neurofibromatosis type 1 in adulthood. *Brain* 1999;122:473–481.
30. Cummings TJ, Provenzale JM, Hunter SB, et al. Gliomas of the optic nerve: histological, immunohistochemical (MIB-1 and p53), and MRI analysis. *Acta Neuropathol* 2000;99: 563–570.
31. Deliganis AV, Geyer JR, Berger MS. Prognostic significance of type I neurofibromatosis (von Recklinghausen disease) in childhood optic glioma. *Neurosurgery* 1996;38:1114–1118.
32. Lee AG, Dutton J. A practice pathway for the management of gliomas of the anterior visual pathway: an update and an evidence-based approach. *Neuro-Ophthalmology* 1999;22:139–155.

33. Dunn DW, Purvin V. Optic pathway gliomas in neurofibromatosis. *Dev Med Child Neurol* 1990;32:820–824.
34. Dutton JJ. Gliomas of the anterior visual pathway. *Surv Ophthalmol* 1994;38:427–452.
35. Imes RK, Hoyt WF. Magnetic resonance imaging signs of optic nerve gliomas in neurofibromatosis. *Am J Ophthalmol* 1991;111:729–734.
36. Jans AJ, Grundy R, Caan A, et al. Optic pathway and hypothalamic/chiasmatic gliomas in children younger than 5 years with a 6-year follow-up. *Cancer* 1995;75:1052–1059.
37. Jenkin D, Angyalfi S, Becker L, et al. Optic glioma in children, surveillance or irradiation? *Int J Radiat Oncol Biol Phys* 1993;25:215–225.
38. Friedman JM, Birch P. An association between optic glioma and other tumours of the central nervous system in neurofibromatosis type I. *Neuropediatrics* 1997;28:131–132.
39. Gayre GS, Scott IU, Feuer W, et al. Long-term visual outcome in patients with anterior visual pathway gliomas. *J Neuro-Ophthalmol* 2001;21:1–7.
40. Grill J, Couanet D, Cappelli C, et al. Radiation-induced cerebral vasculopathy in children with neurofibromatosis and optic pathway glioma. *Ann Neurol* 1999;45:393–396.
41. Kestle JRW, Hoffman HJ, Mock AR. Moya moya phenomenon after radiation for optic glioma. *J Neurosurg* 1993;79:32–35.
42. Fuss M, Hug EB, Schaefer RA, et al. Proton radiation therapy (PRT) for pediatric optic pathway gliomas: comparison with 3D planned conventional photons and standard photon technique. *International J Radiat Oncol Biol Phys* 1999;45:1117–1126.
43. Dutton JJ. Optic nerve gliomas and meningiomas. *Neurol Clin* 1991;9:163–177.
44. Dutton JJ. Optic nerve sheath meningiomas. *Surv Ophthalmol* 1992;37:167–183.
45. Cunliffe IA, Moffat DA, Hardy DG, Moore AT. Bilateral optic nerve sheath meningiomas in a patient with neurofibromatosis type 2. *Br J Ophthalmol* 1992;76:310–312.
46. Fayaz I, Gentili F, MacKenzie IR. Optic nerve sheath meningioma. *J Neurol Neurosurg Psychiatry* 1999;67:408.
47. Garrity JA, Trautmann JC, Bartley GB, et al. Optic nerve sheath meningoceles. Clinical and radiographic features in 13 cases with a review of the literature. *Ophthalmology* 1990;97:1519–1531.
48. Turbin RE, Thompson CR, Kennerdell JS, et al. A long-term visual outcome comparison in patients with optic nerve sheath meningioma managed with observation, surgery, radiotherapy, or surgery and radiotherapy. *Ophthalmology* 2002;109:890–899; discussion 899–900.
49. Goldsmith BJ, Wara WM, Wilson CB, Larson DA. Postoperative irradiation for subtotally resected meningiomas. A retrospective analysis of 140 patients treated from 1967 to 1990. *J Neurosurg* 1994;80:195–201.
50. Goldsmith BJ, Wara WM, Wilson CB, et al. Postoperative irradiation of subtotally resected meningiomas. *J Neurosurg* 1994;80:195–201.
51. Lundsford LD. Contemporary management of meningioma: radiation therapy as an adjuvant and radiosurgery as an alternative to surgical removal? *J Neurosurg* 1994;80:187–190.
52. Lee AG, Woo SY, Miller NR, et al. Improvement in visual function in an eye with a presumed optic nerve sheath meningioma after treatment with three-dimensional conformal radiation therapy. *J Neuro-Ophthalmol* 1996;16:247–251.
53. Mafee MF, Goodwin J, Dorodi S. Optic nerve sheath meningiomas. Role of MR imaging. *Radiol Clin North Am* 1999;37:37–58.
54. Moyer PD, Golnik KC, Breneman J. Treatment of optic nerve sheath meningioma with three-dimensional conformal radiation. *Am J Ophthalmol* 2000;129:694–696.
55. Muci-Mendoza R, Arevalo JF, Ramella M, et al. Optociliary veins in optic nerve sheath meningioma. Indocyanine green videoangiography findings. *Ophthalmology* 1999;106:311–318.
56. Newman SJ. Meningiomas: a quest for the optimum therapy. *J Neurosurg* 1994;80:191–194.
57. Wroe SJ, Thompson AJ, McDonald WI. Painful intraorbital meningiomas. *J Neurol Neurosurg Psychiatry* 1991;54:1009–1010.
58. Zimmerman CF, Schatz NJ, Glaser JS. Magnetic resonance imaging of optic nerve meningiomas. Enhancement with gadolinium-DTPA. *Ophthalmology* 1990;97:585–591.
59. Camera A, Piccirillo G, Cennamo G, et al. Optic nerve involvement in acute lymphoblastic leukemia. *Leuk Lymphoma* 1993;11:153–155.
60. Park KL, Goins KM. Hodgkin's lymphoma of the orbit associated with acquired immunodeficiency syndrome. *Am J Ophthalmol* 1993;116:111–112.
61. Nakajima T, Kumabe T, Jokura H, Yoshimoto T. Recurrent germinoma in the optic nerve: report of two cases. *Neurosurgery* 2001;48:214–218.
62. Lee AG, Phillips PH, Newman NJ, et al. Neuro-ophthalmologic manifestations of adenoid cystic carcinoma. *J Neuro-Ophthalmol* 1997;17:183–188.
63. Kattah JC, Chrousos GC, Roberts J, et al. Metastatic prostate cancer to the optic canal. *Ophthalmology* 1993;100:1711–1715.
64. Newman, NJ, Grossniklaus, HE, Wojno TH. Breast carcinoma metastatic to the optic nerve. *Arch Ophthalmol* 1996;114:102–103.
65. Aarabi B, Haghshenas M, Rakeii V. Visual failure caused by suprasellar extramedullary hematopoiesis in beta thalassemia: case report. *Neurosurgery* 1998;42:922–925.
66. Schaffler GJ, Simbrunner J, Lechner H, et al. Idiopathic sclerotic inflammation of the orbit with left optic nerve compression in a patient with multifocal fibrosclerosis. *Am J Neuroradiol* 2000;21:194–197.
67. Belden CJ, Hamed LM, Mancuso AA. Bilateral isolated retrobulbar opticneuropathy in limited Wegener's granulomatosis. *J Clin Neuro-Ophthalmol* 1993;13:119–123.
68. Chen YR, Breidahl A, Chang CN. Optic nerve decompression in fibrous dysplasia: indications, efficacy, and safety. *Plast Reconstr Surg* 1997;99:22–30.
69. Botella C, Orozco, M, Navarro J, Riesgo P. Idiopathic chronic hypertrophic craniocervical pachymeningitis: case report. *Neurosurgery* 1994;35:1144–1149.
70. Chandra S, Vashisht S, Menon V, et al. Optic nerve cysticercosis: imaging findings. *AJNR Am J Neuroradiol* 2000;21:198–200.
71. Balch K, Phillips PH, Newman NJ. Painless orbital apex syndrome from mucormycosis. *J Neuro-Ophthalmol* 1997;17:178–182.
72. Johnson TE, Casiano RR, Kronish JW, et al. Sino-orbital aspergillosis in acquired immunodeficiency syndrome. *Arch Ophthalmol* 1999;117:57–64.
73. Gurha N, Sood A, Dhar J, Gupta S. Optic nerve cysticercosis in the optic canal. *Acta Ophthalmol Scand* 1999;77:107–109.
74. Hutnik CML, Nicolle DA, Munoz DG. Orbital aspergillosis. A fatal masquerader. *J Neuro-Ophthalmol* 1997;17:257–261.
75. Hao SP. Mucocele of the sphenoid sinus with acute bilateral blindness: report of two cases. *J Formosan Med Assoc* 1994;93:519–521.
76. Brown P, Demaerel P, McNaught A, et al. Neuro-ophthalmological presentation of non-invasive *Aspergillus* sinus disease in the non-immunocompromised host. *J Neurol Neurosurg Psychiatr* 1994;57:234–237.
77. Aylward GW, Sullivan TJ, Garner A, et al. Orbital involvement in multifocal fibrosclerosis. *Br J Ophthalmol* 1995;79:246–249.
78. Bland LI, Marchese MJ, McDonald JV. Acute monocular blindness secondary to fibrous dysplasia of the skull: a case report. *Ann Ophthalmol* 1992;24:263–266.

79. Weisman JS, Hepler RS, Vinters HV. Reversible visual loss caused by fibrous dysplasia. *Am J Ophthalmol* 1990;110:244–249.
80. Michael CB, Lee AG, Patrinely JR, et al. Visual loss associated with fibrous dysplasia of the anterior skull base. Case report and review of the literature. *J Neurosurg* 2000;92:350–354.
81. Katz BJ, Nerad JA. Ophthalmic manifestations of fibrous dysplasia. A disease of children and adults. *Ophthalmology* 1998; 105:2207–2215.
82. Joseph MP. Commentary on Papay FA, Morales L Jr, Flaharty P, et al. Optic nerve decompression in cranial base fibrous dysplasia. *J Craniofac Surg* 1995;6:11–13.
83. Edelstein C, Goldberg RA, Rubino G. Unilateral blindness after ipsilateral prophylactic transcranial optic canal decompression for fibrous dysplasia. *Am J Ophthalmol* 1998;126:469–471.
84. Amrith S, Baratham G, Khoo CY, et al. Spontaneous hematic cysts of the orbit presenting with acute proptosis. *Ophthalmic Plast Reconstr Surg* 1990;6:273–277.
85. Moorthy RS, Yung CW, Nunery WR, et al. Spontaneous orbital subperiosteal hematomas in patients with liver disease. *Ophthalmic Plast Reconstr Surg* 1992;8:150–152.
86. Kazim M, Kennerdell JS, Rothfus W, Marquardt M. Orbital lymphangioma. Correlation of magnetic resonance images and intraoperative findings. *Ophthalmology* 1992;99: 1588–1594.
87. Wright JE, Sullivan TJ, Garner A, Wulc AE, Moseley IF. Orbital venous anomalies. *Ophthalmology* 1997;104:905–913.
88. Dutton JJ, Tse DT, Anderson RL. Compressive optic neuropathy following use of intracranial oxidized cellulose hemostat. *Ophthalmic Surg* 1983;14:487–490.
89. Carter K, Lee AG, Tang RA, et al. Neuro-ophthalmologic complications of sinus surgery. *Neuro-Ophthalmology* 1998;19: 75–82.
90. Buus DR, Tse DT, Farris BK. Ophthalmic complications of sinus surgery. *Ophthalmology* 1990;97:612–619.

8

Ultrasonography in Orbital Differential Diagnosis

Amin M. Nasr and Grace Abou Chacra

Ultrasonography is a noninvasive imaging technique that is essential in the evaluation of orbital diseases. Ophthalmic ultrasonography employs high-frequency sound waves that provide the high resolution required for ocular diagnosis. A lower frequency of 8 MHz is used to obtain the penetration needed to reach the orbital apex.[1] The orbit is evaluated with A- and B-mode scanning (Figure 8.1). Lesions located in the posterior two thirds of the orbit are detected through a transocular examination; lesions in the anterior third of the orbit are detected through a paraocular examination.[2,3]

The acoustic inner texture of an orbital lesion can be correlated with its histologic features. The contents of a normal orbit and lacrimal fossa show high reflectivity and marked sound attenuation owing to the presence of large collagenous connective tissue septae, fat globules, blood vessels, and nerves.[4,5] Most orbital pathologies display less coarse and heterogeneous structures than the normal orbit, hence, usually have lower reflectivity. This is in contrast to intraocular pathology, which usually shows higher reflectivity than the normal standard baseline displayed by the clear vitreous body.

ASSESSMENT OF ORBITAL LESIONS

Primary Orbital Lesions

Cystic Lesions

Epithelial and Dermoid Cysts

The most common developmental cysts occurring in the orbital and periorbital region and having a predilection for the superotemporal quadrant, are the epithelial and dermoid cysts. Dermoid cysts contain one or more epidermal appendages such as hair follicles, sweat glands, and sebaceous glands; epithelial cysts contain only stratified squamous cell epithelium. Echographically, epithelial and dermoid cysts appear on B scans as smoothly rounded, echolucent lesions with good sound transmission (Figure 8.2A,B). However, some dermoid cysts show low internal amplitude echoes depending on the number of hair shafts and other appendages within the lesion, which invariably cause partial sound attenuation. On A scan, epithelial cysts are low reflective. Dermoid cysts are medium to low reflective with occasional high reflective spikes that indicate the presence of certain coarse structures such as fine hairs or cartilaginous remnants.[4,5]

Congenital Cystic Eye

Congenital cystic lesions contain protrusions through defects present in the walls of microphthalmic eyes. A congenital cystic eye results from failure in the invagination of the primary optic vesicle and lack of differentiation into its adult components. Echographically, the cystic portion shows typical roundish, echolucent B-scan characteristics with very low internal reflectivity on A scan. The microphthalmic globe, on the other hand, is highly dense on B scan with marked shadowing. A-scan echography shows a high reflective structure (typical of condensed tissue structures) with marked sound attenuation almost consistent with calcific structures.

Hematocele

A hematocele is a cystic lesion (Figure 8.2C,D) that results from spontaneous accumulation of blood. Invariably it occurs without preexisting orbital vascular disease.

Vascular Lesions

Infantile Hemangioma

A benign vascular tumor (Figure 8.3), infantile hemangioma usually appears during the first few months of life. The majority of these lesions enlarge in size within the first 2 years and in approximately 70% of the cases undergo spontaneous involution by the age of 7 years. The tumor is generally unilateral (although bilaterality has been reported),[6] and it occurs most commonly in the superior nasal quadrant in otherwise healthy children.

Cavernous Hemangioma

The most common primary benign orbital tumor of adults (Figure 8.4A–C), cavernous hemangioma usu-

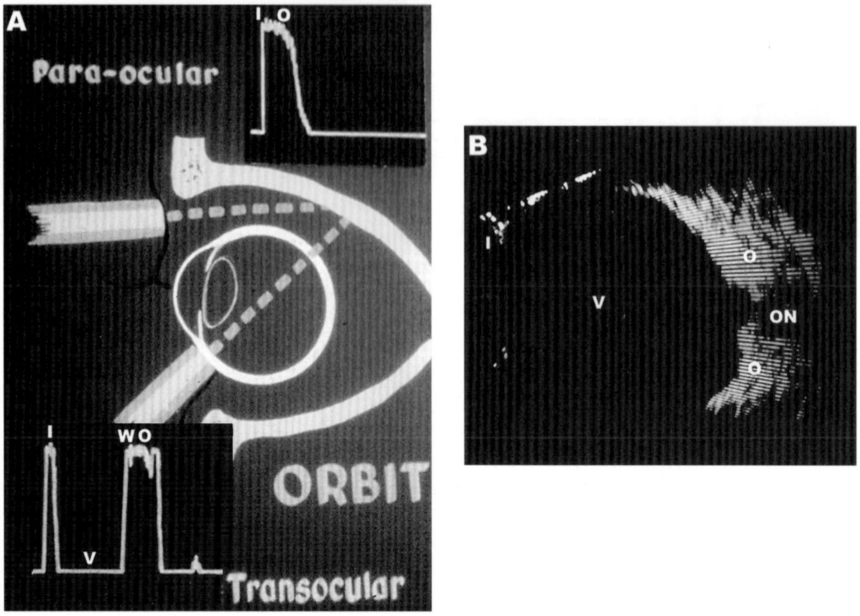

FIGURE 8.1. Transocular and paraocular display of normal orbit. A-scan transocular examination of a normal orbit (A, bottom) reveals the following echospikes from left to right: the initial spike (I), which has no clinical significance and represents echoes generated at the tip of the probe (dead zone of the ultrasound probe); the baseline, which is a horizontal line and represents the vitreous cavity (V); the ocular wall spikes (W), which are high reflective echospikes; and the orbital spikes (O), which are multiple high reflective echo spikes (~100%) with marked attenuation because of the coarse, dense structures within the orbit. (B) B-scan transocular examination of a normal orbit reveals the following areas from left to right: an echogenic area (initial line, I), which has no clinical significance and represents echoes at the tip of the probe (dead zone of the ultrasound probe); a clear or echolucent area representing the vitreous cavity (V); and an echogenic area that represents the posterior ocular wall and the orbital tissues (O) behind it. This normal retrobulbar echo pattern is derived from the orbital fat globules, which are triangular; the pattern is indented by a V-shaped, echolucent area that represents the optic nerve (ON). The display in paraocular examination (A, top) is similar to that of transocular examination, except for the presence of the cystic structure of the globe. However, the echographic criteria are comparable.

ally appears in the third to fifth decades of life. The tumor is characteristically unilateral and solitary, although multifocal lesions have been reported.[7,8] It is most commonly found within the muscle cone, resulting in slowly progressive proptosis of the globe. On gross examination, cavernous hemangiomas are well-encapsulated, round to ovoid masses with violet hue reflecting the stagnation of poorly oxygenated

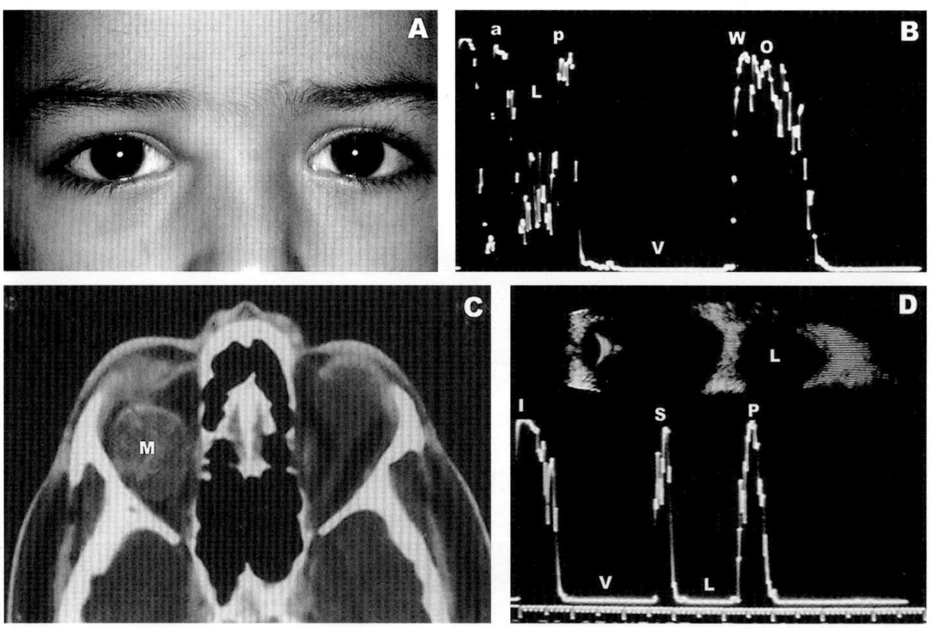

FIGURE 8.2. Cystic lesions (A,B) dermoid cyst and (C,D) hematocele. (A) Clinical photograph of a child with right anterior, medial orbital mass. (B) Transocular A scan shows an anterior low reflective lesion (L) shown within smooth high reflective echo spikes that delineate the anterior (a) and the posterior (p) wall of the cystic structure. V, vitreous cavity; W, ocular wall spike; O, orbital tissue spikes. (C) Axial CT scan shows well-delineated round mass (M) in the right orbit. (D) B scan (top) displays a round echolucent orbital lesion (L). A scan (bottom) shows low reflectivity of the lesion (L) with high posterior surface spike (P) from the cyst wall. Occasionally, there are moderately high reflective, dispersed spikes representing lines of clotted blood. I, initial spike; V, vitreous cavity; S, sclera or ocular wall; O, orbital tissue.

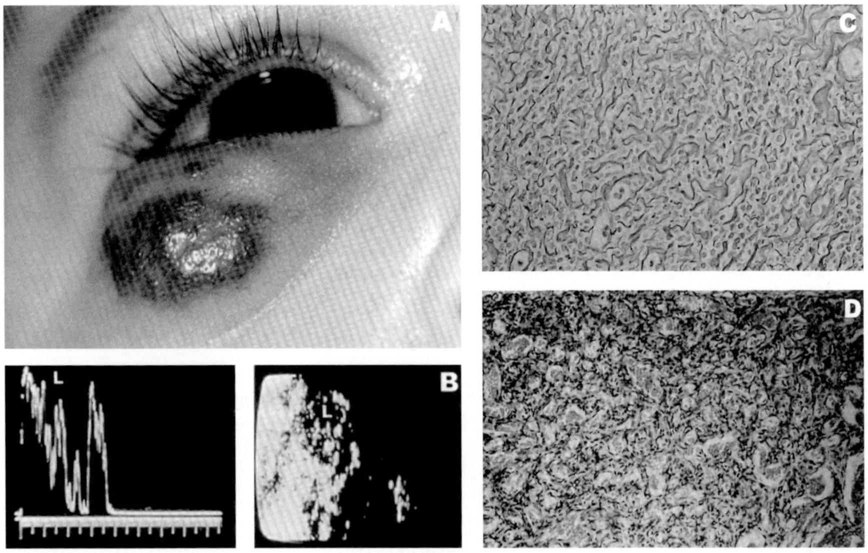

FIGURE 8.3. Infantile hemangioma. (A) Clinical photograph of a child with right lower lid hemangioma. (B) B-scan echogram (left) displays an irregular echogenic lesion (L) with variable degrees of sound attenuation. A-scan (right) shows areas of moderate to high reflectivity representative of the cavernous spaces. The capillary portions of the lesion are typically low reflective with intense, diffuse vascularity (dynamic echography). Color Doppler imaging provides an overview of the significant blood flow representative of an active arterial blood supply.[5] Histopathology shows (C) proliferation of endothelial cells with numerous small capillaries and (D) areas of cavernous spaces. The intermixing of capillaries and lobulated structures provides the heterogenic components of these lesions.

blood within the tumor. Microscopically, the tumor consists of large, dilated venous spaces lined by thin, flattened endothelial cells, along with pericytes and smooth muscle cells that are separated by irregular fibrous connective tissue septae.

LYMPHANGIOMA

Lymphangioma is a benign vascular tumor diagnosed in early childhood (Figure 8.4D–F). Unlike infantile hemangioma, lymphangioma enlarges progressively during the growing years. The lymphangioma is noncapsulated, often diffuse, with the capability of infiltrating normal tissues. The tumor occurs most commonly in the extraconal space. Spontaneous bleeding within the lesion is a frequent complication. Microscopically, lymphangiomas are formed by endothelium-lined, lymph-filled vascular channels separated by loose connective tissue septae that are high reflective. The latter contain fine blood vessels that are responsible for the spontaneous bleeding. Unlike cavernous hemangiomas, pericytes and smooth muscle cells are not present.

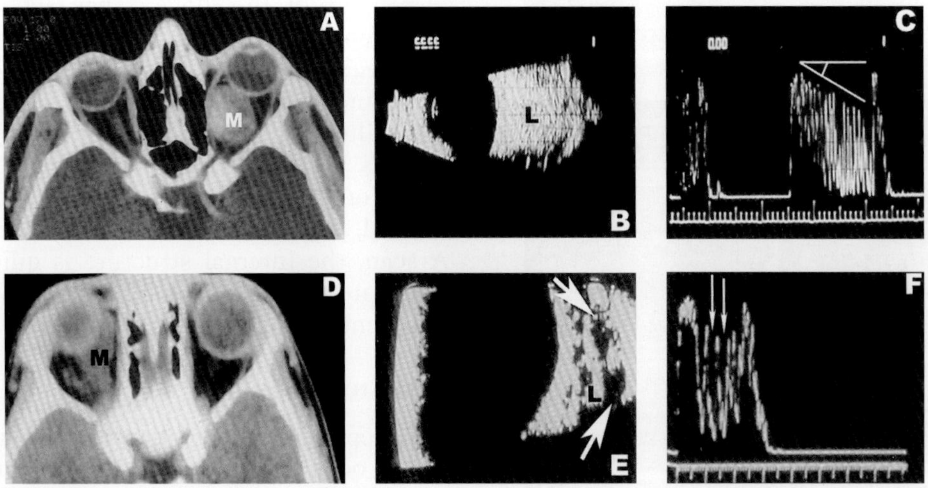

FIGURE 8.4. Vascular lesions: (A–C) cavernous hemangioma and (D–F) lymphangioma. (A) Axial CT scan shows well-delineated intraconal mass (M) in the left orbit. (B) B scan displays a well-defined round to ovoid echogenic lesion (L). (C) A-scan reveals multiple, regular, highly reflective echo spikes with the descending edges reaching a medium reflectivity indicating the presence of blood within the venous spaces and the abundant connective tissue septae.[9] Sound attenuation is moderate (angle $\kappa = 45°$). Color Doppler imaging shows little or no evidence of blood flow attributable to the stagnant blood within the vascular spaces.[10] (D) Axial CT scan shows an irregular mass (M) in the right orbit. (E) B scan displays an irregular, large lesion (L) with multiple, dilated lymph-filled spaces (arrows).[2,11] (F) A scan reveals a regular, heterogeneous pattern with highly reflective echo spikes separated by low reflective, dilated lymphatic spaces. In contrast to cavernous hemangiomas, the presence of clear fluid instead of blood in the wider intracavernous spaces of lymphangiomas provides ample time for the ultrasound beam to reach lower reflective levels (arrows).[5] Sound attenuation is moderately low (angle κ <30°).

Hemangiopericytoma

Hemangiopericytoma is a vascular tumor originating from the pericytes of blood vessels; consequently, it may develop wherever capillaries are present (Figure 8.5).[12] Orbital hemangiopericytomas are rare, slow-growing, unilateral tumors with a predilection to the superior orbit. They occur at any age, although the majority appear in adulthood. Microscopically, the tumor consists of spindle-shaped cells packed around thin-walled blood vessels that are lined by endothelial cells. The tumor is classified as sinusoidal, solid, or mixed depending on the degree of vascularity between the tumor cells.[13] Cystic changes within the tumor may develop secondary to zones of necrosis.

Orbital Varices

Primary orbital varices (Figure 8.6A,B) are congenital venous malformations that usually become symptomatic in the second to fourth decade of life. The patient presents with a history of intermittent, positional proptosis. Microscopically, an orbital varix represents an enlarged, dilated vein. The lesion is characterized by a stagnant blood flow that may result in thrombus formation.

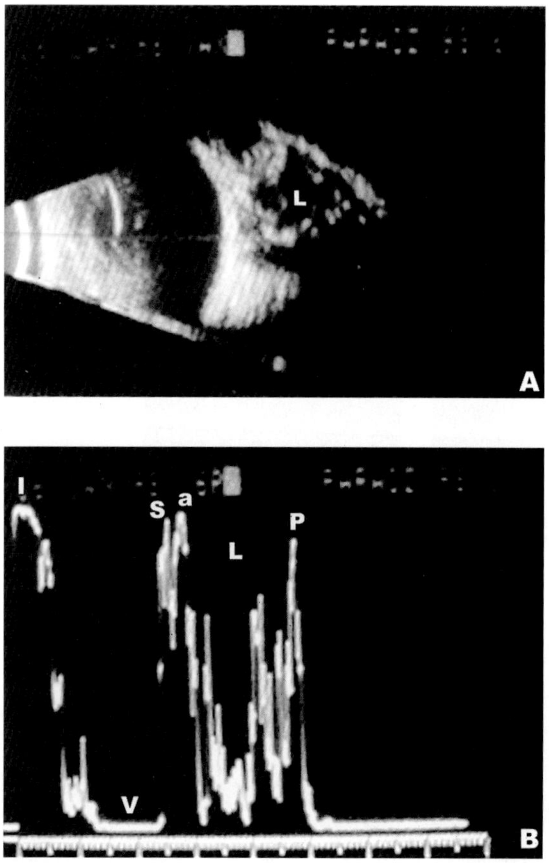

FIGURE 8.5. Hemangiopericytoma. (A) B-scan echogram displays a well-defined round to oval lesion (L).[13,14] The internal structure of the tumor can be irregular, showing solid and cystic components depending on its histopathology. (B) On A scan, the internal reflectivity of the tumor ranges from low (as illustrated) to medium with the latter representing tumor of a mixed nature.[14] I, initial spike; V, vitreous cavity; a, anterior and P, posterior surface spikes of the lesion (L); S, sclera. Color Doppler imaging reveals high-velocity blood flow.

Fast-Draining Carotid Cavernous Fistula

In fast-draining carotid cavernous fistula, there is a direct communication between the internal carotid artery and the cavernous sinus. This results in dilation of the superior ophthalmic vein (Figure 8.6C,D) with arterialization of blood flow. The patient usually has a history of head trauma and presents with pulsating exophthalmos, a bruit over the globe, dilated and tortuous episcleral vessels, and restriction of motility.

Peripheral Nerve Lesions

Neurofibroma

A benign peripheral nerve tumor, neurofibroma is characterized histopathologically by the proliferation of Schwann cells, peripheral nerve axons, endoneural fibroblasts, and perineural cells. Echographically, neurofibromas are diffuse, irregular lesions with dense internal vascularity that closely resemble infantile hemangiomas. However, the clinical appearance is quite different and is more periorbital with less bluish discoloration.

Schwannoma (Neurilemoma)

Schwannoma is a benign peripheral nerve tumor characterized by pure proliferation of Schwann cells. It usually becomes apparent in young to middle-aged adults and is found in 1.5% of patients with neurofibromatosis type 1. The patient generally presents with painless progressive proptosis with downward displacement of the globe, since schwannomas arise more commonly from the supraorbital and supratrochlear nerves. Histologically, schwannomas show a mixture of two patterns.[19] The Antoni type A (dense and cellular pattern) and the Antoni type B (loose, edematous pattern forming cystic spaces). Echographically, on B scan, schwannoma appears as a well-defined, roundish, internally echolucent lesion.[20] On A scan, the internal structure is quite regular with moderate to low internal reflectivity with the latter representing the Antoni type B areas.

Pseudotumor

An idiopathic orbital inflammatory disorder, pseudotumor occurs mostly in the third to fifth decades of life. The inflammation can be diffuse or localized resulting in periscleritis, sclerotenonitis, tendonitis, myositis, dacryoadenitis, or perioptic neuritis. The patient presents with a sudden onset of unilateral eye pain, redness, chemosis, proptosis, and diplopia.[21] Some cases may present with severe chronic inflammation that eventually leads to progressive fibrosis of orbital tissues and results in a frozen globe. Micro-

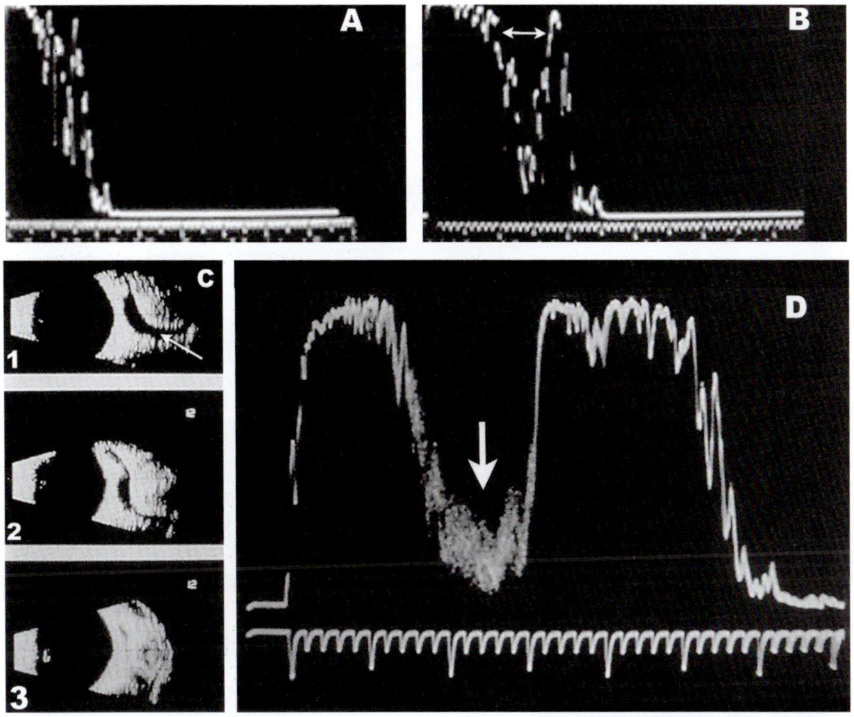

FIGURE 8.6. Vascular lesions: (A,B) orbital varices and (C,D) fast-draining carotid cavernous fistula. (A). Paraocular A scan shows low internal reflectivity with expansion of the lesion during Valsalva maneuver[15] (arrow). (B) On B scan, orbital varices are linear, channeled lesions with echolucent internal structure.[5] Sound attenuation is minimal. Color Doppler imaging shows nonpulsatile blood flow with apparent change in dimensions during respiration.[16] (C) B scan shows a large, dilated superior ophthalmic vein (B1, *arrow*) which is typically meandering on sagittal topography.[5,17] With dynamic echography, the size of the venous structure changes with the arterial pulsations from a near collapsed size (B3) to a widely dilated channel (B1). (D) A scan shows blurred, low reflective spikes from fast flowing blood (*arrow*). Sound attenuation is minimal, and color doppler imaging shows a pulsatile, arterial-type blood flow pattern in the superior ophthalmic vein.[18]

scopically, there is infiltration of the involved orbital tissues by inflammatory cells consisting of lymphocytes, plasma cells, and eosinophils. Echographic findings of pseudotumor depend on the involved tissue.

Scleritis

In scleritis the B scan shows an echolucent area between the anterior and the posterior scleral wall. In most cases it is associated with a linear echolucent area in the retroscleral space representing edema in Tenon's space (T-sign). On A scan, the high scleral spikes are wider than normal and invariably show abnormal thickening. In episcleritis, the similar A- and B-scan characteristics can be seen but in the immediate retroscleral space with a distinct echolucent rim between the sclera and the rest of the orbital tissues; a low reflective A-scan pattern indicates the edematous space that usually exists in this condition.

Myositis

In myositis there is usually a diffuse thickening of the involved muscle including the inserting tendon to the globe with echolucency on B scan and low reflectivity on A scan (Figure 8.7). Comparative assessment with other muscles, especially the counterpart of the other orbit, is quite revealing for the condition.

Orbital Pseudotumor

An orbital pseudotumor is invariably a diffuse condition with significant low reflectivity from the internal structure of the involved area. Lacrimal gland involvement is invariably unilateral and follows the same characteristic pattern but is localized to the area of the lacrimal gland. (Other lacrimal gland conditions are discussed under lacrimal gland lesions.)

Rhabdomyosarcoma

The most common primary malignant orbital tumor in children is rhabdomyosarcoma. It arises from undifferentiated mesenchymal cells that have the ability to differentiate into striated muscle cells. The patient presents with rapid, progressive proptosis. The tumor can involve any part of the orbit with a predilection to the superior portion. The echographic findings of rhabdomyosarcoma (Figure 8.8A,B) are quite similar to those of orbital inflammatory disease (pseudotumor).[22] However, the age group, the clinical presentation, and the ultrasonography and CT findings are usually diagnostic of this condition.

Secondary Orbital Lesions

Lymphoproliferative Disease

Lymphoid tumors of the orbit occupy a wide spectrum of diseases ranging from the benign pseudolymphomas (pseudotumors) to the atypical lymphoid hyperplasias to the malignant lymphomas. Echographically (Figure 8.8C,E), lymphoid tumors share the same characteristics. The patient's age is important in the interpretation of the ultrasound findings especially with pseudotumor, rhabdomyosarcoma, and lymphoma, for which

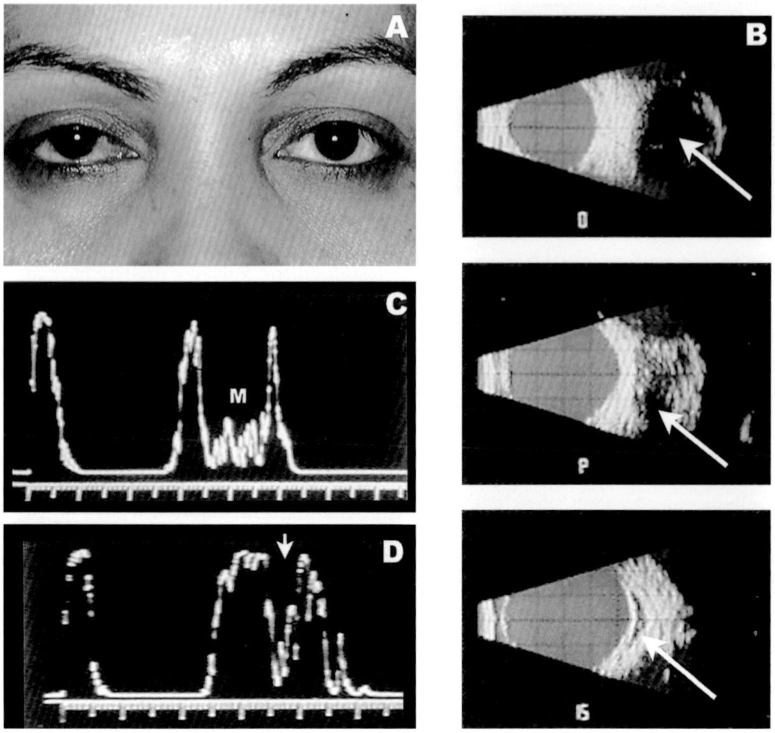

FIGURE 8.7. Myositis. (A) Clinical photograph of a young woman shows right eye injection. (B) B-scan echogram shows enlarged right medial rectus muscle (upper and middle) with thickened insertion (lower) (*arrows*). A-scan echograms show (C) low reflectivity of the enlarged muscle belly (M) and (D) low reflective thickened insertion (*arrow*).

these findings are similar. Also, unilateral low reflective infiltrates in an adult is suggestive of pseudotumor while bilaterality supports a diagnosis of lymphoma.

Metastatic Tumors

The orbit, devoid of lymphatic channels, is reached by metastatic tumors via the hematogenous route. The most common source of metastatic tumor to the orbit in adults is the breast followed by lung, prostate, skin melanoma, and gastrointestinal tract in decreasing order of frequency. In children, neuroblastoma is the most common source of metastatic tumor to the orbit occurring in about 40% of cases. The disease may be bilateral and presents with a sudden onset of proptosis accompanied by lid ecchymosis (Figure 8.9).

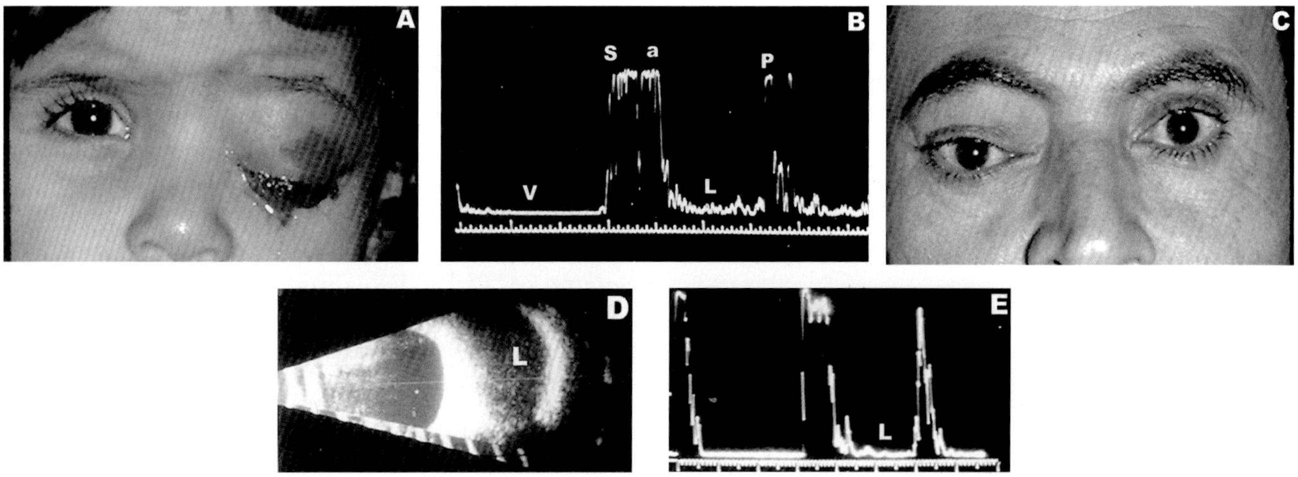

FIGURE 8.8. (A,B) Rhabdomyoarcoma. (C–E) Lymphoproliferative disease. (A) Clinical photograph of a child shows left eye proptosis. (B) A-scan echogram shows diffuse, low-reflective lesion (L). Occasionally, there is active vascularity displayed on dynamic echography. On B-scan the lesion is echolucent with minimal sound attenuation. V, vitreous cavity; S, sclera; a, anterior and P, posterior surface spikes of the lesion. (C) Clinical photograph of an adult man shows right eye proptosis and downward displacement of the globe. (D) B-scan echogram shows large, diffuse echolucent orbital lesion (L), which had low internal reflectivity on A scan (E).

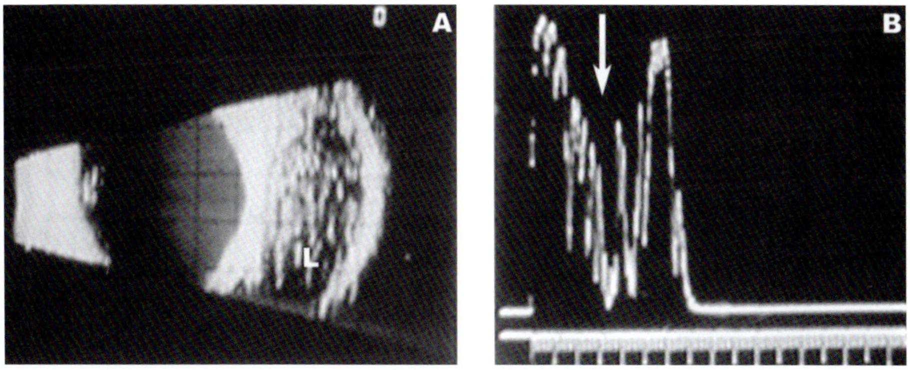

FIGURE 8.9. Metastatic carcinoma. (A) B-scan echogram displays a poorly defined diffuse lesion (L) with varying echogenicity. (B) On A scan, the internal structure is quite irregular with the internal reflectivity ranging from low[23] to moderately high. The characteristic "V" pattern (*arrow*) results from a central zone of dense cellular infiltrates that become more lobulated toward the periphery (hence, the higher ascending limbs of the lesions).[5,22]

Mucocele

Mucocele is a cystic lesion filled with mucoid secretions and epithelial debris that arises from the paranasal sinuses. Orbital invasion occurs more commonly from either frontal or ethmoidal mucoceles. Mucoceles usually develop in adults and produce progressive proptosis, diplopia, or ptosis. Echographically, mucoceles present a distinct characteristic pattern almost pathognomonic of the condition (Figure 8.10).

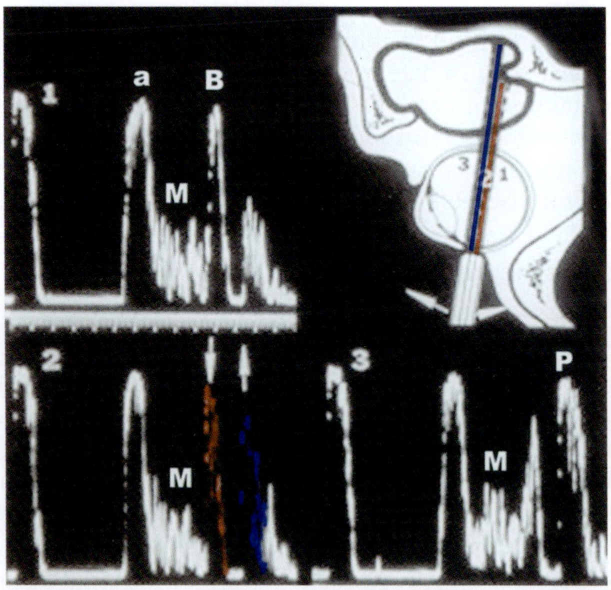

FIGURE 8.10. Mucocele. (1) A-scan echogram shows a highly reflective anterior surface (anterior wall of the lesion, a) followed by an echolucent low-reflective internal structure representing the mucocele, M; B, orbital bone.[24] Sound beam directed through intraorbital portion of the mucocele. (2) The beam is moved slightly and hits the edge of bone defect (red) and posterior wall of the sinus (blue). When scanning the lesion from the intraorbital to the intrasinus site, the posterior wall of the mucocele shifts from the intraorbital normal area into a deep intrasinus part (shifting posterior high reflective sinusoidal pattern). (3) Sound beam is directed entirely through bone defect. P, posterior bony wall of sinus.

Assessment of Thickening of Extraocular Muscles

Thyroid Eye Disease

The most common cause of extraocular muscle thickening, thyroid eye disease, usually entails multiple, bilateral, and asymmetrical muscle involvement (see Chapter 28). Clinically, the inferior rectus muscle is most often involved, followed by the medial, the superior, and the lateral rectus muscles. However, echographically, the superior rectus/levator complex is most commonly enlarged followed by the medial, the inferior, and lateral rectus muscles.[22] Microscopically, there is perivascular infiltration by lymphocytes and plasma cells with increased deposition of hydrophilic mucopolysaccharides in the muscle belly, sparing the tendon. Topographically, there is enlargement of the belly of the involved extraocular muscle with the acquisition of internal tissue echoes reflecting the histological changes.[9,25] On A scan, the internal structure is slightly irregular with medium internal reflectivity (Figure 8.11).

Orbital Inflammatory Disease (Pseudotumor) and Lymphoma

Refer to the preceding section on pseudotumor and lymphoproliferative disease.

Metastatic Tumors

Metastatic lesions to the extraocular muscles are usually unilateral with invariably a single muscle involvement (see Chapter 24).[26] There is a slow, progressive, painless increase in the size of the muscle with late onset diplopia (in contrast to the rapid, painful, acute myositis with early diplopia). Ultrasonography shows echolucency in the belly of the muscle with low internal reflectivity similar in pattern to

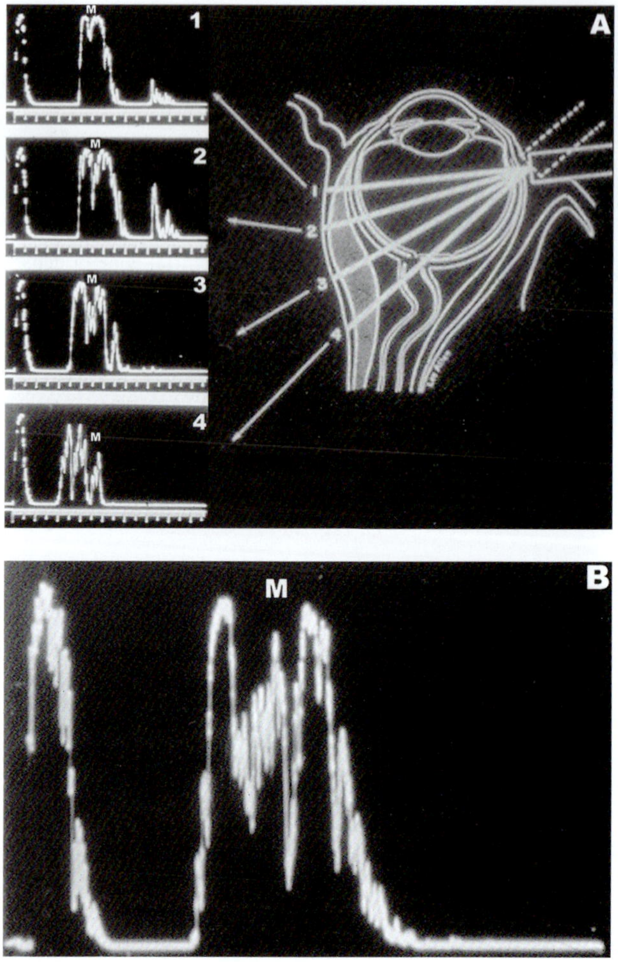

FIGURE 8.11. (A) Dynamic A-scan examination of normal rectus muscle (M). 1, Probe is directed anteriorly toward the muscle insertion, which produces a small defect adjacent to the scleral spike. As the probe is angled more posteriorly (2–4), the sound beam shifts toward the muscle belly, which produces a wider defect that moves from left to right. (B) A-scan echogram of an enlarged rectus muscle (M) in thyroid eye disease showing slightly irregular internal structure with medium reflectivity.

the orbital inflammatory pseudotumor category but, in contrast, the tendon of the muscle is not involved.

Slow-Draining Carotid Cavernous Fistula

In slow-draining carotid cavernous fistula, there is an indirect communication between the cavernous sinus and the internal or external carotid arteries through their meningeal branches. The patient presents with prominent episcleral vessels, but minimal proptosis. The small fistula results in low-flow, low-pressure shunting that causes increase in episcleral venous pressure and enlargement of extraocular muscles on the involved side. Ultrasonography reveals diffuse enlargement of the muscles in the involved orbit when compared to the counterpart muscles of the normal orbit. The belly of the muscles shows a slight increase in width with a tendency of the internal reflectivity to shift from a medium to a lower pattern owing to the vascular congestion present in such a condition. Occasionally, the superior ophthalmic vein (which is usually difficult to isolate and measure in the normal orbit) shows widening and more echographic prominence than the other orbit. This finding is far less significant than the enlarged hyperdynamic superior ophthalmic vein detected in the active carotid cavernous fistula condition.

OPTIC NERVE ASSESSMENT

Thyroid Eye Disease

Optic neuropathy (Figure 8.12A, B, and C) occurs in about 5% of thyroid-associated orbitopathy patients. It is caused by direct compression of the optic nerve or its blood supply at the orbital apex by the enlarged extraocular muscles. Topographically, the optic nerve shadowing is enlarged with duplication of the nerve sheaths.[27–29]

Optic Neuritis

Optic neuritis is an inflammatory or demyelinating disorder of the optic nerve. Clinically, it is divided into retrobulbar neuritis, papillitis, and neuroretinitis. On ultrasonographic examination the perineural sheath thickening shows a low reflective internal structure (in contrast to the high reflectivity of a tumorous condition such as meningioma). However, there is no shifting of fluid visible on dynamic echography such as that seen in cerebrospinal fluid retention (thyroid, pseudotumor cerebri). Also, the thickening of the intersheath space, although significant in comparison to the normal state, is far less than that found in other orbital disorders.

Optic Nerve Lesions

Optic Nerve Glioma (Juvenile Pilocystic Astrocytoma)

A benign, slow-growing tumor (Figure 8.12D), optic nerve glioma arises from astrocytes within the optic nerve. The median age of onset is about 5 years of age, with a slight preponderance for females. Neurofibromatosis type 1 occurs in about 10% of cases and is characterized by bilateral involvement of the optic nerve. The patient presents with progressive proptosis and visual loss.

Optic Nerve Sheath Meningioma

Optic nerve sheath meningioma is a benign tumor (Figure 8.12E) that arises from the meningoendothelial cells of the arachnoid layer. The tumor usually affects middle-aged women. Neurofibromatosis type 1 is found in about 16% of cases. Presentation is with slowly progressive proptosis and unilateral visual loss. Ultrasonography shows a dif-

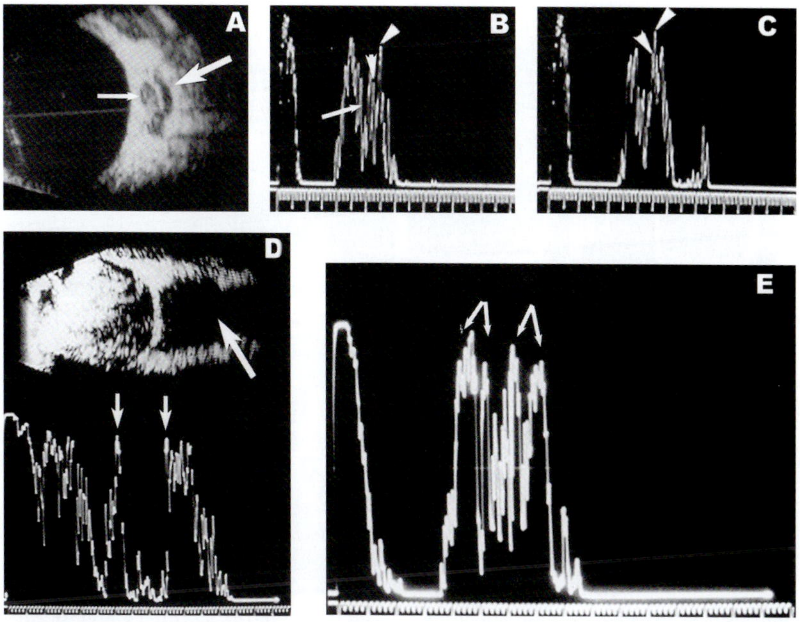

FIGURE 8.12. Optic nerve disorders (A–C) thyroid optic neuropathy, (D) optic nerve glioma, and (E) optic nerve meningioma. (A) B-scan echogram shows crescent sign (*large arrow*) due to accumulation of subarachnoid fluid around the optic nerve (*small arrow*). (B) A-scan echogram reveals double-peaked borders representing a perineural enlargement (*between arrowheads*) between the optic nerve parenchyma (*arrow*) and the perineural sheaths. Upon lateral gaze, retrograde "milking" of cerebrospinal fluid in this perineural enlargement occurs, with secondary collapse of the subarachnoid space shown on dynamic A-scan echography as almost visual adherence of the two spikes (*between arrowheads*). (C) The change of thickening of the intersheath space indicates a fluid retention condition rather than tumefaction of the perineural sheaths. (D) Optic nerve glioma. Echographically, there is widening of the internal lumen of the nerve (nerve proper) showing fusiform topographic pattern (*arrow*) (upper). The perineural sheath normal double spikes on A-scan are invariably touching (*arrows*), giving the appearance of a thick, single spike with a double head (lower). (E) Optic nerve meningioma. On A scan, the optic nerve proper appears thinner than normal (owing to meningeal compression), while the intersheath space is significantly wider (*connected arrows*) with a high-reflective internal structure between the inner and the outer perineural sheaths. Measurement of the intersheath space is possible and indicative of the pathologic thickening.

fuse thickening of the optic nerve following its meandering structure.

Pseudotumor Cerebri

Benign intracranial hypertension or pseudotumor cerebri is characterized by raised intracranial pressure in the absence of an intracranial mass lesion or meningeal cancer. It occurs more commonly in young, overweight women. The patient presents with headache, neck stiffness, nausea, vomiting, and blurring of vision. Examination reveals bilateral papilledema. Topographically, there is duplication of the optic nerve sheaths with significant widening of the double-peaked borders on A scan, reflecting the expansion of the perioptic subarachnoid space.

LACRIMAL GLAND LESIONS

Pleomorphic Adenoma (Benign Mixed Tumor)

Pleomorphic adenoma is a benign tumor that accounts for 50% of epithelial tumors of the lacrimal glands.[30] Pleomorphic adenomas usually arise from the orbital lobe and grow posteriorly, but in rare cases they may affect the palpebral lobe.[31] Presentation is typically in adults as a slowly progressive, nontender, firm mass in the superotemporal quadrant and proptosis. On gross examination, the tumor is encapsulated with nodular irregularities on the surface. Histopathology shows the tumor to be composed of both epithelial and mesenchymal elements.[32] The epithelial elements form ducts, acini, and irregular tubules that are dispersed throughout a matrix of mucoid, myxoid, and chondroid tissue. Topographically (Figure 8.13A), pleomorphic adenoma appears as a well-defined round to ovoid echogenic lesion in the lacrimal gland fossa.

Lymphoid Tumors of the Lacrimal Gland

Lymphoid tumors of the lacrimal gland range from pseudotumors to reactive lymphoid hyperplasia to malignant lymphomas of various types. They tend to involve the orbital and palpebral lobes of the lacrimal gland, resulting in anterior and posterior extension. Lymphoid tumors share similar acoustic characteristics.[35] Topographically, there is diffuse enlargement of the lacrimal gland with quite regular internal structure and low reflectivity on A scan. Sound attenuation is minimal.

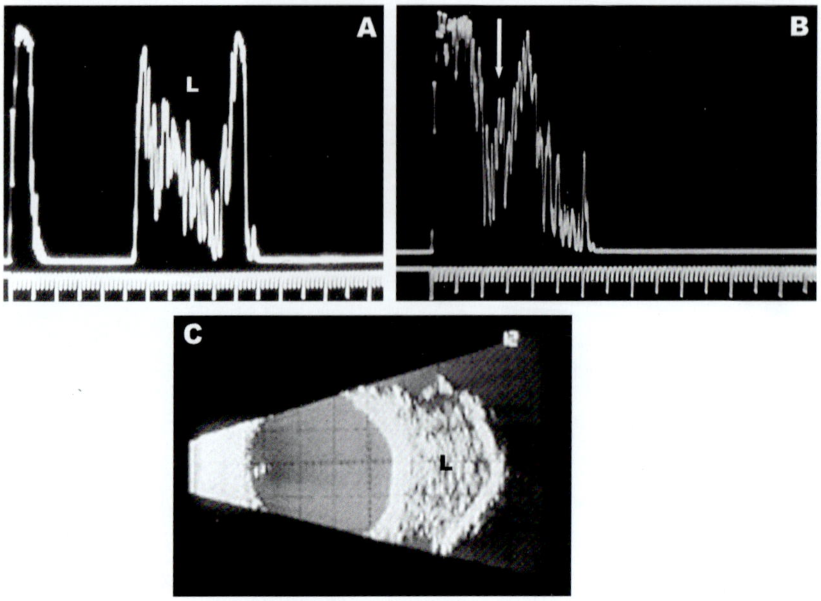

FIGURE 8.13. Lacrimal gland lesions. (A) Pleomorphic adenoma. A-scan echogram displays a regular internal structure with high reflectivity that relates histologically to the multiple contiguous tubular structures embedded in the dense connective tissue.[33] L, lesion. Sound attenuation is moderate (angle $\kappa = 45°$). These acoustic characteristics of pleomorphic adenomas are similar to those seen in cavernous hemangiomas. Since most cavernous hemangiomas occur within the muscle cone, the location and the clinical presentation of the tumor clearly are important diagnostic clues.[5,34] (B) Carcinoma of the lacrimal gland. In the early development of these tumors, the echographic finding shows a V-shaped pattern on A scan, where the anterior and posterior parts of the lacrimal gland retain the normal high-reflective character while the central portion representing the carcinoma site is less reflective because of the condensed cellularity; hence the V-shaped pattern (*arrow*). With an increase in the size of the tumor, the central portion of the V area becomes less reflective. (C) Dacryoadenitis. B-scan echogram shows an enlarged lacrimal gland (L) with moderate echolucency.

Carcinoma of the Lacrimal Gland (Adenocarcinoma and Adenoid Cystic Carcinoma)

Primary carcinomas (Figure 8.13B) account for about 50% of epithelial tumors of the lacrimal gland; adenoid cystic carcinoma is the most common primary malignant tumor. These tumors usually occur in middle-aged adults. The patient presents with unilateral progressive proptosis, pain, tenderness, ptosis, and diplopia. On gross examination, carcinomas of the lacrimal gland are poorly encapsulated, irregular, solid masses. Histopathologically, they are divided into adenoid cystic carcinoma, pleomorphic adenocarcinoma, and mucoepidermoid carcinoma.

Dacryoadenitis

Acute dacryoadenitis is a rare condition, seen most often in children as a complication of mumps, measles, or influenza. The patient presents with pain, swelling, and injection over the temporal aspect of the upper eyelid, resulting in S-shaped deformity. Topographically (Figure 8.13C), there is enlargement of the lacrimal gland with moderate echolucency. The A-scan exam is quite similar to that of the normal gland, retaining the high reflectivity with widening of the high septated internal pattern. In contrast to the chronic lacrimal gland inflammatory disease (lymphoproliferative disorders), the internal reflectivity of these conditions is low, as discussed earlier.

Acknowledgment The authors greatly appreciate the professional assistance provided by Mr. Hcitham A. Abdul-Baki, who is a third-year medical student at the American University of Beirut, in the preparation of the photographs for this chapter.

References

1. Coleman DJ. Reliability of ocular and orbital diagnosis with B-scan ultrasound. *Am J Ophthalmol* 1972;74:704–718.
2. Shammas HJ. Ultrasonography of the orbit. In: Smith B, et al, eds. *Ophthalmic Plastic and Reconstructive Surgery*. St Louis: CV Mosby, 1987:1025–1039.
3. Byrne SF. Standardized echography. I. A-scan examination procedures. *Int Ophthalmol Clin* 1979;19:267.
4. Dallow RL. Ultrasonography of the orbit. *Int Ophthalmol Clin* 1986;26:51–76.
5. Levine RA. Orbital ultrasonography. *Radiol Clin North Am* 1987;25:447–469.
6. Wheeler DT, Nasr AM. Aggressive orbital infantile hemangioma. Simulation of malignancy. *Orbit* 1996;15:237–247.
7. Johnson T, Nasr AM, Nalbandian R. Enschondromatosis and hemangioma (Mafucci syndrome) with orbital involvement. *Am J Ophthalmol* 1990;110:153–159.
8. Harris GJ, Jakobiec FA. Cavernous hemangioma of the orbit: a clinicopathologic analysis of sixty-six cases. In: Jakobiec FA, ed. *Ocular and Adnexal Tumors*. Birmingham, AL: Aesculapius Publishing; 1978.

9. Ossoinig KC. Standardized echography: Basic principles, clinical applications and results. *Int Ophthalmol Clin* 1979;19:127.
10. Aburn NS, Sergott RC. Orbital colour Doppler imaging. *Eye* 1993;7:639–647.
11. Coleman DJ, Jack RL, Franzen LA. B-scan ultrasonography of orbital lymphangiomas. *Br J Ophthalmol* 1973;57:193.
12. Bose B. Hemangiopericytoma: a clinicopathologic and ultrastructural study. *World J Surg* 1981;5:863–871.
13. Croxatto JO, Font RL. Hemangiopericytoma of the orbit: a clinicopathologic study of 30 cases. *Hum Pathol* 1982;13:210–218.
14. Karcioglu ZA, Nasr AM, Haik BG. Orbital hemangiopericytoma: clinical and morphologic features. *Am J Ophthalmol* 1997;124:661–672.
15. Nasr AM, Huaman AM. Anterior orbital varix presenting as a lacrimal sac mucocele. *Ophthalmic Plast Reconstr Surg* 1998; 14:193–197.
16. Lieb W, Merton D, Shields J, et al. Colour Doppler imaging in the demonstration of an orbital varix. *Br J Ophthalmol* 1990; 74:305–308.
17. Valencak E, Ossoinig K. Arterio-venous fistulas of the orbit in A and B-mode echograms. *Neurochirurgie* 1968;4:549.
18. Flaharty PM, Lieb WE, Sergott RC, et al. Colour Doppler imaging: a new noninvasive technique to diagnose and monitor carotid cavernous fistulas. *Arch Ophthalmol* 1991;109:522–526.
19. Jackobiec FA, Font RL, Iwamoto T. Diagnostic ultrastructural pathology of ophthalmic tumors. In: Jakobiec FA, ed. *Ocular and Adnexal Tumors.* Birmingham, AL: Aesculapius Publishing; 1978.
20. Byrne BN, Van Heuven WAJ, Lawton AW. Echographic characteristics of benign orbital schwannomas (neurilemomas). *Am J Ophthalmol* 1988;106:194–198.
21. Chavis RM, Garner A, Wright JE. Inflammatory orbital pseudotumor. *Arch Ophthalmol* 1978;96:1817–1822.
22. Byrne SF, Green RL. *Ultrasound of the Eye and Orbit.* St Louis: CV Mosby; 1992.
23. Nasr AM, Teichmann K, Dabbagh N, et al. Metastatic pancreatic islet cell carcinoma to the orbit: a case report. *Orbit* 1998;17:55–62.
24. Coleman DJ, Jack RL, Franzen LA. B-scan ultrasonography of orbital mucoceles. *Eye Ear Nose Throat Mon* 1972;51:207.
25. Hodes BL, Stern G. Contact B-scan echographic diagnosis of ophthalmic Grave's disease. *J Clin Ultrasound* 1975;3:255.
26. Slamovits TL, Burde RM. Bumpy muscles. *Surv Ophthalmol* 1988;33:189.
27. Abramson DH, Coleman DJ, Franzen LA. Ultrasonography of optic nerve lesions. *Bibl Ophthalmol* 1975;83:231.
28. Shalka HW. Perineural optic nerve changes in endocrine orbitopathy. *Arch Ophthalmol* 1978;96:468.
29. Shammas HJ, Minckler DS, Ogden C. Ultrasound in early thyroid orbitopathy. *Arch Ophthalmol* 1980;98:277.
30. Sanders TE, Ackerman LV, Zimmerman LE. Epithelial tumors of the lacrimal gland. A comparison of the pathologic and clinical behavior with those of the salivary glands. *Am J Surg* 1962;104:657–665.
31. Auran J, Jakobiec FA, Krebs W. Benign mixed tumor of the palpebral lobe of the lacrimal gland—clinical diagnosis and appropriate surgical management. *Ophthalmology* 1988;95:90.
32. Jakobiec FA, Font RL. Orbit. In: Spencer WH, Font RL, Green WR, et al, eds. *Ophthalmic Pathology. An Atlas and Textbook.* Philadelphia: WB Saunders; 1986.
33. Byrne SF. Standardized echography in the differentiation of orbital lesions. *Surv Ophthalmol* 1984;29:226.
34. Ossoinig KC, Keeman TP, Bigar F. Cavernous hemangioma of the orbit: a differential diagnosis in clinical echography. *Bibl Ophthalmol* 1975;83:236–244.
35. Ossoinig KC. Quantitative echography: the basis of tissue differentiation. *J Clin Ultrasound* 1974;2:33–46.

9

The Basics of Orbital Imaging

Paul Rosel

Computed tomography (CT) and magnetic resonance imaging (MRI) are performed for the detection and definition of orbital space-occupying lesions. Both studies are highly sensitive for lesion detection and are frequently complementary in generating a differential diagnosis. Imaging guidelines are well established via protocols dedicated to orbital imaging.[1] This chapter reviews quality imaging, highlighting goals and limitations of both modalities. Basic anatomy of the orbit related to imaging is also reviewed.

COMPUTED TOMOGRAPHY

The basis of CT is the measurement of different tissue absorption values, following exposure to x-rays. The tissue absorption values are defined arbitrarily by Hounsfield units (HU). Water is assigned an HU of zero. HU values ranging from −1000 (air) to +1000 (bone) are obtained in the region of orbit and periorbital tissues. What is important in routine CT examinations is the relative absorption value of a given tissue to neighboring structures. This relativity in tissue density is usually described with the terms "isodense," "hypodense," and "hyperdense." Normal brain tissue, which usually appears gray, is said to be isodense; hypodensity is seen in tissues with high water content, as in edema, and appears dark gray to black; hyperdensity represents tissues with high absorption of x-rays, such as cartilage and bone, and appears white (Table 9.1).

Computed tomography was the first modality that allowed high quality imaging of orbital contents.[2] There has been continuous improvement of CT since its introduction. Today's CT studies have evolved to a spiral (helical) technique with multiple detectors or a rotating detector system.[3,4] This technique allows one to scan in only a single plane, usually axial. Thin slice, high-resolution images can then be reformatted or reconstructed in any plane allowing very revealing views of essential orbital structures. The patient receives approximately 35 mGy of radiation for single slice spiral CT.[5] On the other hand, for conventional CT done under the biplane (axial and coronal) protocol, the patient receives approximately 75 mGy. The new, multidetector spiral CT is capable of obtaining multiple, very thin sectioned scans within minutes and can reformat the data in any plane required.[3] For routine orbital scanning purposes, sliced thicknesses of 2 to 3 mm are used, and standard imaging protocols are followed for axial and coronal views.[2] In axial scanning, the slices are acquired parallel to the infraorbitomeatal line; the coronal images are obtained perpendicular to the axis of the orbit (i.e., the axial cut). The window selected for orbital studies should be appropriate for orbital tissue absorption properties, with a width of 350 to 400 HU and a level of 80 to 100 HU. For better examination of the bone, a window wider than 1000 HU is necessary; this is called a *bone window*. The apex of the orbit is very crowded and therefore difficult to define. For this area, 1 mm slices, parallel to a line from the posterior foramen magnum to the hard palate, are utilized. Pre- and postcontrast scanning are essential for full evaluation of orbital lesions; this is most useful in suspected vascular lesions. Specifics of a given study are usually summarized on the films, which offer valuable information (Figure 9.1 and Box 9.1).

The images depicted in this chapter are examples of the capabilities of spiral CT with multidetector scanning.[4] The extraocular muscles are well defined in the axial and coronal views. The extraocular recti muscles outline the intraconal compartments well (Figure 9.2A,B). The muscles themselves are best identified in the coronal plane. Parasagittal reconstructions can show detailed views of the entire optic nerve within the orbit and through the optic canal, all the way to the optic chiasm (Figure 9.2C). The optic chiasm is best viewed on the coronal reconstruction (Figure 9.2D). The lacrimal gland is also best seen in the coronal view (Figure 9.2E).

Lesions affecting the orbital and extraorbital fat can be well visualized in almost any plane with reconstructions. Tumors involving the globe with or without orbital extension may also be depicted with CT, but MRI serves this purpose better. If bony involvement is clinically suspected, bone algorithm reconstruction is the study of choice (Figure 9.3). Algorithms for bone represent an artificially enhanced edge contrast and are applied as filters during reconstruction. CT is also very sensitive for detecting calcifications within orbital lesions, which can be very help-

TABLE 9.1. Commonly Encountered Absorption Values in Orbital CT.

Hounsfield unit	*Fluid or tissue*
−1000	Air
−70 to −100	Fat
0	Water
4–10	Cerebrospinal fluid
35–45	Brain
+1000	Bone

BOX 9.1. CT Imaging Parameters for Orbits

High resolution orbits
0.63 mm axials
Pitch 1
Table speed 1.25 cm/s
Intravenous contrast medium
Field of view 13 cm

ful in generating a differential diagnosis (Figure 9.4).[6–8] For orbital tumors with bony involvement, CT is superior to all other modalities (Box 9.2).

The main advantages of CT are availability and speed. With spiral scanning and multidetector machines, images can be obtained in a single plane virtually in moments, and reconstructions can be performed in any plane. CT does, however, present some risks to patients.[9–18] The main disadvantage of CT over other imaging modalities is that CT uses ionizing radiation (Table 9.1).[11–13] Radiation dose is related to CT technique, but 5 rads to the orbit and lens is common. This is well below a dose that could induce cataracts.[18] There is some risk of subsequent tumor induction to the patient, particularly in the pediatric age group.[14–17] This risk is, however, very small. With the use of intravenous contrast medium, the possibility of an allergic reaction is always present. The risk can be reduced with the use of nonionic contrast materials and prophylaxis if allergy is a consideration. Allergy is usually addressed with nonionic contrast material and a combination of steroids, Benadryl, and a histamine (H_2) blocker such as Zantac. Diabetics or patients with borderline renal function are at risk for contrast-induced renal failure.[9,10] The risk of contrast material-induced renal failure is higher in patients with renal failure, multiple myeloma, and other hyperviscosity syndromes and dehydration. In patients with a serum creatine value higher than 1.5 mm/dl, a nonionic contrast agent should be used. In patients with known hyperthyroidism, iodized contrast agents should be avoided.

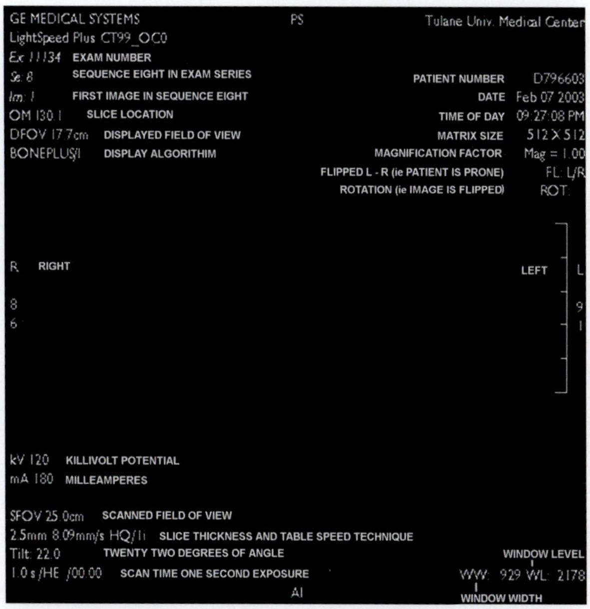

FIGURE 9.1. Sample CT scan parameters.

CT Artifacts

Artifacts of CT studies (Figure 9.5A–G) include high density foreign bodies such as a shotgun pellet in the right orbit and face causing streak artifact (Figure 9.5C). More significant metallic streak artifacts can be seen from dental fillings (Figure 9.5A). By viewing the image at bone window, most of that artifact can be reduced (Figure 9.5B). Circular or ring-type artifacts are usually related to detector problems. Figure 9.5D is an axial CT scan that was performed on a machine with a detector failure. Motion can degrade the quality of imaging and introduce artifacts at the time of scanning (Figure 9.5G). Positioning artifacts can also be misleading. On occasion, one may get the impression of proptosis due to an artifact. For example, a positioning artifact (Figure 9.5E,F) makes the left globe appear to be proptotic. The normal position of the globe in adults is 9.4 mm behind the interzygomatic line (range, 5.9–12.8 mm).[18] Other artifacts include partial voluming, where the scanning voxel will include tissues of two widely different densities such as cerebrospinal fluid and brain. When these two densities are averaged together they may create the illusion of a lesion. Beam-hardening artifact (Hounsfield artifact), which is mostly seen in the posterior fossa in the middle cranial fossa and orbit, represents increased attenuation of the x-ray beam due to the density and thickness of bone in these areas. The beam-hardening artifacts present a problem, particularly in the apex of the orbit and the optic canal.

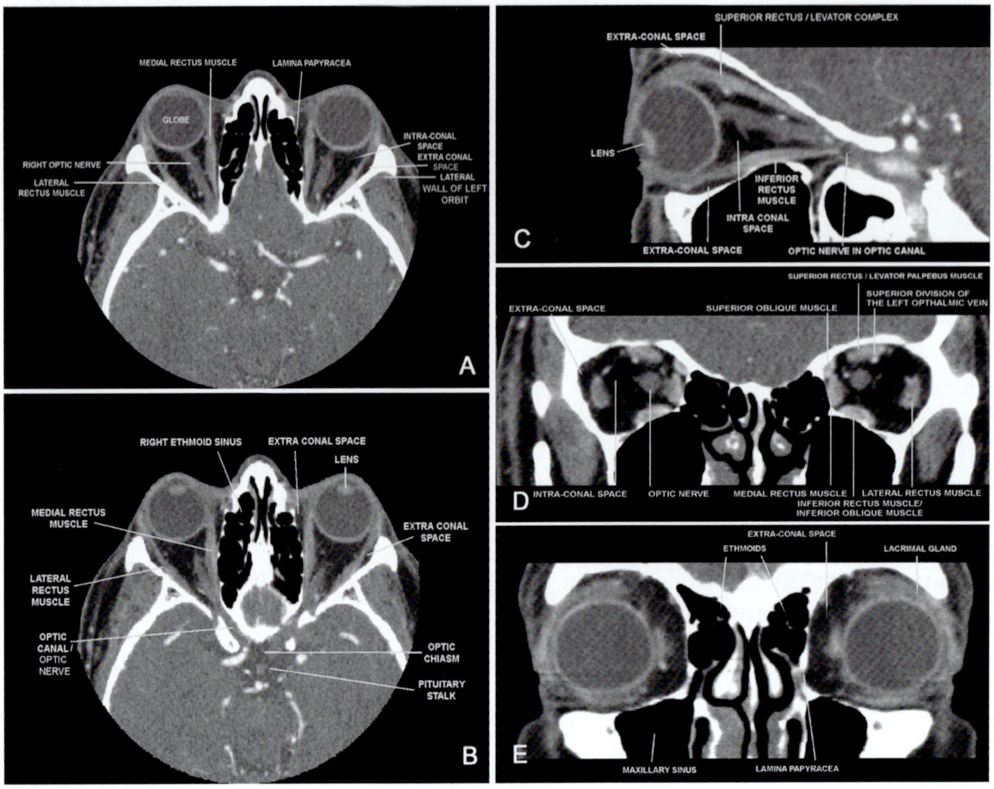

FIGURE 9.2. Axial orbital CT images with contrast (A) at level of the optic nerve and (B) showing the optical canal. (C) Parasagittal reconstruction of orbital CT along the course of the optic nerve. (D) Orbital coronal reconstruction of the orbits at midlevel. (E) Coronal orbital reconstruction with contrast at the equator level of the globe.

MAGNETIC RESONANCE IMAGING

MRI is also very useful for detecting and evaluating orbital mass lesions because of its excellent tissue resolution.[19–21] This technique allows one to generate cross-sectional images of the tissues without using x-rays. It is based on a physical phenomenon called the nuclear magnetic resonance effect on the atomic nuclei, primarily hydrogen atoms of water molecules within human tissues. When an external, static magnetic field is applied to the tissues, the random distribution of the atomic dipoles is distorted, and they tend to align in the direction of the field. When the applied radiofrequency pulse is discontinued, the macroscopic, magnetic field returns to its original state by emitting electromagnetic waves with precisional frequencies. The waves emitted during the reformation of the magnetic status (relaxation) are measurable and represent contrast values, corresponding to the brightness of the individual pixels, which, in turn, construct the images with the use of mathematical algorithms.

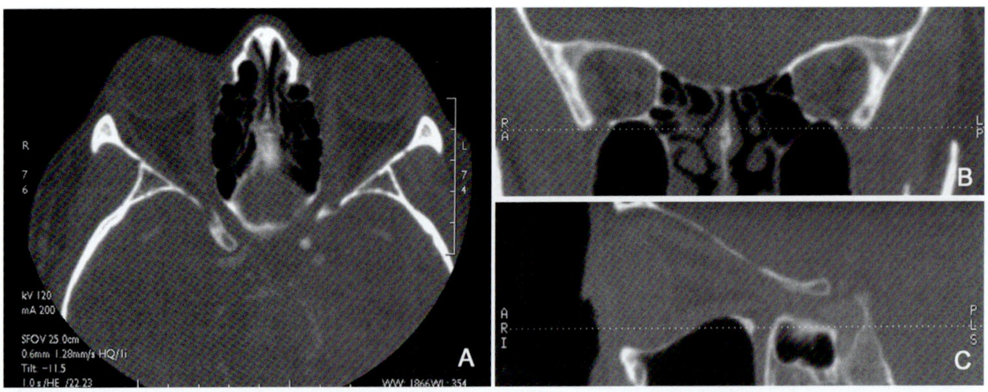

FIGURE 9.3. Bone windows: (A) normal axial CT, (B) normal coronal reconstruction, and (C) normal sagittal reconstruction.

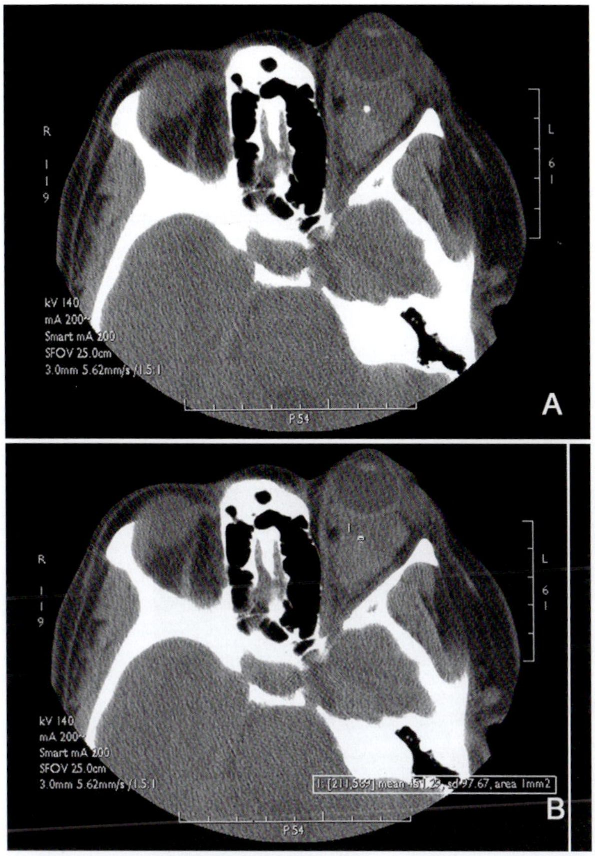

FIGURE 9.4. Orbital mass with focal density. (B) The CT number, shown as 451.29, is consistent with calcification, which is evidence of a phlebolith in a lymphangioma.

There are two types of relaxation: longitudinal (T1) relaxation and transverse (T2) relaxation. During the T1 relaxation, the excess energy is transferred from the nuclei to the environment. The T2 form, which is also termed spin–spin relaxation, represents the decay of the signal vector perpendicular to the strong magnetic field. These signals, which are obtained from biological tissues, depend on the water concentration of tissues, which can be excited. The degree of this excitation depends on the relaxation characteristics of the protons in water molecules of the tissues being examined. The water reveals a high concentration of excitable protons and a slow relaxation. In contrast, protons bound to macromolecules would reveal a fast relaxation. The relaxation times are therefore determined by the composition of the MRI characteristics of different types of tissues. A summary of signal characteristics of orbital tissues listed in Table 9.3 and Figure 9.6 gives MRI nomenclature and parameters, respectively. Orbital MRI examinations are also performed and interpreted according to predetermined neuroradiology protocols (Box 9.3).[20] MRI first became widely available in 1986 and gadolinium contrast enhancement in 1988.[21]

Currently MRI is most often done with a 1.5-tesla unit using either a head coil or a specially designed surface coil. Fast spin-echo sequences greatly reduce scan time over what is possible with traditional spin-echo techniques. Studies should include pre- and postcontrast T1-weighted axial and coronal images of the orbits extending through the optic chiasm. Fat suppression is done on postcontrast images, to increase lesion conspicuity by removing high-signal fat. Following intravenous administration of contrast agents, such as gadopentate, dimeglumine (Gd-DPTA), a different take-up by the tissues is seen in MRI studies. The axial pre- and postcontrast images should also be interlaced to optimize imaging of the optic nerves (Figure 9.7A–C). This is done with 100% gap or an interlace technique. T2-weighted images should also be obtained routinely through the orbits and optic nerves (Figure 9.7D). Many protocols also include a routine brain scan consisting of precontrast T1-weighted axial and sagittal images, diffusion axial, T2-weighted axial, FLAIR (fluid attenuation inversion recovery), and postcontrast T1-weighted axial, sagittal, and coronal images of the brain. MRI is also very sensitive for detection of intra- and extraconal orbital lesions. The optic nerve and chiasm are also very well defined. Optic nerve lesions that are not detected with CT may be well delineated with MRI. MRI offers tissue resolution superior to that available from CT scanning, allowing better detection of

BOX 9.2. Indications for CT and MRI

CT	MRI
Orbitocranial trauma	Detection of orbital masses
Orbitocranial hemorrhage	Evaluation of orbital and ocular masses
Detection of orbital masses	Evaluation of sinuses
Evaluation of orbital bones	Evaluation of optic pathway
Evaluation of sinuses	Orbital changes secondary to ocular tumors
Detection of calcification	Orbitocranial hemorrhage

TABLE 9.2. Advantages and Disadvantages of CT and MRI.

	Advantages	*Disadvantages*
CT	Availability and fast examination time Evaluation of bony involvement	Ionizing radiation Contrast reaction Beam-hardening and other artifacts
MRI	Detects virtually all lesions of the orbit except trauma No ionizing radiation	Motion and other artifacts Missile and thermal injuries Incompatible with a number of medical devices and metal implants Longer scanning times Overweight and claustrophobic patients cannot be accommodated

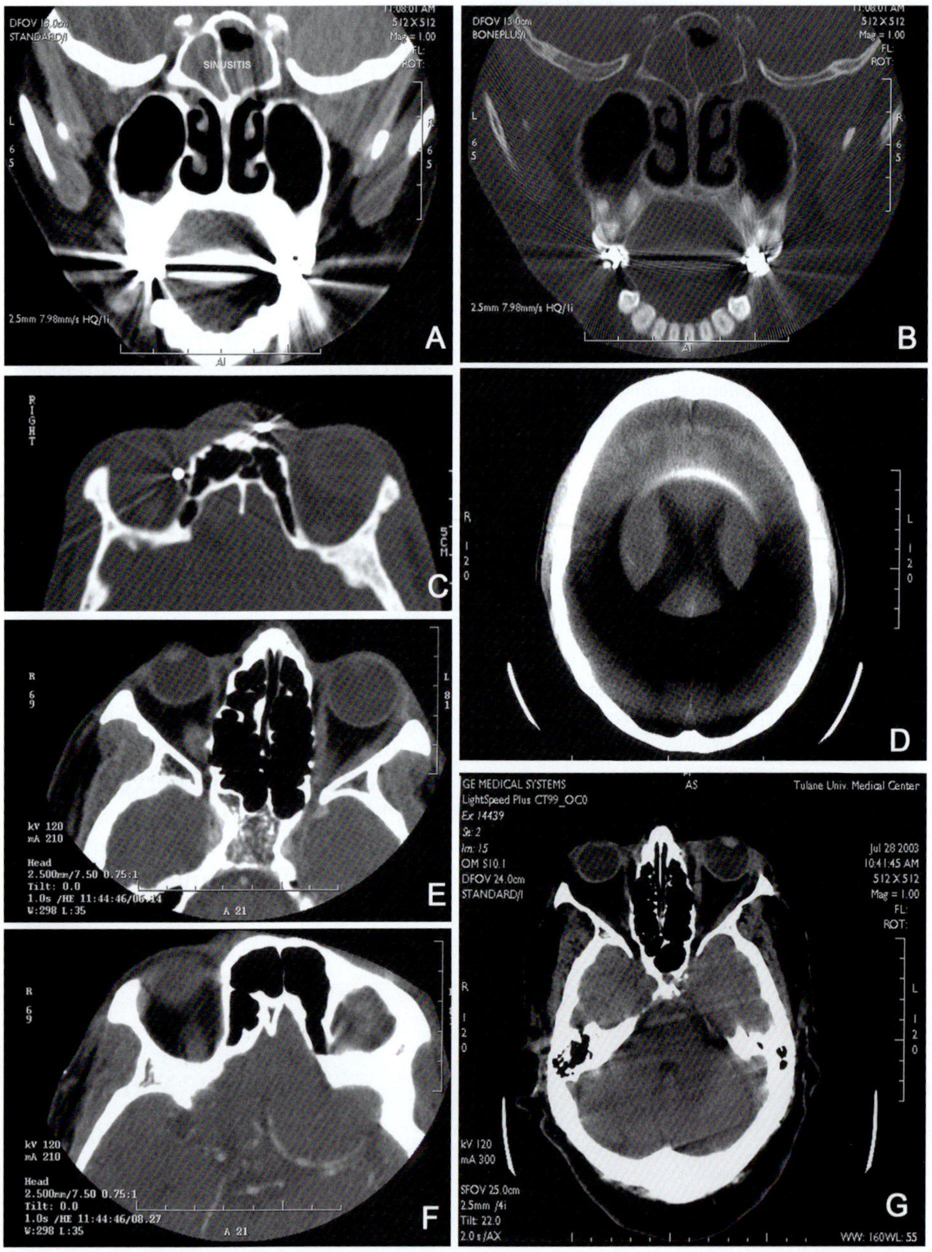

FIGURE 9.5. CT artifacts. (A) Dental fillings causing streak artifacts. (B) Artifact in the patient shown in (A) is reduced in bone windows. (C) Shotgun pellets causing streak artifacts. (D) Detector artifact. (E,F) Positioning artifacts. (G) Distortion due to patient motion.

TABLE 9.3. Commonly Encountered Signal Types in Orbital MRI.

	Signal type		
Tissue type	***Tl-weighted***	***T2-weighted***	***Fat suppression***
Globe	Hypo (dark gray)	Hyper (white)	Hypo (dark gray)
Fat	Hyper (white)	Hypo (white)	Intermediate (gray)
Extraocular muscle	Hypo (dark gray)	Hypo (light gray)	Hyper (white)
Optic nerve	Hyper (light gray)	Hypo (light gray)	Hyper (light gray)
Cerebrospinal fluid	Hyper (dark gray)	Hyper (white)	Hypo (dark gray)
Bone	Void (black)	Void (black)	Void (black)
Vessels	Void (black)	Void (black)	Void (black)

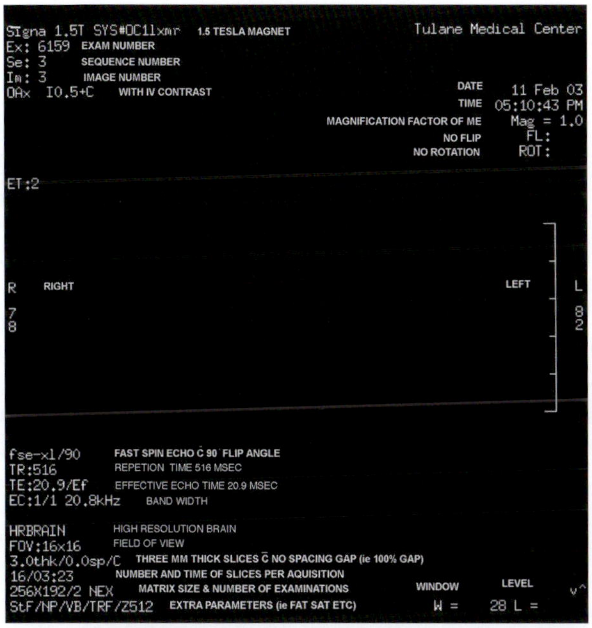

FIGURE 9.6. Sample MRI parameters.

BOX 9.3. MRI Parameters for Orbital Study

Axial T1-weighted: 3 mm with 100% gap
Coronal T1-weighted: 3 mm with 100% gap
Coronal T1-weighted: 3 mm with 10% gap
Postcontrast fat-saturated T1-weighted axial and coronals: 3 mm with 100% gap
A routine brain scan is often included.

small lesions. Changes of the globe, such as retinal or choridal detachment and scleral compression, which may happen secondary to orbital tumors, also are properly evaluated with MRI. Furthermore, tissue characterization by MRI is useful in leading to a differential diagnosis of the space-occupying lesions in the orbit.

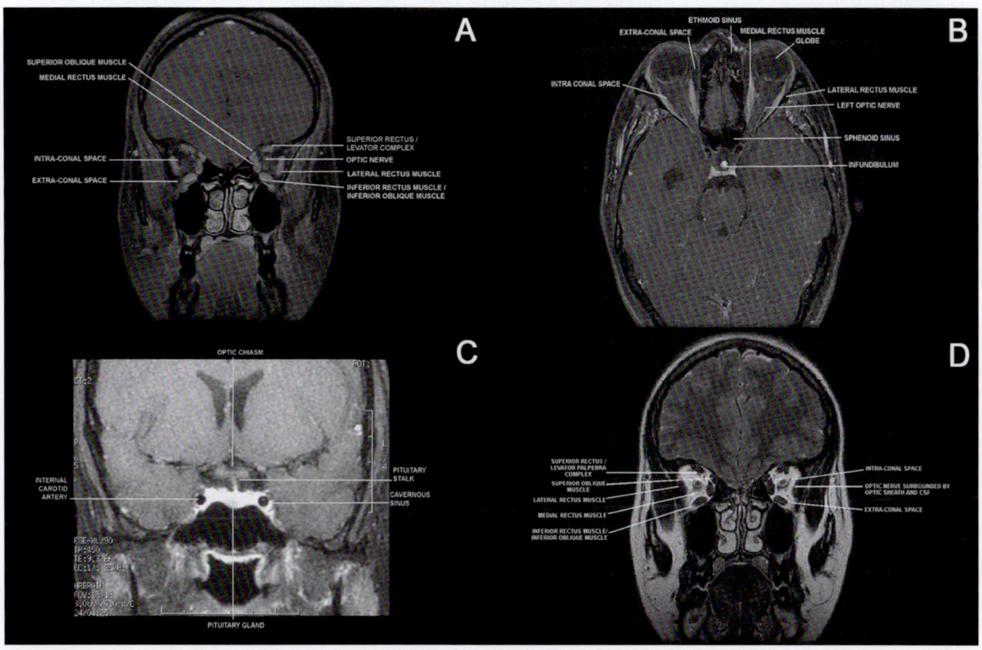

FIGURE 9.7. Fat-saturated postgadolinium images: (A) coronal image through posterior orbit, (B) axial image through optic nerve, and (C) coronal T2-weighted image through the optic chiasm. (D) Direct coronal T2-weighted image at midorbit.

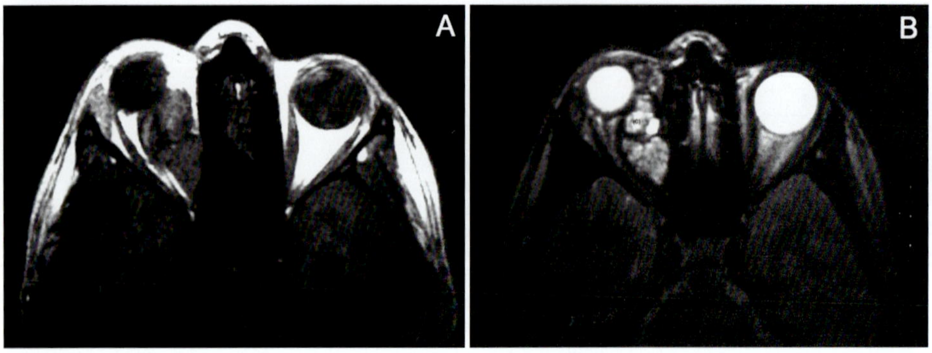

FIGURE 9.8. (A) Coronal T1-weighted image of a relatively homogeneous mass in right orbit, isointense to the ocular muscles. (B) This T2-weighted image shows a multicompartment cystic mass with high signal indicating fluid. The lesion was a lymphangioma.

TABLE 9.4. MRI Artifacts.

Artifact	*Cause*
Wrap around	Wrong field of view
Bioinhomogeneity	Magnetic field distortion by metal objects
Motion	Patient motion during procedure
Flow or pulsation	Misregistration with resulting artifacts
Chemical shift	Usually related to fat protons' resonating at a frequency different from water protons
Partial volume	Related to two different tissues being measured in a single voxel, the resultant display is an average of the two tissues

In particular, cystic or vascular lesions are better characterized on MRI and its multisequenced parameters.[5–7] For example, a lymphangioma of the orbit can be suggested with a high level of confidence based on the T1- and T2-weighted relaxation characteristics (Figure 9.8).[6]

Since the MRI does not use ionizing radiation, it does not pose any significant patient risk. Because MRI utilizes high-strength magnetic fields, however, injuries can occur. The deflection of aneurysm clips or other metallic devices can cause injury to the pa-

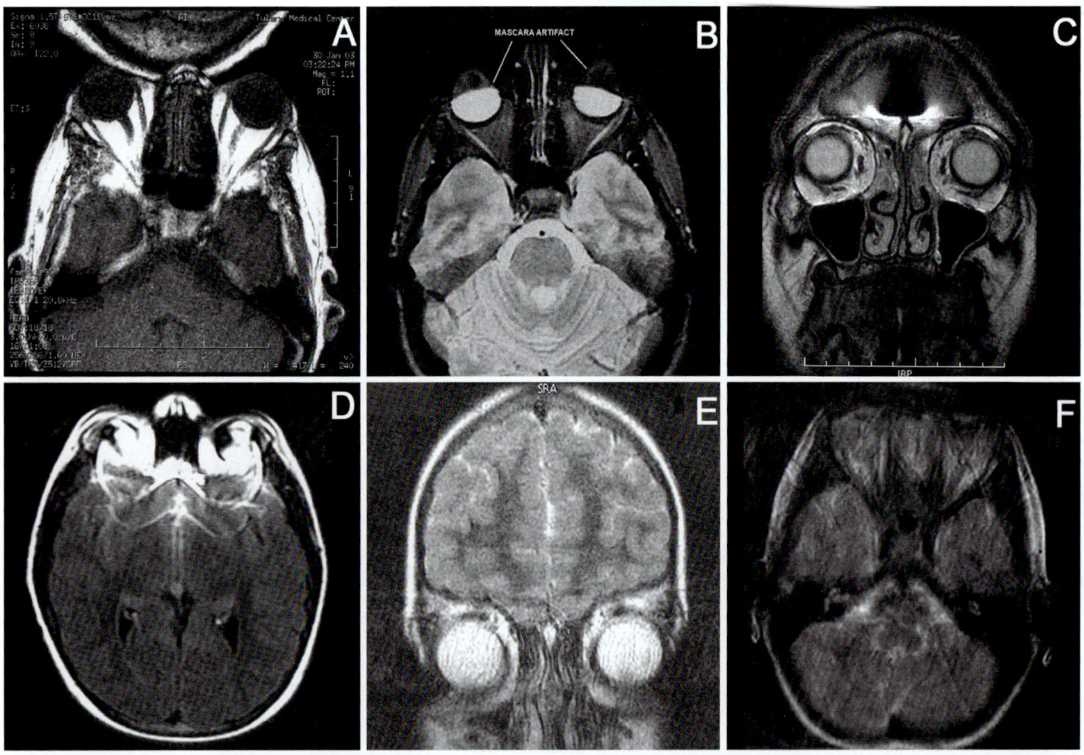

FIGURE 9.9. MRI artifacts. (A) Wraparound artifact due to wrong field of view. (B) Distortion because of the iron pigment in patient's mascara. (C) Surgical clip results in distortion or shielding of magnetic field. (D) Metal artifact (dental hardware). (E) Ghosting from orbital motion. (F) Distortion due to head motion.

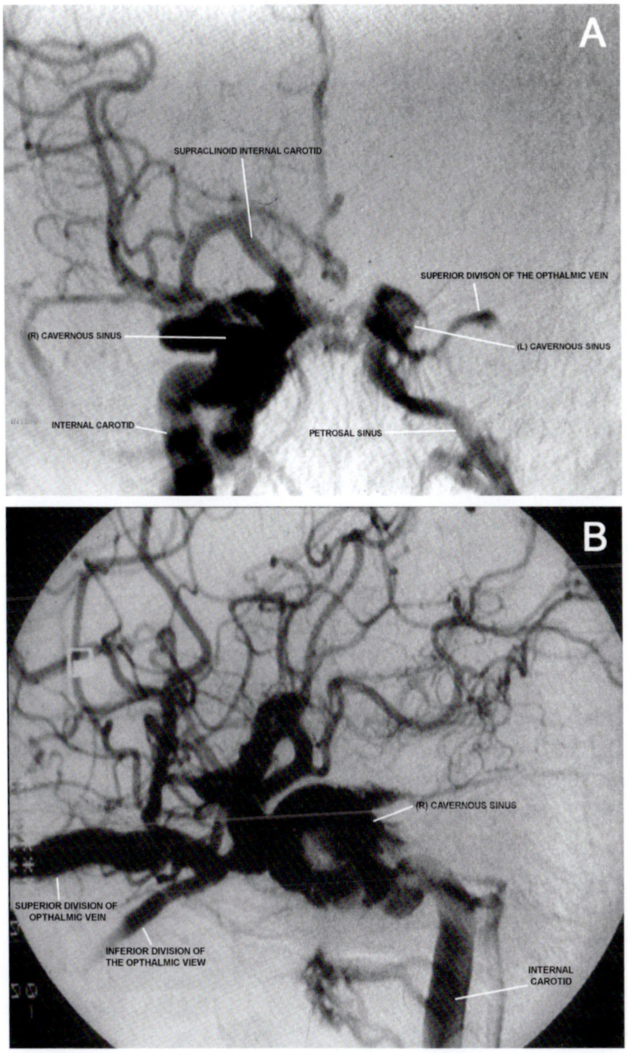

FIGURE 9.10. Radiographs from views of a right internal carotid angiogram. (A) Anterior–posterior (AP) view shows a typical high-flow fistula from the right carotid artery to the cavernous sinus. (B) Lateral view: typically type A fistulas are treated endovascularly from the arterial side.

tient.[22,23] In addition, there are case reports of ocular injuries due to deflection of small metallic fragments present in the orbits of sheet metal workers when these patients were placed in the magnet.[24] Thermal injuries can occur with pacing or monitoring wires that form a loop adjacent to the skin.[25]

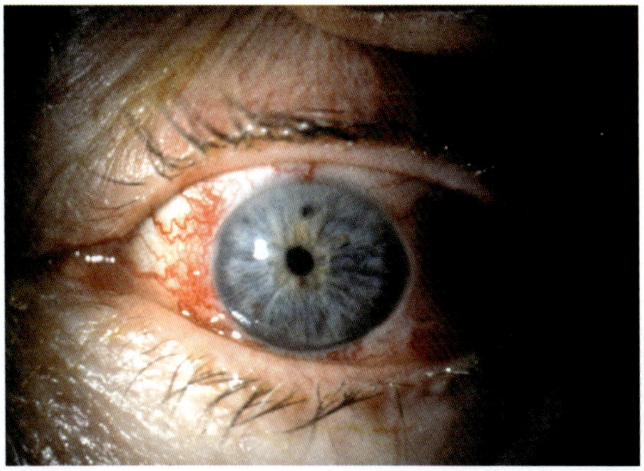

FIGURE 9.12. Proptosis with chemosis, congestion, and tortuosity of the conjunctival vessels in a carotid cavernous fistula.

MRI Artifacts

MRI artifacts far outnumber CT artifacts.[26–30] The main cause of this is the prolonged acquisition time for MRI: the longer the time, the greater the extent of motion artifacts because of eye movements. Some of the common MRI artifacts are listed in Table 9.4 and shown in Figure 9.9.

ANGIOGRAPHY AND ORBITAL INTERVENTIONS

With the development of magnetic resonance angiography (MRA) and computed tomographic angiography (CTA), the use of catheter diagnostic angiography has diminished dramatically. Catheter diagnostic angiography is not commonly used for orbital tumor diagnosis other than for vascular lesions. This imaging technique, however, remains the examination of choice for evaluating some of the vascular pathologies, particularly carotid cavernous fistula. The cath-

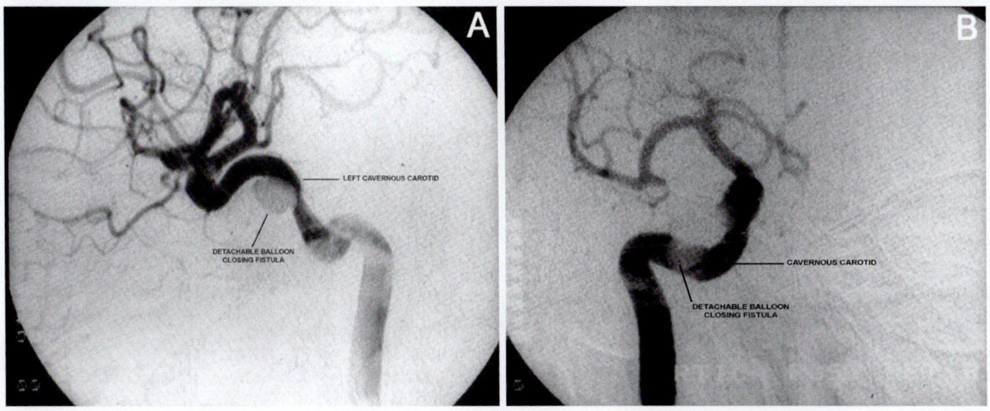

FIGURE 9.11. Angiograms of a right internal carotid artery after placement of a detachable balloon: (A) AP view and (B) lateral view.

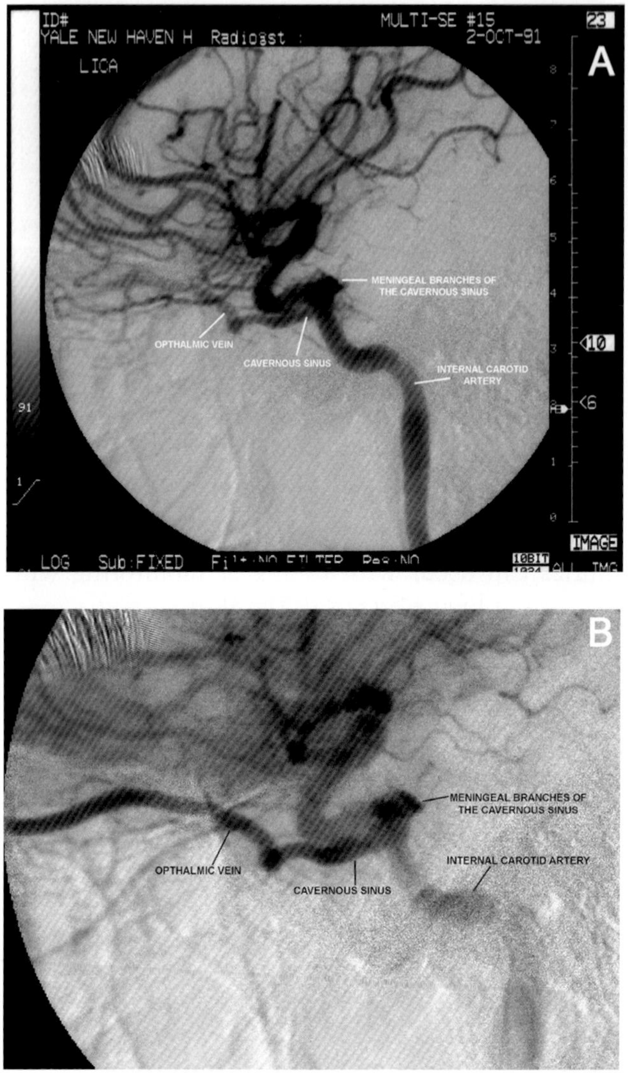

FIGURE 9.13. A type B fistula: (A) lateral angiogram and (B) enlarged lateral angiogram.

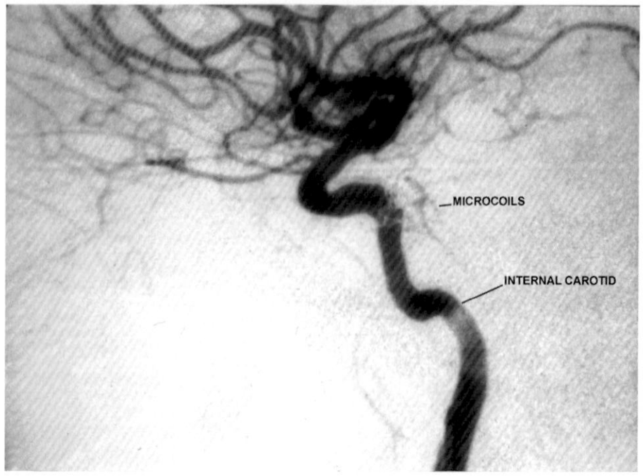

FIGURE 9.15. Tip of microcatheter in cavernous sinus; microcoils at level of fistula.

eter angiogram is essential to classify the arteriovenous fistula and also determines the best treatment option.[31,32] Angiography is briefly reviewed in this chapter because of its limited role in differential diagnosis of lesions occupying orbit–cranial space. Barrow and coworkers classify spontaneous carotid cavernous fistulas as follows:[31]

Type A: Direct high flow fistula between the internal carotid artery and the cavernous sinus (Figures 9.10, 9.11, and 9.12)

Type B: Dural shunts between meningeal branches of the internal carotid artery and the cavernous sinus (Figures 9.13, 9.14, and 9.15)

Type C: Dural shunts between meningeal branches of the external carotid and the cavernous sinus

Type D: Dural shunts between the meningeal branches of both the internal and external carotid arteries and the cavernous sinus

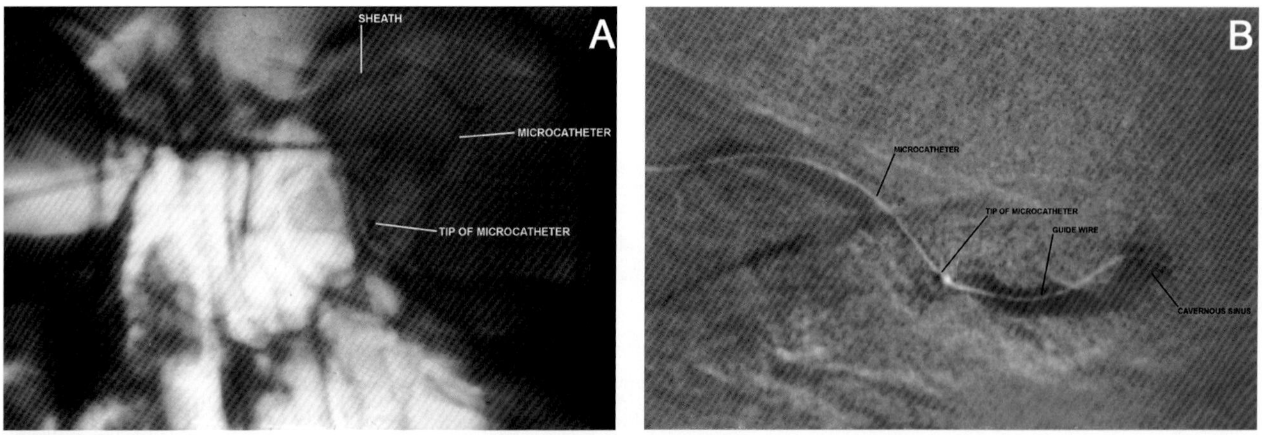

FIGURE 9.14. (A) Sheath placed into the superior ophthalmic vein. (B) Lateral view of microcatheter and contrast injection into the superior ophthalmic view and cavernous sinus. Radiographs of a right internal carotid angiogram after placement of a detachable balloon in the cavernous sinus to seal the fistula; the balloon was introduced from the arterial side.

References

1. Som PM, Cutin HD. *Head and Neck Imaging*. 4th ed. St. Louis: CV Mosby, 2003:451–452.
2. Muller-Forell WS. Computed tomograpy. In: Muller-Forell WS, ed. *Imaging of Orbital and Visual Pathway Pathology*. Berlin: Springer-Verlag; 2002:15–17.
3. Hu H, He HD, Foley WD, Fox SH. Row helical CT: image quality and volume coverage speed. *Radiology* 2000;215:55–62.
4. Jones R, Kaplan RT, Lane B, et al. Single versus multi-detector row CT of the brain: quality assessment. *Radiology* 2001; 219:750–755.
5. Lakitis A, Prokesch R, Scholda CH, et al. Helical and conventional CT in the imaging of metallic foreign bodies in the orbit. *Acta Ophthalmol Scand* 2000;789:79–83.
6. Graeb DA, Rootman J, Robertson WD, et al. Orbital lymphangiomas: clinical, radiologic and pathologic considerations. *Radiology* 1990;175:417–421.
7. Gunalp I, Gündüz K. Cystic lesions of the orbit. *Int Ophthalmol* 1997;20:273–277.
8. Savoiardo M, Stradas L, Passerini A. Cavernous hemangioma of the orbit: value of CT, angiography and phlebography. *Am J Neuroradiol* 1983;4:741–744.
9. American College of Radiology Committee of Drugs and Contrast Media. *Manual on Contrast Media*. 4th ed. 2001.
10. Katzbert RW. Urography into the 21st century: new contrast, renal handling, imaging characteristics and nephrotoxicity. *Radiology* 1997;204:297–312.
11. Barns E. Studies shed doubt on low level radiation dangers. 2003. www.auntminnie.com
12. Rehani MM. CT: caution on radiation dose. *Indian J Radiol Imag* 2000;10:19–20.
13. Hidajat N, Wolf M, Nunnerman, et al. Survey of conventional and spiral CT doses. *Radiology* 2001;218:395–401.
14. Donnely LF, Emery KH, Brody AS, et al. Minimizing radiation dose for pediatric body applications of single-detector helical CT: strategies at a large children's hospital. *AJR Am J Roentgenol* 2001;176:303–306.
15. Brenner DJ, Elliston CD, Hall EJ, Berdon WE. Estimates of the cancer risks from pediatric CT radiation are not merely theoretical: comment on "point/counterpoint: in x-ray computed tomography, technique factors should be selected appropriate to patient size against the proposition." *Med Phys* 2001;28: 2387–2388.
16. Paterson A, Frush DP, Donnelly LF. Helical CT of the body: are the settings adjusted for pediatric patients? *AJR Am J Roentgenol* 2001;176:297–301.
17. Rodgers L. Taking care of children: check out parameters used for helical CT. *AJR Am J Roentgenol* 2001;176:287.
18. Maclennan AC, Hadley DM. Radiation dose to the lens from computed tomography scanning in a neuroradiology department. *Br J Radiol* 1995;68:19–22.
19. Wichmann W. Magnetic resonance imaging (MRI). In: Muller-Forell WS, ed. *Imaging of Orbital and Visual Pathway Pathology*. Berlin: Springer-Verlag; 2002:18–23.
20. Ettl A, Kramer J, Daxer A, et al. High resolution magnetic resonance imaging of neurovascular orbital anatomy. *Ophthalmology* 1997;104:869–877.
21. Wichmann W, von Ammon K, Fink V, et al. Aneurysm clips made of titanium: magnetic characteristic and artifacts in MR. *AJNR Am J Neuroradiol* 1997;18:939–944.
22. Landrigan C. Preventable deaths and injury during magnetic resonance imaging. *N Engl J Med* 2001;345:1000–1001.
23. Dempsy MR, Condon B, Hadley DM. Investigation of the factors responsible for burns during MRI. *J Magn Reson Imaging* 2001;13:627–631.
24. Hornak JP. The basics of MRI. Ch 11. Image artifacts. www.-vibrantljue.com.
25. Tope WD, Shellock FG. Magnetic resonance imaging and permanent cosmetic (tattoos): survey of complications and adverse events. *J Magn Reson Imaging* 2002;15:180–184.
26. Basics of MRI—artifacts. Department of Radiology, Nagasaki University Site. www.med.nagasakiu.ac.Jr/Radiology%20of%20The 20%foot/mri-cnduh/nf-artifacts.html
27. Shellock FG, Kanal E. Aneurysm clips: evaluation of MR Imaging artifacts at 1.5 tesla. *Radiology* 1998;209:563–566.
28. Roeltgen DP. Orbital vascular mass, ability to assess. http://www.shcares.org/services/IRC/CME.
29. Kim DH, Adalsteinsson E, Spielman DM. Spiral readout gradients for the reduction of motion artifacts in chemical shift imaging. *Magn Reson Med* 2004;51:458–463.
30. Chang CJ, Chen YR, Noordhoff MS, et al. Facial bone fracture associated with carotid-cavernous fistula. *J Trauma* 1990;30: 1335–1339.
31. Meyers PM, Halbach VW, Dowd CF, et al. Dural carotid-cavernous fistula: definitive endovascular management and long-term follow-up. *Am J Ophthalmol* 2002;134:85–92.
32. Debrun GM, Vinuela F, Fox AJ, et al. Indications for treatment and classification of B2 carotid-cavernous fistulas. *Neurosurgery* 1998;22:285–289.

10

Imaging in Orbital Differential Diagnosis

Patrick De Potter

As in other disciplines, interpreting computed tomography (CT) and magnetic resonance (MR) scans requires practice and experience. A systemic radiological approach to examining the images is needed to reach a differential diagnosis. The images should be studied for lesion appearance, localization, information on contrast enhancement, bony orbit evaluation, and detection of calcification.

LESION APPEARANCE

In reviewing information about the appearance of an orbital lesion on the CT or MR scans, we may classify a lesion being solid or cystic, well circumscribed or ill defined, and localized or infiltrative.[1–3] Comparing the density of the lesion with that of the vitreous body will help to identify a solid lesion, whose density is higher than that of the vitreous on CT images. The wide range of signal intensities related to the internal structure and proteinaceous or blood content will not always allow us to differentiate a solid from a cystic orbital lesion (Figure 10.1).[2–6]

Information obtained from MR images allows us to identify tissue components such as melanin, methemoglobin, deoxyhemoglobin, ferritin, proteinaceous material, and fibrous tissue.[1,2–7] Therefore, the clinician will derive more information from the appearance of a lesion from MRI than from CT.

LOCALIZATION

The role of CT and MRI in orbital disease is mainly to evaluate the orbital content and the localization of the lesion, particularly if surgery is contemplated. CT gives us about the same information as MRI on the extent of an orbital lesion and its localization in the globe, the intraconal–extraconal space, the orbital apex, the extraocular muscles, or the lacrimal gland. However, CT remains the modality of choice in the evaluation of the bony orbit, paranasal sinuses, and adjacent structures.[3,8–11]

MR imaging is preferred for studying optic nerve and optic nerve sheath lesions.[1,2,12–14] MR imaging offers contrast resolution (tissue discrimination) superior to that available from CT scanning, as well as three-dimensional capability. Hard bone artifacts visible in MR imaging are not seen on CT scans. Contrast-enhanced T1-weighted images will allow us to identify the enhancing lesion within the optic nerve (optic nerve lesion) or surrounding it (optic nerve sheath lesion); in addition, the involvement of the optic nerve can be traced through the optic canal to the chiasm and optic tracts.[1,2,12–14]

Although CT is excellent for bony detail of the lacrimal drainage system, it provides more limited soft tissue detail than MRI and suffers from image degradation in out-of-plane images.[15] New MRI protocols, including topical instillation of gadolinium-DTPA (diethylenetriamine penta-acetic acid) into the conjunctival cul-de-sac (MRDt) or injection of contrast-enhanced saline solution after cannulation (MRDc), three-dimensional gradient-echo T1-weighted acquisition, 2 mm thick images through the nasolacrimal duct, and dynamic acquisition after contrast instillation for timing dye progression, contribute to the physiological study of tear evacuation and appear to be useful in assessing the anatomic and functional lacrimal system.[16,17] No significant difference in sensitivity was found among dacryocystography, CT dacryocystography, MRDt, and MRDc.

CONTRAST ENHANCEMENT

The positive enhancers are strongly paramagnetic proton relaxation agents, the most widely used of which is gadolinium. The most common uses of gadolinium are in the detection of the integrity of the blood–brain barrier and defining the extent of abnormal tissue. Because retrobulbar fat also displays bright signal in T1-weighted images, the use of fat suppression sequences is crucial in demonstrating enhanced tissues within the orbit. In the diagnosis of orbital disorders, abnormalities of the blood–brain barrier are rarely of clinical value.[18]

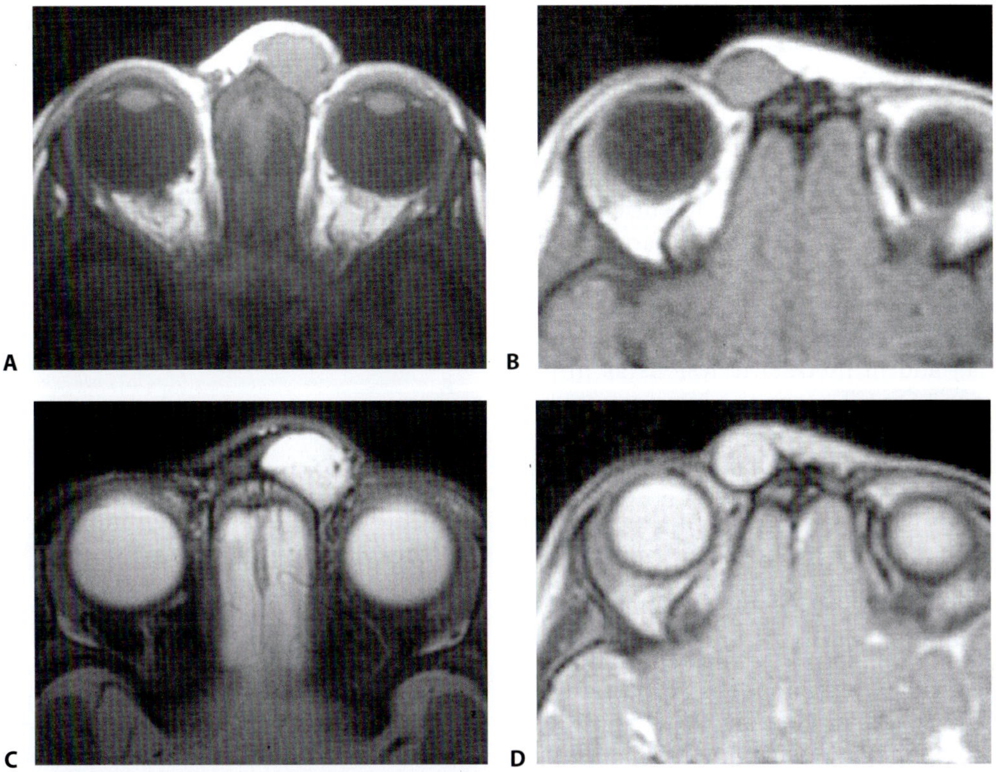

FIGURE 10.1. Axial images of two young patients presenting with swelling of the medial canthal area. (A,B) T1-weighted images; both lesions demonstrate the same signal intensity. (C,D) T2-weighted images; both lesions demonstrate the same signal intensity. Therefore, based only on the precontrast MR characteristics, it is difficult to differentiate the solid (capillary hemangioma, A and C) from the cystic (dermoid cyst, B and D) lesions.

Unlike CT examination, which uses iodinated contrast materials, the enhancement of vascular structures in MR imaging is not uniform, and their visualization depends on the velocity of the flow. As a result, one cannot identify contrast MR images simply by looking at vessels.

In orbital lesions, the degree of contrast enhancement within an orbital lesion or abnormal enhancement of optic nerve and optic nerve sheath tumors may guide the differential diagnosis.[1–3] Moderate to marked contrast enhancement is usually noticed in solid tumors as well as in acute inflammatory orbital lesions.[1–4,19] Minimal contrast enhancement suggests a chronic or sclerosing orbital inflammation, a fibrotic tumor, or posttherapeutic scar tissue.[1–4,19] No enhancement is documented in hemorrhagic process, dense scar tissue, collection of fluid, or the necrotic portion of neoplasms.[5,20] Linear enhancement surrounding a nonenhancing, well-delineated lesion suggests that the tumor is cystic. Well-defined linear or enhancement signal a void within an enhancing lesion may suggest the presence of air, high blood flow vessels (artery or vein), fragments of cortical bone, or foreign bodies.[1,2,4,19]

MRI will give the clinician more information from the enhancement pattern of an orbital lesion than can be obtained by means of CT.

BONE EVALUATION

Bone changes induced by an orbital lesion include cortical bony indentation and molding, bone erosion, bone lysis, and hyperostosis. Although MR scans may give indirect information, it is often difficult to separate the air-containing sinuses from the bone changes induced by an orbital and/or sinus lesion. A CT scan with bone windows, three-dimensional CT, or spiral CT is almost always preferred to assess an orbital disorder suspected to affect the bony orbit as well as congenital orbital disorders and orbital trauma.[9–11,21,22]

Molding of the bone by a well-circumscribed orbital mass is highly suggestive of a congenital lesion (e.g., dermoid cyst, lymphangioma) or a slowly growing benign lesion (e.g., cavernous hemangioma, neurofibroma, neurilemoma, benign lacrimal gland tumor).[1–4] Bone erosion or scalloping is usually seen in a more aggressive inflammatory or neoplastic primary or secondary lesion.[1–3,8]

Bone destruction is found in very aggressive primary or secondary malignant tumors but also in inflammatory lesions (idiopathic orbital inflammation, eosinophilic granuloma) or benign tumors (aneurysmal bone cyst).[1–3,23] The destruction of the cortical bone is visible on CT scans as a loss of the highly dense cortical bone and on MR scans as a discontinuity of the linear signal void produced by the normal cortical bone (Figure 10.2).[1–3,23,24] Osseous spiculation and inhomogeneous density are findings suggestive of malignancy on CT scan. Tumor infiltration of the bony orbit may be identified on MR films by replacement of the cortical bone, which shows discontinuity of its signal void, and of the fatty bone marrow, which loses its low signal intensity.[1–3,24]

Hyperostosis may be seen in benign osseous tumors (meningioma) and malignant bone tumors (osteosarcoma), and in metastatic lesions as in prostate carcinoma.[25] On CT scans the hyperostotic bone appears expanded and less dense than the normal osseous orbital wall.[3,11] Occasionally, the tumor may cause an en plaque bony sclerosis with or without soft tissue mass.

DETECTION OF CALCIFICATION

CT is the method best suited for the detection of calcification. Punctate or conglomerate increased densities on CT scans or foci of signal void on MR scans may be seen in trauma, vascular tumors, optic nerve sheath tumors (meningioma), epithelial lacrimal gland tumor (Figure 10.3), and malignant osseous tumors (osteosarcoma).[1–4,11,12,24]

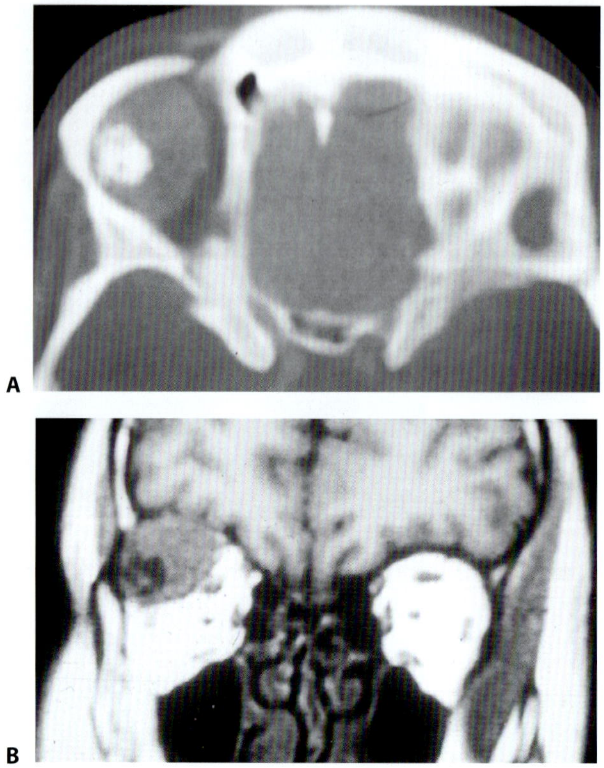

FIGURE 10.3. Adenoid cystic carcinoma of the lacrimal gland. (A) Coronal CT scan (bone window) showing the highly dense calcification within the tumor. (B) Axial T1-weighted image showing the calcified portion of the tumor as signal void.

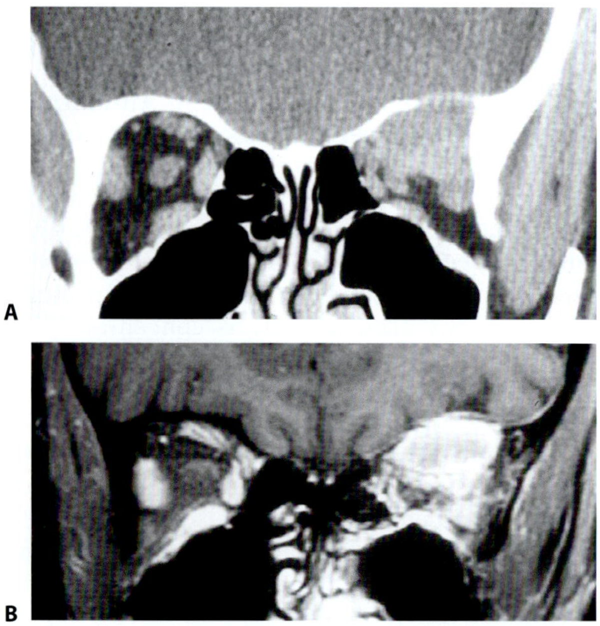

FIGURE 10.2. Images of left orbital metastasis from breast carcinoma. The infiltrative lesion produces bone destruction. (A) Contrast-enhanced coronal CT. Bone destruction is well identified as discontinuity of the cortical bone. (B) Contrast-enhanced coronal T1-weighted image. Bone destruction is suggested by discontinuity of the signal void of cortical bone. Meningeal neoplastic infiltration not seen on CT was identified on postcontrast MR scans.

RADIOLOGICAL DIFFERENTIAL DIAGNOSIS

CT and MR studies give minimal information about the histologic specificity of an orbital tumor. In many situations an accurate histologic diagnosis based on CT and MR characteristics of the tumor is not possible.[1–3] Therefore the radiological differential diagnosis of an orbital lesion will be stated by reviewing all the information provided by the scans, particularly about the appearance of the lesion. Soft tissue lesions may be categorized as well-circumscribed solid lesions, infiltrative/ill-defined solid lesions, or well-circumscribed cystic lesions. The differential radiological diagnosis may also depend on specific tumor location such as the optic nerve, lacrimal gland, or bony orbit.

Well-Circumscribed Solid Orbital Lesions

The most common well-circumscribed orbital tumors are cavernous hemangioma, neurilemoma, neurofibroma, fibrous histiocytoma, and hemangiopericytoma.[1–4,25] Cavernous hemangioma is one of the most common primary orbital tumors in adults and presents on MRI as a well-defined, oval-to-round intraconal orbital mass. On T1-weighted images, cavernous

TABLE 10.1. MR Features of the Most Frequent Well-Circumscribed Orbital Lesions on Spin-Echo Sequences.[a]

	Lesion appearance and signal with respect to vitreous		*Degree of lesion enhancement after Gd-DTPA*
	T1-Weighted image	*T2-Weighted image*	
Cavernous hemangioma	Homo Iso/Hyper	Homo Iso/Hypo	Hetero/Homo (late) +++
Neurilemoma	Hetero Iso/Hyper	Hetero Iso/Hypo	Hetero +/+++
Neurofibroma	Hetero Iso/Hyper	Hetero Iso/Hypo	Hetero +/+++
Fibrous histiocytoma	Hetero Hyper	Hetero Hypo	Hetero ++++
Hemangiopericytoma	Homo Iso/Hyper	Homo Iso/Hypo	Hetero ++++

[a]The abbreviations apply to all tables in this chapter: Homo, homogeneous; Hetero, heterogeneous; Iso, isointense; Hyper, hyperintense; Hypo, hypointense.

hemangioma appears to have a homogeneous, isointense to slightly hyperintense signal with respect to the vitreous, and a hypointense signal with respect to the orbital fat.[4] On T2-weighted images, the tumor has a high signal intensity with respect to the orbital fat (Table 10.1). Heterogeneity in tumor signal may be related to the presence of calcified phleboliths, which produce signal void on T1- and T2-weighted images and may mimic vessels with high blood flow. Other well-circumscribed solid lesions that can conceivably have identical MR characteristics include neurilemoma, neurofibroma, fibrous histiocytoma, and hemangiopericytoma.[4,6,26] However, less common well-circumscribed orbital lesions such as lymphoproliferative disorder, metastasis from skin melanoma or carcinoid tumor, capillary hemangioma, orbital varix, rhabdomyosarcoma, and extraocular extension of intraocular malignancies may also present with the same nonenhancing MR features as cavernous hemangioma (Table 10.2).[4,7,27–30] Gradient echo images are most helpful in differentiating calcification from intrinsic blood vessels.

Well-circumscribed solid orbital lesions usually demonstrate heterogeneous moderate to marked enhancement after gadolinium-DTPA administration (Tables 10.1 and 10.2).[4,8,26–29] However, unlike other orbital lesions, cavernous hemangioma shows increasing homogeneous enhancement on delayed images, owing to the pooling of the contrast medium within the tumor (Figure 10.4). Tumor enhancement and delineation are best evaluated on Gd-DTPA-enhanced T1-weighted images by means of fat suppression (frequency-selective presaturation) techniques.

Orbital CT will give less information than MRI regarding spatial location or tissue components.[3] All solid well-circumscribed lesions demonstrate higher density than those in the vitreous body, as well as variable degree of enhancement after contrast administration.[3,8] Calcified phleboliths are occasionally seen as highly dense foci within a cavernous hemangioma.[3]

The age of the patient, the clinical presentation, and the anatomic location of the lesion will help the clinician or radiologist in arriving at a differential diagnosis.

Ill-Defined Solid Orbital Lesions

The clinical differential diagnosis of the most common solid ill-defined orbital lesions in children includes capillary hemangioma, lymphangioma, plexiform neurofibroma, idiopathic orbital inflammation, and metastasis.[1–3,25] In adults there can be idiopathic orbital inflammation, metastasis, primary orbital tumor, and lymphoproliferative disorder.[1–3,25]

TABLE 10.2. MR Features of the Less Common Well-Circumscribed Orbital Lesions on Spin-Echo Sequences.

	Lesion appearance and signal with respect to vitreous		*Degree of lesion enhancement after Gd-DTPA*
	T1-weighted image	*T2-Weighted image*	
Lymphoproliferative disorders	Homo Iso/Hyper	Homo Iso/Hypo	Homo +++
Capillary hemangioma	Homo/Hetero Iso/Hyper	Homo/Hetero Iso/Hypo	Homo/Hetero +++
Orbital varix	Homo/Hetero Iso/Hyper	Homo/Hetero Iso/Hypo	Homo/Hetero ++++
Thrombosed varix	Hetero Iso/Hyper	Hetero Iso/Hypo	Hetero −/+
Orbital metastasis (skin malignant melanoma carcinoid)	Homo Iso/Hyper	Homo Iso/Hypo	Homo +/+++

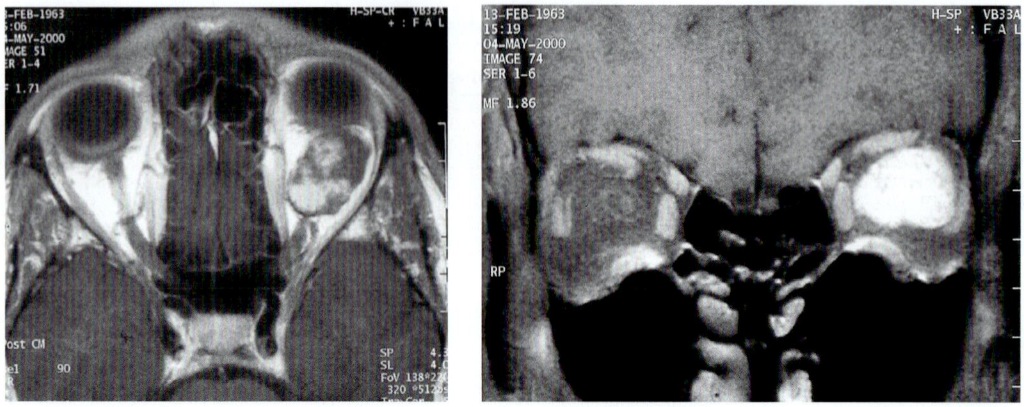

FIGURE 10.4. Orbital cavernous hemangioma. (A) Axial postcontrast T1-weighted image. This well-circumscribed lesion demonstrates heterogeneous enhancement shortly after contrast injection. (B) Fat-suppressed coronal postcontrast T1-weighted image. Fifteen minutes later, the lesion shows marked homogeneous enhancement owing to the pooling of the contrast agent.

Solid ill-defined orbital lesions usually present on MR studies as a diffuse, infiltrating, nonencapsulated pattern that often involves the extraocular muscles, the lacrimal gland, and sometimes the bony orbit. Idiopathic orbital inflammation has a homogeneous isointense to slightly hyperintense signal with respect to the vitreous and a hypointense signal with respect to the orbital fat on T1-weighted images.[19] On T2-weighted images, the lesion may appear isointense to hypointense with respect to the vitreous.[19] The increased signal of an inflammatory process is related to its acute stage and its high concentration of free water.[18] Other differential diagnoses that can conceivably have identical MR characteristics most often include capillary hemangioma, plexiform neurofibroma, metastasis, lymphoproliferative disorder, and rhabdomyosarcoma (Table 10.3, Figure 10.5).[1–4,27–29] Malignant processes and occasionally inflammatory lesions may produce bone changes as disruption of the regular signal void of the adjacent cortical bone or replacement of the high signal of the fat marrow by the hypointense lesions.[1–4,27–29]

After administration of Gd-DTPA, these solid, ill-defined orbital lesions demonstrate diffuse moderate to marked enhancement on T1-weighted images. This enhancement as well as the extent of the lesion is best delineated on fat-suppressed scans. Minimal and heterogeneous enhancement is usually seen in the sclerosing type of idiopathic orbital inflammation, and marked enhancement is actually seen in the acute type, making its radiologic differentiation easier (Table 10.3).[19,20]

MRI does not provide sufficient tissue specificity to allow reliable differentiation among benign reactive lymphoid hyperplasia, atypical lymphoid hyperplasia, and malignant non-Hodgkin or Hodgkin lymphoma and between lymphoproliferative disorders and idiopathic orbital pseudotumor.[19,28] The main role of MRI in evaluating an ill-defined orbital lesion is to delineate the extent of the lesion if surgery is contemplated.

There are no specific CT features of ill-defined orbital mass that can help the clinician or the radiologist to identify the histologic nature of the lesion.[3] CT may give some information regarding the malignancy or chronic behavior of the lesion if bone changes are identified on bone window scans.[3,23] Radiolucent areas within the tumor may suggest necrotic changes. The age of the patient, the clinical presentation, and

TABLE 10.3. MR Features of the Most Common Ill-Defined Orbital Lesions on Spin-Echo Sequences.

	Lesion appearance and signal with respect to vitreous		*Degree of lesion enhancement after Gd-DTPA*
	T1-Weighted image	*T2-Weighted image*	
Metastasis	Homo/Hetero Hyper	Homo/Hetero Hypo	Homo/Hetero +/+++
Primary orbital tumor	Homo/Hetero Hyper	Homo/Hetero Hypo	Homo/Hetero +/+++
Lymphoid proliferative disorder	Homo Hyper	Homo Hypo	Homo +++
Capillary hemangioma	Homo/Hetero Iso/Hyper	Homo/Hetero Iso/hypo	Homo/Hetero +++
Acute idiopathic inflammation	Homo Iso/Hyper	Homo Iso/Hypo	Homo +++
Chronic idiopathic inflammation (sclerosing type)	Homo Iso/Hyper	Homo Hypo	Homo/Hetero −/+

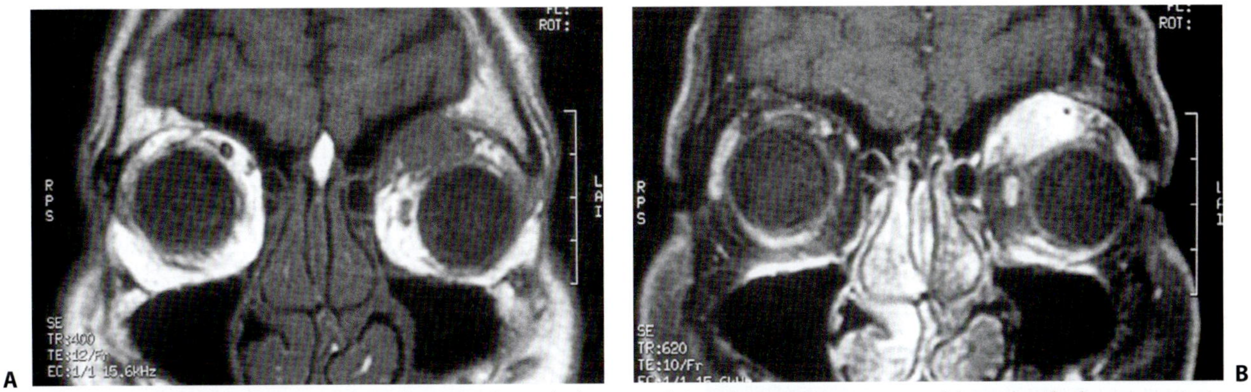

FIGURE 10.5. Ill-defined infiltrative orbital lesion with a radiological differential diagnosis including idiopathic orbital inflammation, metastasis, and malignant lymphoma. (A) Coronal precontrast and (B) postcontrast T1-weighted images show an infiltrative lesion involving the superior rectus and levator palpebrae superioris muscles and the surrounding orbital fat. Incisional biopsy confirmed the diagnosis of B-cell malignant lymphoma.

the anatomic location of the lesion will help the clinician or radiologist in this differential diagnosis.

Well-Circumscribed Cystic Lesions

The most common clinical differential diagnosis of cystic orbital lesions includes dermoid cyst, colobomatous cyst, teratoma, meningoencephalocele, lymphangioma, acquired inclusion cyst, chronic hematic cyst (cholesterol granuloma), mucocele, subperiosteal hematoma, and parasitic cyst.[25] On MRI these lesions appear as well-defined, round to oval lesions with variable signal intensity depending on the composition of their content (Table 10.4).[1,2,5,31]

Dermoid cyst may have an homogeneous or heterogeneous, isointense to hyperintense signal with respect to the vitreous on T1-weighted images.[5] On T2-weighted images, the cyst may appear isointense or hypointense to the vitreous.[5] Dermoid cyst may have a characteristic dumbbell configuration.[5,25] The varying intensity pattern of dermoid cyst on nonenhanced MR studies may also be seen in the other cystic orbital lesions. However, fat–fluid level is characteristically seen in dermoid cyst.[5] The oily portion of the cyst content appears in the nondependent portion of the cyst and the keratin and water content in the dependent portion of the cyst lumen. A fluid–fluid level is suggestive of subacute hemorrhagic lymphangioma or hemorrhagic cyst.[4,32]

Lymphangioma appears as a well-circumscribed unicystic or multicystic, homogeneous, or heterogeneous mass.[4,32] The lesion may show an isointense or hyperintense signal on T1-weighted images and an isointense or hypointense signal on T2-weighted images with respect to the vitreous (Table 10.4). This MR pattern is likely to be secondary to prominent lymphatic channels containing clear fluid. The tendency of orbital lymphangiomas to present with recurrent hemorrhage makes them ideal for MRI evaluation by demonstrating fluid–fluid levels (Figure 10.6). The superior aspect of the cyst contains the methemoglobin released from the lysed erythrocytes: the dependent portion contains the settled cellular elements of the hemorrhage with intracellular methemoglobin.[4,32]

Mucocele may have a variable signal intensity depending on the chronicity of the cyst. The concentration of proteinaceous secretions increases, as do the viscosity of the secretions and the slow resorption of the water through the mucosa.[5,33]

After Gd-DTPA administration, no enhancement is documented within the lumen of the cyst (Table 10.4).[2,5,31,32] The lack of enhancement within the le-

TABLE 10.4. MR Features of the Most Common Cystic Orbital Lesions on Spin-Echo Sequences.

	Lesion appearance and signal with respect to vitreous		*Degree of lesion enhancement after Gd-DTPA*
	T1-Weighted image	*T2-Weighted image*	
Dermoid cyst	Hetero Iso/Hyper	Hetero Iso/Hypo	–
Epithelial cyst	Homo Iso/Hyper	Homo Iso/Hypo	–
Mucocele	Homo Iso/Hyper	Homo Iso/Hypo/Hyper	–
Hemorrhagic cyst/lymphangioma	Hetero Iso/Hyper	Hetero Iso/Hypo/Hyper	–/+

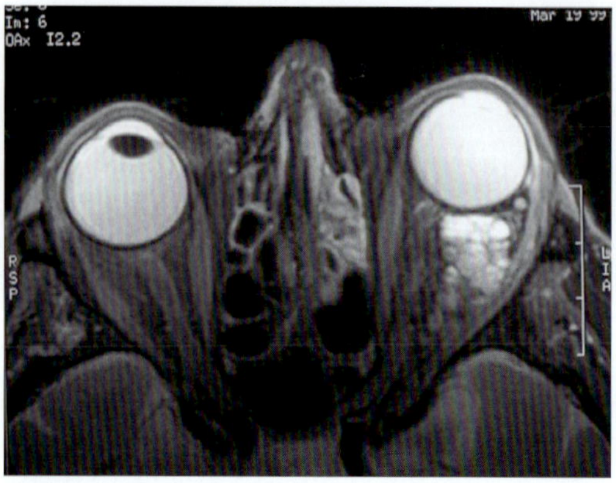

FIGURE 10.6. Recurrent hemorrhagic orbital lymphangioma with fluid–fluid levels. Axial T2-weighted image shows a multicystic lesion with heterogeneous high signal intensities and fluid–fluid levels suggesting lysed and intact erythrocytes.

sion usually rules out a solid neoplastic process. Enhancement may be seen within the capsule and septae surrounding the cystic lesion. On Gd-DTPA-enhanced T1-weighted images, the degree of enhancement of lymphangioma is variable.[2,5,32]

Orbital CT gives excellent information regarding the cystic features of the lesion because its density is similar to that of the vitreous.[3,11,31,33] However cystic lesions with higher density (with a high content of protein, keratinaceous material, or blood products) may simulate solid, well-circumscribed orbital tumor.[3,5,11] MR studies are more specific than CT in identifying tissue component within the cystic mass. The age of the patient, the clinical presentation, and the anatomic location of the cystic lesion will help the clinician or radiologist in the differential diagnosis.

Enlarged Optic Nerve

The pattern of enhancement of an enlarged optic nerve allows us to differentiate an optic nerve lesion from a optic nerve sheath tumor. In optic nerve tumors, the enhancement is seen within the optic nerve. In optic nerve sheath lesions, the enhancement is eccentrically surrounding a hypointense optic nerve.

The most common clinical differential diagnosis of an enlarged optic nerve includes juvenile pilocytic astrocytoma (JPA), malignant glioma, secondary tumor from intraocular tumor (retinoblastoma, uveal melanoma, melanocytoma), central nervous system lymphoma or systemic metastatic disease, and optic neuritis.[25] All may assume a tubular, fusiform, lobular configuration.

The characteristic kinking and buckling of the enlarged optic nerve is highly suggestive of JPA (optic nerve glioma).[2,12–14,34] On precontrast T1-weighted images, JPA appears isointense with respect to the cerebral gray matter. The tumor may be surrounded by reactive arachnoid hyperplasia that shows a slightly hypointense signal. On T2-weighted images, fusiform JPA demonstrates a relatively high signal intensity, whereas large lobulated tumors tend to show a more heterogeneous signal. The peripheral hyperintense portion [perineural arachnoid gliomatosis or arachnoidal hyperplasia or accumulation of cerebrospinal fluid (CSF)] surrounds a central linear core of lower signal intensity (compact proliferation of glial cells).[2,12,35] On postcontrast studies, JPA shows variable enhancement that can be traced through the optic canal to the chiasm and optic tracts when it involves the intracranial portion of the optic nerve.[2,12,35] The nonenhancing peripheral portion of the tumor, which is hyperintense on T2-weighted images, probably represents arachnoidal hyperplasia or an ectatic subarachnoid space around the optic nerve.[2,12,35] The perineural arachnoid gliomatosis shows enhancement. Fat suppression techniques are most helpful in distinguishing the contrast enhancement of the tumor from the bright signal of the orbital fat.[2,12,35]

Involvement of the optic nerve with retinoblastoma or melanoma cells, lymphoproliferative tissue, and metastatic process is best detected on postcontrast MR studies.[12,13] In those cases, the pattern of enhancement within the optic nerve is localized or diffuse. If intraorbital optic neuritis is suspected, T2-weighted images and fat-suppressed postcontrast T1-weighted images are recommended. On these pulse sequences, the intensity of the optic nerve is increased.[12,36,37]

The most common clinical differential diagnosis of an enlarged optic nerve sheath lesion includes meningioma, meningeal spread of tumor, meningitis, arachnoidal cyst, hemorrhage, and CSF expansion, as seen with pseudotumor cerebri or orbital apex compression.[25] The intensity pattern of optic nerve sheath meningioma on precontrast MR studies is variable, and the tumor may appear isointense or hypo- or hyperintense with respect to the optic nerve on T1- and T2-weighted images.[2,12,38] Calcification shows a low signal intensity on T1- and T2-weighted images without enhancing after Gd-DTPA administration. On postcontrast films, the tumor shows a marked enhancement that characteristically presents as a rim or eccentric pattern surrounding the nonenhancing optic nerve.[2,12,38] Detection and delineation of small orbital, or intracanalicular and intracranial, extension of the tumor is best identified on postcontrast T1-weighted images with fat suppression techniques.[2,12,38]

The spectrum intensities of optic nerve sheath hemorrhage reflects the chronicity of the subarachnoidal hemorrhage.[12] Cystic accumulation of CSF shows a high signal intensity on both spin-echo images. However, no enhancement of the optic nerve sheath enlargement secondary to hemorrhage and CSF accumulation is documented after Gd-DTPA administration. Linear enhancement of slightly thickened meninges is highly suggestive of inflammatory process (meningitis) or neoplastic infiltration (carcinomatosis meningitis).

On CT, the tubular or globular enlargement seen with an optic nerve sheath meningioma is nonspecific.[3,11] Tram-tracking, a sign in which the denser and thicker optic nerve sheath outlines a central lucency representing the residual optic nerve, is a characteristic but not specific finding suggestive of optic nerve sheath meningioma.[3,11] Detection and delineation of the intracanalicular and intracranial portions of the optic nerve sheath meningioma are best achieved by contrast-enhanced MR studies.[11,13]

Enlarged Lacrimal Gland

Lacrimal gland lesions may be classified as nonepithelial and epithelial. The nonepithelial lacrimal gland lesions include inflammation and lymphoid tumors. The epithelial lesions include dacryops, pleomorphic adenoma, and malignant epithelial tumors (adenoid cystic carcinoma).[25]

On MRI, among the nonepithelial lesions of the lacrimal gland, an inflammatory process (dacryoadenitis) usually appears more ill defined than a lymphoid infiltrate, which can mold to the globe.[1,2,39] Epithelial tumors of the lacrimal gland usually present as a well-circumscribed mass in the lacrimal gland fossa; these tumors produce scalloping of the frontal bone. Adenoid cystic carcinoma may have an irregular, relatively well-defined, or infiltrative pattern with possible evidence of bone destruction.[1,2,39] The age of the patient and the clinical presentation will help the clinician or radiologist in the differential diagnosis.

On T1-weighted images, inflammatory or neoplastic lacrimal gland lesions may have an isointense to slightly hyperintense signal with respect to the vitreous. On T2-weighted images, the enlarged lacrimal gland shows an isointense to hypointense signal with respect to the vitreous (Table 10.5). An acute dacryoadenitis is easily differentiated from a chronic and/or sclerosing inflammatory process or epithelial tumor by its higher signal intensity on T2-weighted images, which is suggestive of tissue edema. Epithelial tumors of the lacrimal gland and particularly malignant epithelial tumor have a more heterogeneous appearance than nonepithelial lesions.[2,39] Calcification within the enlarged lacrimal gland is highly suggestive of adenoid cystic carcinoma and appears as hypointense areas on T1- and T2-weighted images without enhancement on postcontrast scans.[2,39] Destruction of the orbital roof and lateral walls is evidenced by interruption of the low signal intensity of the cortical bone and possible replacement of the signal of the fat marrow by the infiltrative process. Owing to its high protein content, dacryops shows a high signal intensity on T1- and T2-weighted images.

After Gd-DTPA administration, nonepithelial lacrimal gland lesions demonstrate varying degrees of homogeneous or heterogeneous enhancement.[2,19,28,39] Minimal enhancement is usually seen in the sclerosing form of idiopathic lacrimal gland inflammation. Moderate to marked enhancement is present in acute or subacute form of dacryoadenitis and lymphoproliferative disorders. Epithelial lacrimal gland tumors demonstrate heterogeneous moderate to marked enhancement. The cystic cavity of dacryops is not amenable to enhancement. Delineation of the enlarged lacrimal gland is best accomplished with postcontrast T1-weighted images using fat suppression techniques.

CT characteristics of solid inflammatory or benign neoplastic process of the lacrimal gland are nonspecific with an enlarged lacrimal gland.[3,11,40] Orbital CT is more specific than MRI in detecting calcification within the enlarged lacrimal gland suggestive of adenoid cystic carcinoma and in evaluating bone destruction in the lacrimal gland fossa.

TABLE 10.5. MR Features of Lacrimal Gland Enlargement on Spin-Echo Sequences.

	Lesion appearance and signal with respect to vitreous		*Degree of lesion enhancement after Gd-DTPA*
	T1-Weighted image	*T2-Weighted image*	
Dacryops	Homo Iso/Hyper	Homo Iso/hypo	–
Lymphoid proliferative disorder	Homo Hyper	Homo Hypo	Homo +++
Acute idiopathic inflammation (dacryoadenitis)	Homo Iso/Hyper	Homo Iso/hypo	Homo +++
Chronic idiopathic inflammation (sclerosing type)	Homo Iso/Hyper	Homo Hypo	Homo/Hetero –/+
Pleomorphic adenoma (benign mixed tumor)	Homo Iso/Hyper	Homo Iso/hypo	Homo +++
Adenoid cystic carcinoma	Homo/Hetero Hyper	Homo/Hetero Hypo	Homo/Hetero +/+++

Bony Orbit

Because cortical bone has a signal void, bone can be demarcated from adjacent tissues. Good contrast is therefore available between bone and orbital fat, muscle, and brain. However, cortical bone may not be clearly defined when it lies adjacent to structures in which signal is not generated such as air, rapidly flowing blood, dura, or calcification.

The presence of bone scalloping, deformity, hyperostosis, expansion, and bone marrow invasion can all be demonstrated with MR.[1,2,8,24] However, the degree of bone destruction cannot always be easily assessed by MR techniques. CT remains the modality of choice for the evaluation of bone abnormalities as well as for osseous, fibro-osseous, and fibrous tumors.[3,10,11,21,24]

Benign osteoma shows a low signal intensity on both T1- and T2-weighted images without enhancement after Gd-DTPA administration.[2,24] Osteosarcoma appears as an ill-defined mass with a heterogeneous, hyperintense signal with respect to the vitreous and gray matter on T1-weighted scans.[2,24] On T2-weighted images, the tumor has a heterogeneous lower signal intensity with respect to the vitreous.[2,24] After Gd-DTPA injection, osteogenic sarcoma demonstrates heterogeneous enhancement. Replacement of the cortical bone and fat marrow as well as orbital and cranial extension are best identified on postcontrast fat-suppressed, T1-weighted images.[2,24] CT scans demonstrate an irregular, invasive, and destructive tumor with lytic and sclerotic changes associated with focal areas of calcification.[3,11,24]

The orbital bones affected by fibrous dysplasia appear to be thickened, with a very low signal intensity, on T1- and T2-weighted images.[2,24] The less calcified portion of the tumor may not appear as hypointense as the bony lesion itself. Depending on the histologic features of the lesion, the fibrous stroma may enhance, but the mature calcified portion of the lesions does not enhance. Orbital CT scans demonstrate a lesion with a sclerotic, homogeneous, dense, ground-glass appearance, but alternate areas of lucency and increased density can be observed.[3,11,24]

Aneurysmal bone cysts of the orbit appear as multicystic, loculated masses associated with bone destruction and possible extension to the adjacent sinuses.[24,25,41] These tumors have a heterogeneous signal intensity, and fluid–fluid levels are usually present. The spectrum of signal intensities noted in aneurysmal bone cyst reflects the various stages of evolution of the hemorrhagic content of the cystic portion of the lesion.[24,41] Orbital CT scans show irregular expansion and destruction of bone associated with a mildly enhancing loculated cystic mass.[3,11,24,41]

The major role of MR studies in secondary orbital tumors from the paranasal sinuses is to delineate the extent of the infiltrative tumor process within the orbit, the sinuses, and the brain.[2,42] These malignant neoplasms are fairly cellular and usually show a low signal intensity on T1-weighted images and increased signal on T2-weighted images with respect to orbital fat. The bony wall of the orbit can be evaluated if there is suspicion of orbital invasion. The lack of signal void produced by orbital walls between the tumor and the orbital tissue or the brain indicates either thinning or destruction of the bone.[2,42] After Gd-DTPA administration, the tumor usually shows moderate to marked enhancement. Fat suppression techniques are useful in differentiating tumor margins from orbital fat.[2,42]

CONCLUSIONS

Orbital MRI is indicated as a first imaging step to evaluate the following aspects of orbital lesions:

1. Localization and extent of orbital process
2. Orbital, intracanalicular, and prechiasmal optic pathways
3. Sudden proptosis (a hemorrhagic rather than a neoplastic process)
4. Progressive bluish lid swelling (capillary hemangioma versus lymphangioma)
5. Progressive proptosis, looking for true neoplastic growth, fibrosclerotic changes, mucinoid/cystic degeneration, and hemorrhagic process
6. Tumor response after radiotherapy or chemotherapy
7. Anophthalmic socket when orbital tumor recurrence is suspected
8. Orbital trauma when ferromagnetic material is excluded
9. Identification of fibrovascular ingrowth within the biocompatible sphere when drilling is contemplated

Orbital CT is indicated as a first imaging step to evaluate orbital lesions in the following situations:

1. A patient with proptosis with suspicion of osseous, fibro-osseous, or fibrous lesions
2. A patient with clinical diagnosis of lacrimal gland lesion
3. Orbital trauma
4. Contraindication for MRI

References

1. De Potter P, Flanders AE, Shields CL, Shields JA. Magnetic resonance imaging of orbital tumors. *Int Ophthalmol Clin* 1993;33:163–173.
2. Bilaniuk LT, Zimmerman RA, Newton TH. Magnetic resonance imaging: orbital pathology. In: Newton TH, Bilaniuk LT, eds. *Radiology of the Eye and Orbit. Modern Neuroradiology.* Vol 4. New York: Raven Press; 1990: Chap 5.

3. Sobel DF, Salvolini U, Newton TH. Computed tomography: ocular and orbital pathology. Radiological aspects. In: Newton TH, Bilaniuk LT, eds. *Radiology of the Eye and Orbit. Modern Neuroradiology.* Vol 4. New York: Raven Press; 1990: Chap 9.
4. De Potter P, Dolinskas C, Shields CL, Shields JA. Vascular tumors. In: De Potter P, Shields JA, Shields CL, eds. *Magnetic Resonance Imaging of the Eye and Orbit*. Philadelphia: JB Lippincott; 1995:159–181.
5. De Potter P, Shields JA, Shields CL. Acquired cystic lesions. In: De Potter P, Shields JA, Shields CL, eds. *Magnetic Resonance Imaging of the Eye and Orbit*. Philadelphia: JB Lippincott; 1995:131–143.
6. Foroozan R, Shields CL, Shields JA, et al. Congenital orbital varices causing extreme neonatal proptosis. *Am J Ophthalmol* 2000;129:693–694.
7. Ezzadin EM, Liu D, Al-Rashed W, Jacquemin C. Bilateral orbital hemorrhage in a newborn. *Am J Ophthalmol* 2000;129:531–532.
8. De Potter P, Shields CL, Shields JA, et al. The CT and MRI features of an unusual case of isolated orbital neurofibroma. *Ophthalmic Plast Reconstr Surg* 1992;8:221–227.
9. Klevansky A. The efficacy of multiplanar reconstructions of helical CT of the paranasal sinuses. *AJR Am J Roentgenol* 1999;173:493–495.
10. De Potter P. Advances in imaging in oculoplastics. *Curr Opin Ophthalmol* 2001;12:342–346.
11. Maya MM, Heier LA. Orbital CT: current use in the MR era. *Neuroimaging Clin North Am* 1998;8:651–683.
12. De Potter P, Shields JA, Shields CL. Optic nerve and meningeal tumors. In: De Potter P, Shields JA, Shields CL, eds. *Magnetic Resonance Imaging of the Eye and Orbit*. Philadelphia: JB Lippincott; 1995:193–212.
13. McCaffery S, Simon EM, Fischbein NJ, et al. Three-dimensional high resolution magnetic resonance imaging of ocular and orbital malignancies. *Ophthalmology* 2002;120:747–754.
14. Barnes PD, Robson CD, Robertson RL, Poussaint TY. Pediatric orbital and visual pathway lesions. *Neuroimaging Clin North Am* 1996;6:179–198.
15. Rubin PED, Bilyk JR, Shore JW, et al. Magnetic resonance imaging of the lacrimal drainage system. *Ophthalmology* 1994;101:235–243.
16. Manfrè L, de Maria M, Todaro E, et al. MR dacryocystography: comparison with dacryocystography and CT dacryocystography. *Am J Neuroradiol* 2000;21:114–150.
17. Pariselle J, Froussart F, Sarrazin JL, et al. Apport de l'IRM dans l'étude dynamique des voies lacrymales d'excrétion. *J Fr Ophtalmol* 1999;22:628–634.
18. Millar WS. Basic principles. In: De Potter P, Shields JA, Shields CL, eds. *Magnetic Resonance Imaging of the Eye and Orbit*. Philadelphia: JB Lippincott; 1995:3–17.
19. De Potter P, Shields CL, Shields JA. Inflammatory diseases. In: De Potter P, Shields JA, Shields CL, eds. *Magnetic Resonance Imaging of the Eye and Orbit*. Philadelphia: JB Lippincott; 1995:145–158.
20. Schaffler GJ, Simbrunner J, Lechner H, et al. Idiopathic sclerotic inflammation of the orbit with left optic nerve compression in a patient with multifocal fibrosclerosis. *Am J Neuroradiol* 2000;21:194–197.
21. Rhea JT, Rao PM, Novelline RA. Helical CT and three-dimensional CT of facial and orbital injury. *Radiol Clin North Am* 1999;37:489–513.
22. Zonneveld FW, Vaandrager JM, van der Meulen JHC, Koornneef L. Three-dimensional imaging of congenital disorders involving the orbit. *Radiol Clin North Am* 1998;36:1261–1279.
23. Daumerie CH, De Potter P, Godfraind C, et al. Orbital metastasis as primary manifestation of thyroid carcinoma. *Thyroid* 2000;10:189–192.
24. De Potter P, Shields CL, Shields JA. Fibrous tissue, osseous, and fibrous osseous tumors. In: De Potter P, Shields JA, Shields CL, eds. *Magnetic Resonance Imaging of the Eye and Orbit*. Philadelphia: JB Lippincott; 1995:213–221.
25. Shields JA, Shields CL. *Atlas of Orbital Tumors*. Philadelphia: Lippincott, Williams & Wilkins, 1999.
26. De Potter P, Dolinkas C, Shields JA, Shields CL. Peripheral nerve tumors. In: De Potter P, Shields JA, Shields CL, eds. *Magnetic Resonance Imaging of the Eye and Orbit*. Philadelphia: JB Lippincott; 1995:183–191.
27. De Potter P, Dolinkas C, Shields JA, Shields CL. Metastatic tumors. In: De Potter P, Shields JA, Shields CL, eds. *Magnetic Resonance Imaging of the Eye and Orbit*. Philadelphia: JB Lippincott; 1995:237–243.
28. De Potter P, Dolinkas C, Shields CL, Shields JA. Lymphoproliferative and histiocytic disorders. In: De Potter P, Shields JA, Shields CL, eds. *Magnetic Resonance Imaging of the Eye and Orbit*. Philadelphia: JB Lippincott; 1995:245–253.
29. De Potter P, Dolinkas C, Shields JA, Shields CL. Myogenic tumors. In: De Potter P, Shields JA, Shields CL, eds. *Magnetic Resonance Imaging of the Eye and Orbit*. Philadelphia: JB Lippincott; 1995:223–226.
30. De Potter P, Shields JA, Shields CL. Modified enucleation via lateral orbitotomy for choroidal melanoma with orbital extension. A report of two cases. *Ophthalmic Plast Reconstr Surg* 1992;8:109–113.
31. De Potter P, Kunin AW, Shields CL, et al. Massive orbital cyst of the lateral rectus muscle after retinal detachment surgery. *Ophthalmic Plast Reconstr Surg* 1993;9:292–297.
32. Bond JB, Haik BG, Taveras JL, et al. Magnetic resonance imaging of orbital lymphangioma with and without gadolinium contrast enhancement. *Ophthalmology* 1992;99:1318–1324.
33. Van Tassel P, Lee YY, Jing BS, De Penna CA. Mucoceles of the paranasal sinuses. MR imaging with CT correlation *AJNR Am J Neuroradiol* 1989;10:607–612.
34. Haik BG, Saint Louis L, Bierly J, et al. Magnetic resonance imaging in the evaluation of optic nerve glioma. *Ophthalmology* 1987;94:709–717.
35. Seiff SR, Brodsky MC, MacDonald G, et al. Orbital optic glioma in neurofibromatosis. Magnetic resonance diagnosis of perineural arachnoidal gliomatosis. *Arch Ophthalmol* 1987;105:1689–1692.
36. Guy J, Mancuso A, Quisling RG, et al. Gadolinium-DTPA-enhanced magnetic resonance imaging in optic neuropathies. *Ophthalmology* 1990;97:592–600.
37. Guy J, Mao J, Bidgood D, et al. Enhancement and demyelination of the intraorbitaloptic nerve. Fat suppression magnetic resonance imaging. *Ophthalmology* 1992;99:713–719.
38. Elster AD, Challa VR, Gilbert TH, et al. Meningiomas: MR and histopathological features. *Radiology* 1989;170:857–862.
39. De Potter P, Dolinskas C, Shields JA, Shields CL. Tumors of the lacrimal gland. In: De Potter P, Shields JA, Shields CL, eds. *Magnetic Resonance Imaging of the Eye and Orbit*. Philadelphia: JB Lippincott; 1995:227–235.
40. Mafee MF, Haik BG. Lacrimal gland and fossa lesions: role of computed tomography. *Radiol Clin North Am* 1987;25:767–780.
41. Patel BC, Sabir DI, Flaharty PM, Anderson RL. Aneurysmal bone cyst of the orbit and ethmoid sinus. *Arch Ophthalmol* 1993;111:586–587.
42. De Potter P, Shields JA, Shields CL. Secondary orbital tumors. In: De Potter P, Shields JA, Shields CL, eds. *Magnetic Resonance Imaging of the Eye and Orbit*. Philadelphia: JB Lippincott; 1995:255–268.

11

New Concepts in Orbital Imaging

Michael D. Abramoff

When a patient presents with exophthalmos, the ophthalmologist will take the history, perform a complete examination, and then will likely request a computed tomography (CT) scan. If the scan reveals a space-occupying lesion, diagnosis and management will be determined based on the history, the patient's signs and symptoms, and the features of the tumor on CT; a biopsy procedure may be performed to confirm the diagnosis. Additional imaging procedures may be done later to evaluate the effectiveness of the treatment.

A DIAGNOSTIC PARADIGM

The common sequence just outlined requires orbital imaging for three distinct purposes:

1. To confirm that the patient's signs and symptoms could be explained by an orbital tumor. This is the *is-there-a-tumor* use of orbital imaging.
2. The nature of the tumor, such as its malignant potential, tissue type, and extension into other tissues, can be decided on the basis of specific radiologic features (e.g., the smoothness of the lesion's boundary or its relationship to other orbital tissues). This is the *which-tumor-is-it* use of orbital imaging, needed to help decide how to manage the tumor.
3. The use of follow-up imaging to monitor treatment. This may be termed the *how-is-it-doing* use.

Current orbital CT techniques are very good at answering the *is-there-a-tumor* question; it is usually unnecessary to order a different imaging modality, such as a magnetic resonance imaging (MRI) scan, to confirm the existence of a lesion. However, CT may be inadequate for the *which-tumor-is-it* question. Frequently, other studies such as MRI are needed to decide on tissue type or malignancy; often only biopsy and histopathology results acquired from the specimen can provide a definitive answer. Consequently, the management of orbital tumors is based on a combination of clinical experience, history, radiologic features on imaging studies, histopathology of the biopsy specimen, and other factors to decide *which tumor is it?*

The distinction among the clinical imaging applications for the *is-there-a-tumor, which-tumor-is-it, how-is-it-doing* paradigm may seem artificial. The localization of the tumor on imaging studies combined with the clinical course of its signs and symptoms often suffices to determine management of cavernous hemangiomas, for example. If an excisional biopsy will be curative, knowing the exact type of tumor before surgery is also less important. Nevertheless, the distinction is worthwhile, especially in judging the value of new developments in orbital imaging. In view of the enormous effectiveness of current CT, MRI, and ultrasonographic orbital tumor imaging techniques, with their ability to resolve even tumors only a few millimeters in size, will new orbital imaging techniques really influence the way orbital tumors are diagnosed and managed?

Many new techniques show promise in better answering the *which-tumor-is-it* and *how-is-it-doing* questions. Such new techniques have already helped decide the malignancy potential of soft tissue tumors, the tissues in which orbital inflammatory pseudotumors originate, and the histopathology of lymphomas. Ideally, one day, "in vivo histopathology" may circumvent the need for most biopsies. After all, the orbital biopsy procedure remains risky and can result in visual loss and blindness if complications occur during or after the procurement of the specimen.

STATE OF THE ART OF ORBITAL TUMOR IMAGING

Ultrasonography

Ultrasonography was widely employed in the diagnosis of orbital tumors in the late 1960s, before the advent of the CT. An early review was written by Howard.[1] Orbital tumor imaging by ultrasonography has recently seen a number of innovations, including three-dimensional imaging[2] and vascular imaging, called color Doppler imaging, because it uses the Doppler signal from the blood flow. Ultrasonography is flexible because the patient does not need to be inside a scanner. However, it is limited by the requirement for skilled operators and because penetration of the deeper regions of the orbit at energy levels acceptable for the retina cannot be achieved. Since the advent of the CT, ultrasonography has been largely superseded for determining the presence of a tumor. It is difficult to differentiate normal from abnormal tissue by means of ultrasonography, and there are no studies of the relationship between reflectivity and histopathology in the orbit. However, ultrasonography has been shown to be effective in specific cases.[3] For example, it was found to be superior to CT in detecting extraocular extension of melanoma.[4] Color Doppler ultrasonography may be able to differentiate meningioma from glioma of the optic nerve,[5] and it may be effective in confirming the diagnosis of orbital varix.[6] As far as orbital imaging is concerned, ultrasonography probably cannot be developed further simply because improved imaging would necessitate prohibitively high energy levels at the level of the retina.

Computed Tomography

CT was first described in 1973[7]; the first description of its use in orbital tumor imaging dates from 1977.[8] Notwithstanding the advent of MRI in other specialties, it is still the most important imaging modality for the diagnosis of orbital tumors.[9] It is especially effective in determining the presence of tumors, even those a few millimeters in diameter.

However, CT is less useful in identifying the type of tumor once the presence of a growth has been confirmed. Although studies that really correlate orbital CT features with histopathology after biopsy are rare, in existing studies there is a lack of correlation between tumor type and radiological features in neck metastases[10] and optic nerve sheath tumors[11]. Still, specific radiological features of tumors are commonly thought to relate to specific diagnoses, such as the localization of the tumor relative to other orbital structures, smoothness and delineation of the boundary of the tumor, associated calcifications or bone destruction, and homogeneity of contrast enhancement. For tumors of some types, such as orbital inflammatory pseudotumors and cavernous hemangiomas, the combination of clinical course and features such as those just named usually suffices for diagnosis, even without a biopsy.[12,13]

Magnetic Resonance Imaging

Although potentially a noninvasive method of in vivo neuropathology, MRI is still far from being sufficiently specific, since dissimilar lesions often look the same despite the use of refined imaging protocols. The first MRI prototypes were tested on clinical patients in 1980, and the first report on the use of MRI in imaging tumors in the orbit dates from 1984.[14] Even in this early report, the question of whether CT or MR is the better orbital imaging technique was posed. This discussion has been continuing ever since, though currently most clinicians favor CT over MR as the initial modality to settle the *is-there-a-tumor* issue for suspected orbital tumors.[9]

MRI has the advantage of high soft tissue contrast, large imaging depth (depending on the type of coil), and the absence of radiation load; however, image acquisition is usually slower than CT scanning, commonly on the order of minutes. Subjects need to fixate during this period and are not allowed to blink.[15] Nevertheless, MRI was found to be superior to CT and ultrasonography in helping to identify tumors, for example, in classifying lacrimal gland tumors,[16] diagnosing cavernous hemangioma,[17] and differentiating solitary fibrous tumors.[18] However, it was found to be ineffective in differentiating lymphoma from pseudotumor[19] and fibrous histiocytoma from fibrous tissue tumors.[20]

CT, MRI, and ultrasonography usually suffice to determine whether a tumor is present. Current imaging techniques have an impact in differentiating the tumor (*which-tumor-is-it*), but new developments in imaging have potential in this regard.

NEW DEVELOPMENTS IN IMAGING

A large number of new imaging techniques have developed since the advent of CT, MRI, and ultrasonography. Some developments are essentially improvements of established techniques, such as spiral CT, which offers faster acquisition, lower exposure to ionizing radiation, and higher resolution than conventional CT. Especially in the MRI field, there has been a constant search for better and faster imaging algorithms and stronger magnetic fields to decrease noise and increase resolution. MRI magnetic field strengths, measured in teslas, have improved from 0.3 T 20 years ago to 1.5 T as the current standard for clinical imaging. These developments will gradually improve the quality of orbital imaging.

However, other new orbital imaging techniques represent real innovations that may become important in orbital tumor diagnosis and management. Although in vivo histopathology imaging of orbital tumors is not yet feasible, what can be imaged is the change in function of the orbital structures that are the result of the presence and growth of a tumor. Functional imaging, defined as that range of imaging techniques in which the aim is to extract quantitative information about the physiological function of tissues, is different from the CT, ultrasonography, and (current) MRI techniques, which all show the spatial relationships of tissues to each other. The functional changes can be either macroscopic or microscopic and are specific to a particular type of tumor. In malignant tissue, examples of microscopic functional changes are an increased ratio of cells to extracellular matrix, increased ratio of apoptotic to normal cells, increased concentration of the amino acid choline, oxygen perfusion, and increased capillary flow. Changes in all these variables have been imaged successfully in patients, and some of them in the orbit. Examples of macroscopic functional changes in the orbit are changes in tissue motion, or increased attachments to other tissues caused by scarring or invasive growth, which have also been imaged successfully in the orbit.

Some of the "new" techniques, such as positron emission tomography (PET) and single-photon emission computed tomography (SPECT), have been around for decades but are new to orbital imaging and thus deserve mention.

MR-Based Techniques

MRI imaging is the most active research area for new techniques. Some of these techniques, especially diffusion imaging, are already being used by neurosurgeons to discriminate tumor types. Others, such as magnetic resonance spectroscopy (MRS) and functional MRI (BOLD), were thought to be promising in tumor characterization in the past, but have not been shown to be really effective in clinical studies. This section focuses on three techniques: diffusion imaging, MRS, and dynamic color mapping. These are particularly attractive because they do not require new hardware and can be performed on current clinical MR scanners. In contrast, other interesting "new" techniques discussed in this chapter, such as PET and SPECT, typically require large investments in scanners and nuclide instrumentation.

Diffusion-Weighted MR Imaging

Diffusion-weighted MRI, which is similar to regular MRI and employs the same scanner, measures the potential of water molecules to move and is based on the random, microscopic movement of water molecules in tissue. As water molecules collide, they spread out (diffuse). Normally (e.g., in normal brain gray matter), this motion is unrestricted, which leads to spin dephasing and attenuation of the MR signal. However, if the motion is restricted, which can happen if the tissues consist of parallel fibers, such as nerves or skeletal muscles, or if there is a restricted extracellular space, such as in high-cellularity tumors, the MR signal will be less attenuated. Diffusion-weighted images are MR images in which the signal intensity shows the MR attenuation caused by diffusion. On these images high diffusion is shown as black and low diffusion (the optic nerve and extraocular muscles) as white. The resulting MR signal can be normalized in several ways, leading to images of different "diffusion signals," known by acronyms such as TDC (true diffusion coefficient), ADC (apparent diffusion coefficient) or D_{av} (average diffusion constant), which are not discussed here.

Diffusion imaging measures function on a microscopic scale. Diffusion in tissue is largely determined by microscopic features such as density and type of cells and intracellular matrix, since these structures impede the free movement of water molecules to a greater or lesser extent; compare this with the common forms of MRI such as T1, T2, and proton imaging, which measure processes on the atomic scale. Theoretically, changes in diffusion may more directly reflect changes occurring within and between cells.

In brain gliomas, diffusion-weighted imaging was found to differentiate between high and low cellularity as found on histopathological examination (different ADCs) in a prospective study.[21] Cellularity is an important histologic determinant of glioma malignancy. Histopathological cellularity of lymphomas was found to be predictable by means of diffusion imaging.[22] In a prospective study of brain meningiomas, diffusion-weighted imaging was found to differentiate between aspecific and malignant meningiomas on the one hand and benign meningiomas on the other, with malignant and aspecific meningiomas showing low D_{av} on imaging.[23] In a prospective study of soft tissue tumors, diffusion imaging could predict the malignancy of soft tissue tumors as determined by histopathology, with benign tumors (such as leiomyoma and schwannomas) showing high TDC and malignant tumors (such as liposarcoma and leiomyosarcoma) showing low TDC.[24]

Magnetic Resonance Spectroscopy

Magnetic resonance spectroscopy uses the same concepts as MRI, but instead of imaging the spatial relationships of tissues, the concentrations of specific chemical compounds within the tissue are imaged. The radiofrequency pulse sequence of the scanner produces a signal decay, the amount of which is ultimately determined by the chemical relationships in the tissue. These series of signals can be transformed into a spectrum, where the concentration of different chemical compounds is imaged via different color intensities. By using MRS, it is possible to image the concentration of different compounds in a particular region of interest such as the brain or the orbit. The most interesting compounds for tumor characterization are choline, creatine, *N*-acetyl aspartate, and *N*-acetylaspartyl glutamate.[25] Choline and creatine are present in most cells, whereas *N*-acetyl aspartate and *N*-acetylaspartyl glutamate are localized predominantly in neurons. The ratios between these compounds help to indicate the type of tissue in the tumor. The proliferative capacity of gliomas as measured

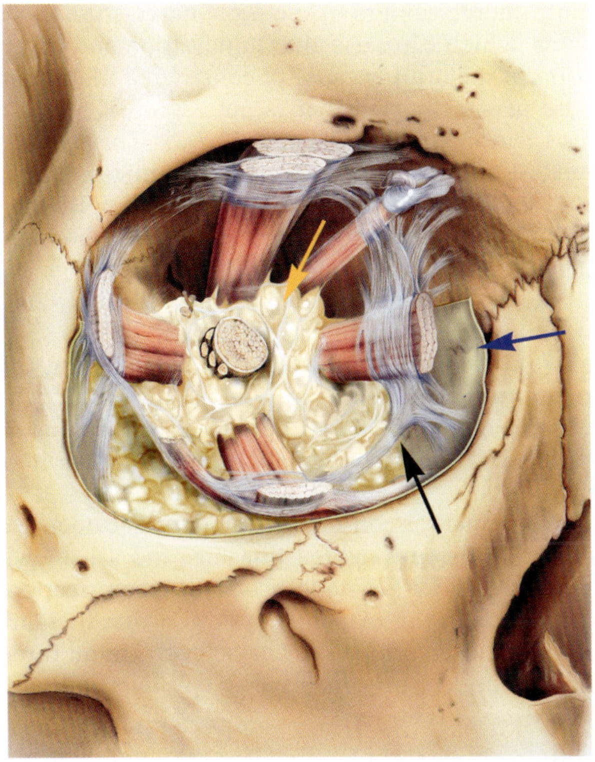

FIGURE 11.1. Anatomy of the right orbit showing the results of new research. The orbit has been opened, and the globe and Tenon's capsule have been removed. In the superior part of the orbit, the extraconal fat and the periorbital have been removed. The pulleys (faintly bluish fibers) insert on the orbital walls via the periorbital (blue arrow) but are stable because of their interconnections (black arrow) even when the pulley insertions are removed from the wall. The intraconal fat (yellow arrow) has fluidlike behavior, even though it is part of the same connective tissue network as the pulleys. (With permission from M. D. Abrámoff, "Objective Measurement of Motion in the Orbit" [Ph.D. thesis]. Transatlantic Publishing, New York, 2001.)

by histopathology and response to treatment was found to correspond to the choline/creatine level in a prospective study.[26] Medium to high ratios of choline to creatine have been used as a marker for the presence of actively proliferating tumor cells, whereas decreases in the overall levels of choline, creatine, and *N*-acetyl aspartate, as well as increases in lipid/lactate proton resonances, were found to correspond to necrotic processes.[27]

MR Dynamic Color Mapping

MR dynamic color mapping uses a specific property of the orbit.[28] All tissues in the orbit are involved in motion during gaze changes, and changes in tissues change the motion of these tissues (Figure 11.1). For example, a tumor originating in a rectus muscle will move along the same trajectory as that muscle, even when it is spreading through other tissues. Once it has grown invasively into another tissue, however, the motion of the tumor starts to mimic the motion of the invaded tissue. If a tissue is adjacent to another tissue, it may or may not have similar motion, but the more connected the tissues become, the more their motion becomes similar.

Dynamic color mapping involves two stages: a stage of cinematic MR, where sequences of MR images are acquired with the eyes moving along different gaze positions, and a second stage, during which the motion fields in these image sequences are computed and imaged. Though MRI is able to image real-time motion (called dynamic MRI), it is at present too slow to do so in the comparatively small orbit at acceptable resolution.[15] Therefore, motion imaging uses *cine* acquisition. Here, the tissues are allowed to move over the full range of motion with small increments. After every increment (stop), a new image is acquired (shoot). The result is a sequence of images (Figure 11.2). The difference between dynamic and cine acquisition is relative, not absolute, because in the limit where the time increments are very small, cine acquisition is the same as dynamic acquisition. The term cine derives from "cinematic": the stop–shoot technique is comparable to cartoon animation.

Cine acquisition has been used to image the role of connective tissue in determining extraocular muscle paths,[29–31] the role of connective tissue ligaments in eyelid motion,[32] and the optic nerve path.[33] The motion in the anophthalmic socket has also been studied.[34] Cine MR requires gaze sequencing to allow the patient to gaze over the specified range. An example is the Snow White machine (Figure 11.3), consisting of a transparent acrylic half-pipe fitted snugly in the scanner bore. On the inside is a row with nine fixa-

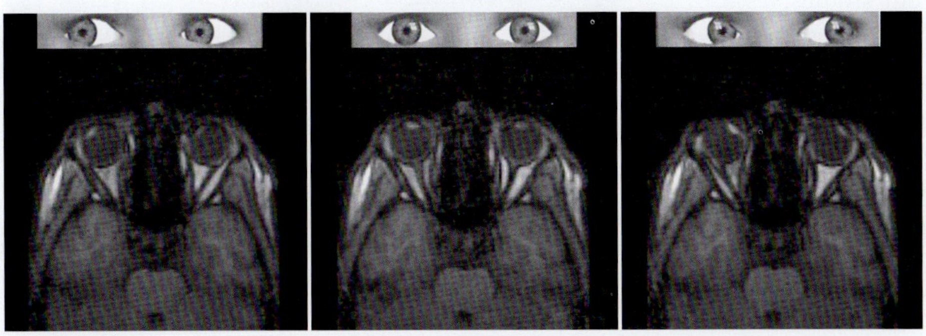

FIGURE 11.2. Typical frame of an orbital cine MRI sequence. The corresponding position of the eyes is shown. (With permission from M. D. Abrámoff, "Objective Measurement of Motion in the Orbit" [Ph.D. thesis] Transatlantic Publishing, New York, 2001.)

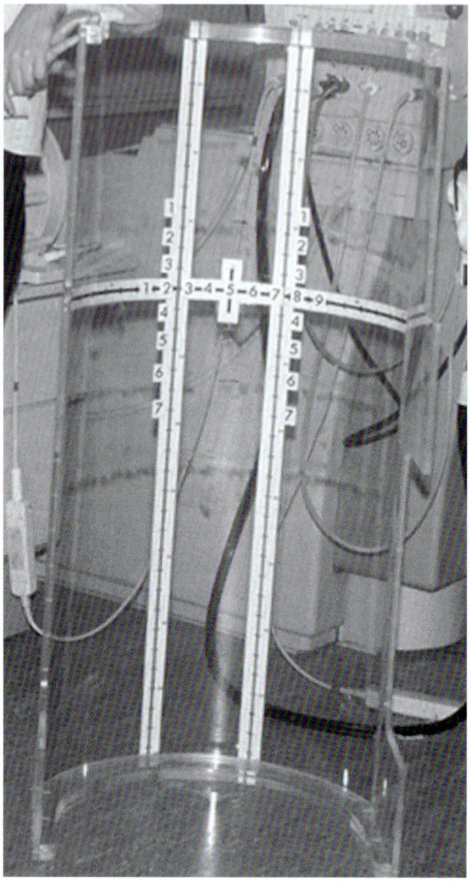

FIGURE 11.3. Snow White machine fixation aid. (With permission from M. D. Abrámoff, "Objective Measurement of Motion in the Orbit" [Ph.D. thesis] Transatlantic Publishing, New York, 2001.)

tion marks indicated with numbers 1 through 9. This sequence is horizontal, and the marks are 8° apart if the rotational centers of the eyes are 200 mm from the device. There are also two rows, vertical with respect to the patient's face, one 20° to the left and one at 20° to the right of the straight-ahead fixation mark. The Snow White machine was left transparent to minimize reactions of claustrophobia (Figure 11.4). To compute and visualize the two- and three-dimensional motion of the orbital tissues, there are specific computer algorithms.[35,36] The resulting images use colors to specify the direction of the moving tissues and also the magnitude of the motion (Figure 11.5). These images have been validated in recent studies.[35–37]

The use of two- and three-dimensional MR dynamic color mapping revealed that the orbit behaves similarly to the organ of gaze and that the so-called soft tissue in the orbit is actually quite rigid in the anterior, forming a skeleton, while the soft tissue in the posterior part of the orbit is almost fluidlike.[38,39] The cause of ocular motility changes after some forms of decompression surgery were also found.

MR dynamic color mapping has been used in the orbit to discover microscopic neuromas, small and painful nerve tumors in the optic nerve stump. Neuromas, which can arise after enucleation and implantation in the orbit because of constricted motion, can cause persistent pain that is not responsive to other treatment (Figures 11.6 and 11.7).[40] These tumors were suspected because the MR dynamic color mapping showed restricted motion of the optic nerve stump and attachment of the stump to the scleral cover of the implant.

MR dynamic color mapping may also help in determining the origin of orbital tumors, as was shown in two patients in whom the tumor was found to be originating in the rectus muscle because it moved in the same direction and at the same magnitude as that muscle and not with the optic nerve to which it was adjacent.[37]

In summary, a considerable amount of evidence exists for diffusion-weighted imaging, and a somewhat lesser amount for magnetic resonance spectroscopy and MR dynamic color mapping, to suggest that these may be promising techniques to characterize orbital tumors and help decide the *which-tumor-is-it* question.

Radionuclide Imaging

PET and SPECT are techniques that image the uptake of radioactively labeled compounds into tissue; these labeled compounds are called radiotracers and are usually injected intravenously. The subsequent tissue uptake of the radiotracer is measured over time and used to make a series of images. Although PET and SPECT rely on similar principles to produce their images, important differences in instrumentation and, especially, clinical use necessitate separate discussion.

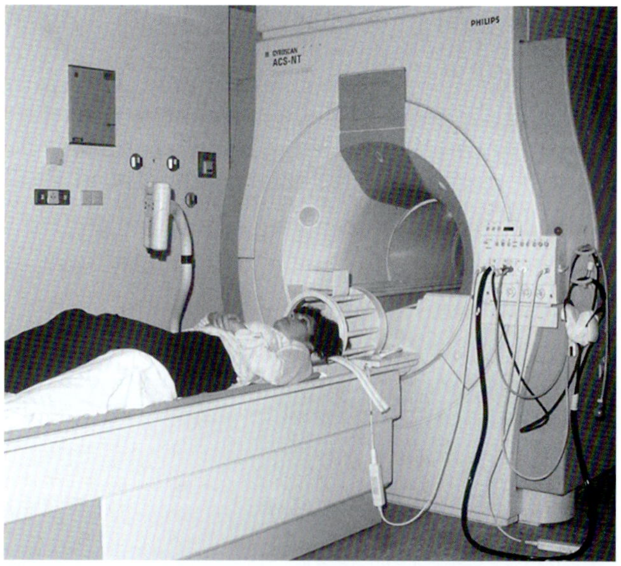

FIGURE 11.4. Patient being slid into the scanner; the Snow White machine is in place. (With permission from M. D. Abrámoff, "Objective Measurement of Motion in the Orbit" [Ph.D. thesis] Transatlantic Publishing, New York, 2001.)

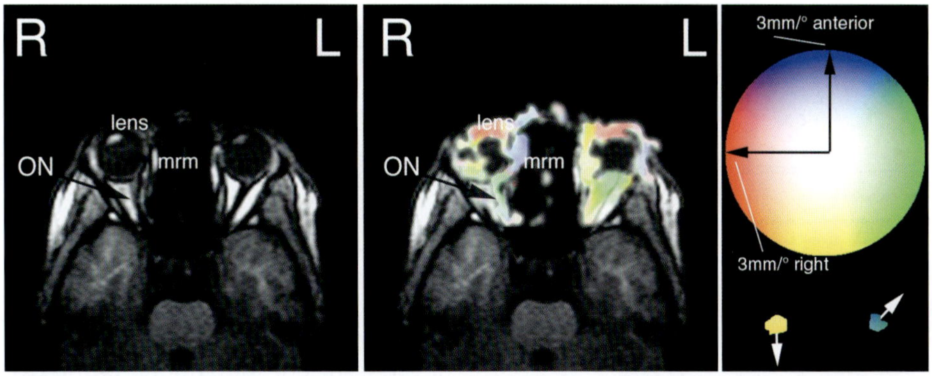

A B C

FIGURE 11.5. Normal orbital soft tissue motion imaged by MR dynamic color mapping. (A) Static MR image from the sequence. MRI images are as viewed from below. (mrm, medial rectus muscle; ON, optic nerve.) (B) MR dynamic color map. The subject gazes from left to right. Wherever the flow is zero or cannot be measured reliably, the original MR image is visible. (C) The circle serves as an aid to relate a particular color to orientation and motion. The arrowheads on the perimeter of the circle indicate motion of 0.3 mm/deg directed anteriorly and left, respectively. Blobs that move in the orientation indicated by the white arrows (posteriorly and left-anteriorly) at 0.3 mm/deg are included as examples. (With permission from M. D. Abrámoff, "Objective Measurement of Motion in the Orbit" [Ph.D. thesis] Transatlantic Publishing, New York, 2001.)

Positron Emission Tomography

A PET scanner is similar to a CT scanner in appearance. Instead of imaging the transparency of tissues to x-rays, however, PET scanners measure the emission of positrons (photons) from the radiotracer that has been injected intravenously. Because of the amount of radioactivity thus introduced into the body, individuals are limited to approximately five scans per year. After injection, multiple scans are made over several hours. Among the most commonly used positron-emitting nuclides are 11-carbon (^{11}C) and 18-fluorine (^{18}F). These nuclides replace the normal, nonemitting atoms in medically interesting compounds to obtain a labeled compound that is taken up into the tissue of interest. Thus, 18-fluorine replaces normal fluorine in fluoridated glucose, resulting in the labeled compound [2-^{18}F]fluoro-2-deoxy-D-glucose, usually known as FDG.

FDG PET takes advantage of the increased glycolytic activity associated with neoplastic disease. FDG PET has been shown to be superior to MR in the detection of squamous cell carcinoma head/neck metastases in a prospective study, although neck dissection and biopsy of lymph nodes remained necessary.[41] FDG PET has also been found to be superior to gallium scanning in the staging of lymphoma (Hodgkin's, indolent non-Hodgkin's, or aggressive non-Hodgkin's), with four patients reclassified to a higher stage, necessitating a change in treatment.[42]

When 11-carbon replaces 12-carbon, the resulting radiotracer compound is referred to as ^{11}C PK11195 (1-[2-chlorphenyl]-*N*-methyl-*N*-[1-methyl-propyl]-3-isoquinoline carboxamide). This compound binds specifically to peripheral benzodiazepine receptors on macrophages, and, in the absence of blood-borne inflammatory cells, on the surface of activated microglia.[43] Activated microglia proliferation is a marker

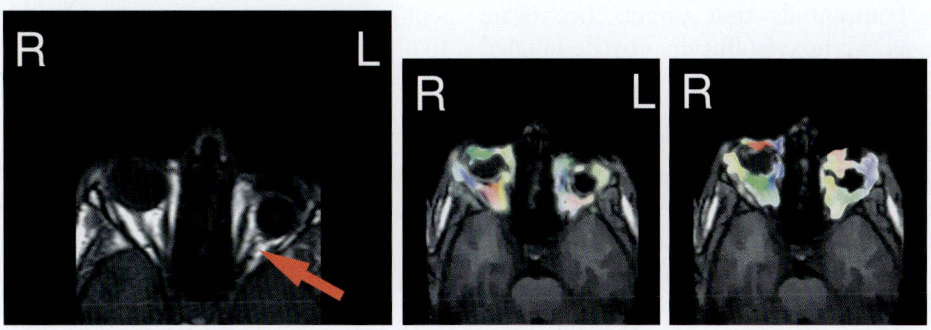

A B C

FIGURE 11.6. (A) Static transversal MR scan of the face of a patient who had persistent pain after enucleation with implant, optic nerve attached. (B) MR dynamic color mapping with patient gazing from left to right. (C) Same with patient gazing from right to left. The implant on the left shows decreased motion compared to the healthy right orbit (0.14 mm/deg) but moves concurrently with the stump. Shear is absent, and the optic nerve is continuous with the implant. (With permission from M. D. Abrámoff, "Objective Measurement of Motion in the Orbit" [Ph.D. thesis] Transatlantic Publishing, New York, 2001.)

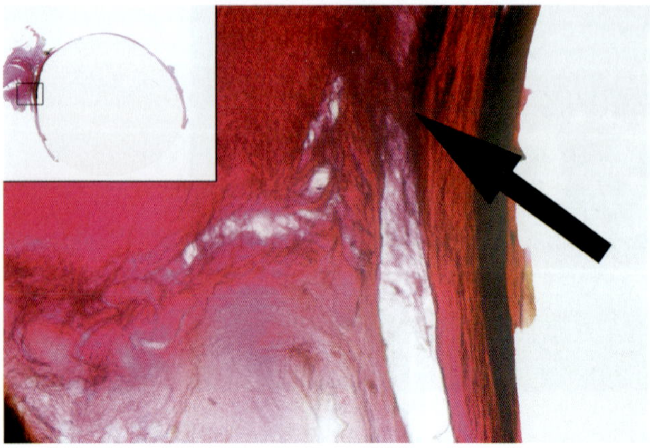

FIGURE 11.7. Histological section of surgically removed implant of patient who had persistent pain after enucleation and abnormal MR dynamic color mapping. The scleral cover on the right is connected to the stump of the optic nerve on the left by a mass of collagen fibers forming a pseudodisk (black arrow). *Inset*: Macroscopic aspect of the removed implant with the optic nerve including the remnant of the central retinal artery attached to it (hematoxylin–eosin, original magnification × 0.8. (With permission from M. D. Abrámoff, "Objective Measurement of Motion in the Orbit" [Ph.D. thesis] Transatlantic Publishing, New York,

of inflammation of and damage to neural tissue. Binding of ^{11}C PK11195 is minimal in normal nerve tissues and increases significantly in cases of neuronal damage or inflammation; the compound has been used to visualize activation of microglia in patients with stroke, multiple sclerosis, facial nerve lesion, and Rasmussen's encephalitis.[44] The suitability of ^{11}C PK11195 PET to detect inflammation in the orbit and along the optical tract is under investigation by the author.

Single Photon Emission Computed Tomography

In SPECT, a scanner is used to image the number of γ-rays coming from the tissue being studied. Therefore, different radioactive labels that emit γ-rays are needed, such as 123-iodine (^{123}I), the long-lived nuclide 99m-technetium (^{99m}Tc), and indium-111 (^{111}In). Just as in PET, these γ-ray-emitting labels can be incorporated into compounds that target the tissue of interest, such as methoxyisobutylisonitrile labeled with 99m-technetium (^{99m}Tc-MIBI), *N*-isopropyl-*p*-[^{123}I] iodoamphetamine (^{123}I-IMP), and [^{111}In]-DTPA-octreotide (^{111}INOCT). ^{123}I-IMP SPECT has been found to be sensitive and specific in differentiating uveal melanomas from nevus, as determined by histopathology of the melanoma specimen and follow-up of nevus eyes by ultrasonography and funduscopy.[45] ^{111}INOCT SPECT can differentiate the origin of mucosa-associated lymphoid tissue (MALT) lymphoma, including lymphomas in the orbit, as gastric or extragastric, as shown in a prospective study that used SPECT imaging to compare the histopathology of biopsy specimens.[46]

The radiotracer ^{99m}Tc-MIBI, probably a marker for mitochondrial activity, was found to be successful in differentiating malignant from benign orbital masses.[47]

Although not directly related to tumor imaging, SPECT imaging of Graves orbitopathy activity has been found to be effective: ^{111}INOCT SPECT was able to predict the response of Graves orbitopathy to immunosuppressive therapy and radiotherapy in 22 patients in a prospective study.[48]

The radionuclide imaging techniques are meanwhile well established in oncology. However, because of the issues of ionizing radiation exposure and cumbersome instrumentation needs, among others, they are still not available in many clinics, precluding their widespread use in orbital imaging.

CONCLUSIONS

The natural history of new imaging techniques usually starts with a first stage of amazement at the results of initial studies, with the new technique promising to answer a multitude of questions and clinicians clamoring for it. This period is commonly followed by the emergence of larger studies showing that the technique is not as universally applicable and effective as initially thought. Finally, balance is achieved when the new technique has become established and is known to be useful in a limited number of applications. The new techniques discussed in this chapter are probably somewhere in the first or second stage. Only future prospective studies of orbital tumors can show whether these techniques are really effective in managing orbital tumors and improving outcome, and whether they will be helpful in achieving "in vivo histopathology."

Newer, more exotic techniques offer great promise; however, there is not yet enough evidence from clinical trials to warrant their consideration for widespread use. Among the most promising new techniques is nanoparticle MR imaging.[49] Monocrystalline iron oxide nanoparticles (MIONs) can be made to bind (conjugate) to specific peptides that bind, for example, to a specific receptor. These nanoparticles are capable of responding to a radiofrequency pulse in a magnetic field, so that they light up in MRI. MRI can thus specifically image the concentration of the receptor to which the MION–peptide conjugate binds. If a receptor is chosen that binds to specific tumor cells, tumor-specific imaging is possible, similar to antibody-specific staining in histopathology. Currently, the emphasis in nanoparticle imaging is on searching for useful peptides that also bind to the nanoparticle.[50]

It is important to realize that good results from tumor imaging in other tissues such as the brain may not necessarily apply to orbital tumor imaging, especially in different types of MR imaging, such as diffusion imaging and MRS, because the orbit is surrounded by air-filled spaces, the sinuses. The air can lead to susceptibility artifacts. In addition, the scale of orbital pathology is usually much smaller than in the brain, partly because of the constricted space in the orbit; tumors often present earlier and at smaller size. Imaging techniques that can discriminate tumor tissue types in tumors 10 cm in diameter may not be able to do so in orbital tumors typically no larger than a few centimeters.

It is clear that a single technique for "in vivo histopathology" is not yet feasible. Instead, a large number of different techniques are available, all of them suitable to a greater or lesser degree for specific tumor types in a specific context. Since the techniques are so specific, it is very important to ask the right question. This implies that history and clinical examination in addition to *is-there-a-tumor* imaging techniques will remain essential in the foreseeable future, since they help decide which imaging technique should be employed to further confirm, rule out, or stage a lesion.

References

1. Howard GM. The orbit. *Arch Ophthalmol* 1968;80:667–680.
2. Downey DB, Nicolle DA, Levin MF, Fenster A. Three-dimensional ultrasound imaging of the eye. *Eye* 1996;10(pt 1):75–81.
3. Itani KM, Frueh B, Nelson C. The value of orbital echography in orbital practice. *Ophthalmic Plast Reconstr Surg* 1998;14:432–435.
4. Scott IU, Murray TG, Hughes JR. Evaluation of imaging techniques for detection of extraocular extension of choroidal melanoma. *Arch Ophthalmol* 1998;116:897–899.
5. Jacquemin C, Bosley T, Mullaney P. Orbital color Doppler imaging of optic nerve tumors. *Int Ophthalmol* 1999;23:11–15.
6. Wildenhain PM, Lehar SC, Dastur KJ, Dodd GD III. Orbital varix: color flow imaging correlated with CT and MR studies. *J Comput Assist Tomogr* 1991;15:171–173.
7. Hounsfield GN. Computerized transverse axial scanning (tomography). 1. Description of system. *Br J Radiol* 1973;46:1016–1022.
8. Peeters F, Kroger R, Verbeeten B Jr, Verteege C. The value of computer tomography, orbital venography and carotid angiography in the diagnosis of exophthalmos. *Radiol Clin (Basel)* 1977;46:430–438.
9. Maya MM, Heier LA. Orbital CT. Current use in the MR era. *Neuroimaging Clin N Am* 1998;8:651–683.
10. Stuckensen T, Kovacs AF, Adams S, Baum RP. Staging of the neck in patients with oral cavity squamous cell carcinomas: a prospective comparison of PET, ultrasound, CT and MRI. *J Craniomaxillofac Surg* 2000;28:319–324.
11. Dervin JE, Beaconsfield M, Wright JE, Moseley IF. CT findings in orbital tumours of nerve sheath origin. *Clin Radiol* 1989;40:475–479.
12. Rubenstein WA, Gray G, Auh YH, et al. CT of fibrous tissues and tumors with sonographic correlation. *AJR Am J Roentgenol* 1986;147:1067–1074.
13. Wenig BM, Mafee MF, Ghosh L. Fibro-osseous, osseous, and cartilaginous lesions of the orbit and paraorbital region. Correlative clinicopathologic and radiographic features, including the diagnostic role of CT and MR imaging. *Radiol Clin North Am* 1998;36:1241–1259, xii.
14. Han JS, Benson JE, Bonstelle CT, et al. Magnetic resonance imaging of the orbit: a preliminary experience. *Radiology* 1984;150:755–759.
15. Demer JL, Miller JE. Orbital imaging in strabismus surgery. In: Rosenbaum AL, Santiago AP, eds. *Clinical Strabismus Management*. Philadelphia: WB Saunders; 1999:84–98.
16. Lemke AJ, Hosten N, Grote A, Felix R. Differentiation of lacrimal gland tumors with high resolution computerized tomography in comparison with magnetic resonance tomography [in German]. *Ophthalmologe* 1996;93:284–291.
17. Thorn-Kany M, Arrue P, Delisle MB, et al. Cavernous hemangiomas of the orbit: MR imaging. *J Neuroradiol* 1999;26:79–86.
18. Gigantelli JW, Kincaid MC, Soparkar CN, et al. Orbital solitary fibrous tumor: radiographic and histopathologic correlations. *Ophthalmic Plast Reconstr Surg* 2001;17:207–214.
19. Cytryn AS, Putterman AM, Schneck GL, et al. Predictability of magnetic resonance imaging in differentiation of orbital lymphoma from orbital inflammatory syndrome. *Ophthalmic Plast Reconstr Surg* 1997;13:129–134.
20. Dalley RW. Fibrous histiocytoma and fibrous tissue tumors of the orbit. *Radiol Clin North Am* 1999;37:185–194.
21. Kono K, Inoue Y, Nakayama K, et al. The role of diffusion-weighted imaging in patients with brain tumors. *AJNR Am J Neuroradiol* 2001;22:1081–1088.
22. Guo AC, Cummings TJ, Dash RC, Provenzale JM. Lymphomas and high-grade astrocytomas: comparison of water diffusibility and histologic characteristics. *Radiology* 2002;224:177–183.
23. Filippi CG, Edgar MA, Ulug AM, et al. Appearance of meningiomas on diffusion-weighted images: correlating diffusion constants with histopathologic findings. *AJNR Am J Neuroradiol* 2001;22:65–72.
24. van Rijswijk CS, Kunz P, Hogendoorn PC, et al. Diffusion-weighted MRI in the characterization of soft-tissue tumors. *J Magn Reson Imaging* 2002;15:302–307.
25. Castillo M, Kwock L. Clinical applications of proton magnetic resonance spectroscopy in the evaluation of common intracranial tumors. *Top Magn Reson Imaging* 1999;10:104–113.
26. Shimizu H, Kumabe T, Shirane R, Yoshimoto T. Correlation between choline level measured by proton MR spectroscopy and Ki-67 labeling index in gliomas. *AJNR Am J Neuroradiol* 2000;21:659–665.
27. Preul MC, Caramanos Z, Villemure JG, et al. Using proton magnetic resonance spectroscopic imaging to predict in vivo the response of recurrent malignant gliomas to tamoxifen chemotherapy. *Neurosurgery* 2000;46:306–318.
28. Abrámoff MD. *Objective Measurement of Motion in the Orbit* [PhD thesis]. New York: Transatlantic Publishing; 2001.
29. Miller JM. Functional anatomy of normal human rectus muscles. *Vis Res* 1989;29:223–240.
30. Miller JM, Robins D. Extraocular muscle forces in alert monkey. *Vis Res* 1992;32:1099–1113.
31. Demer JL, Miller JM. Magnetic resonance imaging of the functional anatomy of the superior oblique muscle. *Invest Ophthalmol Vis Sci* 1995;36:906–913.
32. Goldberg RA, Wu JC, Jesmanowicz A, Hyde JS. Eyelid anatomy revisited—dynamic high-resolution MRI images of Whitnall's ligament and upper eyelid structures with the use of a surface coil. *Arch Ophthalmol* 1992;110:1598–1600.
33. Smiddy WE, Michels RG, Kumar AJ. Magnetic resonance imaging of retrobulbar changes in optic nerve position with eye movement. *Am J Ophthalmol* 1989;107:82–83.
34. Ghabrial R, Potts MJ, Harrad RA, et al. Assessment of the anophthalmic socket with dynamic cine-MRI. *Orbit* 1997;16:207–216.
35. Abrámoff MD, Niessen WJ, Viergever MA. Objective quantification of the motion of soft tissues in the orbit. *IEEE Trans Med Imaging* 2000;19:986–995.
36. Abrámoff MD, Viergever MA. Computation and visualization

of three-dimensional soft tissue motion in the orbit. *IEEE Trans Med Imaging* 2002;21:296–304.
37. Abrámoff MD, Van Gils AP, Jansen GH, Mourits MP. MRI dynamic color mapping: a new quantitative technique for imaging soft tissue motion in the orbit. *Invest Ophthalmol Vis Sci* 2000;41:3256–3260.
38. Abrámoff MD, Kalmann R, de Graaf ME, et al. Rectus extraocular muscle paths and decompression surgery for Graves orbitopathy: mechanism of motility disturbances. *Invest Ophthalmol Vis Sci* 2002;43:300–307.
39. Abrámoff MD, Volker-Dieben HJ, et al. Three-dimensional motion of intraorbital fatty tissue measured with 3-D MRI dynamic color mapping [ARVO abstract]. *Invest Ophthalmol Vis Sci* 2001;42:936.
40. Abrámoff MD, Ramos LP, Jansen GH, Mourits MP. Patients with persistent pain after enucleation studied by MRI dynamic color mapping and histopathology. *Invest Ophthalmol Vis Sci* 2001;42:2188–2192.
41. Jabour BA, Choi Y, Hoh CK, et al. Extracranial head and neck: PET imaging with 2-[F-18]fluoro-2-deoxy-D-glucose and MR imaging correlation. *Radiology* 1993;186:27–35.
42. Wirth A, Seymour JF, Hicks RJ, et al. Fluorine-18 fluorodeoxyglucose positron emission tomography, gallium-67 scintigraphy, and conventional staging for Hodgkin's disease and non-Hodgkin's lymphoma. *Am J Med* 2002;112:262–268.
43. Tagawa H, Okada A, Furukawa H, et al. Effect of topical timolol on the blood velocity of the iris microcirculation and aqueous veins in human subjects [in Japanese]. *Nippon Ganka Gakkai Zasshi* 1995;99:435–439.
44. Ishai A, Sagi D. Common mechanisms of visual imagery and perception. *Science* 1995;268:1772–1774.
45. Goto H, Usui M, Ishii I. Efficacy of (123)*N*-isopropyl-*p*-[(123)I]-iodoamphetamine single photon emission computed tomography for the diagnosis of uveal malignant melanoma. *Am J Ophthalmol* 2001;132:937–939.
46. Raderer M, Traub T, Formanek M, et al. Somatostatin-receptor scintigraphy for staging and follow-up of patients with extraintestinal marginal zone B-cell lymphoma of the mucosa associated lymphoid tissue (MALT)-type. *Br J Cancer* 2001;85:1462–1466.
47. Alonso O, Nunez M, Canepa J, et al. Evaluation of ocular tumors with technetium-99m-MIBI: planar pinhole technique or SPECT? *J Nucl Med Technol* 2000;28:85–87.
48. Gerding MN, van der Zant FM, van Royen EA, et al. Octreotide-scintigraphy is a disease-activity parameter in Graves' ophthalmopathy. *Clin Endocrinol (Oxford)* 1999;50:373–379.
49. Hogemann D, Josephson L, Weissleder R, Basilion JP. Improvement of MRI probes to allow efficient detection of gene expression. *Bioconjug Chem* 2000;11:941–946.
50. Hogemann D, Ntziachristos V, Josephson L, Weissleder R. High throughput magnetic resonance imaging for evaluating targeted nanoparticle probes. *Bioconjug Chem* 2002;13:116–121.

12

Orbital Biopsy

Zeynel A. Karcıoglu and Luis E. Remus III

Biopsy of a mass lesion implies tissue sampling for histopathologic examination. Tissue sampling can be done with different methodologies.[1–5] Orbital biopsy techniques include excisional, incisional, core, and aspiration biopsies and intraoperative biopsy with frozen section and Mohs methods; sentinel node biopsy is also utilized occasionally for staging purposes of certain tumors. Final diagnosis of any disease process is based on its histopathologic features. Most of the anteriorly located and well-delineated tumors can be excised in toto and provide ample tissue material to be examined histopathologically. Incisional biopsy material provides a moderate amount of tissue for pathological examination which is usually obtained from mid- or posterior orbit. Infiltrating tumors can be sampled by multiple incisional biopsies. It is easier to reach the mid- and posterior orbit with core or fine-needle aspiration biopsy (FNAB) techniques, but these methods provide a limited amount of tissue material.

All biopsies should be performed using appropriate sterile techniques and protective clothing and local or general anesthesia. Orbital biopsy techniques with their advantages and disadvantages are summarized in Table 12.1.

EXCISIONAL BIOPSY

Somewhat of a misnomer, "excisional biopsy" means histopathologic examination following total surgical removal of a mass lesion. Although this is not exactly a biopsy, "excisional biopsy" is a time-honored term that is commonly used among surgeons. This type of procedure offers a large tissue sample (Figure 12.1) to provide dependable diagnosis in a great majority of cases. It is important that the specimens be properly labeled before they are submitted to pathology (Figure 12.1).

INCISIONAL BIOPSY

Incisional biopsy is partial tissue excision from a mass lesion for histopathologic studies without complete removal of the tumor. This type of biopsy affords an adequate tissue sample under direct visualization. Furthermore, if there is any doubt about whether the sample is representative, a frozen section can be performed intraoperatively; if that sample is not satisfactory, additional tissue can be obtained. Incisional biopsy must be performed as a surgical procedure and most of the time as an orbitotomy under general anesthesia.

The surgeon should be confident that the biopsy material is representative of the clinically abnormal tissue and should ensure that it is not crushed or cauterized during its removal. Therefore, wedge biopsy samples and tissue plugs of the tumor should be obtained expeditiously. The hemostasis of the area should be accomplished with pressure after the removal of the biopsy sample. In frozen sections, the cauterization of the base of the biopsy site should be done once it is certain that no other specimens from the same area will be obtained. Fragile tumors of certain types, such as lymphomas and soft mesenchymal tumors, are more prone to crush artifacts and therefore should be handled very gently with the forceps.

It is important for biopsy samples to be processed expeditiously by the circulating OR nurse, pathologist, or technician, particularly if any additional special procedures such as special tissue stains, immunohistochemistry, cultures, gene studies, and flow cytometry are required. Most samples from incisional and excisional biopsies can be adequately evaluated by conventional histopathological methods of formalin fixation and staining with hematoxylin and eosin (H&E) and offer extra tissue for additional studies. However, in certain instances the clinical presentation, or a previous biopsy or frozen section diagnosis, may suggest to the surgeon and the pathologist the necessity of special studies. In these cases, it is wise to save fresh frozen tissue for future special studies. For example, if sebaceous gland carcinoma is suspected, the pathologist should be alerted at the time of the biopsy that a fat stain (oil red-O) may be needed and that a piece of fresh tissue for fat staining should be saved. Unfixed tissue must also be saved for the flow cytometry, molecular studies, and certain types of immunohistochemistry preparation. Most of the immunohistochemistry studies, however, can be done on formalin-fixed, paraffin-embedded tissue material. If numerous special studies are to be ordered from a single biopsy specimen, the on-service pathologist should be so advised and the tissue submitted "fresh,"

TABLE 12.1. Dos and Don'ts in Orbital Biopsy.

Biopsy	*Comment*
Excisional	Advise the pathologist and the radiologist if the lesion presents with atypical clinical features. Do a quick frozen section on an unknown mass before it is totally submitted in formalin; fresh tissue may be needed for special studies and cultures. Excise cystic lesions intact; a well-formed cystic lesion may be helpful for histopathologic examination. Do not cauterize small mass lesions and do not let them dry out before fixation; cauterization and drying artifact may interfere with histopathologic evaluation.
Incisional	Communicate with the pathologist. Try to obtain a representative piece of the mass. Do not cauterize the biopsy site or the bed of the biopsy site; cauterization artifact should be avoided if additional tissue is obtained. Try to obtain at least a 2.5 cm segment of temporal artery for biopsy purposes, and let the pathologist know that the entire specimen should be serially sectioned.
Core	Communicate with the pathologist. Do not use large trephines through the skin, only through conjunctiva. Make a small cut before using trephine/stylet complex through the skin. Place firm pressure onto the orbit after the biopsy procedure, followed by ice compress for 24 hours.
Fine-needle aspiration biopsy	Communicate with the radiologist/cytologist. Be sure that enough tissue sample is obtained for all pathology studies. If imaging reveals that the lesion is vascular, do not make too many passes with the needle and do not apply too much suction. Place firm pressure onto the orbit following the biopsy procedure followed by ice compress for 24 hours.
Frozen section	Communicate with the pathologist; invite him/her to the operating room and/or examine the frozen section in the lab with the pathologist when necessary. Orient the pathologist to the margins carefully, particularly on repeat tissues obtained from margins. Do not use the Mohs technique in orbit cases; it is easy to lose track of the specimens while mapping a three-dimensional surgical field. In recurrent tumor excisions, ask the pathologist to review previously removed tissues (if available). Do not undertake major procedures (e.g., enucleation, exenteration) based on diagnosis of frozen sections; remember the limitation of the technique.

that is, in a sterile specimen container *without* formalin or any other fixative.

If margins of the tumor excision are to be determined on permanent sections, it is absolutely essential to devise a labeling scheme with numbers or letters to mark multiple biopsy specimens very carefully, and to list every single one on the pathology request slip (as specimen #1: inferior margin, specimen #2: inferior lateral margin, etc.).

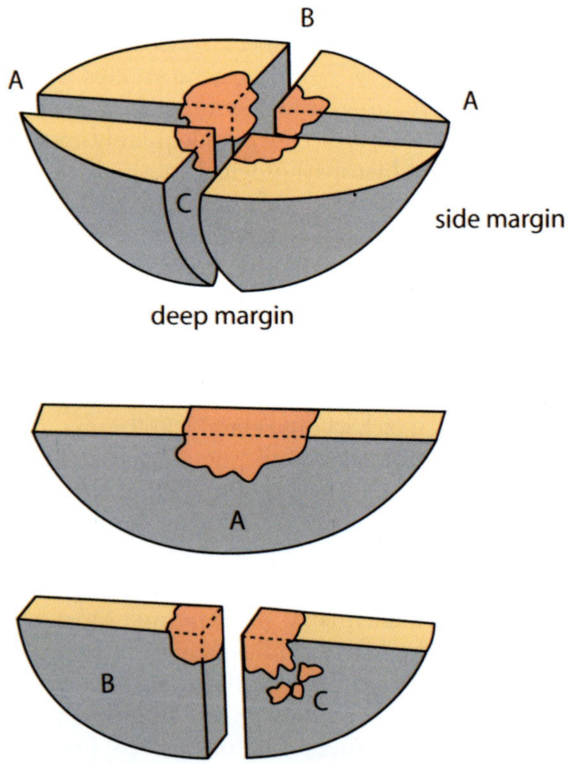

FIGURE 12.1. Sampling skin ellipse: The conventional way of sampling of a skin tumor for frozen and permanent sections.

CORE BIOPSY

Lidocaine 1% with epinephrine (1:100,000) should be injected subcutaneously and into the orbit in the region of the tumor approximately 15 to 20 minutes before a fine-needle aspiration or core biopsy. This amount of time offers not only good local anesthesia but also sufficient hemostasis within the orbit. Compression onto the globe and the biopsy site should be applied by hand for approximately 2 minutes after the procedure to ensure hemostasis.

Core biopsy can be performed with different types of instrument consisting of a trephine needle and an obturator (stylet) that fits inside the trephine needle. It is important to use a sharp needle with a stylet properly fixed by a locking device that does not move the needle. The needle harboring the stylet is then introduced into the orbit. When the approximate area of the tumor is reached, the needle is pushed into the tumor with a slight rotary motion. It is difficult to feel soft and partially necrotic tumors, but when firm tumors are penetrated, the surgeon feels a distinct yielding sensation. After the penetration, the stylet is removed and the needle is advanced approximately 0.5

to 1.0 cm, depending on the size of the tumor. The needle is rotated a few times clockwise and then a few times counterclockwise. The thumb is then placed on the hub of the needle, which is extracted with slight lateral movements. With gentle boring and suction application, a considerable amount of tissue can be collected within the chamber of the needle. If the attempt at the biopsy is not successful, the procedure should be repeated from the same entry site. If the second biopsy attempt is also unsuccessful, ultrasound or CT monitoring should be used on the third try.

In some instruments, a spiral fixator that fits into the needle is used instead of negative pressure to bore

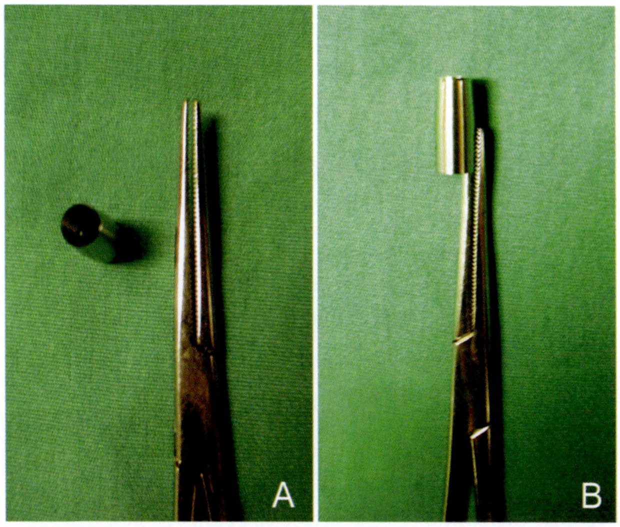

FIGURE 12.3. A pediatric corneal trephine (A) can be attached to a straight hemostat to create a useful tool (B) for sampling tumors located in the anterior and mid orbit.

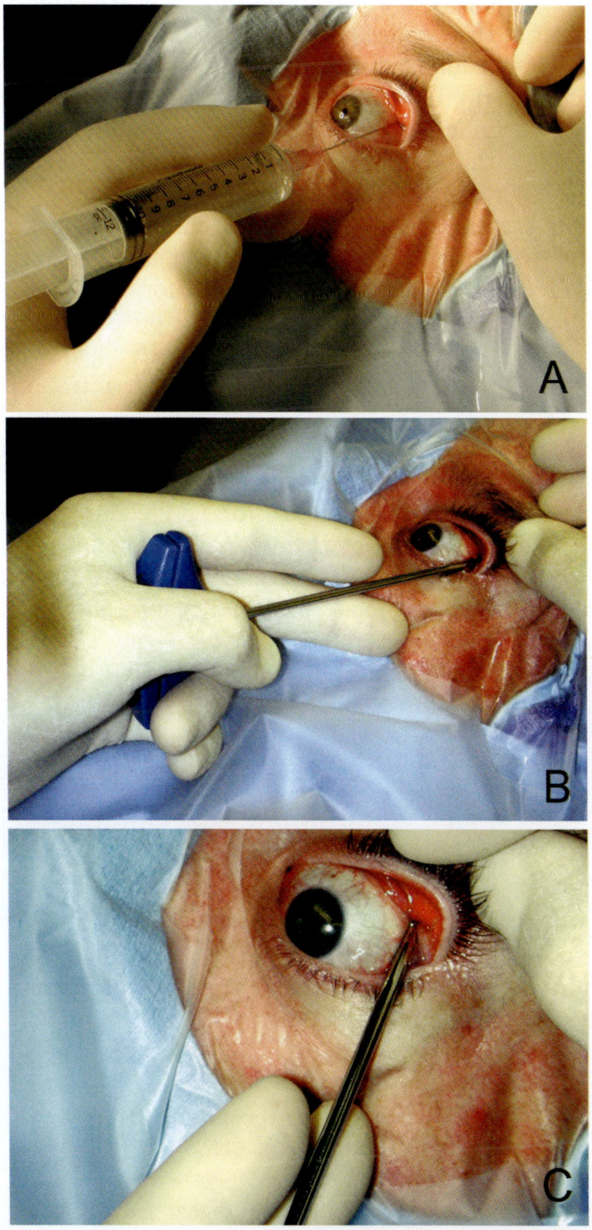

FIGURE 12.2. Core biopsy being performed with Jamshidi needle following local anesthesia. The Jamshidi needle's shaft distends slightly toward the tip to allow a generous tumor sample to be pulled into the needle.

into the tumor and pull tissue into the needle shaft. The author prefers to perform core biopsies with a Jamshidi bone marrow biopsy needle (Figure 12.2); because of the slight distention at the end of the needle, more tissue can be pulled into the shaft of the instrument.

If the lesion is anteriorly located and covered with a conjunctival surface, core biopsies can be performed with a disposable cutaneous punch or a small-diameter corneal trephine that easily bores into the lesion through the conjunctiva (Figure 12.3). The advantage of the core biopsy over the incisional biopsy is that the former can be done under local anesthesia without elaborate surgical exposure. However in some instances (e.g., fibrotic or nectotic tumors), tissue may not be representative for histopathologic examination, and core biopsy may cause bleeding more readily than FNAB, particularly after several passes. Most of the core biopsy instruments can be utilized under ultrasound or CT guidance (Figure 12.4).[2,3]

FINE-NEEDLE ASPIRATION BIOPSY

The main advantage of the FNAB over the other biopsy techniques is that it can be performed with simple local anesthesia or, in some cases, even without anesthesia in a rapid fashion in the clinic. The principal disadvantage is that if postbiopsy orbital hemorrhage occurs, the closed orbit may make management more difficult. Another disadvantage from the standpoint of tissue sampling is that the material obtained is usually scanty and can be examined only by cytopathology, ruling out histopathology. Furthermore, the material obtained with FNAB would be insufficient in most cases for other studies including

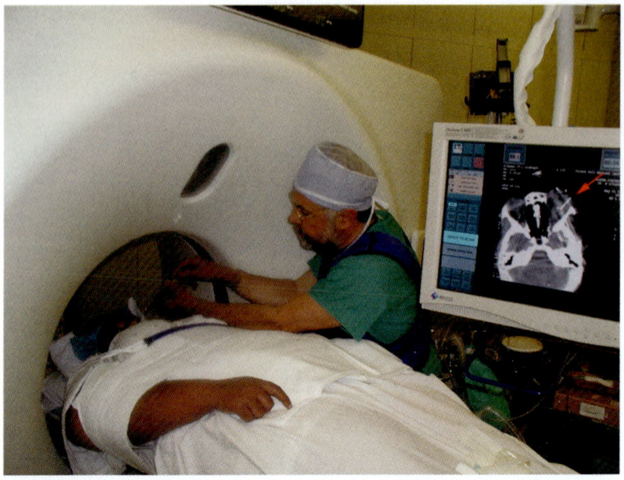

FIGURE 12.4. An FNAB procedure performed under CT guidance. Note that the position of the needle can easily be followed on the monitor.

flow cytometric studies, immunophenotyping, and electron microscopy.

Martin and Ellis are the first investigators credited with performing tumor biopsy, using a small gauge needle.[6] The procedure, although it was initiated in the United States during the 1930s, failed to be adapted universally. Instead it became popular in Europe among the hematologists and oncologists during the late 1950s and early 1960s.[7,8] In the 1970s interest in cytopathology and FNAB was revitalized in the United States, and more and more cytopathologists were trained in this subspecialty.[9] Furthermore, advances in radiologic imaging techniques, including ultrasonography, computed tomography (CT), and fluoroscopy, opened the door for surgeons and radiologists to perform FNAB.[10] The first use of FNAB in orbital tumors was by Schyberg.[11] In the United States, however, it was popularized by Kennerdell and coworkers in the late 1970s and early 1980s.[4,5]

Technique

Aspiration of anterior and midorbit lesions that can be palpated is easy. However, core biopsies, and in some instances incisional biopsies, offer better tissue material in these regions. Most of the lesions that require FNAB are located posteriorly in the orbit and cannot be readily palpated or visualized. Therefore, the surgeon needs to rely on information obtained from imaging studies. In the orbit, depending on the location, it may be easier to do the FNAB with or without an aspiration syringe pistol (Box 12.1). In many instances, it is possible to insert the needle through the conjunctiva, then advance it slowly into the mass. The positioning of the needle into an orbital mass is much easier when the biopsy is performed under imaging guidance. Once one is comfortable that the tip of the needle is within the tumor, the syringe may be moved back and forth with short quick strokes. To ensure that the specimen contains more diagnostic cells than blood, the needle should stay in the same axis to minimize bleeding. Although the range of the strokes vary with the size of the tumor mass, it should not exceed 10 mm, and the direction of the needle should not be changed significantly; one should always keep the anatomic limitations of the orbit in mind. Once the surgeon feels that the tumor is penetrated, suction should be applied to the aspirating syringe, usually about a third of the length of the barrel, and the junction of the needle and the hub of the syringe should be watched for the appearance of any blood or specimen.

When the sample is recognized, the vacuum in the syringe should be equated to normal by releasing the trigger of the syringe pistol. When the pressure in the syringe is equalized, the needle should be withdrawn from the orbit, following a curved path around the globe to avoid any scleral damage. The needle should not be withdrawn from the mass before the pressure in the syringe has been equalized; with residual vacuum, the small sample may be sucked into the syringe where it is difficult to recover and even if recovered may be dry and not suitable for examination. When the biopsy needle is out, gentle pressure should be applied onto the globe and orbit with a gauze pad, similar to pressure applied following a retrobulbar block.

If too much suction is applied to vascular lesions, particularly to lymphoid lesions, bleeding may take place that produces a poor sample. If bleeding continues following the biopsy, there may be a serious complication such as intraorbital hematoma (see Chapter 31).[12] Therefore, biopsy procedures for lesions that show significant vascularity with imaging should be performed with minimum suction and with limited needle passes into the tumor.

BOX 12.1. Equipment and Supplies Needed for FNAB

1. 10 or 20 mL disposable syringe with straight or Luer-Lok® tip or butterfly needle.
2. 21 to 25 gauge, 0.6 to 1 mm external diameter disposable needles
3. Aspiration handle (e.g., Cameco® syringe pistol, or Aspir-Gun®)
4. Vials of 50% alcohol, tissue culture transfer medium, glutaraldehyde, etc.
5. Alcohol spray fixative
6. Alcohol and Betadine sponges, gauze pads, etc.

Smear Preparation

Most cytopathologists, radiologists, and even general ophthalmologists are reluctant to perform FNAB in the orbit; the procedure is usually performed by ocular oncologists and orbital surgeons who are not well trained for the preparation of tissue material for the smears.

Smear preparation should be done immediately after the completion of the aspiration. The needle is detached from the syringe, and the syringe pistol is pulled back to fill the syringe with air. The needle is reattached to the syringe, and the tip of the needle is placed on the center of a glass slide, touching its surface.

Then a small amount of the needle contents is expressed onto as many glass slides as possible. Next, a second plain glass slide is positioned over each aspiration sample, and the two slides are pulled apart in a single gentle motion to achieve spreading. When all the smears have been completed, slides are fixed with appropriate fixatives, in most cases with 95% ethyl alcohol; a few smears are air-dried instead.

Smear preparation is an essential part of the FNAB. It should be done by an experienced person, not by a surgeon who does FNAB occasionally. It is important that aspirated material not be splattered onto the surface of the slide; it should be smeared thinly, occupying only a small area of the slide.

FNAB Interpretation

As it was commented in 1933, "Aspiration biopsy is as good as the combined intelligence of the clinician and the pathologist" (quoted in ref. 13). This statement is particularly true for orbital FNAB, since the procedure is usually performed by a surgeon and interpreted by a cytopathologist. Therefore, success will depend on the close working relationship between these individuals. The cytopathologist or an experienced technician, who will prepare the smears, should be with the surgeon during the performance of the biopsy. If a technician prepares the smears, the surgeon should contact the pathologist to offer information about the patient and the tumor that was aspirated. The information should include the clinical history of the patient, a detailed description of the location of the mass, and its consistency during aspiration. The surgeon's differential diagnosis is extremely helpful for the interpretation of the smear; therefore, it should be conveyed to the pathologist accurately. If the final cytologic diagnosis does not fit the clinical presentation of the patient, this should also be communicated to the pathologist with a request for another review of the slides or a repeat biopsy. The limitations of the FNAB in the diagnosis should always be kept in mind. Major therapeutic decisions should not be based on cytology findings alone, particularly when the cytology does not fit the clinical presentation of the patient.[14]

FNAB of orbital masses yields tissue material in 80 to 90% of cases and obviates the need for the open biopsy in approximately 50% of cases.[15,16] Char and coworkers reported that 15 of 17 (88%) of metastatic orbital cases were diagnosed accurately with FNAB.[16] The cytology examination may reveal a false negative result, primarily in tumors containing a considerable amount of fibrous tissue. In the series of Char and coworkers, FNAB was negative in one scirrhous carcinoma of the breast and in one lung carcinoma with fibrosis. Posteriorly located small lesions contiguous to vital structures of the apex are usually difficult to aspirate.

When the FNAB is undertaken with CT or ultrasound guidance, or with electromyography control, the yield may be better and the procedure may be safer.[17] However, in most cases, no significant morbidity is associated with this procedure. Another approach is to perform FNAB in the operating room, exposing the field with the mass lesion. The main advantage of this approach is that accurate sampling is obtained with minimum damage to adjacent normal structures of the orbit. Also multiple biopsies may be done with this method.

In another series, by Tijl and Koornneef, FNAB was performed with a 23-gauge needle without local anesthesia; positive cytopathology diagnosis was obtained in 43 out of 46 biopsies. Twenty-six of these patients later had incisional biopsies and the accuracy of FNAB based on the comparison of histopathological and cytopathological diagnosis was determined to be 57%.[18] Karohel et al. reported only 47% accuracy in FNAB performed under direct visualization.[19] Karohel et al. had rather low FNAB accuracy; however, most of their patients' lesions did not lend themselves to aspiration biopsy. Zadjela, Tarkanen, and Kennerdell, and coworkers reported much higher FNAB accuracy, reaching to 100% in some series.[15,20,21]

FNAB is a simple and safe diagnostic biopsy technique that provides information by establishing or excluding the diagnosis of neoplasm without any significant alteration to the natural behavior of the tumor.[22] Some authors advocate not using FNAB for masses anterior to the orbital septum; however, others consider it to be applicable to any orbital tumor because it is easy to perform and less invasive than other biopsy techniques.[5,18] It is also no more painful than a venipuncture; therefore, there is no need for local anesthesia. Because of this, the anatomy of the biopsy site is minimally distorted, and the tissue artifact secondary to an anesthetic injection is avoided.

The sampling error of FNAB is higher than the other biopsy techniques because of the indirect approach to the tumor and because of the small amount of tissue recovered as a sample. The diagnosis of pseudotumors and lymphomas is particularly difficult with FNAB.[4,5] Furthermore, inflammatory mass lesions masquerading as neoplasms such as Wegener's granulomatosis may be misleading with FNAB.[23] Furthermore, the sampling error increases in small lesions located at the orbital apex, tumors containing a significant amount of fibrous tissue, and lymphoproliferative lesions.

Complications

Complications of FNAB elsewhere in the body are not many; most of them are directly related to the needle size. A complication rate of less than 0.03% has been reported in large series when aspiration needles of finer gauge than 20 are utilized.[24] When minor complications such as discomfort or a small hematoma occur, they are of little consequence elsewhere in the body. However, in the orbit, a small but persistent hematoma may lead to significant clinical problems, particularly if it is located toward the apex of the orbit. In most instances, tumor seeding and tissue damage are not significant issues in systemic FNAB practice. In the orbit, however, tumor tissue seeding may lead to serious consequences. For example, if a superior lateral orbital mass undergoes biopsy with a presumed diagnosis of a lymphoma and turns out to be a pleomorphic adenoma of the lacrimal gland, the violation of the capsule with the needle may lead to recurrent tumors in the future. If a small dermoid tumor is aspirated and the contents leak into the adjacent soft tissues of the orbit, leakage may trigger an acute inflammatory process, which would make surgical removal of the lesion much more difficult. Therefore, the orbital mass lesions subjected to FNAB should be carefully selected.

Even when serious complications are not encountered, failure to obtain a representative specimen is higher in orbital tumor FNAB than in other parts of the body because of the difficulty in locating deep orbital lesions.[25]

Although FNAB is minimally invasive and quite safe in a great majority of instances, it has complications. A survey done among 202 ophthalmic/orbital surgeons indicated interesting but distressing results. In this study, 152 patients were divided into two groups. On the first group of 138 patients, FNAB was performed by an oculoplastic/orbital surgeon, and complications were reported in 10 cases (7 orbital hemorrhages, 1 extraocular muscle hemorrhage, 1 ptosis, and 1 cutaneous scar). In the second group, with 14 patients, the biopsies were done by other physicians who were not oculoplastic/orbital surgeons. This group had many complications including 3 orbital hemorrhages, 2 perforated globes, 1 motility disturbance, and ptosis. Three of the patients became blind and another 3 died. The deaths were attributed to direct injury of the brain during the biopsy procedure, to meningitis, and to brain abscess.[26]

INTRAOPERATIVE BIOPSY (FROZEN SECTION)

The use of intraoperative biopsy with a frozen tissue sectioning method originated in the late nineteenth century after the invention of the freezing microtome.[27] This technique was initially very slow, and it was not until the early 1900s that diagnosis during surgery with the frozen section method was accepted as a routine procedure. Even after the improvement of the frozen section technique, many surgeons and pathologists were reluctant to utilize it for decades.[28] Over the years, many of the technical difficulties were resolved and the anxieties that plagued the surgeon and pathologist when the technique was unfamiliar have been put aside. Intraoperative biopsy with frozen section technique is now available throughout the world and is utilized in all surgical disciplines.

Indications

The main purpose of an intraoperative biopsy processed as a frozen section is to enable the surgeon to make decisions that may change the therapeutic course of action during surgery.[29,30] Two primary reasons for frozen section in tumor-containing orbits and adnexa are to provide histopathologic diagnosis for the clinically abnormal tissue and to determine the surgical excision margins of tumor specimens to ensure the adequacy of the excision.[31,32] Lesser indications for the frozen section technique include the following: to confirm the adequacy of the tissue amount and/or nature for permanent processing; to identify inadvertent excision of a normal structure such as the lacrimal gland, peripheral nerve, or sinus mucosa; and to confirm the appropriateness of the tissue obtained for ancillary studies such as electron microscopy, immunohistochemistry, or molecular genetic studies.[33] Another very useful application of frozen section in the orbit is to differentiate inflammatory lesions from neoplastic ones. Once the lesion has been determined to be an inflammatory or infectious process, specimens are obtained for cultures, polymerase chain reaction (PCR), and other studies, and the surgery is completed.

Technique

To obtain the maximum amount of information from the frozen section biopsy, the tissue orientation must be accurately known. First, the pathologist must be familiar with ophthalmic/orbital tissues so that the identification of the tissue types (conjunctiva, lacrimal gland, lacrimal sac, etc.) does not present any difficulty. A critical step in tissue orientation is communication between the surgeon and the pathologist. It is beneficial if clinical information and intraoperative findings are shared with the pathologist; even better, the pathologist can physically walk into the operating room to observe the procedure and specimen collection as a means of orienting himself or herself to the anatomy and gross pathology. It is also helpful in many instances for the surgeon to walk to the laboratory and examine the frozen section specimen with the pathologist. This communication also is very useful to decide on further pathological procedures (e.g., molecular genetic studies or immunohistochemistry) and to ensure that the pathologist apportions the specimen accordingly. If there is any shortage of tissue, this advice could be relayed to the surgeon while the surgical field is still open. In complicated cases, particularly in recurrent tumor excisions, it is helpful if the pathologist can study the histopathologic sections obtained prior to the frozen section. For reporting purposes, direct communication via telephone or intercom is ideal; however, if the patient is under local anesthesia, communication by intercom should be done discreetly.

No fixative is needed for frozen section specimens; tissue should be placed on a piece of cardboard or gauze and kept wet with a few drops of saline or borate-buffered saline prior to delivery to the frozen section laboratory. In frozen sections intended for excisional margin analysis, labeling of tissue should be done meticulously and immediately at the time of excision. The tissue specimen from the margin may be placed on a piece of cardboard with its excision margin facing down. The direction of the excision margin should be clearly written on the requisition slip to guide the pathologist in determining the proper orientation. A simple diagram drawn on the same piece of cardboard helps to orient the pathologist.[34]

The conventional approach to excisional margin analysis is to remove the tumor and label the specimen accurately and let the pathologist obtain samples from the margins in the laboratory for frozen section purposes (see Figure 12.5). A more surgeon-friendly approach is to obtain the tumor bulk for permanent section processing and then sample and label the excision margins (e.g., M1, M2, etc. for the medial eyelid margins of an eyelid tumor; L1 and L2, etc. for the lateral margins) (Figure 12.6). In this approach, the pathologist should be oriented to the cut surface of the specimen and needs to know whether the cut surface of the specimen is placed up or down on the piece of cardboard.

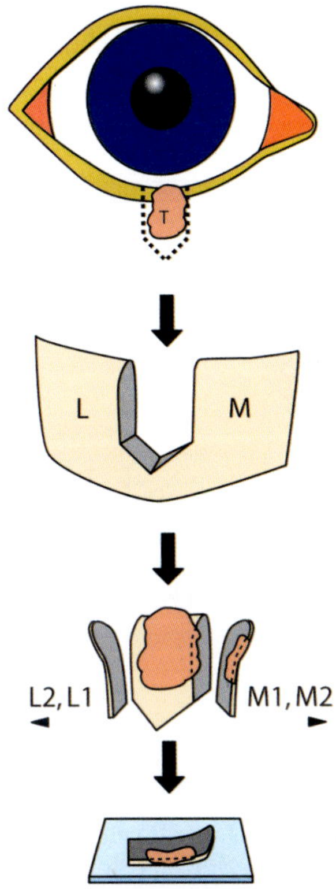

FIGURE 12.6. Orientation and labeling of the samples (M1, L2, etc.) for frozen section to monitor the margins of excision of an eyelid tumor (T). Note that the excision margin of the sample is positioned face down on a piece of cardboard. M: medial; L: lateral.

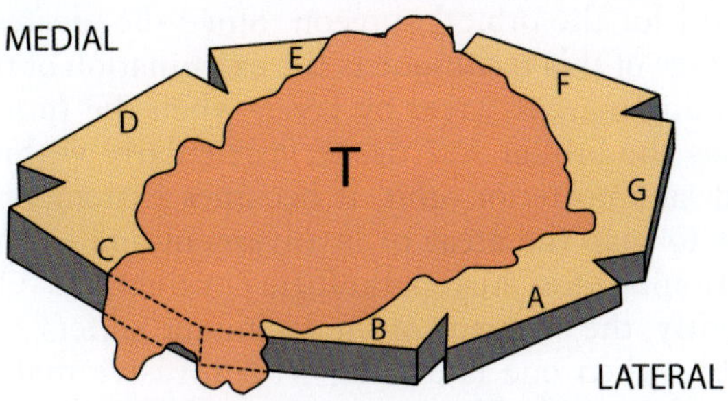

FIGURE 12.5. Diagram of the sampling technique from the margins of an excisional biopsy of an irregular tumor (T). The labeling of the margins should be marked meticulously at the time of excision to ensure accurate results from the frozen section. If the margins are not accurately labeled, the entire exercise is useless and may be misleading if tumor-containing margins are left behind.

The advantage of the conventional approach is that the pathologist has full control of the specimen and the deeper margins can be sampled easily. The advantage of the latter approach is that the surgeon will be better oriented to the margins with a list to hand and a simple diagram on the drapes. Such information is very useful, particularly if repeated margins turn out to be positive, since the surgeon knows exactly at what point the margin becomes negative (Figure 12.7). This method, which is the premise of Mohs micrographic surgery, can also be effectively utilized in conventional frozen section sampling.

To obtain the most accurate results from the frozen section, the labeling of the margins should be done meticulously at the time of excision. The labeling should be short and simple and clearly understandable

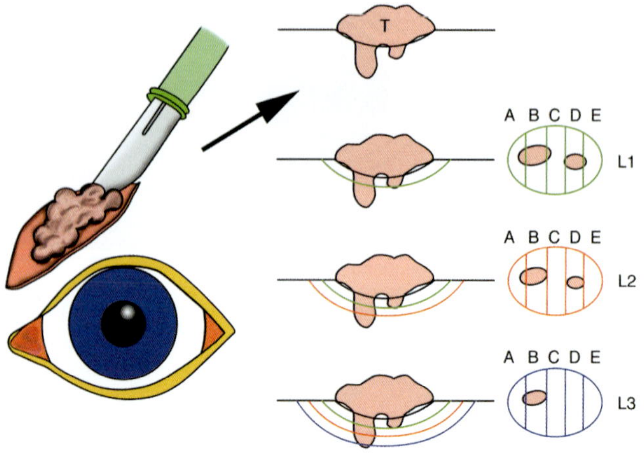

FIGURE 12.7. Diagram of the labeling technique for multiple frozen sections obtained from different levels of the tumor (T) excision; this is the main principle behind the Mohs microsurgical technique.

to the pathologist. Tissue removed for frozen section should be handled delicately to avoid crush artifacts at the time of excision and transportation. Most of the samples in ophthalmic surgery consist of small pieces of tissue. Even the slightest handling can result in crush artifacts, which in turn may produce misleading results. A point commonly overlooked by the surgeon who is unfamiliar with the frozen section procedure is that the margins of tissue remaining around an area of tumor involvement should not be cauterized until the tissue or frozen section submitted earlier has been proven to be free of tumor. This is because cautery artifacts would make it difficult to interpret the adjacent layer of tissue from questionable margin. Maintaining marginal integrity is particularly important with the deep margins of the excision, which usually involve the subcutaneous adipose tissue.

Frozen section diagnosis in ophthalmology is most commonly utilized in eyelid and conjunctival tumors rather than orbital lesions. For most of the localized presentations of basal and squamous cell carcinomas of the eyelids, the conventional sectioning of the skin ellipse (Figure 12.1) or the pentagonal eyelid excision (Figure 12.6) would reveal satisfactory information about surgical excision margins. If the margins are free, the primary closure takes place. If, on the other hand, one or all margins are found to be involved with the tumor, additional full-thickness frozen sections from the area of concern are submitted for further study. If the deep surgical margin happens to be involved with the tumor, additional specimens are obtained from the base. At this point it is helpful to map the base of the excision and code the deeper layers of tissues with numbers and/or letters (Figure 12.7). Thus the areas of residual tumor are marked on the diagram, and only those areas will be excised. Mapping identifies the exact location of residual tumor, and therefore uninvolved tissue can be spared; surgical excision is continued until the margins are histopathologically proven to be tumor free. This histographic frozen section technique is the basis of Mohs micrographic surgery.[35,36]

Mohs Microsurgical Technique

The original Mohs technique utilized tissue fixation, which facilitated the histopathologic examination but was toxic to the external eye. To avoid the toxicity, Mohs developed the fresh tissue technique, by which tissues are anesthetized and excised in the unfixed state. The Mohs technique, intended particularly for eyelid lesions,[35,36] has proven to offer very good cure rates for epithelial malignancies of the skin when the lesions happen to be located in flat areas. In a series of 7000 basal cell carcinomas and over 2500 squamous carcinomas of the skin treated with micrographic surgery, Mohs reported 5-year survival rates of 99.3 and 99.4%, respectively.[36] The reliability of the Mohs technique in the excision of eyelid carcinomas was attested by a 5-year nonrecurrence rate of 99% in 1773 cases of basal cell carcinoma and of 98.1% in 213 cases of squamous cell carcinoma.[37,38]

There is no doubt that the Mohs technique has helped to improve the prognosis after the surgical treatment of skin tumors, as well as eyelid malignancies, and has decreased morbidity and mortality. However, the great majority of periocular lesions, particularly lower lid tumors, can be effectively excised under conventional frozen section control. This point was eloquently summarized in Cook and Bartley's study: "When performed by a collaborative ophthalmic surgeon-pathologist team, results of excision with frozen section control may equal or surpass those from the Mohs micrographic technique."[39] Although Mohs microsurgery is a valuable adjunct, it should not be presented as dogma; it is important to select the surgical approach that best fits each individual case.

The Mohs technique is most useful for the morphea type of basal cell carcinoma and superficially invasive squamous cell carcinoma; in many cases of nodular tumors it is not necessary. It is also not very useful for the orbital surgeon. Since the greatest advantage of this technique is the examination of the remaining margins layer by layer, when the tumor invades the orbital soft tissue, particularly within the mid- and posterior orbit, it becomes extremely difficult to map the areas of involvement and orient the sectioning for histopathologic evaluation. Consequently, the accuracy of the technique suffers considerably when one is dealing with invasive malignancies of the orbit. The limitations of frozen sections in orbit tumor surgery should be kept in mind, and no major procedure should ever be based on frozen section diagnosis. In the orbit, the usefulness of the excisional margin analysis is less than the eyelid tumors;

however, frozen section becomes very valuable in the identification of tumor types such as lymphoma, rhabdomyosarcoma, and other sarcomas.

Interpretation of Frozen Sections

Since the main advantage of the frozen section is to offer intraoperative decision-making flexibility to the surgeon, the turnaround time for the diagnosis should be as short as possible. The average acceptable time is 10 minutes for simple margin assessment and 15 to 20 minutes for diagnostic biopsies.[31,40] However, turnaround times longer than 20 minutes may be encountered when technical problems arise or if several pathologists are reviewing a complex case. Even in the fastest hands, at least 5 to 7 minutes should be allowed per frozen section processing. If three or four frozen sections are requested to control the margins of a moderate-sized specimen, the surgery time can easily be prolonged by submitting tissue for frozen section study. Frozen section could occasionally add about an hour to surgical time. The patient and the anesthesiologist should be informed about this prior to surgery. The surgeon should keep the time element in mind and not order frozen sections casually, particularly if the permanent sections are going to be available within a day or two. Furthermore, if the frozen tissue is the only sample to be submitted for permanent processing, the freezing artifact may prove to be a disadvantage in the interpretation of paraffin-embedded tissue. It is a waste of valuable time to order a frozen section and then to close the field prior to knowing the results.

The surgeon and the pathologist should always keep in mind that frozen section preparations contain artifacts in comparison with permanent, paraffin-embedded sections. Frozen sections contain more wrinkles, folds, staining condensations, and distortions of cellular detail due to sectioning and/or staining defects. Frozen section diagnosis usually offers an accuracy rate of approximately 95% despite the limitations of the process.[31,41]

Discrepancies between frozen and permanent diagnosis can be put into two main groups: (1) sampling errors by the surgeon and the pathologist and (2) interpretation errors by the pathologist. Inaccurate diagnosis based on poor sampling is common. A common scenario is to leave the site of pathology outside the sample; therefore false negative results are more frequent than false positives.[32] This is also true regarding the interpretation errors. Tumor cell clusters that can easily be discovered in better quality permanent sections may not appear or may be overlooked in frozen section counterparts of the same block. It is, therefore, not advisable to undertake major surgical procedures such as orbital exenteration based on frozen section diagnosis.

Because of all these limitations, for a certain percentage of frozen sections, those interpreting the results cannot come to a conclusion and the diagnosis must be deferred until the permanent sections can be reviewed. Average deferral rate is approximately 4% to 5% in general surgical pathology practice; the exact percentage of deferrals in ophthalmic surgical practice is not known.[42]

SENTINEL NODE BIOPSY

Sentinel lymph node (SLN) biopsy is a technique that allows the early detection of metastasis within a clinically negative regional lymphatic drainage basin. The rationale behind SLN biopsy is to identify the patients who develop microscopic lymph node metastasis at the time of initial diagnosis and are most likely to benefit from lymph node dissection to avoid distant metastasis.[43,44]

The application of this technique to ocular and adnexal tumors was recently introduced by Esmaeli and coworkers.[45–47] The technique of mapping sentinel lymph nodes begins with lymphoscintigraphy of ^{99m}Tc sulfur colloid and isosulfan blue dye (Figure 12.8). Identification of the positive lymph nodes is done with a handheld gamma probe during lymphoscintigraphy, and the lymph nodes to be harvested for histopathologic examination are marked on the skin as soon as they have been identified. Skin incisions are made over the positive lymph nodes, and the lymph nodes that are stained with blue dye are identified and removed for histopathologic examination.

The harvested lymph nodes are submitted for routine formalaldehyde-fixed and paraffin-embedded sections; the entire node should be serially sectioned at 2 mm intervals for H&E staining. Depending on the

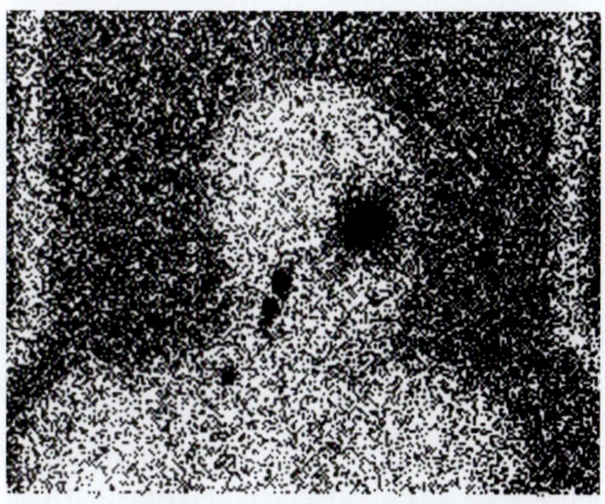

FIGURE 12.8. Sentinel lymph node biopsy: lymphoscintigraphy showing tumor-positive satellite lymph nodes in the region of a conjunctival/orbital melanoma. (Courtesy of Dr. Bita Esmaeli, Houston, TX.)

TABLE 12.2. Antibody Panels Commonly Used in Flow Cytometric Analyses of Hematologic Disorders.

	Cluster designations									
Diagnosis	*CD5*	*CD10*	*CD19*	*CD20*	*CD23*	*CD79b*	*FMC-7*	*CD25*	*CD11c*	*CD103*
SLL/CLL	+	−	+	+(w)	+	−	−	−/+	+/−	−
Mantle cell lymphoma	+	−	+	+	−	+	+	−	−	−
Follicle center lymphoma	−	+	+	+	−/+	+/−	+/−	−	−	−
Marginal zone lymphoma	−	−	+	+	−	+/−	+/−	−/+	+	−
Hairy cell leukemia	−	−	+	+	−	+/−	+/−	+/−	+	+
MALToma	−	−		+	−					

SLL/CLL, small lymphocytic lymphoma/chronic lymphocytic leukemia; +, positive; −, negative; +/−, often positive; −/+, occasionally positive; w, weak expression; FMC, Flander's Medical Center; MALToma, B-cell lymphoma of mucosa-associated lymphoid tissue.

tumor type, certain immunohistochemical stains can be used (e.g., S-100 and HMB-45 for melanoma, cytokeratin for squamous cell carcinoma).

Although with proper patient selection SNL biopsy is useful in the clinical management of early conjunctival and eyelid tumors, its application to orbital tumor management is limited and its significance in the staging of orbital tumors warrants further study.[48–50]

METHODS USED IN TISSUE DIAGNOSIS

From the time physicians are exposed to clinical medicine, the mantra echoing down the hall from the surgical pathology laboratory has been "If you want to know what pathology you are dealing with, bring a piece of sick tissue." Over the past two centuries, the histology laboratory has been propelled by numerous critical developments. Among these have been the improvement of reliable fixatives, manageable embedding materials, and, particularly, the invention of the microtome, which allows for preparation of thin sections with subsequent display on the traditional slide. One recent critical development was the introduction of synthetically prepared dyes or stains that enhanced the morphological characteristics of the tissue under study. Today we have made such significant progress in the diagnostic arena that we are no longer dependent on morphologic descriptions of multicolored tissue sections alone. Like many other fields in medicine, today's surgical pathology laboratory daily exploits the discoveries and developments coming out of research into the workings of the immune system. The use of specific antibodies directed toward specific antigenic sites allows for fuller elucidation of the biological characteristics of neoplasms. The application of flow cytometric techniques allows for the close monitoring of therapeutic intervention in hematologic diseases as well as enhanced correlation with surgical biopsy specimens.

We turn now to a brief and directed review of the varied techniques that are used to arrive at a tumor diagnosis; we discuss the methodologies and provide specific examples.

Immunohistochemical Stains

Special stains have historically been limited to little more than the use of natural and synthetic dyes to display or enhance specific morphologic characteristics of the tissue in question.[51] For example, a reticulin stain might be used on a suspected hemangiopericytoma specimen to enhance the morphology and evaluate the clustering of tumor cells. The immunohistochemical (IHC) stain utilizes specific antibodies that have been prepared by means of specific antigens isolated from a given neoplasm (Tables 12.2, 12.3, and 12.4).[52–56] Once prepared, the antibody is conjugated with a "tag" that serves to localize the antibody and thus the antigen in question. In the majority of cases, the tag shows up as a brown stain on a blue background. The use of a "panel" of antibodies allows the identification of a specific lesion (Table 12.3). Figure 12.9 is a composite photograph that shows some possible histopathology for a space-occupying lesion of the orbit: lacrimal gland tumor, inflammatory infiltrate, and large-cell lymphoma. From the clinical standpoint, any of the three histological biopsies could be representative of the neoplastic process. The sticking point is that two of the three diagnoses have potentially poor prognosis for the patient. Historically, the pathologist would study the tissue section(s) under various magnifications of light microscopy looking for various specific morphologic characteristics to arrive at a final diagnosis. The great majority of these preparations are stained with H&E stain. In current

TABLE 12.3. Antibody Panels Commonly Used for Study of Paraffin-Embedded Tissues.

Neoplasm	*Antibody panel*
Carcinoma	Carcinoembryonic antigen epithelial membrane antigen, neuron-specific enolase (NSE), and cytokeratin (CK) antibodies: CK-7, CK-20, panCK, and high and low molecular weight CK
Sarcoma	Actin, CD-31, CD-34, desmin, CD-68/KP-1, myoglobin, S-100, vimentin
Neuroendocrine	Chromogranin, NSE, synaptophysin, panCK

TABLE 12.4. IHC Cell Markers Commonly Used in Differential Diagnosis of Orbital Tumors.

Markers	*Tumors that react positively*
Muscle Cell Markers	
Actin	Smooth and skeletal muscle tumors
Desmin	Smooth and skeletal muscle tumors
Vimentin	Melanoma, hemangiopericytoma, most sarcomas, neurofibroma
Endothelial Markers	
CD 34	Hemangioma, hemangiopericytoma, Kaposi sarcoma, neurofibroma
CD 31	Hemangioma, Kaposi sarcoma
Neural and Neuroendocrine	
S-100 protein	Schwannoma, neurofibroma, glioma, melanoma, lacrimal gland tumors (+/−), Langerhans and non-Langerhans cells, histiocytoses
Neuron-specific enolase	Carcinoid, neuroblastoma, paraganglioma, Merkel cell carcinoma
Neurofilament proteins	Carcinoid, neuroblastoma, paraganglioma
Chromogranin	Carcinoid, neuroblastoma, paraganglioma
Glial fibrillary acidic protein	Glioma, glial tissue in encepholocele cells, teratoma
Melanocyte Markers	
Melan A	Primary melanoma, metastatic melanoma (+/−), lymphangioma (+/−)
HMB45	Primary melanoma (normal melanocytes are HMB45 negative), lymphangioma, metastatic melanoma (+/−)
Tyrosinase	Metastatic melanoma
Histiocyte Markers	
Lysozyme	Juvenile xanthogranuloma (JXG), Langerhans cell histiocytoses, lacrimal tumors (+/−)
Factor XIIIa	Fibrous histiocytoma, JXG, sarcomas, schwannoma, melanoma, granular cell tumor
Keratins (K) (cytokeratins)	Squamous cell carcinoma (K14, 17, 19), Merkel cell carcinoma (K8, 18, 20), basal cell carcinoma (+/−), lacrimal gland carcinoma (+/−), sarcomas (+/−), hemangioma (K18), metastatic melanoma (K8, K18)
Epithelial Membrane Antigen	Meningioma, sarcomas (+/−)
Metastatic Carcinoma Markers	
BRCA 225	Breast, lung (+/−)
ERs + PRs	Breast
CA 19 − 9	Gastrointestinal tract, breast (+/−), lung (+/−)
PSA, PSAP	Prostate
TTF_1	Lung, thyroid

practice, additional tools are available to the pathologist to facilitate the diagnosis—IHC is used almost reflexively. Routinely, tissue specimens are embedded in paraffin. Other techniques include the use of alternative embedding materials (e.g., celloidin, epoxy resin, and acrylics) and electron microscopy (transmission and scanning).[57,58]

The use of IHC, plastic embedding, and transmission electron miscroscopy as an adjunct to routine paraffin embedding with H&E staining gives the pathologist more tools to arrive at the proper diagnosis. In the case shown in Figure 12.10, the use of IHC revealed that the patient had intermediate-grade large B-cell lymphoma of the lacrimal orbit.

In the examination of other neoplastic processes that may be found in the orbit, be they primary or metastatic, the same use of IHC staining serves strictly as an adjunct to routine histologic study. Figures 12.11, 12.12, 12.13, and 12.14 show algorithms for using IHC to arrive at a final diagnosis. In all the algorithms, the starting point is the examination of the routine H&E stained slide. After the pathologist has made the initial morphologic diagnosis, these algorithms can be used to generate a final diagnosis.

Perhaps the most important point to remember is that communication between the surgeon and the pathologist is essential if a correct and appropriate diagnosis is to be reached. For example, most tissues fixed in 10% formalin are amenable to IHC staining when embedded in paraffin. However, this is not an absolute. On occasion the special staining will require fresh tissue, or the tissue will have to be prepared in a fixative other than routine formalin. One other consideration is that a specific amount of tissue might be required. Conversations with the pathologist will minimize potential diagnostic pitfalls.

Flow Cytometry

Flow cytometry (FC) is an analytical technique that again utilizes specific antibodies.[59,60] FC differs from IHC in that whereas IHC utilizes formalin-fixed, paraffin-embedded soft tissue, FC makes use of suspensions of live cells. The cells may be leukocytes isolated from

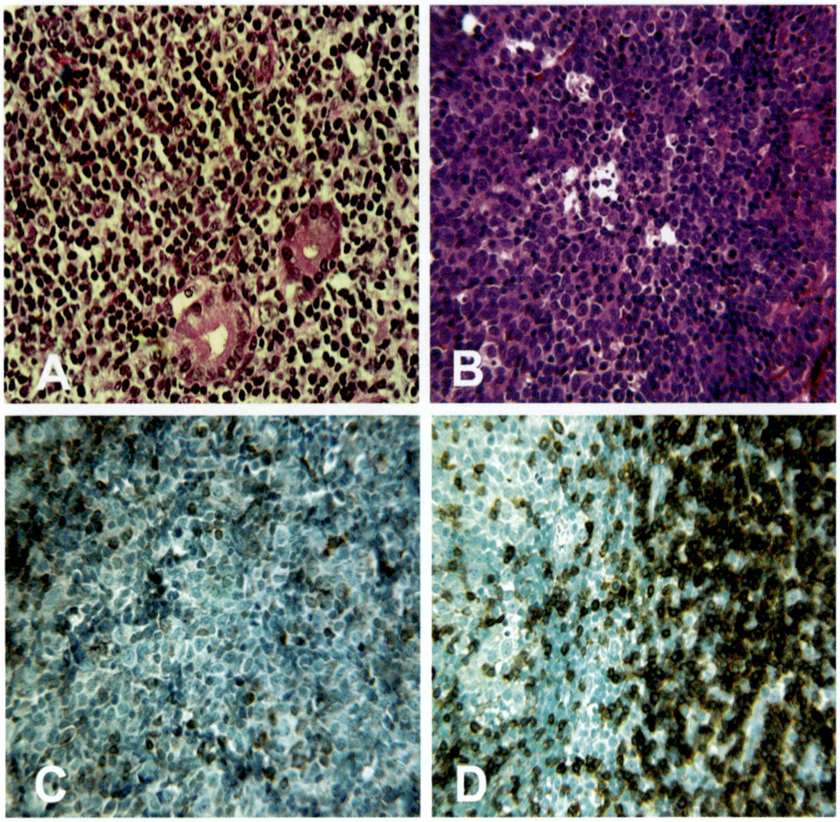

FIGURE 12.9. Combination of routine and ancillary testing. For the superior lateral orbital lesion shown, the clinical differential diagnosis included lacrimal gland tumor, inflammatory infiltrate, and lymphoma. (A) Intraoperative frozen section analysis showed that the lesion is not an epithelial tumor. (B) The paraffin-embedded sections were more compatible with one of the latter two diagnoses. (C) The combination of flow cytometry results [CD19 (+), CD20 (+), with κ-chain restriction–B-cell lymphoma], morphologic study of the routine H&E sections (mixture of small and large lymphocytes), along with IHC staining of the paraffin tissue (CD3 (+), CD10 (−), and bcl-2 (−) generated a final diagnosis of an intermediate-grade large B-cell lymphoma of the orbit.

the peripheral blood, a cell suspension derived from a solid lymph node, or cells obtained from a fine-needle aspiration. Regardless of the source, the cells are ultimately incubated with labeled/tagged antibodies. Once prepared, the cells are analyzed on an instrument called a cell sorter.

The data produced from this analysis allow for the differentiation and relative enumeration of the cells. For example, analysis of leukocytes from the peripheral blood would produce a graphic distribution as shown in Figure 12.15. The distribution of the data signals generated is based on two concepts: forward scatter and side scatter. Forward scatter varies depending on the size of the cell, mature lymphocytes being the smallest leukocyte and the monocyte/granulocyte lineage being larger. The second concept, that of side scatter, is a reflection of the cytoplasmic complexity of the cells.

Just as in IHC, the concept of analytical panels is utilized in FC. Because it uses antibodies that are reactive to specific cellular surface antigens, the FC profile, again, when coupled with a surgical biopsy specimen (e.g., a bone marrow core biopsy of bone), will allow for a much more specific diagnosis. Some of the more routinely used antibody panels in FC are listed in Table 12.2.[52,53,61,62]

DNA Sequencing and Antibody/Gene Microarray

The human genome can now be manipulated to such an extent that single nucleic acid substitutions are es-

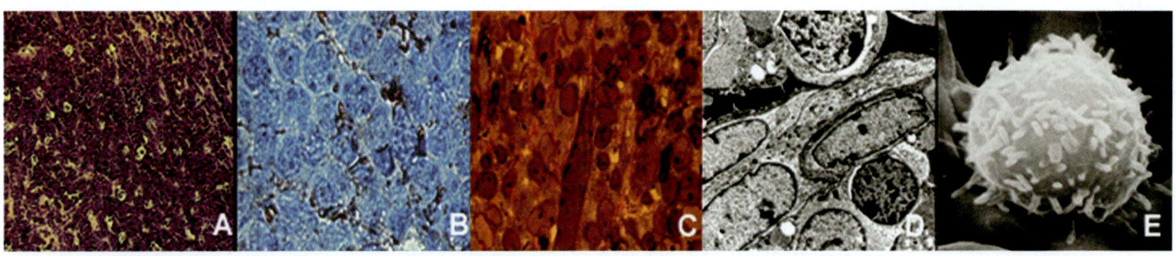

FIGURE 12.10. Alternative embedding and staining techniques: (A) paraffin-embedded H&E stain, (B) paraffin-embedded IHC staining, (C) celloidin embedding, (D) transmission electron microscopy, and (E) scanning electron microscopy.

37. Mohs FE. Micrographic surgery for microscopically controlled excision of eyelid cancers. *Arch Ophthalmol* 1986;104:901–909.
38. Anderson RL. Mohs micrographic technique. *Arch Ophthalmol* 1986;104:818–819.
39. Cook C, Bartley G. Treatment options and future prospects for the management of eyelid malignancies: an evidence-based update. *Ophthalmology* 2001;108:2088–2098.
40. Novis DA, Zarbo RJ. Interinstitutional comparison of frozen section turnaround time. *Arch Pathol Lab Med* 1997;121:559–567.
41. Ferreiro JA, Mayers JL, Bostwick DJ. Accuracy of frozen section diagnosis in surgical pathology: review of a one-year experience, 24,880 cases at Mayo Clinic. *Mayo Clin Proc* 1995;70:1137–1141.
42. Zarbo RJ, Hoffman GG, Howanitz PJ. Interinstitutional comparison of frozen section consultation. CAP Q-Probe Study of 79,647 consultations in 297 North American institutions. *Arch Pathol Lab Med* 1991;115:118–194.
43. Bostick P, Essner R, Sarantou T, et al. Intraoperative lymphatic mapping for early stage melanoma of the head and neck. *Am J Surg* 1997;174:536–539.
44. Morton DL, Wen DR, Foshag LJ, et al. Intraoperative lymphatic mapping and selective cervical lymphoidectomy for early-stage melanomas of the head and neck. *J Clin Oncol* 1993;11:17–56.
45. Esmaeli B, et al. Advances in the management of malignant tumors of the eyelid and conjunctiva. *Int Ophthalmol Clin* 2002;42:151–162.
46. Esmaeli B. Sentinel lymph node mapping for patients with cutaneous and conjunctival melanoma. *Ophthalmic Plast Reconstr Surg* 2000;16:170–172.
47. Esmaeli B. Sentinel node biopsy as a tool for accurate staging of eyelid and conjunctival malignancies. *Curr Opin Ophthalmol* 2002;13:317–323.
48. Naderi A, Hidajil, et al. *Arch Opthalmol* 2002;120:646–648.
49. Solorzano MJ, Ross M, Mansfield P, et al. Role of sentinel node biopsy in Merkel cell carcinoma patients. *Proc Am Soc Clin Oncol* 2001;20:358–361.
50. Cochran AJ. Surgical pathology remains pivotal in evaluation of sentinel lymph nodes. *Am J Surg Pathol* 1999;23:1169–1172.
51. Bancroft JD, Gamble M. *Theory and Practice of Histological Techniques*. 5th ed. New York: Churchill Livingstone; 2002.
52. Miettinen M. *Diagnostic Soft Tissue Pathology*. New York: Churchill Livingstone; 2003.
53. Weiss, SW, Goldblum, JR,. *Enzinger and Weiss's Soft Tissue Tumors*. 4th ed. St Louis: CV Mosby; 2001.
54. Swanson PE, Wick MR. Soft tissue tumors. In: Colvin RB, Bhan AK, McCluskey RT, eds. *Diagnostic Immunopathology*. New York: Raven Press; 1995:599–631.
55. Ordonez NG. Application of immunocytochemistry in the diagnosis of soft tissue sarcomas: a review and update. *Adv Anat Pathol* 1998;5:67–85.
56. Miettinen M. Immunohistochemistry of soft tissue tumors. *J Histotechnol* 1999;22:219–227.
57. Erlandson RA, Woodruff JM. Role of electronmicroscopy in the evaluation of soft tissue neoplasms with emphasis on spindle cell and pleomorphic tumor. *Hum Pathol* 1998;29:1372–1981.
58. Ordonez MG, Mackay B. Electron microscopy in tumor diagnosis: Indications for its use in the immunohistochemical era. *Hum Pathol* 1998;29:1403–1411.
59. Stewart CC, Stewart, SJ. Cell preparation for the identification of leukocytes, In: Darzynkiewicz, Z, Robinson, JP, Crissman, GA, eds. *Flow Cytometry*. 2nd ed. San Diego, CA: Academic Press; 1994.
60. Keren, DF, McCoy, JP, Carey, JL. *Flow Cytometry in Clinical Diagnosis*. 3rd ed. Chicago: American Society for Clinical Pathology Press; 2001.
61. Dabbs, DJ. *Diagnostic Immunohistochemistry*. New York: Churchill Livingstone; 2002.
62. O'Leary, TJ. *Advanced Diagnostic Methods in Pathology: Principles, Practice, and Protocols. Philadelphia: WB Saunders; 2003.*
63. Adams, M, Fields, C, Venter, J. *Automated DAN Sequencing and Analysis*. San Diego, CA: Academic Press; 1994.
64. Brown, TA. *DNA Sequencing: The Basics*. Oxford: IRL Press; 1994.
65. Causton HC, Quackenbush J, Brazma A. *Microarray Gene Expression: A Beginner's Guide*. Edinburgh: Blackwell; 2003.
66. Jordan, B. *DAN Microarrays: Gene Expression Applications*, New York: Springer-Verlag; 2001.
67. Strachan, T, Read, AP. *Human Molecular Genetics*. 2nd ed. New York: Wiley-Liss; 1999.
68. Sharara N, Holden JT, Wojon TH, et al. Ocular adnexal lymphoid proliferations. *Ophthalmology* 2003;110:1245–1254.
69. Lenkins C, Rose GE, Bunce C, et al. Histological features of ocular adnexal lymphoma (REAL classification) and their association with patient morbidity and survival. *Br J Ophthalmol* 2000:84:907–913.
70. Couplan SE, Krause L, Delecluse HJ, et al. Lymphoproliferative lesions of the ocular adnexa: analysis of 112 cases. *Ophthalmology* 1998;105:1430–1441.
71. The Nobel Foundation. http://www.nobel.se/medicine/laureates/1959
72. Mullis K, Faloona F, Scharf S, et al. Specific enzymatic amplification of DNA in vitro: the polymerase chain reaction. *Cold Spring Harbor Symp Quant Biol* 1986;51:263–273.
73. Mullis KB, Faloona F. Specific synthesis of DNA in vitro via a polymerase-catalyzed chain reaction. *Methods Enzymol* 1987;155:335–350.
74. Brock TD. *Brock Biology of Microorganisms*. Upper Saddle River, NJ: Prentice Hall, 2002.
75. Leonard DGB. *Diagnostic Molecular Pathology*. Philadelphia: WB Saunders; 2003.

PART THREE

Primary Tumors of the Orbit

13

Orbital Lymphoma

Bita Esmaeli and Misha Faustina

Malignant lymphomas are neoplastic transformations of cells that reside predominantly within lymphoid tissues. Lymphoid tumors are the most common primary orbital malignancy in adults,[1,2] yet they constitute only about 2% of all lymphomas.[3] Many studies have described the clinical and histopathologic features of primary orbital lymphomas.[1–4] However, the advent and popularity of more sophisticated diagnostic tests such as positron emission tomography (PET) and gastrointestinal endoscopy will often lead to discovery of lymphoma elsewhere in the body of a patient who has orbital or ocular adnexal lymphoma. This chapter discusses the classification and staging workup for primary orbital lymphomas as well as the characteristics and course of systemic non-Hodgkin's lymphoma (NHL), which may secondarily spread to the orbit or present with involvement of the orbit at the time of initial diagnosis of systemic lymphoma.[5,6] The section entitled Management reviews the treatment options currently available for orbital lymphoma. The majority of published reports focus on the use of external-beam radiation therapy or systemic chemotherapy for treatment of orbital lymphoma.[7–11] In addition to these modalities, more recent treatment options are discussed, such as immunotherapy (monoclonal antibody therapy), which may be effective in the treatment of low-grade non-Hodgkin's lymphoma of the orbit.[12]

CLINICAL FEATURES

Lymphoid tumors are the most common primary orbital malignancy,[1,2] constituting approximately 10% of all orbital tumors and 40 to 60% of lymphoproliferative disease in the orbit.[5] The majority of orbital lymphomas are non-Hodgkin's type and are seen primarily in adults in the 50- to 70-year age group.

Orbital lymphomas are usually unilateral but may involve both orbits and demonstrate a predilection for the lacrimal gland. Patients with orbital lymphoma usually present with a painless proptosis of insidious onset, downward displacement of the globe, eyelid edema, a palpable nontender orbital mass, and ptosis (Figure 13.1). Imaging studies usually confirm the presence of a mass, most commonly in the superior and anterior orbit but less commonly deep in the orbital apex (Figure 13.2).

The distinction between "primary" and "secondary" orbital lymphoma is somewhat arbitrary. Primary lymphomas are thought to be isolated to the orbit, with the orbit as the only extranodal site of involvement of lymphoma. Thus, by definition, "primary" orbital lymphomas are stage I. Secondary orbital lymphomas are those in which the orbit is a secondary extranodal site of involvement either where there was a previously diagnosed NHL or where the orbital lymphoma is diagnosed simultaneously with the discovery of systemic lymphoma. Given the more recent sensitive tools such as PET for detecting small foci of lymphoma and the routine use of bone marrow biopsies as part of the staging workup, we suspect that the incidence of truly "primary" orbital lymphoma is lower than suggested in most textbooks. Table 13.1 compares some features of what have been termed primary versus secondary orbital lymphomas, although these distinctions are somewhat arbitrary and not applicable to every patient with orbital lymphoma.[6]

MORPHOLOGIC FEATURES

Accurate histopathologic evaluation is the most critical diagnostic step in the management of orbital lymphomas. Open incisional biopsy or fine-needle aspiration of an orbital mass that is suspected to be a lymphoma is often necessary to establish the diagnosis and guide management. Tissue should arrive at the pathology department fresh (without preservatives) and sterile. Care should be taken to avoid excessive crushing or manipulation to preserve the tissue architecture. Under the hood in the pathology laboratory, touch preps and permanent and frozen sections can be prepared. Additional fresh tissue is reserved for special lymphoma studies.[13,14]

Malignant lymphoma is diagnosed when diffusely arranged population of immature and mitotically active lymphocytes are found in the orbit.[15,16] Histologic hallmarks of this disease are monoclonal populations of B cells confirmed by immunohistochemical studies, with prominent nucleoli, chromatin margination

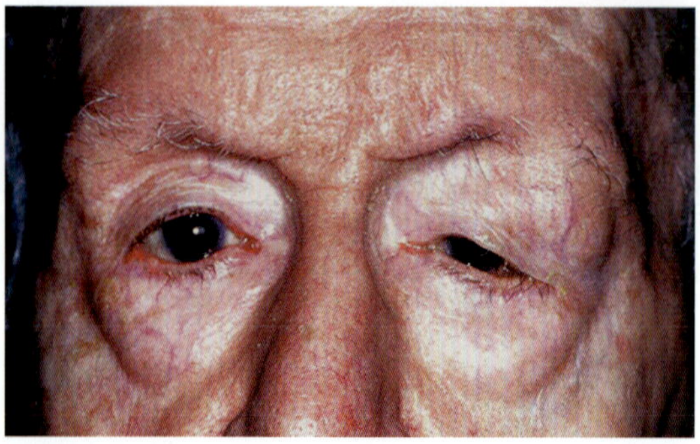

FIGURE 13.1. Patient with a left lacrimal gland mass causing mechanical ptosis of the left upper eyelid.

at the nuclear membrane, nuclear membrane irregularities, and cellular atypia.

In addition to sections prepared with standard hematoxylin eosin stain, lymphoma studies currently utilized include the following:

- Immunohistochemistry: a sensitive technique to identify antigenic expression of lymphoma cells, which can aid in the histologic classification of lymphomas. The numerous target antigens characterized thus far include CD20 for mature B lymphocytes, CD10 for precursor B lymphocytes, and many others that help classify the lymphoma.
- Flow cytometry: measures cellular parameters while a suspension of sampled cells flows through a laser beam. Clonality of lymphocytes can be rapidly determined with flow cytometry.
- Cytogenetics studies: evaluate chromosomal deletions, additions, and translocations by gene karyotyping and are useful in evaluating tumors with characteristic chromosomal abnormalities.
- Molecular studies of the biopsied tissue: can provide additional information that may help characterize the type of lymphoma. The polymerase chain reaction can amplify the DNA or RNA, allowing for detection of minute genetic aberrations.

Approximately 85 to 90% of orbital lymphomas are low-grade, diffuse proliferations of small, monoclonal B-cell lymphocytes (Figure 13.3). The remaining 10 to 15% have follicular or nodular characteristics. Lesions displaying high mitotic activity are most likely associated with extraorbital disease. Follicular lesions with germinal centers are more likely indicative of localized disease.

CLASSIFICATION

Histologic classification of lymphoma has evolved and improved as newer techniques are utilized to elucidate the antigenic expression, cytogenetic features, and molecular characteristics of lymphomas. In the past, the most commonly used system of classification for lymphoma was the National Cancer Institute's Working Formulation, which divided lymphomas into low, intermediate, and high grades based on their histologic characteristics and morphologic features (Box 13.1). The availability of monoclonal antibodies, which identify surface antigens on lymphoid cells, has helped the classification of lymphomas based on their immunophenotype. The chromosomal and molecular characteristics of lymphomas are now studied routinely and correlated with their clinical behavior. The Revised European–American Classification of Lymphoid Neoplasms (REAL) is the most recently and widely used pathology classification system based on morphology, immunophenotype, genotype, and clinical features of the lymphoma (Box 13.2).[17] In this classification, lymphomas are categorized as indolent, aggressive, or highly aggressive. In addition to the histologic subtypes included in the earlier classification schemes, several new entities, such as the peripheral T-cell lymphomas, are included in REAL.[18]

INVESTIGATION

As with lymphomas in other sites, detailed investigation is necessary to determine the stage of the disease before a definitive treatment plan is established.[19] A thorough staging workup is necessary to identify patients with orbital lymphoma who may harbor additional foci of lymphoma throughout the body, thus requiring systemic or combined-modality treatment.

A complete history and physical examination may provide evidence of systemic, although clinically silent, disease or presence of constitutional signs. In addition to a usually painless and nontender orbital

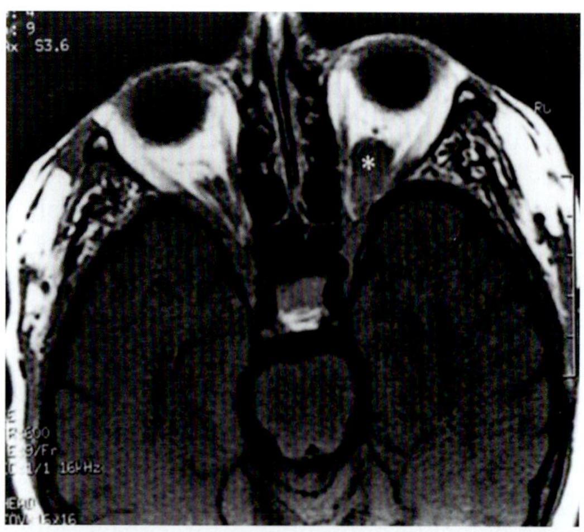

FIGURE 13.2. Axial noncontrast, T1-weighted magnetic resonance image of an intraconal lymphoma in the posterior left orbit (asterisk).

TABLE 13.1. Primary vs Secondary Orbital Lymphomas.

	Primary lymphomas	*Secondary lymphomas*
Characteristics	Isolated, extranodal, orbit is often the first site of lymphoma involvement	Disseminated, systemic involvement, may appear late as part of generalized relapse
Location	Usually unilateral	Usually unilateral
Age	Most common in 50- to 70-year-old age group	Most common in 50- to 70-year old age group, but younger patients more likely to have high-grade lymphomas
Sex	M = F	M = F
Histology	Low-grade, indolent, small lymphocytic, follicular, or MALT	More often intermediate- or high-grade (diffuse mixed or large cell type) but low-grade secondary orbital lymphomas also common

mass, which may be palpable or visible during the examination, there may be visual loss due to compressive optic neuropathy, a condition revealed by a thorough ophthalmic examination.

Box 13.3 summarizes the recommended staging workup for orbital lymphomas. An imaging study of the orbit is critical in delineating the extent of orbital involvement. A characteristic diffuse to moderately well-defined orbital mass with molding to the globe, optic nerve, and orbital bones strongly suggests the diagnosis of orbital lymphoma (Figure 13.4). On computed tomography, lymphomas appear homogenous in texture and isodense to muscle, showing mild enhancement with contrast.

Fine-needle cytology or open biopsy of orbital and adnexal masses is often necessary to confirm the diagnosis and help with the histologic classification of orbital lymphomas.

Imaging studies of the abdomen, thorax, and pelvis are performed to rule out disseminated disease. A bone marrow aspiration is performed to rule out marrow involvement. Upper GI tract endoscopy and barium studies are done to detect gastrointestinal involvement and are particularly important for certain subtypes of orbital lymphoma, such as mantle cell lymphoma with a predilection for gastrointestinal involvement.

PET is replacing bone and gallium scans for detecting small foci of lymphoma throughout the body.

A

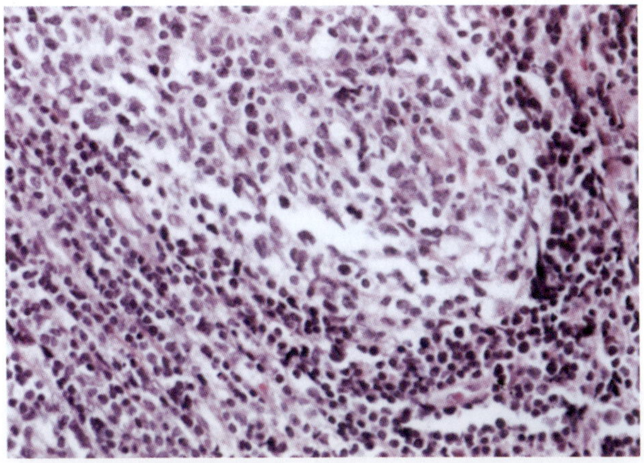

B

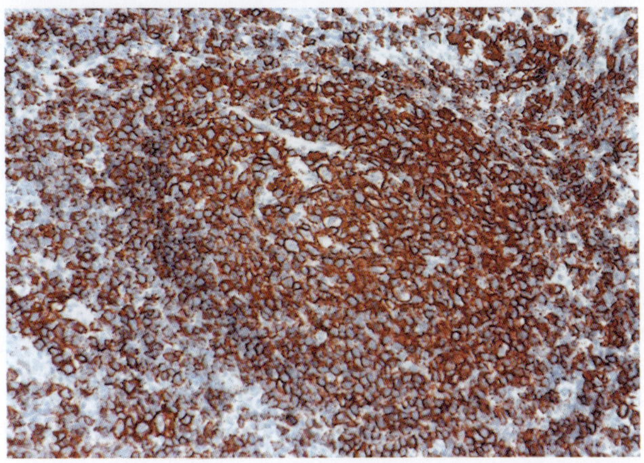

FIGURE 13.3. Histologic findings for the lacrimal gland mass shown in Figure 13.1. (A) Histologic section (with H&E stain) demonstrates a mostly follicular lymphoma with areas of diffuse infiltration by a mixture of small cleaved and large noncleaved lymphoid cells. (B) Immunohistochemical staining of paraffin-embedded tissue sections demonstrates that the lymphoma cells are positive for CD20, confirming B-cell lineage.

BOX 13.1. U.S. National Cancer Institute Working Formulation of Non-Hodgkin's Lymphomas

Low-Grade Lymphomas

Small lymphocytic
Follicular, predominantly small cleaved cell
Follicular, mixed, small cleaved cell and large cell

Intermediate-Grade Lymphomas

Follicular, predominantly large cell
Diffuse, mixed, small and large cell
Diffuse, large cell (cleaved and noncleaved)

High-Grade Lymphomas

Diffuse large cell, immunoblastic
Lymphoblastic (convoluted and non-convoluted)
Small noncleaved cell (Burkitt's and non-Burkitt's)

BOX 13.2. Revised European-American Classification of Lymphoid Neoplasms (REAL)

Indolent Lymphomas

Follicular lymphoma
B-chronic lymphocytic leukemia/small lymphocytic lymphoma
Lymphoplasmacytic lymphoma
Marginal zone lymphoma (nodal, extranodal, splenic)
T-cell/natural killer large cell granular lymphocyte leukemia
T-chronic lymphocytic leukemia/ prolymphocytic leukemia

Aggressive Lymphomas

Mantle cell lymphoma
Diffuse large B-cell lymphoma
Peripheral T-cell lymphoma (unspecified)
Peripheral T-cell lymphoma (angioimmunoblastic, angiocentric)
T-cell/natural killer cell, hepatosplenic, intestinal T-cell lymphoma
Anaplastic large cell lymphoma

Highly Aggressive Lymphomas

Precursor T or B lymphoblastic leukemia/ lymphoma
Burkitt's and Burkitt's-like lymphoma
Adult T-cell leukemia/lymphoma

Source: Data from Harris NL, Jaffe ES, Stein H, et al. A revised European–American classification of lymphoid neoplasms: a proposal from the International Lymphoma Study Group. *Blood* 1994;84:1361–1392.

It appears to be sensitive for detecting extranodal sites of involvement, including bone marrow.[20]

The Ann Arbor Staging System is most commonly used to designate a stage for lymphomas and is summarized in Table 13.2.

MANAGEMENT

Most published reports advocate the use of external beam radiotherapy or systemic chemotherapy for the treatment of primary orbital lymphomas.[7,8,21,22] While external beam radiotherapy may be successful in controlling local orbital disease in the majority of patients with low-grade indolent orbital lymphoma, the risk of distant relapse is not insignificant with radiotherapy alone. For more aggressive histologic subtypes of orbital lymphoma for which widespread systemic involvement is likely, systemic chemotherapy or systemic immunotherapy may be more appropriate. In some patients, combining systemic chemotherapy with local radiation treatment is warranted.[11,23] The therapeutic approach chosen for each patient varies according to the stage and histologic classification of lymphoma in addition to other comorbid risk factors.

Radiotherapy

Lymphomas are markedly radiosensitive. Primary radiotherapy for stage I indolent orbital lymphoma can achieve local control in more than 90% of patients, but the rate of distant relapse may be as high as 40% with external beam radiotherapy alone.[21,22] The median total dose of radiation used in external beam radiotherapy for non-Hodgkin's lymphoma of the orbit is 40 Gy (range 20–50 Gy).[22] Low-grade lesions are usually treated with a 30 Gy dose; intermediate-grade lymphomas may be more appropriately treated with higher doses (≤40 Gy). Distant relapse rates have been observed in 20 to 25% of patients with low-grade lymphoma and 40 to 60% for higher grade lymphomas.[21,24]

Field arrangement varies according to tumor location. Most studies of radiotherapy for primary orbital lymphoma have reported minimal acute ocular toxicity, but long-term follow-up can demonstrate common ocular side effects of dry eye syndrome, ocular surface irritation, and, occasionally, cataracts.[24–28] Total dose and length of time between fractions markedly influence the degree of ocular toxicity. A regimen of daily radiation fractions less than 2.25 Gy reduces radiation-induced morbidity. A cumulative dose of 16.5 Gy or higher is likely to lead to lens opacities.[27] Adequate shielding can decrease the risk of cataract formation and the amount of radiation delivery to the

BOX 13.3. Recommended Staging Workup for Orbital Lymphoma

Thorough history and physical examination
Dilated eye examination
Complete blood count and biochemistry profile
Liver function tests
Chest radiography
Computed tomography or magnetic resonance imaging of orbit
Computed tomography of abdomen, thorax, and pelvis
Bone marrow aspiration
Open or fine-needle biopsy of orbital mass
Upper endoscopy and barium studies
Total body positron emission tomography

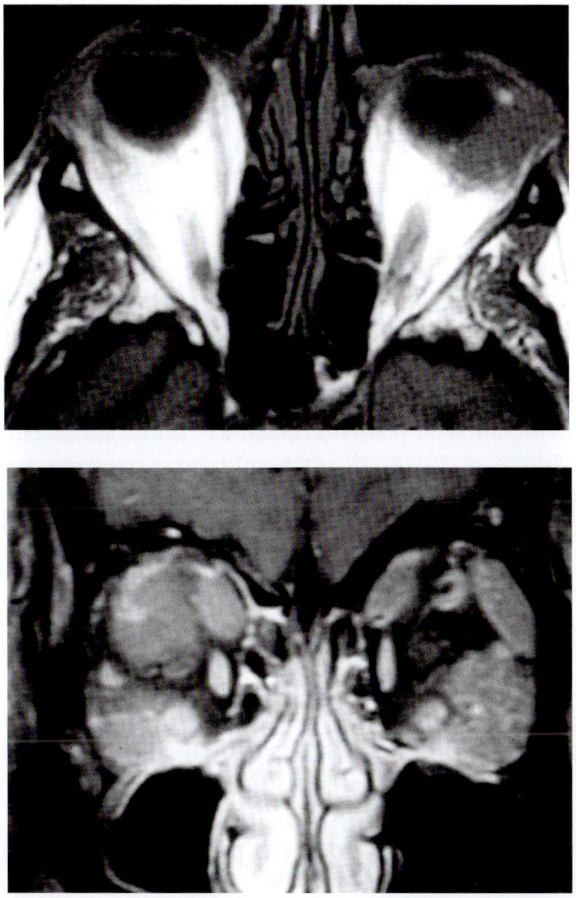

FIGURE 13.4. Magnetic resonance images in a patient with large-cell lymphoma demonstrate multiple intraorbital masses infiltrating the lacrimal gland and the extraocular muscles. (A) Axial noncontrast T1-weighted image. (B) Coronal fat-suppressed, contrast-enhanced T1-weighted image.

corneal surface. Despite shielding, tear film insufficiency and subsequent dry eye syndrome frequently occur after radiation therapy for orbital lymphoma. Significant radiation vasculopathy of the retina and optic nerve does not usually occur with the usual total dose used for orbital lymphoma (< 50 Gy).[28]

Newer approaches in radiation delivery could improve the treatment of orbital tumors in the future. Intensity-modulated conformal therapy, which promises isodose delivery to tumors while sparing the uninvolved neighboring structures, may minimize the ocular toxicity due to radiotherapy.[29]

Systemic Chemotherapy or Combined Modality Therapy

Chemotherapy is usually indicated for the more aggressive histologic subtypes of orbital lymphoma with potential for future systemic involvement or with existing disseminated disease.

Indolent lymphomas are very sensitive to both single-agent and combination chemotherapy. Single-agent therapy is carried out with alkylating agents such as cyclophosphamide. For intermediate- to high-grade lymphomas, initial combination chemotherapy is usually with a doxorubicin-containing regimen such as cyclophosphamide, doxorubicin, vincristine, and prednisone (CHOP) or cyclophosphamide, vincristine, doxorubicin, and dexamethasone (CVAD). The most common life-threatening toxic effect from chemotherapy is myelosuppression, resulting in anemia, infection, and abnormal bleeding. Congestive heart failure secondary to decreased left ventricular function is another significant toxicity of these regimens.

Combined chemotherapy and radiation therapy may be an appropriate option for intermediate- to high-grade lymphomas.[23] The rationale for combined modality therapy originates from observations that systemic extranodal sites of relapse are common following radiation therapy alone. Single-institution and cooperative group series, in which chemotherapy was combined with radiotherapy, have reported 5-year rates of relapse-free survival of 94 to 100% for stage I lymphomas and 72 to 78% for stage II disease.[23,30,31] Furthermore, overall life-threatening toxicity and cardiac toxicity are significantly lower in patients receiving combined chemotherapy and radiation because fewer cycles of chemotherapy may be required.[23]

Aggressive chemotherapy induction regimens followed by stem cell transplantation have been investigated at the M. D. Anderson Cancer Center.[32] Hyper-CVAD, with escalated doses of cyclophosphamide, high-dose methotrexate, and cytarabine followed by autologous or allogenic stem cell transplantation, can result in improved rates of remission for the more aggressive lymphomas.

Immunotherapy and Radioimmunotherapy for Low-Grade Indolent NHL of the Orbit

Although external beam radiotherapy is effective at controlling orbital lymphomas, it is associated with the risk of distant relapse and ocular toxicity. Systemic chemotherapy is an effective treatment for

TABLE 13.2. Ann Arbor Staging System for Lymphoma.

Stage	*Description*
I[a]	Involvement of a single lymph node region or lymphoid structure (e.g. spleen or Waldeyer ring)
II[a]	Involvement of two or more lymph node regions on same side of the diaphragm or localized involvement of an extranodal lymphoid structure and of one or more lymph node region on same side of diaphragm
III	Involvement of lymph nodes on both sides of diaphragm ± extranodal sites
IV	Involvement of two or more extranodal sites or liver or bone marrow

[a]Involvement of an extranodal organ or site is designated with the suffix E (stage IE or stage IIE).

higher grade or more advanced stages of lymphoma, but in the elderly patient the presence of comorbid disease may mitigate against intensive chemotherapy approaches. Thus, new and alternative treatment options for orbital lymphoma may be desirable.

Recent reports have suggested that monoclonal antibody therapy may be effective in the treatment of low-grade NHLs.[33–35] Investigators have characterized the patterns of expression of surface antigens on B cells and have developed targeted therapy with monoclonal antibodies directed against several of these antigens. One of these surface antigens is CD20, which is a hydrophobic phosphoprotein that is expressed on mature B cells and most B-cell malignancies but not on stem cells, pre-B cells, or plasma cells. Rituximab (Rituxan) is a genetically engineered chimeric mouse/human antibody discovered in 1990 by IDEC Pharmaceuticals; it binds with high affinity to cells expressing the CD20 antigen and causes tumor lysis via both complement-dependent and antibody-dependent cellular cytotoxicity.[36] It also can sensitize chemoresistant human lymphoma cell lines and induce apoptosis in vitro. Rituximab was approved by the U.S. Food and Drug Administration in 1997 for the indication of relapsed or refractory CD20-positive B-cell low-grade or follicular NHL. It is the first monoclonal antibody approved for the treatment of cancer and the first single agent approved specifically for therapy of lymphoma. It is administered as an intravenous infusion at a dose of 375 mg/m^2 once weekly for 4 consecutive weeks. Outpatient therapy is feasible and is completed within 22 days (treatment on days 1, 8, 15, and 22). The overall response rate to rituximab is 48% for relapsed low-grade lymphomas. The response rate is somewhat higher for follicular lymphomas (58%).[33–36]

Rituximab is well-tolerated and does not deplete marrow reserves. Most side effects are mild and infusion related, usually occurring with the first infusion. The common reported side effects include transient chills, fever, nausea, fatigue, headache, and pruritis; less frequently there can be bronchospasm, hypotension, rash, or anaphylaxis.

Radioimmunotherapy refers to administration of a monoclonal antibody in combination with a radioactive ligand. Beta particles emitted by commonly used radioisotopes are tumoricidal over a distance of many cell diameters, allowing eradication of antigen-negative tumor cells by radioactive cross fire from neighboring antigen-positive antibody-coated cells. This additional mechanism for tumor lysis leads to a more dramatic treatment effect than the nonradioactive antibody.

IDEC-Y2B8 (Zevalin) is a murine IgG1 κ monoclonal antibody directed against the CD20 antigen that is conjugated to MX-DTPA and bound to the beta-emitting radioisotope yttrium-90.[37] Zevalin is usually given as a single dose following an infusion of rituximab. Radioimmunothearpy with Zevalin in combination with rituximab has shown greater efficacy for treatment of low-grade lymphoma than rituximab alone. Dosimetry has shown that at doses of up to 0.4 mCi/kg, no normal organ, including red marrow, received a radiation dose greater than 14 Gy.[38]

The experience at M. D. Anderson for treating low-grade lymphomas of the orbit with rituximab therapy alone or in combination with Zevalin, its radioactive-liganded counterpart, has been positive.[12] Three patients with low-grade lymphoma of the orbit were treated with four weekly doses of rituximab; two additional patients were treated with one dose of ritux-

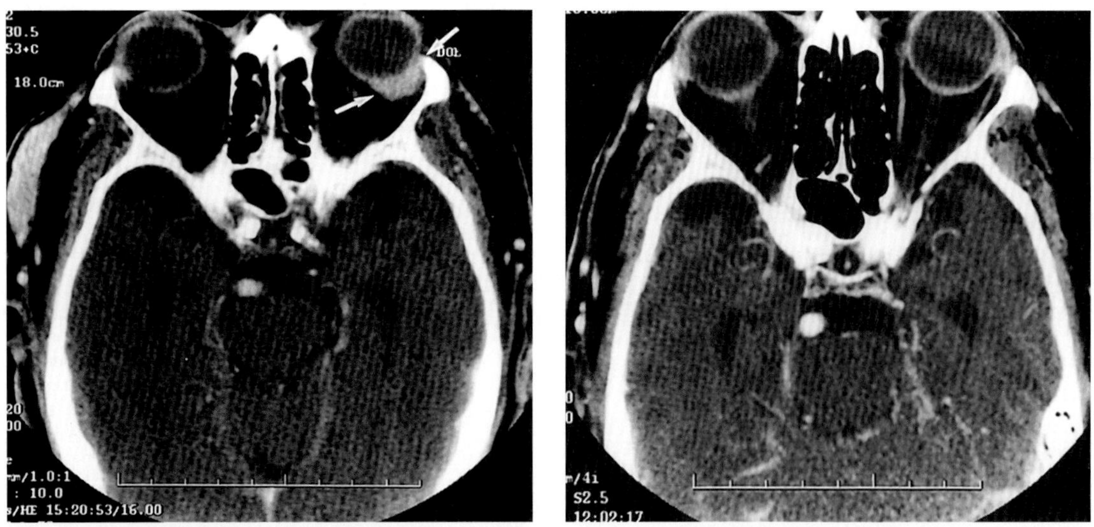

A B

FIGURE 13.5. Computed tomography scans of the orbit in a patient with low-grade follicular lymphoma of the left lacrimal gland. (A) Before monoclonal antibody treatment, a mass was visible in the inferior left orbit (arrows). (B) Two months after administration of rituximab and yttrium-90-labeled ibritumomab tiuxetan, the orbital mass had shrunk considerably.

imab followed by Zevalin. All five patients achieved complete resolution of their orbital lymphoma in response to monocloncal antibody therapy (Figure 13.5). The potential benefits of radioimmunotherapy include fewer side effects than accompany external beam radiation therapy and systemic chemotherapy, repeatability in case of recurrence, and a shorter duration of therapy than is possible with both the other two modalities. If in larger studies monoclonal antibody treatment proves to be as effective as external beam radiotherapy or chemotherapy for the treatment of indolent lymphomas of the orbit, it may indeed be an exciting alternative therapy for orbital lymphomas.

References

1. Jakobiec FA, Font RL. Orbit: lymphoid tumors. In: Spencer WH, Font RL, Green WR, et al, eds. *Ophthalmic Pathology: An Atlas and Textbook*. Vol. 3. 3rd ed. Philadelphia: WB Saunders; 1986:2663–2711.
2. Ellis JH, Banks PM, Campbell RJ, Liesegang TJ. Lymphoid tumors of the ocular adnexa: clinical correlation with the working formulation classification and immunoperoxidase staining of paraffin sections. *Ophthalmology* 1985;92:1311–1324.
3. Hornblass A, Jakobiec FA, Reifler DM, et al. Orbital lymphoid tumors located predominantly within extraocular muscles. *Ophthalmology* 1987;94:688–697.
4. Nikaido H, Mishima HK, Kiuchi Y, et al. Primary orbital malignant lymphoma: a clinicopathology study of 17 cases. *Graefes Arch Clin Exp Ophthalmol* 1991;229:206–209.
5. Bairey O, Kremer I, Rokowsky E, et al. Orbital and adnexal involvement in systemic non-Hodgkin's lymphoma. *Cancer* 1994;73:2395–2399.
6. Esmaeli B, Ahmadi MA, Manning J, et al. Clinical presentation and treatment of secondary orbital lymphoma. *Ophthalmic Plast Reconstr Surg* 2002;18:247–253.
7. Mirabell R, Cella L, Weber D, et al. Optimizing radiotherapy of orbital and paraorbital tumors: intensity-modulated x-ray beams vs. intensity-modulated proton beams. *Int J Radiat Oncol Biol Phys* 2000;47:1111–1119.
8. Letschert JG, Gonzalez DG, Koorneef L, et al. Results of radiotherapy in patients with stage I orbital non-Hodgkin's lymphoma. *Radiother Oncol* 1991;22:36–44.
9. Gordon LI, Harrington D, Anderson J, et al. Comparison of a second-generation combination chemotherapeutic regimen with a standard regimen (CHOP) for advanced diffuse non-Hodgkin's lymphoma. *N Engl J Med* 1992;327:1342.
10. Fisher RI, Gaynor ER, Dahlberg S, et al. Comparison of a standard regimen (CHOP) with three intensive chemotherapy regimens for advanced non-Hodgkin's lymphoma. *N Engl J Med* 1993;328:1002.
11. Hagemeister FB, McLaughlin P, Swan F, et al. Prognostic factors and long-term results with CHOP-bleo and radiotherapy. *Blood* 1991;77:942.
12. Esmaeli B, Murray JL, Ahmadi MA, et al. Immunotherapy for low-grade non-Hodgkin's secondary lymphoma of the orbit. *Arch Ophthalmol* 2002;120:1225–1227.
13. Syed NA, Albert DM. Surgical pathology of ophthalmic plastic surgery. In: Albert DM, ed. *Ophthalmic Surgery: Principles and Techniques*. Edinburgh: Blackwell Science; 1999:1648–1658.
14. Rosai J. In: Rosai J, ed. *Ackerman's Surgical Pathology*. 8th ed. St Louis: CV Mosby; 1996:1–12, 29–62.
15. Jakobiec FA, McLean I, Font R. Clinicopathologic characteristics of orbital lymphoid hyperplasia. *Symp Orbital Dis* 1979;86:948–966.
16. Freedman AS, Nadler LM. Non-Hodgkin's lymphomas. In: Bast RC, Kufe DW, Pollock RE, et al, eds. *Cancer Medicine*. 5th ed. New York: BC Decker; 2000: Sec 36, Ch 130.
17. Harris NL, Jaffe ES, Stein H, et al. A revised European–American classification of lymphoid neoplasms: a proposal from the International Lymphoma Study Group. *Blood* 1994;84:1361–1392.
18. Armitage JO, Weisenburger DD. New approach to classifying non-Hodgkin's lymphomas: clinical features of the major histologic subtypes. *J Clin Oncol* 1998;16:2780–2795.
19. Bennett CL, Putterman A, Bitran JD, et al. Staging and therapy of orbital lymphomas. *Cancer* 1986;57:1204–1208.
20. Carr R, Barrington S, Madan B, et al. Detection of lymphoma in bone marrow by whole-body positron emission tomography. *Blood* 1998;91:3340–3346.
21. Smitt MC, Donaldson SS. Radiotherapy is successful treatment for orbital lymphoma. *Int J Radiat Oncol Biol Phys* 1993;26:59–66.
22. Esik O, Ikeda H, Mukai K, Kaneko A. A retrospective analysis of different modalities for treatment of primary orbital non-Hodgkin's lymphomas. *Radiother Oncol* 1996;38:13–18.
23. Miller TP, Dahlberg S, Cassady JR, et al. Chemotherapy alone compared with chemotherapy plus radiotherapy for localized intermediate- and high-grade non-Hodgkin's lymphoma. *N Engl J Med* 1998;339:21–26.
24. Bessell EM, Henk JM, Wright JE, et al. Orbital and conjunctival lymphoma treatment and prognosis. *Radiother Oncol* 1988;13:237–244.
25. Minehan KJ, Martenson JA, Garrity JA, et al. Local control and complications after radiation therapy for primary orbital lymphoma: a case for low-dose treatment. *Int J Radiat Oncol Biol Phys* 1991;20:791–796.
26. Bolek TW, Moyses HM, Marcus RB, et al. Radiotherapy in the management of orbital lymphoma. *Int J Radiat Oncol Biol Phys* 1999;44:31–36.
27. Henk JM, Whitelocke RAF, Warrington AP, et al. Radiation dose to the lens and cataract formation. *Int J Radiat Oncol Biol Phys* 1993;25:815–820.
28. Stafford SL, Kozelsky TF, Garrity JA, et al. Orbital lymphoma: radiotherapy outcome and complications. *Radiother Oncol* 2001;59:139–144.
29. Dearnaly DF, Khoo VS, Norman AR, et al. Comparison of radiation side-effects of conformal and conventional radiotherapy in prostate cancer: a randomized trial. *Lancet* 1999;353:267–272.
30. Cabanillas F, Rodriguez-Diaz PJ, Hagemeister FB, et al. Alternating triple therapy for the treatment of intermediate grade and immunoblastic lymphoma. *Ann Oncol* 1998;9:511–518.
31. Longo DL, Glatstein E, Duffey PL, et al. Treatment of localized aggressive lymphomas with combination chemotherapy followed by involved-field radiation therapy. *J Clin Oncol* 1989;7:1295–1302.
32. Khouri I, Romaguera J, Kantarjian H, et al. Hyper-CVAD and high-dose methotrexate/cytarabine followed by stem-cell transplantation: an active regimen for aggressive mantle-cell lymphoma. *J Clin Oncol* 1998;16:3803–3809.
33. McLaughlin P, Grillo-Lopez AJ, Liink BK, et al. Rituximab chimeric anti-CD20 monoclonal antibody therapy for relapsed indolent lymphoma: half of patients respond to a four-dose treatment program. *J Clin Oncol* 1998;16:2825–2833.
34. Maloney DG, Grillo-Lopez AJ, White CA, et al. IDEC-C2B8 (rituximab) anti-CD20 monoclonal antibody therapy in patients with relapsed low-grade non-Hodgkin's lymphoma. *Blood* 1997;90:2188–2195.
35. Maloney D, Smith B, Appelbaum F. The anti-tumor effect of monoclonal anti-CD20 antibody (Mab) therapy includes direct

antiproliferative activity and induction of apoptosis in CD20 positive non-Hodgkin's lymphoma cell lines. *Blood* 1996; 88(suppl):637.

36. Leget GA, Czuczman MS. Use of rituximab, the new FDA-approved antibody. *Curr Opin Oncol* 1998;10:548–551.
37. Knox SJ, Goris ML, Trisler K, et al. Yttrium-90-labeled anti-CD20 monoclonal antibody therapy of recurrent B-cell lymphoma. *Clin Cancer Res* 1996;2:457–470.
38. Wiseman GA, White CA, Stabin M, et al. Phase I/II 90Y-Zevvalin (yttrium-90 ibritumomab tiuxetan, IDEC-Y2B8) radioimmunotherapy dosimetry results in relapsed or refractory non-Hodgkin's lymphoma. *Eur J Nucl Med* 2000;27:766–777.

14

Vascular Tumors

Kaan Gündüz and Zeynel A. Karcıoglu

Vascular tumors and malformations of the orbit comprise an important group of orbital space-occupying lesions. Reviews indicate that vascular lesions account for 6.2 to 12.0% of all histopathologically documented orbital space-occupying lesions (Table 14.1).[1–5] There is ultrastructural and immunohistochemical evidence that capillary and cavernous hemangiomas, lymphangioma, and other vascular lesions are of different nosologic origins, yet in many patients these entities coexist. Hence, some prefer to use a single umbrella term, "vascular hamartomatous lesions" to identify these masses, with the qualification that, in a given case, one tissue element may predominate.[6] For example, an "infantile hemangioma" may contain a few caverns or intertwined abnormal blood vessels, but its predominating component is usually capillary hemangioma. This nomenclature does not cover all bases either; it should be noted that although many vascular lesions are made of multiple histopathologic types, all are not. For instance, although caverns lined by endothelial cells are seen in many vascular lesions, no other tissue element is encountered with the classic intraconal "cavernous hemangioma." In this chapter, the time-honored terminology is used to review cavernous hemangioma, capillary hemangioma, lymphangioma, orbital varix, hemangiopericytoma, angiosarcoma, intravascular papillary endothelial hyperplasia, arteriovenous fistulas, vascular leiomyoma, angiolymphoid hyperplasia with eosinophilia, and Kimura disease.

From the standpoint of treatment and predicting prognosis, it is important to determine the predominating tissue element: if a lesion predominantly contains capillary hemangioma, for example, it may sclerose significantly as the patient ages, and, if treated, it may respond well to steroid injections. On the other hand, lesions with predominantly cavernous histology and/or large blood vessel malformations do not regress over the years and do not respond to intralesional steroid injections, even though both these pathologies may be identified as "vascular hamartomatous lesions." In some cases, light-microscopic examination with routine stains may not be sufficient to determine an answer; in these instances immunohistochemistry may help. A number of cellular antigens identify the endothelial cell. These include CD31, CD34, factor VIII related antigen (v,w,f), CV141 (endothelium, mesothelium, and squamous cells), and VEGFR-3 (channels, neovascular endothelium). None of the cell markers is absolutely specific in its application; a combination is recommended in difficult cases. CD31 is the most often used endothelial cell marker, with positive membrane staining pattern in over 90% of capillary hemangiomas, cavernous hemangiomas, and angiosarcomas; CD34 is expressed only in about 50% of endothelial cell tumors. Lymphangioma pattern, on the other hand, is negative with CD31 and CD34, but, it is positive with VEGFR-3. VEGFR-3 expression is also seen in Kaposi sarcoma and in neovascular endothelium. In hemangiopericytomas, the tumor cells are typically positive for vimentin and CD34 and negative for markers of endothelia (factor VIII, CD31, etc.)

Another focus of debate is whether lymphangioma and varix are related lesions. It has been suggested that *orbital venous anomaly* be used for both types of lesion.[7] However, most orbitologists still use *lymphangioma* and *varix* separately. Angiolymphoid hyperplasia with eosinophilia and Kimura disease were once thought to represent the same entity, although differences between the conditions do exist. They no longer are considered to be the same disease.[8]

CAVERNOUS HEMANGIOMA

Cavernous hemangioma is the most common benign orbital tumor in adults. It comprised 3.1 to 9.0% of all histopathologically proven orbital tumors in five series (Table 14.1).[1–5] It most frequently occurs in patients 40 to 60 years old.[3] Rarely, cavernous hemangioma can occur in children. Unlike capillary hemangioma, it is not associated with the presence of hemangiomas elsewhere in the body.

Clinical Features

Orbital cavernous hemangioma can occupy an intraconal or extraconal position in the orbit (Figures 14.1 and 14.2). When the cavernous hemangioma is located intraconally, it leads to a slowly progressive axial proptosis (Figure 14.1). When it is located extraconally in

TABLE 14.1. Frequency of Various Vascular Tumors of the Orbit.

Author	*No. of cases*	*Cavernous hemangioma*	*Capillary hemangioma*	*Lymphangioma*	*Varices*	*Hemangiopericytoma*
Shields et al.[1]	645	20 (3.1%)	7 (1.1%)	4 (0.6%)	2 (0.3%)	5 (0.8%)
Sen[5]	266	16 (6.0%)	5 (1.9%)	4 (1.5%)	—	1 (0.3%)
Günalp and Gündüz[3]	1092	35 (3.2%)	15 (1.3%)	3 (0.3%)	3 (0.3%)	1 (0.1%)
Henderson et al.[2]	1376	60 (4.4%)	30 (2.2%)	18 (1.3%)	4 (0.3%)	16 (1.2%)
Seregard and Sahlin[4]	300	27 (9%)	2 (0.7%)	2 (0.7%)	4 (1.3%)	1 (0.3%)

Author	*Vascular leiomyoma*	*Angiosarcoma*	*Arteriovenous fistula*	*Aneurysm*	*Hamartoma*
Shields et al.[1]	2 (0.3%)	—	—	—	—
Sen[5]	—	—	—	—	—
Günalp and Gündüz[3]	—	3 (0.3%)	3 (0.3%)	—	—
Henderson et al.[2]	1 (0.1%)	—	5 (0.4%)	2 (0.1%)	1 (0.1%)
Seregard and Sahlin[4]	—	—	—	—	—

the orbit, the displacement of the globe is opposite the position of the tumor. Rarely, a cavernous hemangioma presents as a lacrimal gland mass[9] or as an intraosseous tumor.[10,11]

A palpable mass is rarely present. There are usually no significant inflammatory signs such as eyelid edema or conjunctival injection. Visual acuity is usually good unless the cavernous hemangioma compresses the optic nerve. When the tumor is located in the vicinity of the globe, it may induce hyperopia and choroidal folds. It is interesting that the hyperopia and choroidal folds may persist even after complete removal of the cavernous hemangioma (Figure 14.1).[12] Ocular motility may be slightly limited. Amaurosis

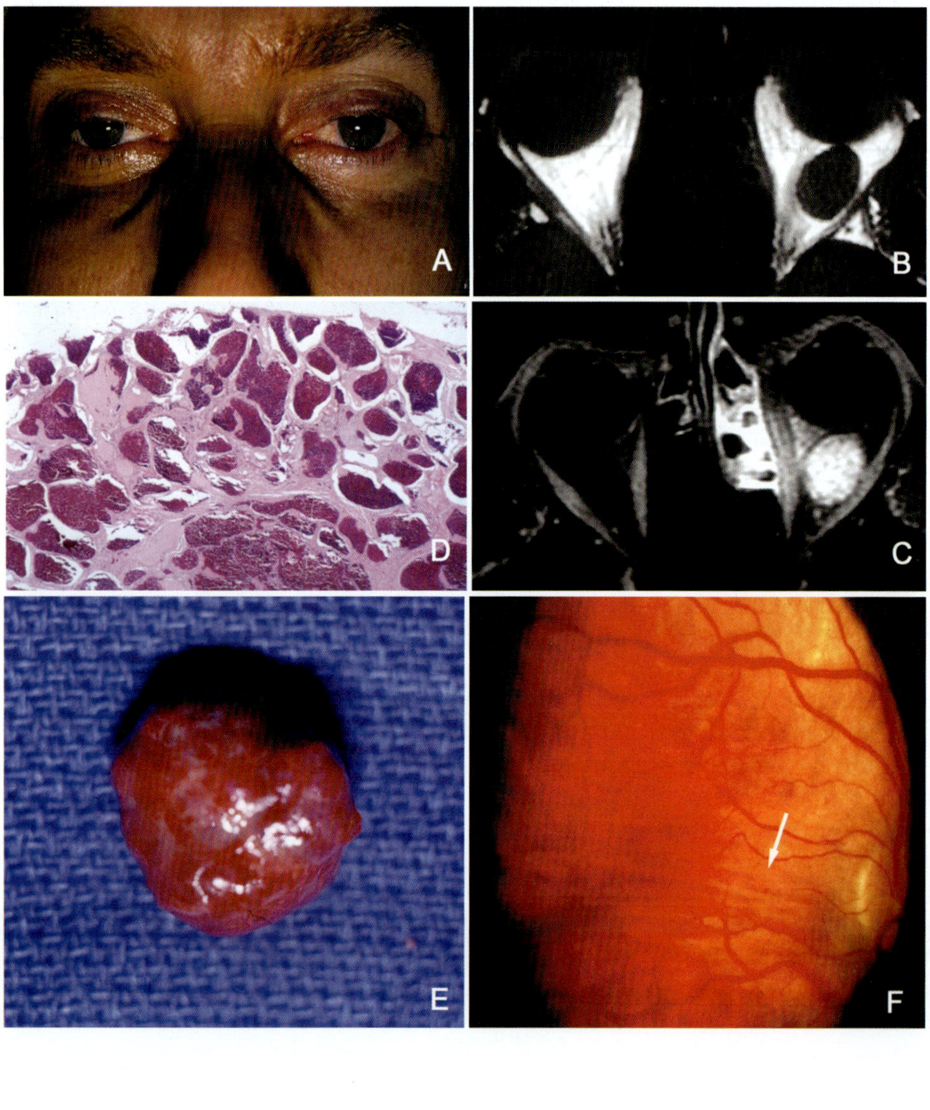

FIGURE 14.1. (A–C) Typical cavernous hemangioma presentation with slowly progressive unilateral proptosis due to an intraconal lesion. (B,C) Axial T1-weighted MR images with and without contrast reveal a well-encapsulated, oval lesion within the cone. (D) Histopathologically, the specimen consists of multiple cavernous spaces separated by fibrous septae; most of the caverns are filled with blood. (E) The gross specimen after surgical excision shows a reddish blue encapsulated lesion. (F) Fundus photograph shows the choroidal folds (arrow) secondary to the compression of the lesion.

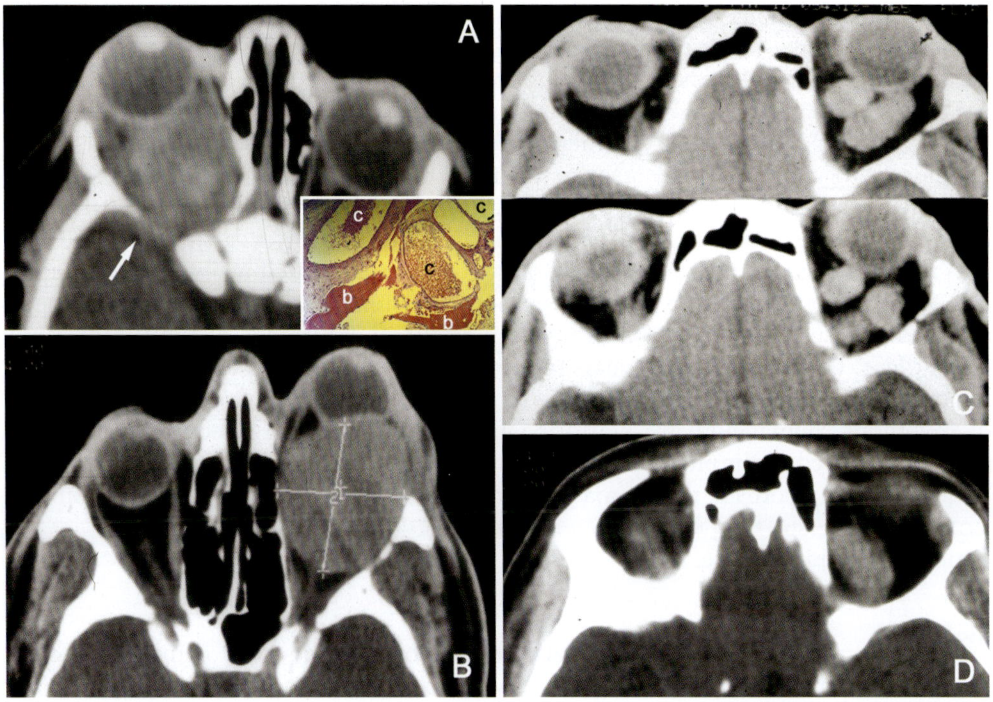

FIGURE 14.2. Axial CTs from three different cavernous hemangiomas. (A) A long-standing, large cavernous hemangioma within and outside of the cone of the right orbit. Note the bony invasion of this lesion into the cranium (white arrow). *Inset*: the cavernous hemangioma (c) invading the bone (b). (B) Large but well-delineated cavernous hemangioma of the orbit causing massive proptosis and compression of the globe. Note that the lesion is larger than the one shown in (A) but is much better circumscribed, without any bony invasion. (C,D) A multilobulated cavernous hemangioma of the left orbit.

fugax, in extreme positions of gaze, is probably related to ischemia of the optic nerve as it is compressed by the retrobulbar mass.[13] The rare occurrence of cavernous hemangioma in a patient with hyperthyroidism has been described.[14]

Ophthalmoscopic findings include choroidal folds, optic disk edema, and optic atrophy.[15] The development of optic atrophy is related to the presence of a long-standing tumor. These tumors have been misdiagnosed in the past as optic neuropathy. Such errors are rare now, since the advent of neuroimaging studies.

Cavernous hemangioma is typically a solitary unilateral tumor. However, rarely bilateral and multiple hemangiomas have been reported in the same patient (Figure 14.2).[16] Multiple orbital cavernous hemangiomas may occur as a sporadic lesion or in association with Maffucci syndrome (multiple enchondromas, soft tissue hemangiomas, and a generalized tendency to neoplasia) and blue rubber bleb nevus syndrome (bluish cutaneous and mucosal hemangiomas, soft tissue hemangiomas, enteric hemangiomas with gastrointestinal bleeding) (see Chapter 16).[17]

Radiologic Features

A-mode ultrasonography demonstrates medium to high internal reflectivity. B-mode ultrasonography shows a regular outline with sharply defined borders and moderate acoustic solidity.[12] CT (computed tomography) and magnetic resonance imaging (MRI) show a well-circumscribed round to ovoid orbital mass usually occupying the intraconal space (Figures 14.1 and 14.2).[15] The cavernous hemangioma usually spares the triangular space in the orbital apex, although exceptions exist.[15] On MRI, which details internal tissue features well, cavernous hemangioma has a heterogeneous structure. The tumor is isointense to the cerebral gray matter and extraocular muscles on T1-weighted images and hyperintense on T2-weighted images. On contrast injection, the cavernous hemangioma shows progressive filling and enhancement. The initial patchy enhancement increases gradually and becomes homogeneous. This pattern is consistent with the pooling of the contrast medium in the caverns within the lesion and is considered to be characteristic of cavernous hemangioma. Other orbital tumors may display similar characteristics.

The differential diagnosis of well-circumscribed orbital lesions on CT and MRI include cavernous hemangioma, schwannoma, fibrous histiocytoma, hemangiopericytoma, and certain metastatic lesions. However, cavernous hemangioma is the most frequently encountered well-circumscribed orbital lesion.

Morphologic Features

Grossly, the orbital cavernous hemangioma is an encapsulated mass. The lesion is purple and has a spongelike consistency. On a cut surface, it displays numerous ectatic vascular spaces (Figure 14.1). Histopathologically, it consists of large, congested vascular channels separated by thin fibrous septae and flattened endothelial cells lining the vascular channels (Figure 14.1). There can be smooth muscle in the wall of blood vessels. There may be a few inflammatory cells and macrophages in the interstitium of the tumor. Foci of lymphocytes are absent or sparse in contrast to lymphangioma where multiple foci of lymphocytes and/or germinal centers are present.[12,15]

It is debated whether capillary and cavernous hemangiomas are related or coexistent tumors. The cavernous type may evolve from a preexisting capillary hemangiomatous progenitor.[12] The lesion may begin as a capillary proliferation. Over an extended period of slow growth, these channels may undergo progressive ectasia and acquire a coat of smooth muscle cells. One other possibility is the coexistence of two tumors. The capillary component represents the growing portion of the tumor. The capillary channels gradually enlarge and turn into cavernous spaces. These areas represent the bosselations observed on the tumor surface. Using transmission electron microscopy, Iwamoto and Jacobiec concluded that capillary and cavernous hemangiomas represented different nosologic entities based on the presence of smooth muscle cells providing support for the endothelial cells in the cavernous type versus the presence of pericytes serving this role in the capillary type.[15a]

Management and Prognosis

The treatment of cavernous hemangioma is surgical excision of the tumor.[12,18] Sometimes an asymptomatic lesion located in the posterior orbit can be observed conservatively for signs of optic nerve compression and visual loss. There are several surgical approaches for the excision of larger symptomatic lesions. A cutaneous or a conjunctival approach can be used. A cutaneous approach may provide better exposure of intraconally located tumors in the mid- and posterior orbits. It is important to use blunt dissection to free the tumor from the surrounding attachments. Sometimes a cryoprobe can be used to assist in the intact removal of the tumor with less bleeding from the surrounding vessels.[19] A Kronlein approach with osteotomy is rarely indicated. However, this approach may be necessary for tumors located near the orbital apex.

Incomplete excision of an orbital cavernous hemangioma can result in recurrence of the tumor many years later.[18] Some of these recurrences can later demonstrate spontaneous regression documented on serial neuroimaging studies. Therefore, recurrence developing in an incompletely excised cavernous hemangioma does not require immediate surgical intervention.

CAPILLARY HEMANGIOMA

Capillary hemangioma is the most common vascular orbital tumor in children. Capillary hemangioma accounted for 0.7 to 2.2% of all histopathologically proven space-occupying lesions in five orbital tumor series (Table 14.1).[1–5] The real frequency of orbital capillary hemangioma is probably higher because many patients do not undergo a biopsy procedure. The clinical courses of eyelid and orbital capillary hemangiomas are similar.

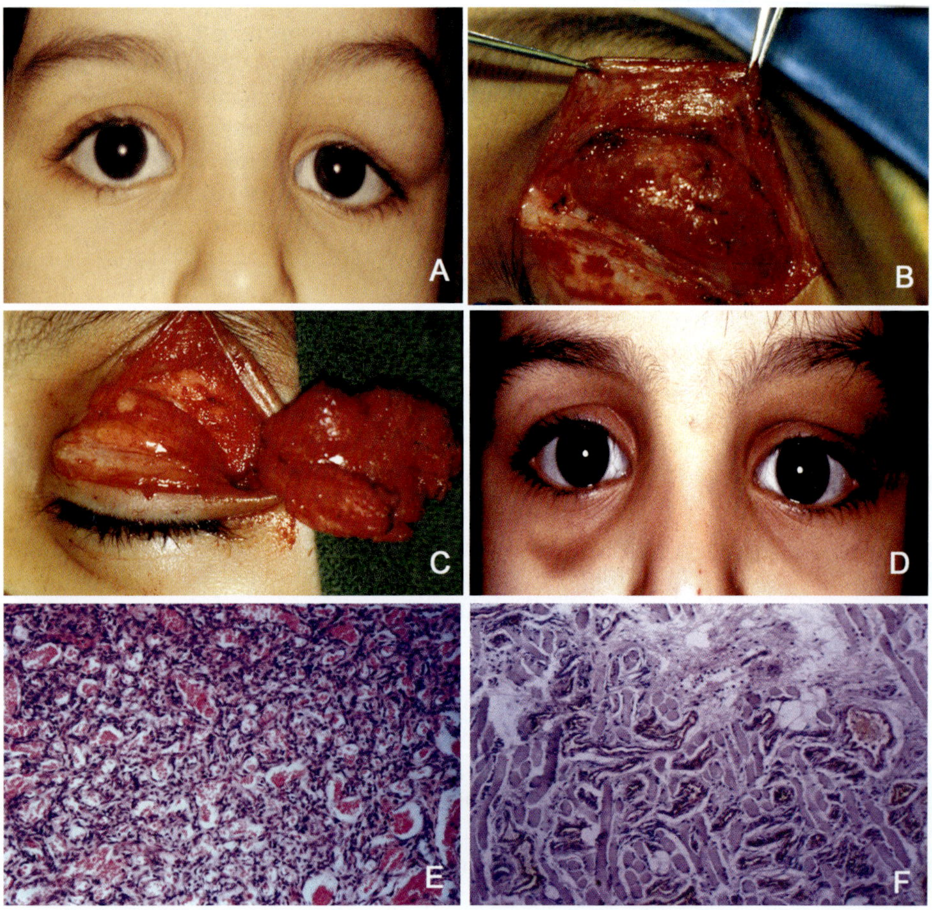

FIGURE 14.3. (A) Preoperative, (B,C) intraoperative, and (D) postoperative photographs of a 5-year-old girl with an upper eyelid hemangioma (E). The lesion was predominantly composed of proliferating endothelial cells but it also contained occasional abnormally formed large blood vessels. (F) Positive immunohistochemical staining (brownish color) with factor VIII depicts tumor components infiltrating into orbicularis muscle.

Clinical Features

Capillary hemangioma of the eyelid or orbit is usually apparent at birth or within the first 8 weeks of life.[15] Females may be affected slightly more often than males.[20,21] About 83% of capillary hemangiomas occur in the anterior orbit. The tumor is usually palpable in the anterior orbit, with or without some extension into the eyelid, giving the appearance of a red cutaneous lesion (Figures 14.3, 14.4, and 14.5). About 17% of capillary hemangiomas occur deep in the orbit (Figure 14.6).[21] When the lesion is confined to the deep orbital structures, a child may show only proptosis and displacement of the globe. Astigmatic and myopic refractive errors can be demonstrated in almost half of the patients with sizable lesions involving the upper eyelid and orbit.[22] Other tumors that should be considered in the differential diagnosis of capillary hemangioma include teratoma, metastatic neuroblastoma, and, rarely, rhabdomyosarcoma.

The capillary hemangioma usually enlarges for several months and then slowly regresses without treatment. Approximately 70% of the capillary hemangiomas regress completely by 7 years of age.[22] The child with eyelid or orbital capillary hemangioma may also have capillary hemangiomas in several visceral (pulmonary, soft tissues, and skin) organs. In the case of extensive visceral hemangiomas, secondary thrombocytopenia, due to entrapment of platelets in the tumor, can lead to extensive hemorrhage, a condition known as Kasabach–Merritt syndrome. Subglottic hemangiomas can result in respiratory distress.[21]

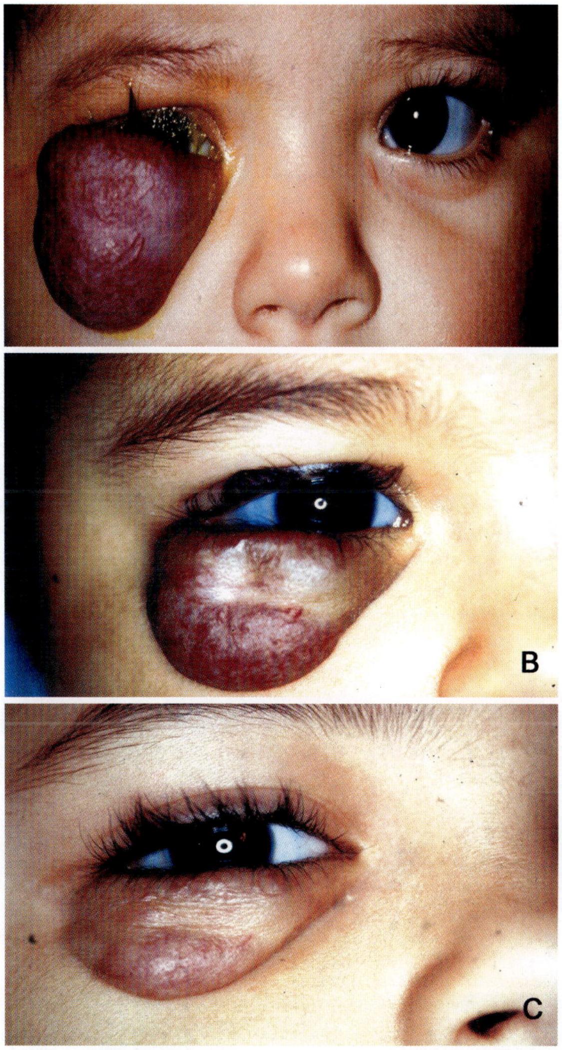

FIGURE 14.5. (A) Large lower eyelid anterior orbit hemangioma photographed before steroid injection. (B,C) Appearance and size of the lesion postoperatively, 8 and 13 months after injection, respectively.

A

B

C

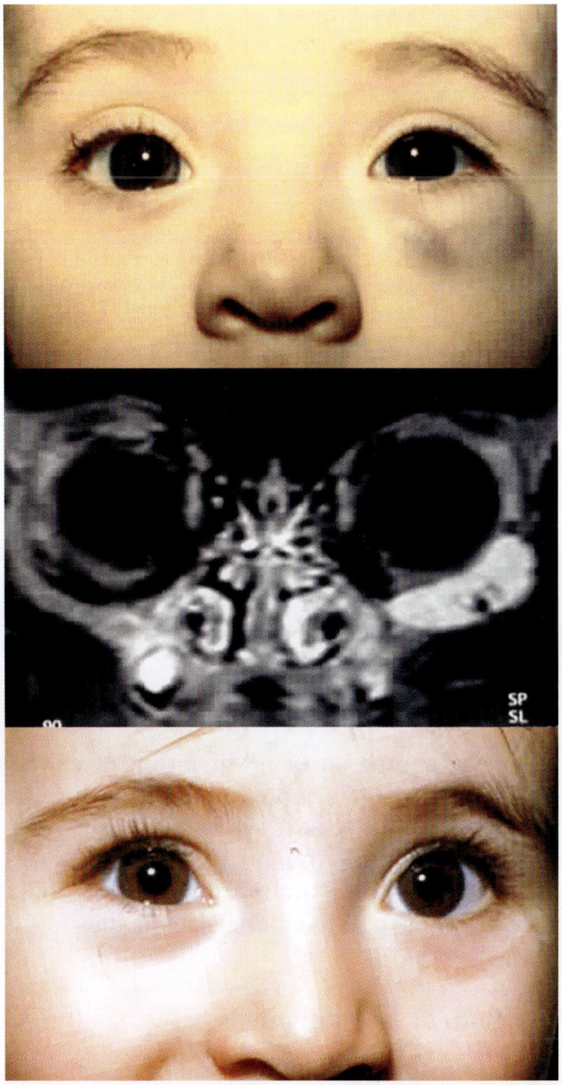

FIGURE 14.4. One-year-old boy with a capillary hemangioma involving the left inferior orbit. (A) Facial photograph showing bluish discoloration, swelling of the left lower eyelid, and upward displacement of the eyeball by the inferiorly located orbital capillary hemangioma. (B) T1-weighted coronal MR image demonstrating the inferiorly located capillary hemangioma with marked contrast enhancement. Note the signal-void areas representative of high flow vessels. (C) Postoperative facial photograph 6 months after excision of the lesion. There is no superior displacement of the globe.

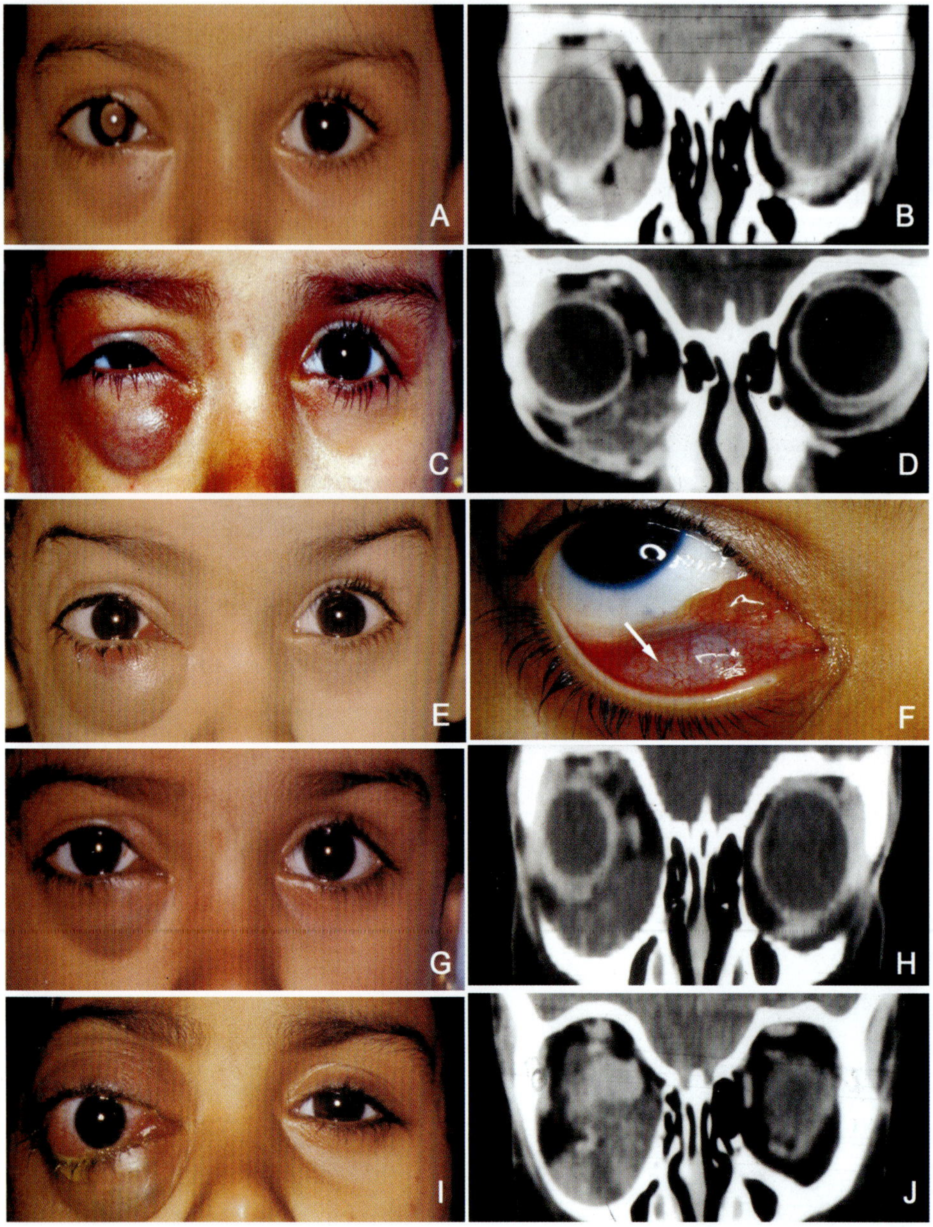

FIGURE 14.6. Facial photographs of a 3-year-old girl with corresponding coronal CTs before and after steroid injection. The lesion proved to be a vascular hamartoma with mixed capillary, cavernous, and lymphangiomatous components that responded well to steroid injection (G) but later developed a spontaneous orbital hemorrhage (I). (A,B) Initial presentation. (C,D) Enlarged lesion prior to injection. (E,F) Three days postinjection, whitish steroid deposits are seen in the slit lamp photo (arrow). (G,H) Four months after injection. (I,J) One year after injection.

Radiologic Features

CT usually demonstrates a well-circumscribed lesion with a heterogenous internal structure. On MRI, capillary hemangioma is isointense to hyperintense on T1-weighted images and hyperintense on T2-weighted images with respect to the extraocular muscle and cerebral gray matter (Figure 14.4). It shows moderate to marked enhancement after contrast injection.[23] MRI shows high blood flow vessels that are characterized as signal-void areas. These signal-void areas are characteristic of capillary hemangioma.[23]

Morphologic Features

Grossly, the lesion is usually red with a multilobulated appearance. Histopathologically, capillary hemangioma is composed of proliferation of endothelial cells (Figure 14.3). There are numerous well-formed or partially formed capillaries in the lesion. With transmission electron microscopy, the endothelial cells are usually found to contain lamellated cytoplasmic structures known as Weibel–Palade bodies.

Management and Prognosis

For orbital capillary hemangioma, the treatment options consist of observation, intralesional corticosteroids, systemic corticosteroids, systemic interferon, and surgical resection. Since capillary hemangioma tends to regress with advancing age, tumors that do not displace the globe or cause refractive errors or amblyopia can be followed with conservative management. Myopic or astigmatic refractive errors should be corrected, and conventional amblyopia treatment with patching of the controlateral eye should be undertaken.[22]

For periocular hemangioma, intralesional corticosteroids can be used. The combination is usually a mixture of a long-acting and a rapid-acting corticosteroid such as triamcinolone diacetate (Aristocort) or acetonide (Kenalog) and betamethasone sodium phosphate and betamethasone acetate (Celestone).[24] The recommended dose is 40 mg of triamcinolone and 6 mg of betamethasone mixed in a single syringe and injected directly into the mass through a 21- to 30-gauge needle.[24–26]

During intralesional injection of corticosteroid into a capillary hemangioma, injection pressures generally exceed the systemic arterial pressures. This causes the embolization of corticosteroid particles into the ocular circulation from retrograde arterial flow.[25,26] When the drug is injected into a terminal artery, the predominant flow is in the direction of least resistance. The resistance to fluid flow in a terminal artery is much less than the resistance in capillaries. Retrograde flow into an arteriole can also occur if the medication is injected at high pressure into a capillary bed.

There are a number of practical guidelines that should be followed to minimize the risk of embolization of corticosteroid into the ocular circulation[25,26]:

1. Before each injection of corticosteroid into the lesion, aspiration into the syringe should be performed to detect the presence of arterial blood. If blood is aspirated into the syringe, the cannula should be withdrawn and repositioned.
2. Multiple areas of the capillary hemangioma should be treated with small volumes of corticosteroid. The individual treatment sites usually receive 0.1 mL of medication. The total volume of corticosteroid is about 0.8 to 1.5 mL for periocular tumors between 4 and 8 mL in volume. The injection volume accounts for approximately 20% of the tumor volume. This is because the injectable space comprising the interstitium and vasculature are assumed to occupy 20 to 30% of the total tumor volume in capillary hemangiomas.
3. The surgeon injecting the corticosteroids should perform indirect ophthalmoscopy and, if there is central retinal artery enucleation, immediate paracentesis of the anterior chamber should be performed and intravenous carbonic anhydrase inhibitors given. Retinal cells survive ischemia for 90 to 100 minutes. Therefore, immediate action should be taken if retinal arterial occlusion is observed on ophthalmoscopy.
4. After the injection, pressure should not be applied to the tumor, and a pressure patch should not be applied. A shield should be placed around the tumor for 24 hours to prevent inadvertent pressure to the lesion.

Rapid involution of the capillary hemangioma starts in 3 days and continues for about 2 weeks. The involution generally lasts for 6 to 8 weeks (Figures 14.5 and 14.6).[24] Many tumors shrink to less than 20% of the original volume, attesting to a successful outcome. If involution is not satisfactory, a second injection can be given 1 to 3 months (average 2 months) after the first injection.[24] Many patients show nearly complete involution with two injections and rarely require additional corticosteroid injection. The effect of intralesional corticosteroids on capillary hemangioma seems to be related to a vasoconstricting effect. The blanching of the lesion 1 or 2 days after intralesional injection supports this hypothesis of the action of corticosteroids.[24]

Potential complications of local corticosteroid injections of capillary hemangioma include subcutaneous fat atrophy,[27] eyelid necrosis,[28] and retinal artery occlusion.[26] Orbital capillary hemangiomas located posterior to the orbital septum should not be injected because of the risk of bleeding or hematoma.[24] However, the lesion can be exposed surgically, partially debulked, and injected intralesionally.

Larger tumors that do not respond to periocular corticosteroid injections can be treated using a tapering dose of oral prednisone or prednisolone (2 to 3 mg/kg/day).[29] The full dose is given in the morning for 4 to 6 weeks and then tapered slowly. If rebound occurs, the lesion usually responds to a higher dose for 2 weeks before tapering again. In time, an alternate-day regimen may be effective. In the past, radiotherapy was occasionally employed in the management of selected orbital and adnexal capillary hemangiomas.[29]

Extensive capillary hemangiomas that do not respond to systemic corticosteriods can be treated with systemic interferon alfa 2a or 2b (Figure 14.7).[30,31] The recommended dose is 1 to 3 million U/day. Treatment is usually started on a lower dose around 1 million U/day and gradually increased to the upper therapeutic level. The drug is expensive and treatment should continue for months to establish a long-lasting remission. Side effects include increased body temperature, elevated serum transaminases, leukocytosis, delay in motor development, flulike syndrome, and congestive heart failure.

Surgical resection can be used for anteriorly located capillary hemangiomas that do not respond to intralesional corticosteroid (Figures 14.3 and 14.4).[32] More posterior lesions can be difficult to debulk in large volumes or to excise totally. Embolization treatment of orbital capillary hemangioma as the sole treatment or prior to surgical resection has also been reported.[33,34] The tumor is more amenable to surgical excision after em-

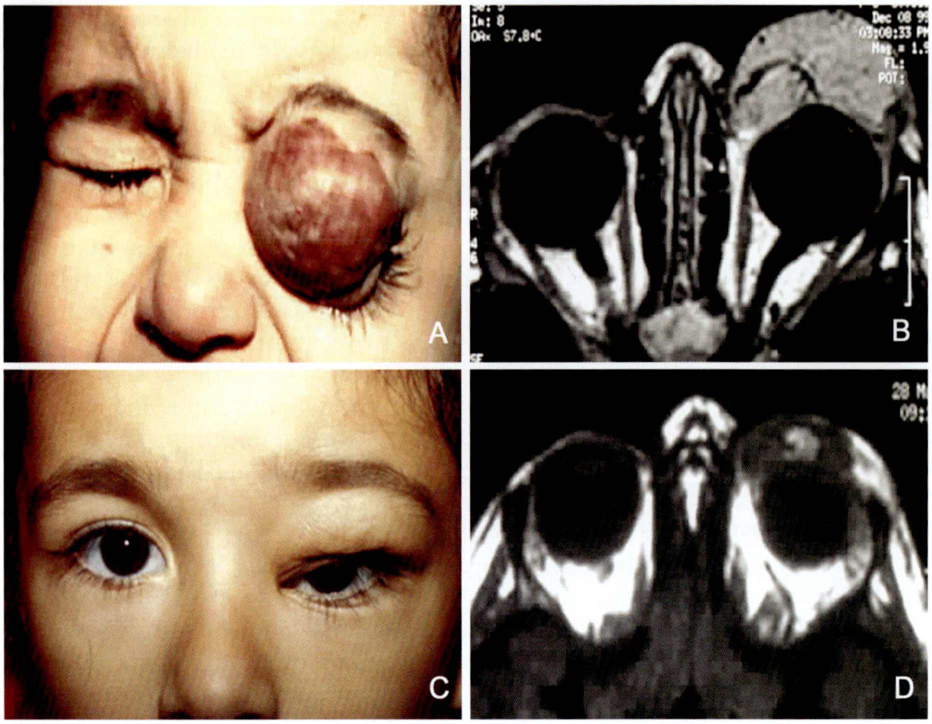

FIGURE 14.7. (A) Facial photograph demonstrating nonregressing extensive left eyelid capillary hemangioma in a 3-year-old girl after several corticosteroid injections. (B) T1-weighted, contrast-enhanced axial orbital MR image showing the hyperintense capillary hemangioma. Note the signal-void high-flow vessels in the lesion. (C) Facial photograph after alfa-2b interferon treatment showing marked regression of the lesion at 1-year follow-up. (D) T1-weighted axial orbital MR image at 1-year follow-up demonstrating the marked resolution of the capillary hemangioma. The tumor is isointense to slightly hyperintense to the extraocular muscle and cerebral gray matter.

bolization and closing of the feeder vessels.[34] Intralesional Nd:YAG laser photocoagulation has also been used in selected cases of periorbital and head and neck hemangiomas and vascular malformations.[35,36]

LYMPHANGIOMA

Lymphangioma is a common vascular tumor in children. This tumor comprised 0.3 to 1.5% of all orbital biopsies in five orbital tumor series (Table 14.1).[1–5] The real frequency may be higher because some asymptomatic and mildly symptomatic cases do not undergo biopsy. Lymphangioma most commonly presents in patients under 10 years of age. However, it is sometimes detected later in life following trauma and intralesional hemorrhage. In such cases, the diagnosis is difficult. In contrast to capillary hemangioma, lymphangiomas do not regress spontaneously. However, they generally become more encapsulated in later years of life as a result of the tendency of the body to form a barrier to further tumor expansion.

When studied with arteriography or venography, lymphangiomas show no demonstrable connections to the venous system.[6] This is in contrast to orbital varices, which usually demonstrate connections to the venous system.

Clinical Features

Clinically, orbital lymphangioma usually presents with a slowly progressive proptosis, globe displacement, ptosis, and eye motility restriction (Figures 14.8 and 14.9).[37] The eyelids may have a bluish discoloration due to subcutaneous involvement of the lymphangioma (Figure 14.8). The conjunctiva may show clear or hemorrhagic lymph channels (Figure 14.8).[38] Rarely, a focal lesion may remain asymptomatic.

Spontaneous hemorrhage is the most dreaded occurrence in a lymphangioma and may lead to eyelid ecchymosis, subconjunctival hemorrhage, and acute proptosis (Figure 14.6). This may create diagnostic difficulty in a patient with a previously undiagnosed asymptomatic lymphangioma. Acute increase in intraorbital pressure can result in compressive optic neuropathy and vision loss.[37,39] In the clinical differential diagnosis of spontaneous orbital hemorrhage, the following possibilities should be considered in addition to lymphangioma: trauma, bleeding disorder, orbital varix, and, rarely, cavernous hemangioma. One characteristic feature of lymphangioma is that the proptosis is exacerbated after trauma or upper respiratory tract infection.[38,40] Under these circumstances, hemorrhage into the channels of the tumor may lead to the development of chocolate cysts.

Orbital lymphangioma may occupy an intraconal or extraconal (Figures 14.9 and 14.10) location.[41] Differential diagnosis of this tumor should include cavernous hemangioma, hemangiopericytoma, fibrous histiocytoma, or neurilemoma and solitary neural tumors.

Orbital lymphangioma can rarely be associated with an orbital and/or intracranial arteriovenous malformation.[42,43] Another rare complication of orbital

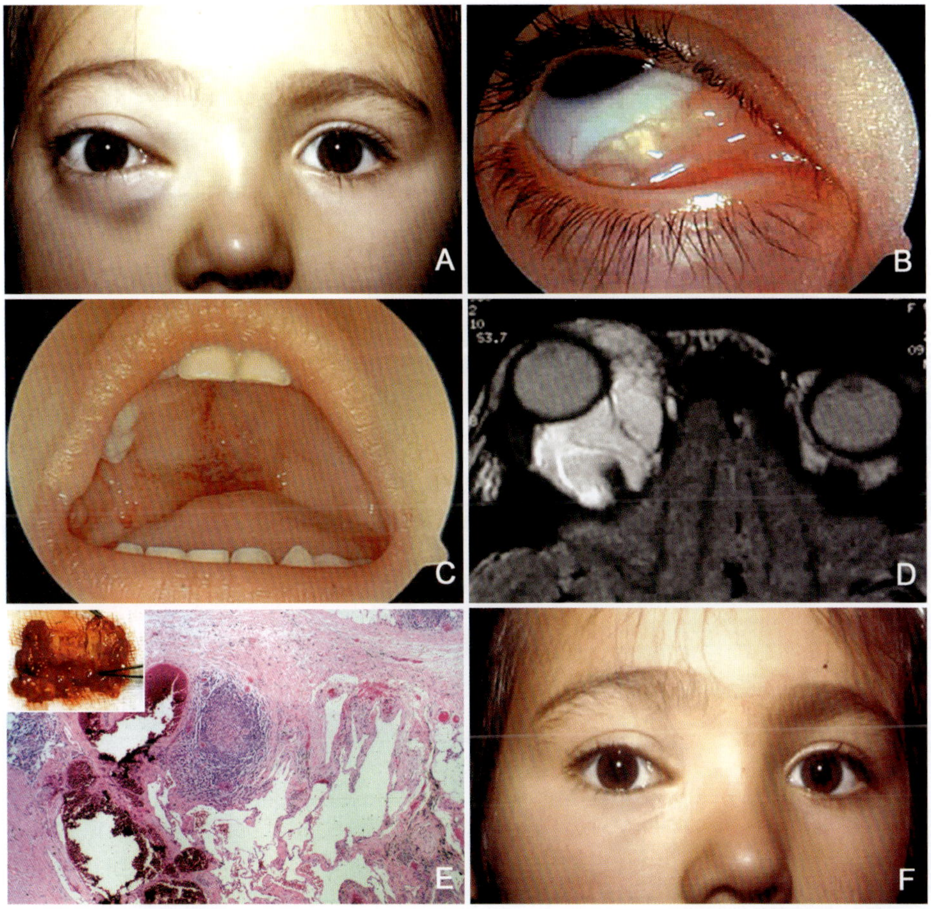

FIGURE 14.8. (A) Facial and (B) slit lamp photographs show swelling of the right periorbital tissues in a 4-year-old girl with right orbital lymphangiomas; note lateral displacement and clear conjunctival lymph channels on the medial conjunctiva. (C) Photograph of the open mouth showing a similar lesion affecting the soft palate. (D) T2-weighted axial MR image demonstrating various lymphatic cysts hyperintense to the extraocular muscle and cerebral gray matter in the right orbit. The cysts contain higher and lower intensity fluid, demonstrating a fluid–fluid level. The higher intensity fluid is due to the release of methemoglobin into the superior portion of the cyst. Histopathologic examination reveals large bloodless ectatic lymph channels lined by thinned endothelial cells. There are lymph follicles within the connective tissue trabeculae. The lymphangioma channels may appear empty, if intralesional hemorrhage has occurred; however, they will contain blood. *Inset*: Gross photograph of the partially excised lymphangioma. (F) Postoperative facial appearance showing complete resolution of right proptosis and eyelid swelling after partial excision of the lesion.

lymphangioma is association with orbital cellulitis. Because of its infiltrating nature, orbital lymphangioma may provide a route of entry for infections into the orbit from otherwise minor infections of the periocular skin and eyelids.[44]

Patients with orbital lymphangioma can have similar lesions in the skin and mucous membranes of the head including the soft palate (Figure 14.8). It is important to examine the skin and soft palate of the patient with orbital lymphangioma.[38]

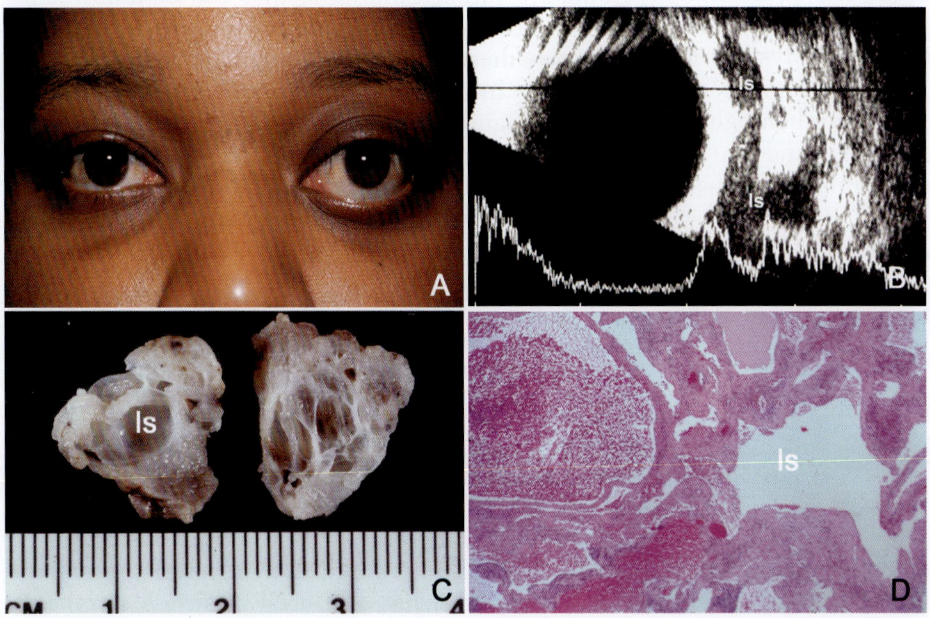

FIGURE 14.9. (A) Lymphangioma in a 24-year-old woman causing marked axial proptosis due to multicystic tumor. The lesion is well depicted in the B-scan ultrasonography (B) gross, and (C) microscopic (D) specimens of the tumor. Photomicrograph shows two cystic lesions within the same area, one filled with blood and the other empty. Note the aggregates of lymphocytes with and without germinal centers within the fibrous skeleton of the tumor (ls, lymphatic space).

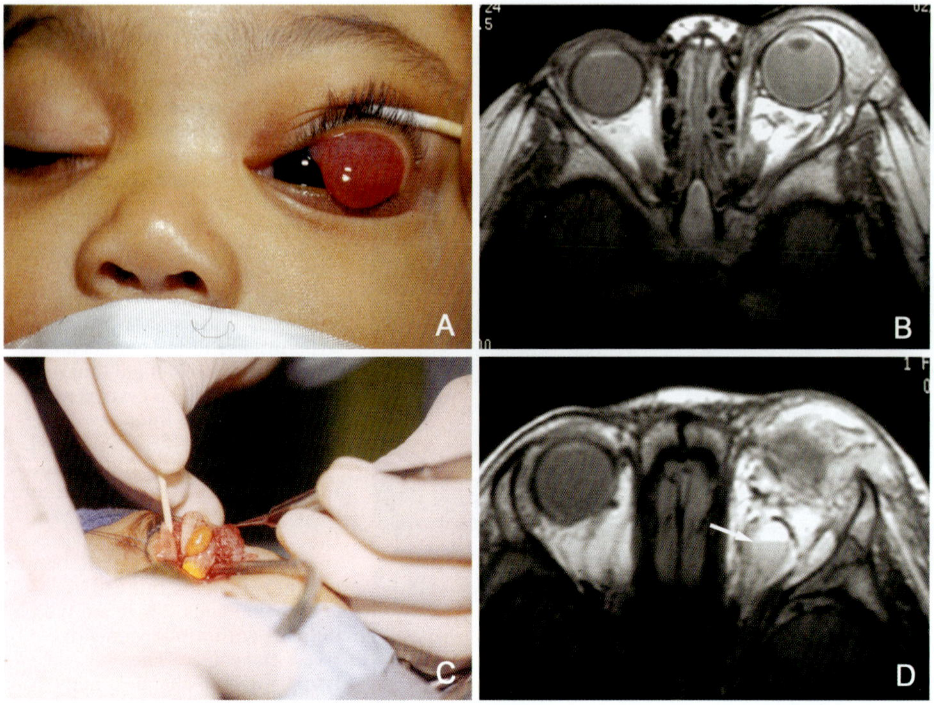

FIGURE 14.10. (A) An eyelid and anterior orbit lymphangioma prolapsing from the superior eyelid with bluish purple glistening surface. The T1-weighted axial MR images (B,D) reveal the multiloculated tumor anterior and posterior to the orbital septum. (C) The multicystic appearance of the tumor is also seen clearly in the intraoperative photograph with yellowish, transparent cystic structures. (D) Some of the cystic structures posterior to the globe show fluid–fluid level (arrow).

Radiologic Features

A-scan and particularly B-scan ultrasonography may help diagnosis by demonstrating the compressibility of large, irregular cystic spaces. The demonstration of multiple spaces differentiate this lesion from a varix.

An irregular mass is demonstrated by CT and MRI. The mass has a multicystic appearance on CT. MRI shows internal tissue features better. Acute hemorrhage in the lesion appears hypointense with respect to the extraocular muscle and cerebral gray matter on T1- and T2-weighted images because of its high concentration of deoxyhemoglobin. As the hemorrhage ages, the tumor demonstrates a hyperintense signal on T1- and T2-weighted images as a result of lysis of red blood cells with release of paramagnetic methemoglobin (Figure 14.8). With aging, the methemoglobin degrades into hemosiderin and ferritin, and the hyperintensity on T1- and T2-weighted images gradually changes to hypointensity.[23,45]

Orbital lymphangioma may demonstrate fluid–fluid levels in the lesion, especially on T2-weighted images. The blood–fluid level is due to the coexistence of higher and lower density fluid (Figure 14.10). The higher density is due to the presence of methemoglobin.[23] In large lymphangiomas, MRI can demonstrate the tumor's blood supply. Such vessels show a flow-void artifact.

Morphologic Features

Grossly, lymphangioma has an ill-defined appearance; the lesion is blue or dark red. Histopathologically, it is composed of bloodless ectatic lymph channels. These spaces are lined by a single layer of flat mesothelial cells (Figures 14.8 and 14.9). Hemorrhage into these spaces produces chocolate cysts. Lymphoid aggregates, with or without germinal centers, are often seen. Fibrosis is present in lymphangiomas with chronic recurrent hemorrhages.[37] Lymphangioma may resemble a cavernous hemangioma or varix microscopically as well as clinically.

Management and Prognosis

The indications for treatment of an orbital lymphangioma are varied. Smaller lesions can be followed serially with neuroimaging studies, provided a presumptive diagnosis of lymphangioma has been made. Surgery is indicated for larger lesions producing cosmetic disfigurement, proptosis and corneal exposure, or signs of optic nerve dysfunction including relative afferent pupillary defect.[46] Therefore, the main indications for surgical intervention in orbital lymphangioma are preservation of visual function and cosmetic appearance.

The treatment of orbital lymphangioma can be challenging. Smaller lymphangiomas can be completely excised. In the case of larger lymphangiomas, the tumor should be treated by debulking or at least partial excision of the anterior part of the lesion.[37,46] Sometimes large blood cysts can be managed by simple aspiration. Electrocauterization has been used to reduce the risk of bleeding at the time of surgical excision. To facilitate surgical removal of a lymphangioma, CO_2 laser has also been used.[47] A number of potential complications, including damage to ciliary nerves producing dilated pupils and symblepharon, can occur with the use of CO_2 laser.

Tunç et al. reported that 15 (58%) of their 26 patients with orbital lymphangioma demonstrated recurrences after initial surgery at a mean follow-up of 9.2 years.[37] They concluded that motility restriction was significantly more frequent at initial examination in patients, who later experienced recurrence than in those without recurrence. This observation attests to the fact that diffuse lymphangiomas causing motility problems are difficult to excise completely and demonstrate more recurrences than focal isolated lesion.[37] Many lymphangiomas are not good candidates for surgical treatment and do not respond well to radiation; therefore, cell-targeted therapies for lymphangioma are under investigation. Esmaeli and coworkers reported promising results with Imatinib Mesylate (Gleevec®) (Bita Esmaeli, M.D. personal communication, 2003).

If a lymphangioma is associated with an orbital arteriovenous malformation, embolization of the arteriovenous malformation should be attempted first to decrease the risk of bleeding at surgery.[42] In the case of intraconal lymphangiomas, if difficulty is encountered in excision of the lesion posteriorly, the surgeon should consider leaving the residual apical component to avoid damage to the major orbital vessels, including the central retinal artery.[41] There has been no report to date on the malignant transformation of a benign lymphangioma.

ORBITAL VARIX

The orbital varix is a rare orbital vascular lesion, which accounted for 0 to 1.3% of all histopathologically proven orbital tumors in five orbital series (Table 14.1).[1–5] The pathogenesis of this lesion is not clearly understood. Weakening of the vein wall may be the initial event in the development of a varix. This leads to stagnant blood flow in the vein. The absence of valves in the orbital veins, as in the veins above the neck, increases the pooling of blood. Both factors, weakening of the vessel wall and pooling of blood, result in thrombosis. After organization, the thrombus recanalizes. However, the sluggish blood flow results in proximal dilation, producing an enlarged varix.[48]

Clinical Features

Orbital varix is usually diagnosed between the ages of 10 to 30 years. However, it can be encountered in every age group, including neonates.[49] This lesion generally involves the superior ophthalmic vein. However, other veins of the orbit can also be affected.

Most patients with an orbital varix develop positional proptosis. This is because the lesion has connections to the systemic venous circulation.[6] The proptosis is exacerbated when the patient assumes a prone position, bends over, or performs a Valsalva maneuver.[50] As the eye becomes more prominent, the palpebral fissure widens if the tumor is in the posterior orbit. Positional proptosis may not be seen in all cases of orbital varix because some small nondistensible varices have minimal or no connection to the systemic venous circulation (Figure 14.11).

Sometimes the lesion can have an acute onset with painful proptosis, compressive optic neuropathy, and decreased visual acuity, probably corresponding to the thrombosis or hemorrhage of the affected vein.[51] Spontaneous orbital hemorrhage is more likely to occur with an orbital lymphangioma than with a varix.

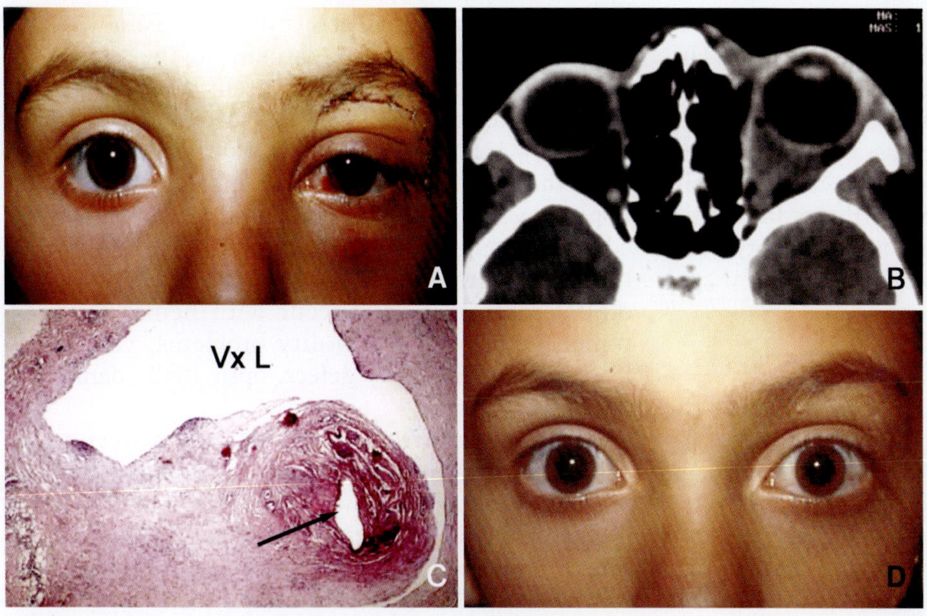

FIGURE 14.11. (A) Facial photograph demonstrating the upper eyelid edema, subconjunctival hemorrhage, and proptosis in a 7-year-old girl who had undergone an orbitotomy for the orbital lesion. The lesion could not be identified during exploration. (B) Axial orbital CT with Valsalva maneuver showing the left orbital varix with ill-defined borders (C). Histopathologic examination of the lesion shows the dilated or ectatic vein with markedly thickened vessel walls. An organized recanalizing thrombus (arrow) is present within the lumen of the varix (VxL). (D) Facial photograph of the child 6 months after surgery shows no residual proptosis or eyelid abnormality.

Orbital varices have been divided into primary or secondary types. A primary orbital varix is confined to the orbit and is unassociated with an orbital or intracranial arteriovenous malformation. The secondary orbital varix develops in association with an intracranial arteriovenous malformation that shunts blood to the orbital venous system, causing the veins to dilate secondarily.[23]

Radiologic Features

Plain x-ray images may demonstrate foci of calcification (phleboliths) in the orbital varix.[50] Venography was a popular method in the demonstration of the orbital varix. Because it is an invasive technique, it is rarely used today.[52] Color Doppler flow imaging has been used in the diagnosis of an orbital varix. The lesion demonstrates increased blood flow during the Valsalva maneuver with color Doppler flow imaging.[53]

CT and MR images show an irregular mass usually located in the posterior orbit (Figure 14.11). CT is superior to MRI in the demonstration of phleboliths. In some cases, the orbital varix may not be visible with routine CT or MR imaging. However, if the patient performs a Valsalva maneuver during the CT or MRI scan, the lesion becomes apparent.[50] If there is no associated hemorrhage or thrombosis, the orbital varix is hypointense on T1-weighted images and T2-weighted images with respect to the extraocular muscles and cerebral gray matter.[23] The lesion demonstrates heterogeneous internal signal intensity consistent with the presence of blood in various stages of degeneration. Hyperintensity on T1- and T2-weighted images is related to the presence of methemoglobin, and hypointensity is related to the presence of deoxyhemoglobin.

Morphologic Features

Grossly, the lesion is dark red. A varix is a dilated vein that has undergone thrombosis and hyalinization. Histopathologic examination reveals that the lesion is composed of irregular vascular channels lined by endothelial cells (Figure 14.11). With the passage of time, there is thickening of the walls of the veins, hemosiderin pigment consistent with chronic hemorrhage, interstitial fibrosis, an infiltration of chronic inflammatory cells, and intraluminal calcification (phleboliths).[48,49]

Management and Prognosis

The treatment of orbital varix is difficult. Usually the anterior portion of the lesion is excised surgically. Alternatively, drainage of the blood clot and electrocauterization of the vessel wall have been done. One problem with surgical excision is that orbital varix is often in a collapsed state when the patient is supine. This may create difficulty in the exposure and dissection of a varix in the posterior orbit. In such cases, surgical management of the lesion is greatly enhanced by the application of jugular compression, placing the patient in the Trendelenburg position or having the anesthesiologist increase the intrathoracic pressure. Intraoperative injection of a hardening substance and subsequent excision of the varix have also been tried. It is seldom possible to remove the entire lesion, especially when it is located posteriorly in the orbit. Most patients with a primary orbital varix have a good prognosis. Although recurrence after subtotal excision is a concern, most patients remain stable without evidence of rebleeding.[48] However, intracranial bleeding may occur secondary to an intracranial arteriovenous malformation.

Endovascular embolization of an orbital varix prior to or as an alternative to surgical removal has also been used.[54] This measure may decrease the risk of bleeding during surgery.

HEMANGIOPERICYTOMA

The orbital hemangiopericytoma is a rare vascular tumor in the orbit. The frequency of hemangiopericytoma in five orbital series[1–5] was 0.1 to 1.2% (Table 14.1). It was first described in 1942 by Stout and Murray.[55] It presumably arises from the fully differentiated pericytes of the orbital blood vessels. In the great majority of patients, the condition becomes clinically apparent between the ages of 20 and 70 years.[56–59] However, hemangiopericytoma can also occur in patients outside this age range.

Clinical Features

The patient with orbital hemangiopericytoma develops a slowly progressive unilateral proptosis with or without pain and visual acuity decrease. Pain was present in 21 to 29% of the patients in two series.[57,59] The majority of these tumors occur superiorly in the orbit and produce downward displacement of the globe (Figure 14.12).[56,57] However, rarely the tumor can occupy the inferior orbit.[60] There may be intermittent upper eyelid swelling resembling angioneurotic edema.[56] Sometimes the skin overlying the tumor is bluish.[56,58] Other manifestations of a space-occupying orbital mass that may occur with hemangiopericytoma include ocular motility problems, visual field loss, afferent pupillary defect, optic disk edema, and choroidal folds.[57]

The slow growth rate of hemangiopericytoma is evident by the long duration of symptoms reported by many patients.[56,58] However, malignant hemangiopericytomas can also demonstrate rapid growth, spanning a few months. In one such case the production of conjunctival chemosis was reported.[61]

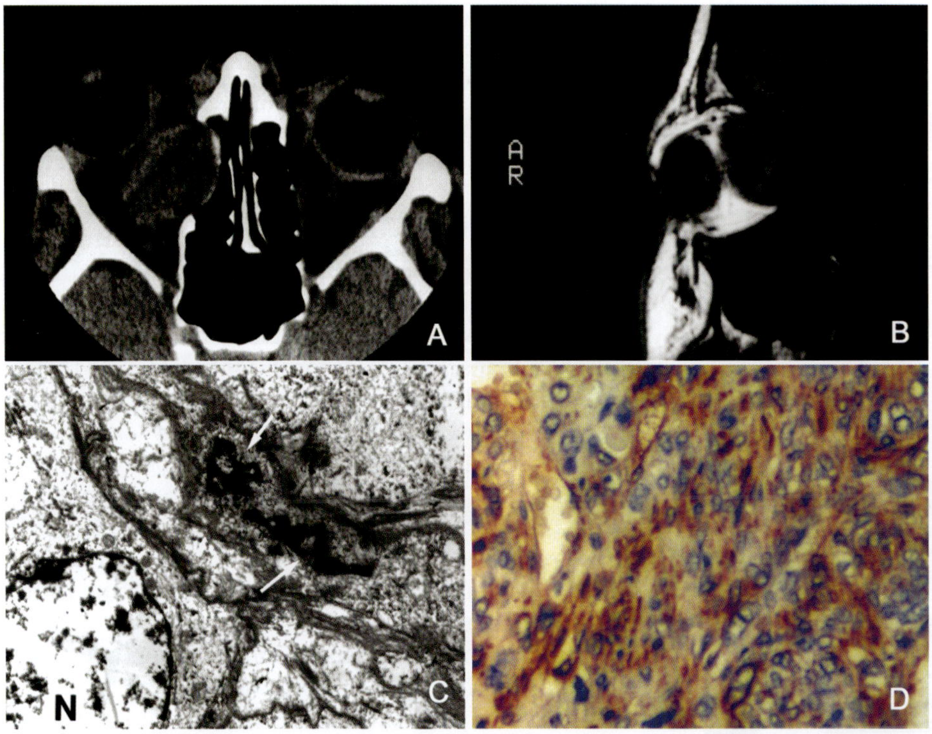

FIGURE 14.12. (A,B) Axial CT and sagittal T1-weighted MR images show a well-delineated vascular tumor within intra- and extraconal space. (C) Histopathologically, the tumor was composed of proliferation of spindle-shaped pericytes with a low mitotic rate; photomicrograph reveals the ultrastructural appearance of a neoplastic pericyte with a rounded nucleus (N) and irregular deposits of basement membrane material (white arrows) in the intercellular matrix between neoplastic cells (C). (D) Immunohistochemical preparation that is markedly CD34 positive (brownish staining).

There have been reports of choroidal,[62] lacrimal sac,[63] and optic nerve[64] involvement by hemangiopericytoma.

Hemangiopericytoma may take a malignant clinical course (Figure 14.13). Malignant hemangiopericytomas tend to undergo local recurrence, invasion into the central nervous system, and metastasis to distant organs, particularly the lungs, bone, and liver. A rare case of hemangiopericytoma metastatic to the breast has also been reported. The biologic behavior of this tumor cannot be predicted from the histopathologic appearance of the lesion.[59] A tumor with benign histopathologic features can demonstrate malignant clinical behavior.

Radiologic Features

A- and B-mode ultrasonography demonstrate, respectively, low–medium reflectivity and acoustic hollowness in the lesion. The reflectivity on A-mode ultrasonography is low in solid tumors and medium in tumors that demonstrate cavitation.[38] Orbital CT and MR images show a well-circumscribed lesion usually located superiorly in the orbit. On CT, orbital hemangiopericytoma can demonstrate calcification in the lesion.[65] Other vascular tumors such as hemangioma, lymphangioma, and varix can also demonstrate calcification in the lesion. Sometimes the hemangiopericytoma can be extensive; involvement of the sinuses and the cranial cavity is best documented on CT and MRI.[57]

MRI discloses that the tumor is isointense with respect to the extraocular muscles on T1-weighted images and hyperintense on T2-weighted images.[57] The tumor demonstrates moderate enhancement after contrast injection. As such, the tumor is indistinguishable from other well-circumscribed orbital lesions by MRI (Figure 14.12). Hemangiopericytoma can develop cavitation and therefore simulate a cystic lesion on neuroimaging studies.[57]

Morphologic Features

Grossly, the hemangiopericytoma is a well-circumscribed lesion. The lesion is red and has an appearance similar to cavernous hemangioma. The tumor may or may not have a capsule surrounding the tumor. Histopathologically, the tumor is composed of pericytes with ill-defined borders, large cytoplasm, and round to oval nuclei. Pericytes usually are ovoid, but spindle cells can also be seen. The histopathologic pattern is mixed and even varies between different zones in a tumor.[57,59] These cells surround the sinusoidal or staghorn-shaped blood channels lined by a single row of flattened endothelial cells. The pericytes are surrounded by a reticulin framework. The reticulin deposits surround individual cells in hemangiopericytoma. This is in contrast to other vascular tumors, in which the reticulin framework surrounds a cluster of cells, not each cell individually.[57]

The pericyte does not react with CD31, factor VIII related antigen, and/or *Ulex europaeus* agglutinin I, which stain the endothelial cells. However, it does react with vimentin and CD34 (Figure 14.12).[66]

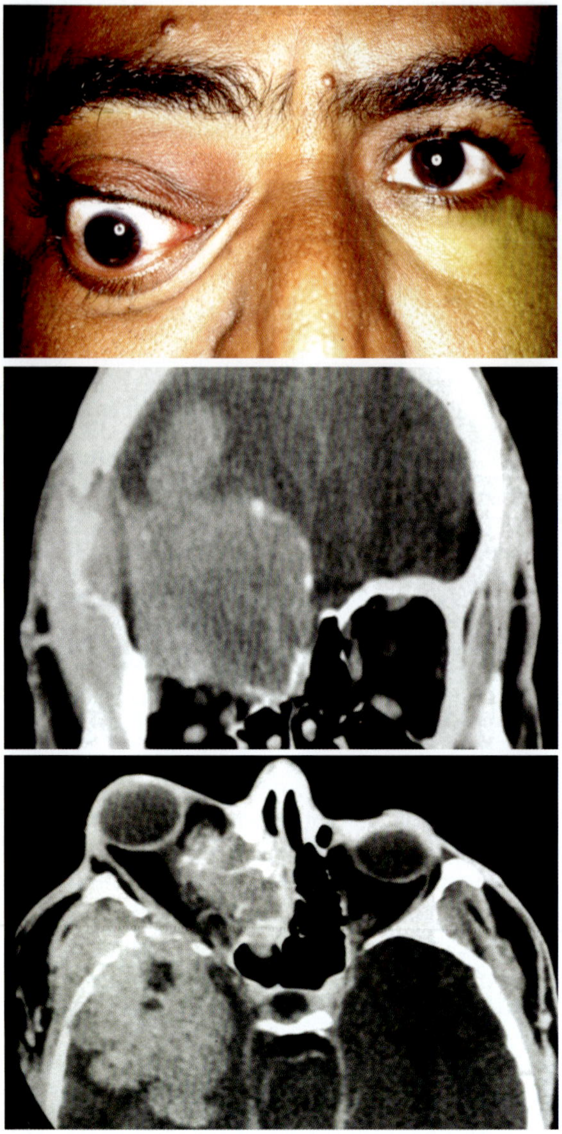

FIGURE 14.13. Massive proptosis and inferior dislocation of the right globe secondary to large hemangiopericytoma extending into the cranium, perinasal sinuses, and nasal cavity. The histopathology revealed sarcomatous changes with high mitotic rate (6 per HPF).

Croxatto and Font counted the number of mitotic figures per 40 high power fields (HPF) and found that in the benign group of tumors there were 4 mitotic figures per HPF and in the borderline group there were 14 mitotic figures per HPF. The malignant tumors averaged 35 mitotic figures per HPF.[59] Hemangiopericytomas that are capable of recurrence and metastasis usually have more than 4 mitotic figures per 10 HPF. However, hemangiopericytomas with fewer than 4 mitotic figures per HPF can also demonstrate malignant potential.[59] Other histopathologic features that may indicate malignant potential are cellular anaplasia, foci of necrosis and hemorrhage, increased cellularity, and scarcity of reticulin fibers.[59] However, the biologic behavior of hemangiopericytoma cannot be reliably predicted from the histopathologic appearance of the tumor.

Ultrastructurally, the hemangiopericytoma demonstrates different cell types. The pericyte-like cell is the type most frequently encountered and is considered to be diagnostic of hemangiopericytoma in transmission electron microscopic studies (Figure 14.12).[57]

Management and Prognosis

Because hemangiopericytoma is usually well circumscribed, the best treatment consists of total excision of the tumor. Tumors that invade the cranial cavity require a transcranial approach for removal of the tumor. External beam radiotherapy[67] and brachytherapy[68] have been used for incompletely excised hemangiopericytoma. A total radiation dose of at least 50 Gy should be delivered to prevent recurrence.[67] If the tumor is histopathologically malignant, some authors prefer to use orbital exenteration and supplemental external beam radiotherapy even if the tumor has been excised completely.

Completeness of initial tumor excision appears to have the greatest impact on the subsequent tumor behavior. Incomplete excision of the tumor is associated with a higher risk of local recurrence and distant metastasis. An incompletely excised orbital hemangiopericytoma can recur many years after initial surgery. In one report, the tumor recurred 33 years after the initial operation. Croxatto and Font noted a 30% recurrence rate and a 15% metastasis-related death rate in their review of 30 orbital hemangiopericytomas.[59] Recurrence is a risk factor for ultimate metastasis (Figure 14.13). In the series by Karcioglu et al., 3 of 7 (43%) patients with orbital hemangiopericytoma eventually died from central nervous system metastasis.[57] Based on these results, orbital hemangiopericytoma does not seem to have a better prognosis than its counterparts elsewhere in the body.

When the tumor shows secondary invasion into the adjacent bones, the sinuses, and the cranial cavity or metastasizes to distant organs, palliative radiotherapy and chemotherapy should be administered. Chemotherapy consisting of doxorubicin hydrochloride, cyclophosphamide, and methotrexate has been reported to be effective.[59]

ANGIOSARCOMA

Angiosarcoma, or malignant hemangioendothelioma, is a very rare tumor of the eyelids and orbit (Table 14.1). It most often develops in the skin and other soft tissues.[69,70] Rarely the deep tissues and viscera may also be involved. Angiosarcoma can also be encountered as a metastatic tumor in the orbit.[71]

The pathogenesis of angiosarcoma is obscure. It develops de novo in most cases, although it has also been reported to arise after irradiation of some vascular tumor or from persistent chronic lymphedema in the extremities (Stewart–Treves syndrome).[72] The tumor may originate from the vascular system, the lymphatic system, or both.

Clinical Features

The majority of tumors arise in the upper part of the face or scalp.[69] The central part of the face, including the eyelids and orbit is involved less often.[73] The lower face, including the mandibular region, is seldom affected. Involvement of the facial skin may present with maculopapular lesions resembling ecchymoses, edema, cellulites, or ulceration, or in a nodular form.[69]

The patient with orbital angiosarcoma usually develops rapidly progressive proptosis and displacement of the globe. The tumor may secondarily invade the orbit from the sphenoid bone[74] and can produce painful ophthalmoplegia, simulating Tolosa–Hunt syndrome.[75] Angiosarcoma is a very aggressive tumor that has the capacity to invade the central nervous system locally and to metastasize to lymph nodes and hematogenously to distant organs such as the liver.[69,76]

Clinically, angiosarcoma is more common in children.[75,76] It is more frequent in the anterior and/or superior orbit and is associated with swelling of the upper eyelid.[76] There is no sex predilection. The tumor seems to have a worse prognosis in adults than in children.[76]

Radiologic Features

CT reveals a well-circumscribed or ill-defined mass in the orbit. The tumor may be located anteriorly or posteriorly.[75,76] It is difficult to differentiate orbital angiosarcoma from other tumors by neuroimaging methods unless there is rapidly expanding bony infiltration.

Morphologic Features

Grossly, the angiosarcoma is usually an ill-defined, reddish-blue mass. Histopathologically, the tumor is composed of cords of pleomorphic atypical endothelial cells lining bizarrely shaped vascular spaces. The vascular spaces intertwine with dense, fibrous connective tissue.[69] A variant with epithelioid metaplasia has also been reported to involve the orbit.[75] The tumor stains positive for CD31, CD34, cytoplasmic factor VIII, and *Ulex europaeus* agglutinin I antigens, proving the endothelial cell origin of this tumor.[66,76] Weibel–Palade bodies, characteristic of endothelial cells, are present in only small numbers in angiosarcoma because of poor differentiation of the cells.[21]

Management and Prognosis

Orbital angiosarcoma is probably best managed with wide surgical excision, including orbital exenteration if necessary. If there is a question of residual tumor, supplemental radiotherapy should be considered. If there is diffuse involvement of the eyelids, wide-field external beam radiation therapy is the best treatment.[73] The prognosis for angiosarcoma of the scalp and face seems to be poor. The 5-year survival rate of face and scalp angiosarcomas is around 12%.[69] However, long-lasting remissions have been reported after total excision and external beam radiotherapy of orbital and spheno-orbital angiosarcomas.[74,76]

INTRAVASCULAR PAPILLARY ENDOTHELIAL HYPERPLASIA

Intravascular papillary endothelial hyperplasia (IPEH) (Masson tumor) is an extremely rare lesion in the orbit. It represents an exuberant proliferation of vascular endothelium as a cellular response to the organization of a thrombus.[77] This condition usually occurs in a varix. However, IPEH can occur as a sequela to thrombus formation in any orbital vascular hamartomatous lesion.

Clinical Features

Intravascular papillary endothelial hyperplasia was first described as an eyelid lesion.[78] Later, orbital cases were diagnosed.[77,79] The patient with orbital IPEH is usually an adult 20 to 55 years old. Ocular findings may include proptosis, chemosis, restricted ocular motility, disk edema, and choroidal folds, depending on the location of the lesion. The onset of proptosis may be acute or progressive. The tumor may occasionally demonstrate invasion into the periocular tissues such as the temporal fossa.[79] The pattern of bone resorption is similar to organizing hematoma of the orbital bone. Another presentation of IPEH is involvement of the superior orbital fissure.[80,81]

Radiologic Features

CT reveals a well-circumscribed or irregular lesion without any pathognomonic features.[77,81]

Morphologic Features

Grossly, the lesion of IPEH appears as a smooth, blue-gray mass that is round or oval. The wall of the vein is in fact the circumscribed wall of the lesion. Microscopically, the tumor consists of papillary fronds lined by single or multiple layers of proliferated endothelial cells with no atypia. Other features such as fibrin deposition, degree of collagenization, and the inflammatory cell component depend on the age of the thrombus.[77,81] The histopathologic differential diagnosis includes angiosarcoma and angiolymphoid hyperplasia with eosinophilia (Kimura disease).[81]

Management and Prognosis

The tumor can usually be managed by total excision.[77] Incomplete excision may lead to recurrence, especially if IPEH originated from a vascular tumor such as a hemangioma or lymphangioma.[38] The prognosis for life is generally good following resection of IPEH. The lesion usually does not undergo malignant transformation.

ARTERIOVENOUS FISTULAS AND MALFORMATIONS

Arteriovenous fistulas affecting the orbit result from some abnormal communication between the arteries and veins. Three basic types of arteriovenous fistula affect the orbit: carotid cavernous fistula, dural cavernous fistula, and orbital arteriovenous fistula. Carotid cavernous fistula develops between the intracavernous internal carotid artery and the cavernous sinus. This type of fistula is usually traumatic but may be caused by rupture of an aneurysm, especially in an atherosclerotic individual. Carotid cavernous fistula has a high flow rate.[82]

Dural cavernous fistula develops between the small meningeal branches of the internal/external carotid artery and the cavernous sinus. These vessels have thin walls and may rupture spontaneously, especially in the hypertensive patient after minor trauma or on straining. This type of fistula usually develops spontaneously and has a low flow rate.[82,83]

Orbital arteriovenous fistula usually results from traumatic rupture of the ethmoidal artery into the orbital venous system. However, it can occur spontaneously. In one case of spontaneous orbital arteriovenous malformation, the communication was between branches of the ophthalmic and facial arteries and the orbital veins.[84] This type of fistula has a low flow rate similar to that of dural–cavernous fistula.

Clinical Features

The primary problem is a rise in the orbital venous pressure. Clinical findings of arteriovenous fistulas include dilation and tortuosity of the conjunctival and episcleral vessels, chemosis, ocular motility problems, proptosis, choroidal detachment,[85] and secondary glaucoma.[86] Secondary acute angle closure glaucoma has also been reported to occur with arteriovenous fistulas.[87] Ocular motility problems can be twofold. Generalized ophthalmoplegia is probably due to congested swollen extraocular muscles.[82] Isolated abduction weakness can also develop in patients with carotid cavernous fistula. The abduction weakness is due to sixth nerve palsy occurring either in the cavernous sinus or more posteriorly near the inferior petrosal sinus.[82] Rarely,

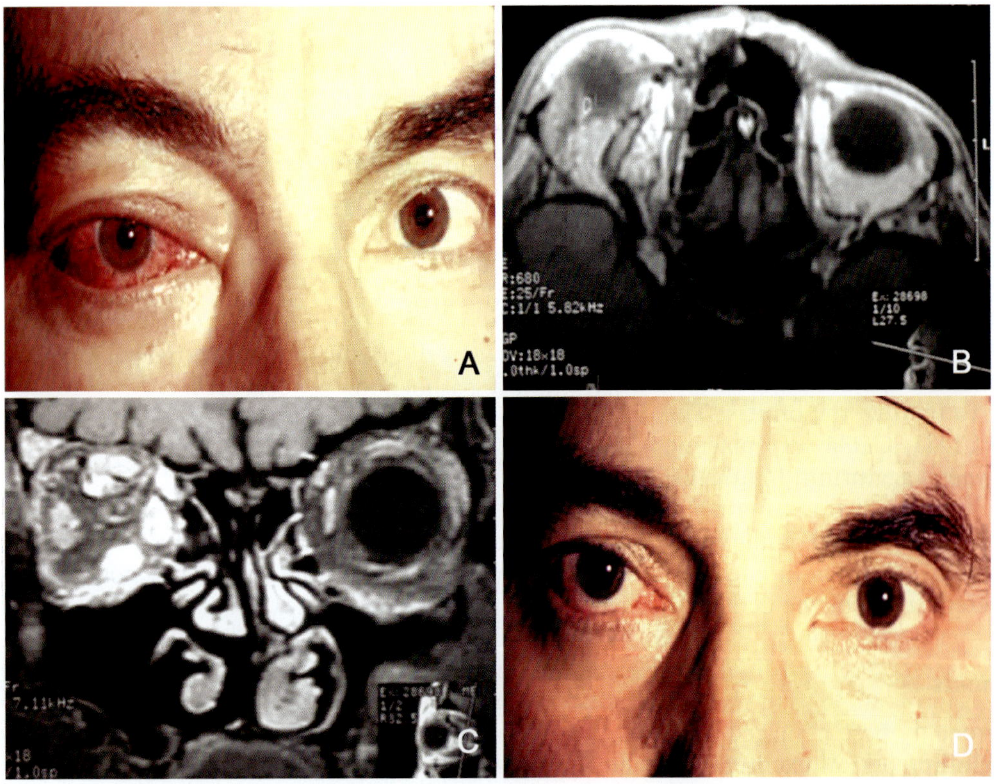

FIGURE 14.14. (A) Facial photograph of a 54-year-old man with carotid cavernous fistula affecting the right eye demonstrates the proptosis of the right eye and conjunctival and episcleral injection. The right eye had secondary glaucoma unresponsive to topical drops. (B) T1-weighted axial orbital MR image showing the dilated superior ophthalmic vein on the right side. (C) T1-weighted contrast enhanced coronal orbital MR image showing the equally enlarged extraocular muscles on the right side. (D) Postoperative appearance of the patient 2 months after balloon catheterization and closure of the fistula.

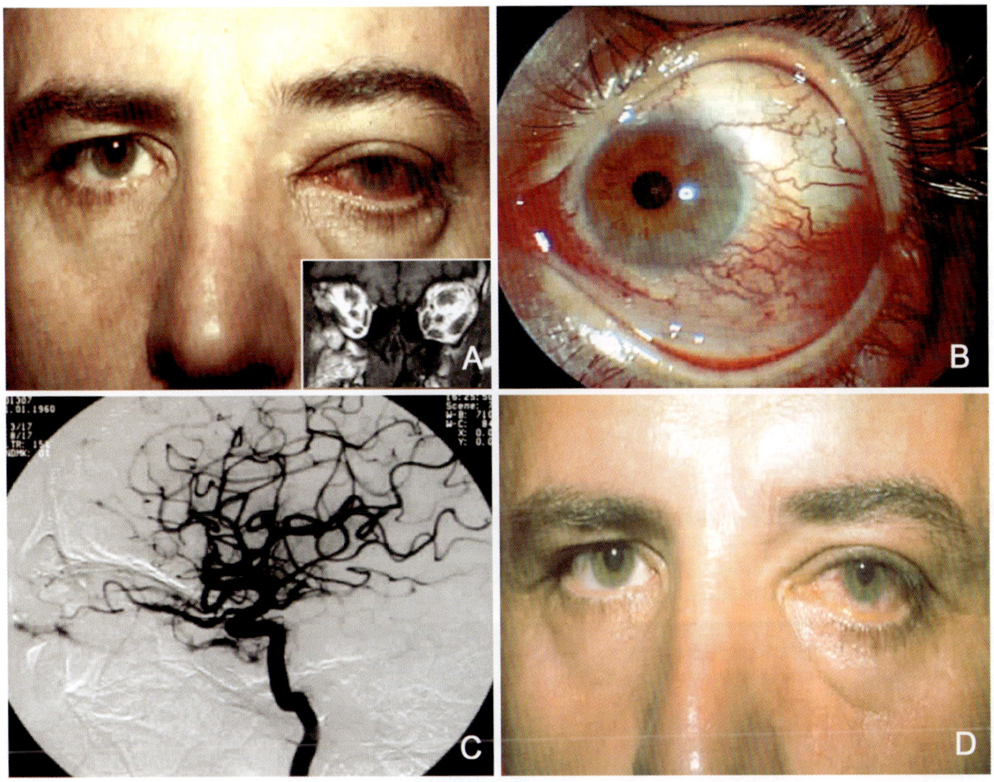

FIGURE 14.15. Photographs of a 40-year-old man with dural cavernous fistula involving the left eye showing (A) proptosis and (B) conjunctival and episcleral injection. *Inset*: T1-weighted coronal orbital MR image depicting the enlarged extraocular muscles on the left side. (C) Cerebral angiogram demonstrating the arteriovenous communication between the meningeal branches of the external carotid artery and the cavernous sinus. (D) Appearance of the patient 2 months after transarterial catheterization and embolization of the fistula.

third or fourth nerve palsy can also be seen in patients with arteriovenous fistulas.[82]

The clinical and radiologic findings are more severe in carotid cavernous fistula than in dural cavernous and orbital arteriovenous fistulas (Figures 14.14 and 14.15).[86] These findings typically occur ipsilateral to the carotid cavernous sinus but may also occur on the contralateral side owing to the presence of connections between the cavernous sinus on both sides.[88] Anomalous intracranial venous drainage such as atresia of sinuses can also lead to a clinical picture similar to arteriovenous fistulas.[89]

Rarely, the anomalous arteriovenous vascular proliferations present within a mass lesion simulating an orbital tumor (Figure 14.16).[90] Some patients experience a severe exacerbation of symptoms before undergoing clinical improvement. This has been correlated clinically with superior ophthalmic vein thrombosis.[91] One report documented an occasion of uncontrolled bleeding at enucleation after penetrating orbital trauma, resulting from an unsuspected carotid cavernous fistula.[92] These anomalous vascular aggregates may or may not have vascular feeder vessels. The presence or absence of a circulatory relationship should be investigated with angiography before surgery.

Radiologic Features

Orbital ultrasonography, CT, and MRI demonstrate enlarged extraocular muscles and a dilated superior ophthalmic vein in arteriovenous fistula (Figure 14.14). An arteriovenous malformation should be suspected in the presence of symmetrically enlarged extraocular muscles.[86] Arteriovenous fistula is seen on CT with contrast enhancement and on MRI with a signal void of the arterialized flow in the superior ophthalmic vein. CT and MR angiography can be used, but these imaging techniques offer information concerning the flow characteristics only, not etiology.[93] Color Doppler flow imaging has also been used to examine the superior ophthalmic vein in arteriovenous fistulas. Color Doppler flow imaging findings correlate well with angiographic findings and can be used to monitor the status of the patient postoperatively.[94] Angiography may be both diagnostic and therapeutic in patients with suspected arteriovenous fistula. Digital subtraction angiography is the examination method of choice in diagnosing arteriovenous fistula. Pathophysiologic classification into high-flow (type A) and low-flow (type B) fistulas is crucial to decide on a management plan.[95]

Morphologic Features

Most patients with an arteriovenous fistula do not undergo a biopsy procedure (Table 14.1). Histopathologically, these malformations consist of abnormally formed arteries and veins with an irregular elastic and muscular layer and secondary endothelial cell proliferation that simulate the appearance of a capillary hemangioma.[96]

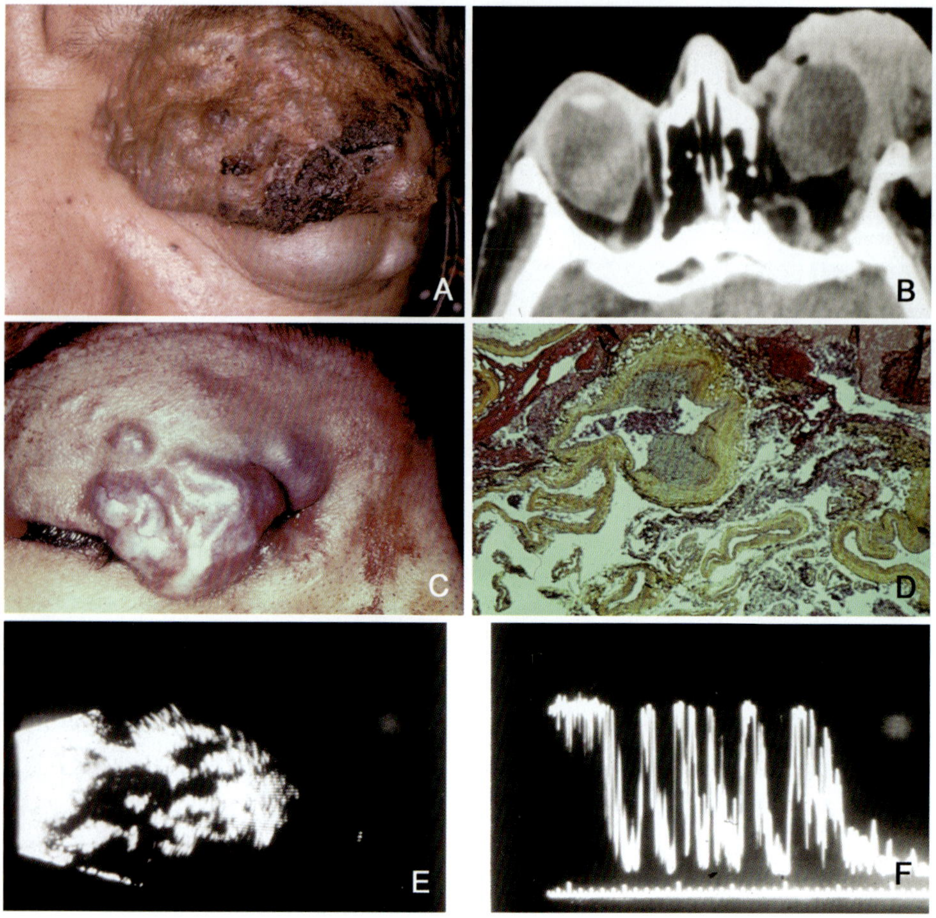

FIGURE 14.16. (A,B) Long-standing vascular malformation of the upper eyelid and the anterior orbit forming a mass lesion without any arterial or venous connections. (C) Another arteriovenous malformation of the upper eyelid that presented as a pulsating mass. (D) The histopathology of the same lesion shows abnormal arterial and venous blood vessels intertwined within a vascular hamartomatous mass. (E,F) The ultrasonographic examination of the lesion reveals multiple cystic spaces with B-mode scan and a marked variation of internal reflectivity with A-mode scan.

Management and Prognosis

The prognosis for life is excellent for any patients with an orbital arteriovenous fistula. However, the angiography techniques used for this condition carry a definitive risk of mortality and morbidity. Therefore, it is best to avoid surgical intervention in many cases of dural cavernous fistulas as long as the patient is not severely symptomatic.[86] The indications for treatment of arteriovenous, mostly carotid cavernous fistulas are visual loss, diplopia, severe headache, severe proptosis leading to corneal exposure, and angle-closure glaucoma.[86]

Extrinsic manual carotid compression has been used to close dural and carotid cavernous fistulas. The patient compresses the carotid artery with his contralateral hand; if he experiences cerebral ischemia, the hand becomes paretic and drops. Successful closure of 30% of dural and 10% of carotid cavernous fistulas with this noninvasive technique has been reported.[86]

In contrast to dural cavernous fistula, carotid cavernous fistulas generally require treatment. The most widely used method in the treatment of carotid cavernous fistula is cerebral angiography and balloon embolization (Figure 14.14). The success of balloon embolization ranges from 70 to 92% for carotid cavernous fistulas.[86] Other procedures that have been combined with angiography include ligation and clipping of small arterial feeders. These procedures are rarely employed today. Potential complications of cerebral angiography include bleeding, persistence of the fistula, cranial nerve palsies, false aneurysm secondary to a prematurely deflated balloon, internal carotid artery occlusion leading to cerebral ischemia and ocular ischemic syndrome, and death from treatment-related complications.

Because of the risks of the surgical procedures through the internal carotid artery trunk, Hanneken et al. developed an alternative approach.[97] These authors surgically expose the superior ophthalmic vein in the orbit, enter the vein by needle puncture, insert a balloon-tipped catheter and pass it into the cavernous sinus, inflate the balloon to close the fistula, and detach the balloon. However, if the superior ophthalmic vein is not dilated or is located deep in the orbit, transorbital venous access may not be possible.

About 25 to 50% of dural carotid sinus arteriovenous fistulas close spontaneously.[86] Therefore, the patients are best followed conservatively without angiography. If the patient becomes severely symptomatic, angiography should be undertaken. The transvenous route is more effective than transarterial access in these cases. The treatment of choice for endovascular surgery is glue or particulate embolization to close the various dural feeders. Clinical improvement or cure is obtained in most embolized dural cavernous fistulas, even those that were incompletely closed by angiography. Goldberg and associates and Benndorf and coworkers reported that cannulation of the superior ophthalmic vein and embolization of the cavernous sinus can also be employed in dural cavernous fistulas either after conventional angiography methods have failed or as a primary treatment.[98,99]

LEIOMYOMA

Vascular leiomyoma is another rare benign tumor of the orbit (Table 14.1). Leiomyoma is believed to arise from the smooth muscle of orbital blood vessels, from pericytes or from Müller's muscle when it is located anteriorly in the orbit.[100,101]

Clinical Features

Orbital leiomyoma can occur as an eyelid or orbital tumor.[100,102,103] In the orbit, leiomyoma can occur in an intraconal or extraconal location, producing slowly progressive proptosis.[103a] It can also occur at the orbital apex and demonstrate intracranial extension through the bony orbital fissures.[103]

Radiologic Features

CT and MRI images show a well-circumscribed lesion in the orbit. On MRI, orbital leiomyoma is isointense with respect to the extraocular muscle and cerebral gray matter on T1-weighted images and hyperintense on T2-weighted images.[103a] The lesion shows moderate enhancement after contrast injection. The MRI features are similar to other well-circumscribed lesions of the orbit including cavernous hemangioma, schwannoma, fibrous histiocytoma, and hemangiopericytoma.

Morphologic Features

Grossly, orbital leiomyoma is a gray-tan, well-circumscribed tumor. There is a well-defined capsule in most cases,[101] but the lesion can also be unencapsulated.[100] Histopathologically, there are two principal patterns: compact bundles and fascicles of spindle cells separated by thin columns of interstitial collagen, or mixed vascular channels and smooth muscle cells with a predominating vascular component.

Studies using Masson trichrome stain and electron microscopy have demonstrated the smooth muscle origin of leiomyoma. Positive immunoreactivity with smooth muscle actin provides the best evidence for the smooth muscle origin of this tumor.[66,100,103a]

Management and Prognosis

Orbital leiomyoma is a benign tumor; the best treatment is complete surgical excision.[101] The prognosis is still excellent for tumors that have been incompletely excised and later, having recurred locally, have been completely excised.

Transformation of an incompletely excised and irradiated orbital leiomyoma into leiomyosarcoma has been reported, but it is quite possible that the high doses of external beam radiotherapy (115 Gy) might have contributed to the development of sarcomatous transformation in that case.[101]

ANGIOLYMPHOID HYPERPLASIA WITH EOSINOPHILIA AND KIMURA DISEASE

Angiolymphoid hyperplasia with eosinophilia (ALHE) and Kimura disease are similar clinical entities. Both conditions are extremely rare in the orbit and periorbital tissues. In the earlier literature, these two conditions were thought to represent the same entity.[104] However, they are now known to be separate entities. They present with dermal or subcutaneous nodules in the head and neck region. Both are associated with eosinophilia. Although Kimura disease has been most frequently described in Asians and ALHE in caucasians, there seems to be no regional or racial predilection. The term "epithelioid hemangioma" has been suggested in place of ALHE.[104]

Clinical Features

Both ALHE and Kimura disease may demonstrate involvement of the orbit,[104–106] eyelids,[107] and lacrimal gland.[106] Both conditions may present with proptosis, eyelid swelling, ocular motility problems, or a palpable mass in the orbit.[105] The rare occurrence of ALHE in relation to an orbital prosthesis has also been reported.[108] Patients with ALHE may have obstructive airway disease.[105]

Radiologic Features

The lesion may appear on CT as a well-circumscribed or ill-defined lesion.[105,106]

Morphologic Features

Grossly, tumors diagnosed as ALHE are yellow to brown and well circumscribed. An ill-defined lesion extending into the adjacent orbital fat occurs rarely. The basic histopathologic feature is a rather exuberant proliferation of small vascular channels lined by enlarged endothelial cells that may form cell clusters extending into the luminal space.[107] In some specimens, medium-sized arteries show fragmentation of their internal elastic membrane and destruction of the smooth muscle cells in their medial layer. Serial sections show intramural neovascularization.[107] Interspersed among the proliferating vessels is a dense infiltrate primarily of eosinophils with varying number of lymphocytes, mast cells, histiocytes, and plasma cells. It is this infiltrate that differentiates the lesion from angiosarcoma and intravascular papillary endothelial hyperplasia, which share the common feature of an abnormal proliferation of endothelial cells.

Lesions diagnosed as Kimura disease are morphologically similar to ALHE. Differentiation between Kimura disease and ALHE is based on the character of endothelial cells. Atypical endothelial cells are not seen in Kimura disease, whereas ALHE is defined by the proliferation of the atypical histiocytoid endothelial cells.[104,106] In Kimura disease, lymphoid follicles and abundant fibrous tissue are present.[104,106] In contrast, ALHE shows a relative scarcity of lymphoid follicles and fibrosis.

Ultrastructurally, some capillaries show prominent multilaminar basement membranes surrounding their walls. The apical surface of the endothelial cells shows broad villous processes protruding into the lumen.[107]

The histopathological and clinical features of Kimura disease are most consistent with an allergic or autoimmune process. Those of ALHE suggest a neoplastic disorder of the vascular endothelium.

Management and Prognosis

The preferred treatment is complete excision of the lesion.[104–107] There are no recurrences among the few orbital cases managed with complete excision.[104–107] Systemic corticosteroid and immunosuppressive treatment can be used for recurrences after initial incomplete excision in patients with ALHE.[105] Both types of lesion respond partially to external beam radiation therapy.

References

1. Shields JA, Bakewell B, Augsburger JJ, Flanagan JC. Classification and incidence of space-occupying lesions of the orbit. *Arch Ophthalmol* 1984;102:1606–1611.
2. Henderson JW, Campbell RJ, Farrow GM, Garrity JA. *Orbital Tumors*. New York: Raven Press; 1994:43–52.
3. Günalp I, Gündüz K. Biopsy-proven orbital lesions in Turkey. A survey of 1092 cases over 30 years. *Orbit* 1994;13:67–79.
4. Seregard S, Sahlin S. Panorama of orbital space-occupying lesions. The 24-year experience of a referral center. *Acta Ophthalmol Scand* 1999;77:91–98.
5. Sen DK. Aetiological pattern of orbital tumors in India and their clinical presentations. A 20-year retrospective study. *Orbit* 1990;9:299–302.
6. Harris GJ. Orbital vascular malformations: a consensus statement on terminology and its clinical implications. *Am J Ophthalmol* 1999;127:453–455.
7. Wright JE, Sullivan TJ, Garner A. Orbital venous anomalies. *Ophthalmology* 1997;104:905–913.
8. Buggage RR, Spraul CW, Wojno TH, Grossniklaus HE. Kimura disease of the orbit and ocular adnexa. *Surv Ophthalmol* 1999;44:79–91.
9. Slem G, Ilcayto R. Hemangioma of the lacrimal gland in an adult. *Ann Ophthalmol* 1972;77–78.
10. Chen YBT, Wornom IL, Whitaker LA. Intraosseous vascular malformations of the orbit. *Plast Reconstr Surg* 1991;87:946–949.
11. Sweet C, Silbergleit R, Mehta B. Primary intraosseous hemangioma of the orbit. CT and MR appearance. *AJNR Am J Neuroradiol* 1997;18:379–381.
12. Harris GJ, Jakobiec FA. Cavernous hemangioma of the orbit. *J Neurosurg* 1979;51:219–228.
13. Brown GC, Shields JA. Amaurosis fugax secondary to presumed cavernous hemangioma of the orbit. *Ann Ophthalmol* 1981;13:1205–1209.
14. Leib ML. Orbital masquerade: hyperthyroidism and cavernous hemangioma of the orbit. *Br J Ophthalmol* 1993;77:676–677.
15. Henderson JW, Campbell RJ, Farrow GM, Garrity JA. *Orbital Tumors*. New York: Raven Press, 1994:89–118.

15a. Iwamoto T, Jacobiec FA. Ultrastructural comparison of capillary and cavernous hemagiomas of the orbit. *Arch Ophthalmol* 1979;97:1144–1153.

16. Sullivan TJ, Aylward GW, Wright JE, et al. Bilateral multiple cavernous hemangiomas of the orbit. *Br J Ophthalmol* 1992;76:627–629.
17. Mojon D, Odel JG, Rios R, Hirano M. Presumed orbital hemangioma associated with the blue rubber bleb nevus syndrome. *Arch Ophthalmol* 1996;114:618–619.
18. Henderson JW, Farrow GM, Garrity JA. Clinical course of an incompletely removed cavernous hemangioma of the orbit. *Ophthalmology* 1990;97:625–628.
19. Hurwitz JJ, Mishkin SK. The value of cryoprobe-assisted removal of orbital tumors. *Ophthalmic Surg* 1988;19:94–97.
20. Haik BG, Jakobiec FA, Ellsworth RM, Jones IS. Capillary hemangioma of the lids and orbit: an analysis of the clinical features and therapeutic results in 101 cases. *Ophthalmology* 1979;86:760–792.
21. Haik BG, Karcioglu ZA, Gordon RA, Pechous B. Capillary hemangioma. *Surv Ophthalmol* 1994;38:399–426
22. Stigmar G, Crawford JS, Ward CM, Thomson HG. Ophthalmic sequelae of infantile hemangiomas of the eyelids and orbit. *Am J Ophthalmol* 1978;85:806–813.
23. Blaniuk LT. Orbital vascular lesions. Role of imaging. *Radiol Clin North Am* 1999;37:169–183.
24. Kushner BJ. Intralesional corticosteroid injection for infantile adnexal hemangioma. *Am J Ophthalmol* 1982;93:496–506.
25. Egbert JE, Paul S, Engel K, Summers G. High injection pressure during intralesional injection of corticosteroids into capillary hemangiomas. *Arch Ophthalmol* 2001;119:677–683.
26. Shorr N, Seiff SR. Central retinal artery occlusion associated with periocular corticosteroid injection for juvenile hemangioma. *Ophthalmic Surg* 1986;17:229–231.
27. Townshend LM, Buckley EG. Linear subcutaneous fat atrophy after a single corticosteroid injection for ocular adnexal hemangioma. *Am J Ophthalmol* 1990;109:102–103.
28. Sutula FC, Glover AT. Eyelid necrosis following intralesional corticosteroid injection for capillary hemangioma. *Ophthalmic Surg* 1987;18:103–105.
29. DeVenecia G, Lobeck CC. Successful treatment of eyelid hemangioma with prednisone. *Arch Ophthalmol* 1970;84:98–102.

30. Loughnan MS, Elder J, Kemp A. Treatment of massive orbito-capillary hemangioma with interferon alfa-2b: short-term results. *Arch Ophthalmol* 1992;110:1366–1367.
31. Chang E, Boyd A, Nelson CC, et al. Successful treatment of infantile hemangiomas with interferon-alpha-2b. *J Pediatr Hematol Oncol* 1997;19:237–244.
32. Aldave AJ, Shields CL, Shields JA. Surgical excision of selected amblyogenic periorbital capillary hemangiomas. *Ophthalmic Surg Lasers* 1999;30:754–757.
33. Kennedy RE. Arterial embolization of orbital hemangiomas. *Trans Am Ophthalmic Soc* 1978;76:266–275.
34. Krastinova-Lolov D, Roddi R. An intracranial/extracranial approach for the surgical management of hemangiomas of the orbit and eyelid. *J Craniomaxillofac Surg* 1989;17:197–205.
35. Burstein FD, Simms C, Cohen SR, et al. Intralesional laser therapy of extensive hemangiomas in 100 consecutive pediatric patients. *Ann Plast Surg* 200;44:188–194.
36. Clymer MA, Fortune S, Reinisch L, et al. Interstitial Nd:YAG photocoagulation for vascular malformations and hemangiomas in childhood. *Arch Otolaryngol Head Neck Surg* 1998;124:431–436.
37. Tunç M, Sadri E, Char DH. Orbital lymphangioma: an analysis of 26 cases. *Br J Ophthalmol* 1999;83:76–80.
38. Shields JA. *Diagnosis and Management of Orbital Tumors.* Philadelphia: WB Saunders; 1989:149–169.
39. Dryden RM, Wulc AE, Day D. Eyelid ecchymosis and proptosis in lymphangioma. *Am J Ophthalmol* 1985;100:486–487.
40. Hemmer KM, Marsh JL, Milder B. Orbital lymphangioma. *Plast Reconstr Surg* 1988;82:340–343.
41. Selva D, Strianese D, Bonavolonta G, Rootman J. Orbital venous-lymphatic malformations (lymphangioma) mimicking cavernous hemangioma. *Am J Ophthalmol* 2001;131:364–370.
42. Coll GE, Goldberg RA, Krauss H, Bateman BJ. Concomitant lymphangioma and arteriovenous malformation of the orbit. *Am J Ophthalmol* 1991;112:200–205.
43. Vaccharajani A, Paes B. Orbital lymphangioma with noncontiguous cerebral arteriovenous malformation, manifesting with thrombocytopenia (Kasabach–Merritt syndrome) and intracerebral hemorrhage. *Acta Paediatr* 2002;91:98–99.
44. Brooks SE, Pillal JJ, Harshivinderjit B. Orbital cellulites due to occult orbital lymphangioma. *South Med J* 2001;94:532–535.
45. Bond JB, Haik BG, Taveras JL, et al. Magnetic resonance imaging of orbital lymphangioma with and without gadolinium contrast enhancement. *Ophthalmology* 1992;99:1318–1324.
46. Wilson ME, Parker PL, Chavis RM. Conservative management of childhood orbital lymphangioma. *Ophthalmology* 1989;96:484–490.
47. Kennerdell JS, Maroon JC, Garrity JA, Abla AA. Surgical management of orbital lymphangioma with the carbon dioxide laser. *Am J Ophthalmol* 1986;102:308–314.
48. Bullock JD, Goldberg SH, Connelly PJ. Orbital varix thrombosis. *Ophthalmology* 1990;97:251–256.
49. Foroozan R, Shields CL, Shields JA, et al. Congenital orbital varices causing extreme neonatal proptosis. *Am J Ophthalmol* 2000;129:693–694.
50. Shields JA, Dolinskas C, Augsburger JJ, et al. Demonstration of orbital varix with computed tomography and Valsalva maneuver. *Am J Ophthalmol* 1984;97:108–110.
51. Shimura M, Kiyosawa M, Aikawa H, et al. Spontaneous orbital hemorrhage in adult females. *Ophthalmologica* 1992;205:149–157.
52. Vignaud J, Clay C, Bilaniuk LT. Venography of the orbit. *Radiology* 1974;110:373–382.
53. Lieb WE, Merton DA, Shields JA. Color Doppler imaging in the demonstration of an orbital varix. *Br J Ophthalmol* 1990;74:305–308.
54. Takechi A, Uozumi T, Kiya K, et al. Embolization of orbital varix. *Neuroradiology* 1994;36:487–489.
55. Stout AP, Murray MR. Hemangiopericytoma: vascular tumor featuring Zimmermann's pericytes. *Ann Surg* 1942;116:26–33.
56. Sullivan TJ, Wright JE, Wulc AE, et al. Hemangiopericytoma of the orbit. *Aust N Z J Ophthalmol* 1992;20:325–332.
57. Karcioglu Z, Nasr AM, Haik BG. Orbital hemangiopericytoma: clinical and morphologic features. *Am J Ophthalmol* 1997;124:661–672.
58. Henderson JW, Farrow GM. Primary orbital hemangiopericytoma. An aggressive and potentially malignant neoplasm. *Arch Ophthalmol* 1978;96:666–673.
59. Croxatto JO, Font RL. Hemangiopericytoma of the orbit. A clinicopathologic study of 30 cases. *Hum Pathol* 1982;13:210–218.
60. Abe M, Hara Y, Ohnishi Y, et al. Case of primary orbital hemangiopericytoma. *Jpn J Ophthalmol* 1983;27:90–95.
61. Shields JA, Shields CL, Rashid RC. Clinicopathologic correlation of choroidal folds: secondary to massive cranioorbital hemangiopericytoma. *Ophthalmic Plast Reconstr Surg* 1992;8:62–68.
62. Papale JJ, Frederick AR, Albert DM. Intraocular hemangiopericytoma. *Arch Ophthalmol* 1983;101:1409–1411.
63. Roth SI, August CZ, Lissner GS, O'Grady RB. Hemangiopericytoma of the lacrimal sac. *Ophthalmology* 1991;98:925–927.
64. Boniuk M, Messmer EP, Font RL. Hemangiopericytoma of the meninges of the optic nerve: a clinicopathologic report including electron microscopic observations. *Ophthalmology* 1985;92:1780–1787.
65. Garrity JA, Kennerdell JS. Orbital calcification associated with hemangiopericytoma. *Am J Ophthalmol* 1986;102:126–127.
66. Miettinen M. Immunochemistry of soft tissue tumors. *J Histopathol* 1999;22:219–227.
67. Setzkorn RK, Lee DJ, Iliff NT, Green R. Hemangiopericytoma of the orbit treated with conservative surgery and radiotherapy. *Arch Ophthalmol* 1987;105:1103–1105.
68. Tijl JWM, Koornneef L, Blank LECM. Recurrent hemangiopericytoma and brachytherapy. *Doc Ophthalmol* 1992;82:103–107.
69. Holden CA, Spittle MF, Jones EW. Angiosarcoma of the face and scalp: prognosis and treatment. *Cancer* 1987;59:1046–1057.
70. Lever WF, Schaumburg-Lever G. Histopathology of the skin. Philadelphia: WB Saunders; 1990:708–711.
71. Burnstine MA, Fruch BR, Elner VM. Angiosarcoma metastatic to the orbit. *Arch Ophthalmol* 1996;114:93–96.
72. Bennett RG, Keller JW, Ditty JF Jr. Hemangiosarcoma subsequent to radiotherapy for a hemangioma in infancy. *J Dermatol Surg Oncol* 1978;4:881–883.
73. Gündüz K, Shields JA, Shields CL, et al. Cutaneous angiosarcoma with eyelid involvement. *Am J Ophthalmol* 1998;125:870–871.
74. Lopes M, Duffau H, Fleuridas G. Primary spheno-orbital angiosarcoma: case report and review of the literature. *Neurosurgery* 1999;44:405–407.
75. Messmer EP, Font RL, McCrary JA, Murphy D. Epithelioid angiosarcoma of the orbit presenting as Tolosa–Hunt syndrome. *Ophthalmology* 1983;90:1414–1421.
76. Hufnagel T, Ma L, Kuo TT. Orbital angiosarcoma with subconjunctival presentation. *Ophthalmology* 1987;94:72–77.
77. Font RL, Wheeler TM, Boniuk M. Intravascular papillary endothelial hyperplasia of the orbit and ocular adnexa. *Arch Ophthalmol* 1983;101:1731–1736.
78. Wolter JR, Lewis RG. Endovascular hemangioendothelioma of the eyelid. *Am J Ophthalmol* 1974;78:727–729.

79. Weber FL, Babel J. Intravascular papillary endothelial hyperplasia of the orbit. *Br J Ophthalmol* 1981;65:18–22.
80. Patt S, Kaden B, Stoltenberg-Didinger G. Intravascular papillary endothelial hyperplasia at the fissura orbitalis superior: a case report. *Clin Neuropathol* 1992;11:128–130.
81. Shields JA, Shields CL, Eagle RC Jr, Diniz W. Intravascular papillary endothelial hyperplasia with presumed bilateral orbital varices. *Arch Ophthalmol* 1999;117:1247–1249.
82. Leonard TJK, Moseley IF, Sanders MD. Ophthalmoplegia in carotid cavernous sinus fistulas. *Br J Ophthalmol* 1984;68: 128–134.
83. Grove AS Jr. The dural shunt syndrome. Pathophysiology and clinical course. *Ophthalmology* 1983;90:31–44.
84. Ohtsuka K, Hashimoto M. Clinical findings in a patient with spontaneous arteriovenous fistula of the orbit. *Am J Ophthalmol* 1999;127:736–737.
85. Guerry DP, Harbison JW, Wiesinger H. Bilateral choroidal detachment and fluctuating proptosis secondary to bilateral dural arteriovenous fistulas treated with transcranial orbital decompression with resolution: report of a case. *Trans Am Ophthalmol Soc* 1975;73:64–72.
86. Keltner JL, Satterfield D, Dublin AB, Lee BCP. Dural and carotid cavernous sinus fistulas. *Ophthalmology* 1987;94:1585–1600.
87. Fourman S. Acute close-angle glaucoma after arteriovenous fistulas. *Am J Ophthalmol* 1989;107:156–159.
88. Bynke HG, Efsing HO. Carotid-cavernous fistula with contralateral exophthalmos. *Acta Ophthalmol* 1970;48:971–978.
89. Tech KE, Becker CJ, Lazo A, et al. Anomalous intracranial venous drainage mimicking orbital or cavernous arteriovenous fistula. *AJNR Am J Neuroradiol* 1995;16:171–174.
90. Busin M, Graefe C, Koch J. Arteriovenous fistula presenting as a tumor of the upper eyelid. *Ophthalmic Surg* 1994;25: 471–473.
91. Sergott RC, Grossman RI, Savino PJ, et al. The syndrome of paradoxical worsening of dural-cavernous sinus arteriovenous malformations. *Ophthalmology* 1987;94:205–212.
92. Purcell JJ. The effect of unsuspected carotid-cavernous fistula in enucleation. *Am J Ophthalmol* 1979;88:946–948.
93. Coskun O, Hamon M, Catroux G, et al. Carotid-cavernous fistulas: diagnosis with spiral CT angiography. *AJNR Am J Neuroradiol* 2000;21:712–716.
94. Costa VP, Molnar LJ, Cerri GG. Diagnosing and monitoring carotid cavernous fistulas with color doppler monitoring. *J Clin Ultrasound* 1997;25:448–452.
95. Debrun GM. Endovascular management of carotid cavernous fistulas. In: Valvanis A, ed. *Interventional Neuroradiology.* Berlin: Springer-Verlag; 1993:23–24.
96. Howard GM, Jakobiec FA, Michelsen WJ. Orbital arteriovenous malformation with secondary capillary angiomatosis treated by embolization with silastic liquid. *Ophthalmology* 1983;90:1136–1139.
97. Hanneken AM, Miller NR, Debrun GM, Nauta HJW. Treatment of carotid-cavernous sinus fistulas using a detachable balloon catheter through the superior ophthalmic vein. *Arch Ophthalmol* 1989;107:87–92.
98. Goldberg RA, Goldey SH, Duckwiler G, Vinuela F. Management of cavernous sinus–dural fistulas. Indications and techniques for primary embolization via the superior ophthalmic vein. *Arch Ophthalmol* 1996;114:707–714.
99. Benndorf G, Bender A, Campi A, et al. Treatment of a cavernous sinus dural arteriovenous fistula by deep orbital puncture of the superior ophthalmic vein. *Neuroradiology* 2001; 43:499–502.
100. Jolly SS, Brownstein S, Jordan DR. Leiomyoma of the anterior orbit and eyelids. *Can J Ophthalmol* 1995;30:366–370.
101. Jakobiec FA, Howard GM, Rosen M, Wolff M. Leiomyoma and leiomyosarcoma of the orbit. *Am J Ophthalmol* 1975;80: 1028–1042.
102. Carrier DA, Mawad ME, Kirkpatrick JB. MR appearance of an orbital leiomyoma. *AJNR Am J Neuroradiol* 1993;14: 473–474.
103. Kulkarni V, Rajshekhar V, Chandi SM. Orbital apex leiomyoma with intracranial extension. *Surg Neurol* 2000;54:327–330.
103a. Gündüz K, Günalp I, Erden E, Erekul S. Orbital leiomyoma: Report of a case and review of the literature. *Surv Ophthalmol* 2004;49:237–242.
104. McEachren TM, Brownstein S, Jordan DR, et al. Epithelioid hemangioma of the orbit. *Ophthalmology* 2000;107:806–810.
105. Sheren SB, Custer PL, Smith ME. Angiolymphoid hyperplasia with eosinophilia of the orbit associated with obstructive airway disease. *Am J Ophthalmol* 1989;108:167–169.
106. Cook HT, Stafford ND. Angiolymphoid hyperplasia with eosinophilia involving the lacrimal gland: case report. *Br J Ophthalmol* 1988;72:710–712.
107. Hidayat AA, Cameron JD, Font RL, Zimmerman LE. Angiolymphoid hyperplasia with eosinophilia (Kimura's disease) of the orbit and ocular adnexa. *Am J Ophthalmol* 1983;96: 176–189.
108. Smith DL, Kincaid MC, Nicolitz E. Angiolymphoid hyperplasia with eosinophilia (Kimura's disease) of the orbit. *Arch Ophthalmol* 1988;106:793–795.
109. Buggage RR, Spraul CW, Wojno TH, Grossniklaus HE. Kimura disease of the orbit and ocular adnexa. *Surv Ophthalmol* 1999;44:79–91.

15

Fibrohistiocytic Tumors

Zeynel A. Karcıoglu

For the sake of simplicity, in this chapter fibrohistiocytic lesions of the orbit are broken down into two major categories: fibromatoses and histiocytoses.

FIBROMATOSES

Fibrohistiocytic tumors include benign and malignant neoplasms as well as a variety of nonneoplastic proliferations that are collectively termed *reactive fibromatoses*. These lesions are currently considered to originate from primitive mesenchyme as a result of its differentiation into multiple cell lines (Figure 15.1).[1,2] Common fibromatoses of the head and neck include desmoid-type fibromatosis, juvenile fibromatosis (aggressive infantile fibromatosis),[3] and nodular fasciitis.[4] Desmoid-type fibromatosis and nodular fasciitis are also known as *aggressive fibromatoses*.[5,6] Most fibromatoses tend to involve fascial tissues of the trunk and extremities. These tumors are rarely seen in the head and neck area, but when they occur in the oronasal cavities, sinuses, and orbit, they are difficult to diagnose and treat. These lesions may seem to be histopathologically benign but are often locally aggressive and have a high rate of recurrence, particularly in relatively restricted anatomic regions such as the orbit. They often lead to the functional compromise of adjacent anatomic structures and in many instances recur postsurgically, requiring further treatment.

Schutz et al. report desmoid-type fibromatosis in a 63-year-old woman who presented with an intraorbital mass with extension toward the apex of the orbit.[5] Although the lesion was histologically classified as fibromatosis, its clinical behavior was aggressive, with invasion of orbital tissues and bone. In view of this and the known tendency for tumor recurrence, the patient's eye was exenterated. Another example of a desmoid-type lesion is described by Henderson in a 5-year-old boy who presented with proptosis and papilledema.[7]

Juvenile fibromatosis of the orbit and periorbital region was reported by Hidayat and Font in six patients ranging from 1 to 11 years of age.[8] The majority of lesions presented in the lower eyelid and inferior orbital area. Extension of three tumors to the underlying periosteum was documented; none metastasized, but two of six lesions recurred after surgical excision.

Nodular fasciitis is another fibroproliferative lesion, sometimes termed *pseudosarcoma*.[4,9] It usually forms a discrete soft tissue mass, partially fixed to adjacent soft tissues; about 10% of all cases occur in the head and neck area. In a large series of 163 pseudosarcomas of the head and neck, 13 were reported in the orbit and periorbital tissues.[9] Most of these lesions develop in the eyelids rather than the orbital cavity.[10] When nodular fasciitis develops within the orbit or periorbital area, it usually presents as a well-circumscribed, painless, firm, and movable tumor. Such lesions are not difficult to excise in toto because they are well delineated, and complete excision of nodular fasciitis is usually curative.[11,12] Histopathologically, the lesion consists of irregular bundles or individual fibroblasts within a myxoid matrix. Although the fibroblastic areas share the same appearance as the fibroblasts of giant cell fibroblastoma (GCF), multinucleated giant cells are rarely seen in nodular fasciitis. While some of these lesions may appear aggressive histopathologically, the overall recurrence rate is reported to range from 1 to 2%.[9]

The neoplastic group is somewhat easier to classify but may be similarly difficult to manage clinically. The two major categories are fibroblastic and fibrohistiocytic tumors. Fibroblastic neoplasms can be benign or malignant and comprise collagen-synthesizing fibroblasts and/or fibrocytes; examples include fibroma, fibromyxoma, solitary fibrous tumor (SFT), GCF, and fibrosarcoma.[13,14] These fibroblastic tumors may occasionally develop in the orbit, but not as often as their fibrohistiocytic cousins, which frequently present as primary orbital tumors. The neoplasms originating exclusively from fibroblasts, namely, fibroma and fibrosarcoma, are the least commonly encountered orbital tumors. Fibromas can be difficult to differentiate from loosely organized fibrous tissue. Fibrosarcoma of the orbit is rare and is primarily encountered as a second malignant neoplasm in hereditary retinoblastoma patients following radiation treatment.[15] Although some fibrosarcomas are well delineated, others infiltrate the orbital tissue haphaz-

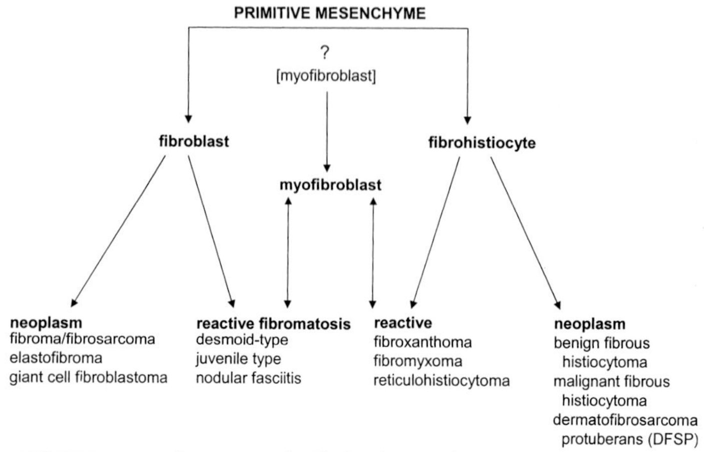

FIGURE 15.1. The origin of cells leading to fibrohistiocytic tumors.

ardly, whether they originate within the orbital cavity as a primary tumor or extend there by contiguity (Figure 15.2).

Fibromyxomas are tumors of primitive mesenchymal cells, composed of a scanty population of spindle cells scattered within a myxomatous matrix of mucin. These benign lesions very rarely develop as solitary tumors in the orbit but more often extend into the orbit secondarily (Figure 15.3). In surgery, even the benign lesions infiltrate to adjacent tissues and therefore are difficult to resect. They tend to recur frequently. It is rare to have a malignant fibromyxoma, but the entire specimen should be examined to rule out focal malignancy.

Fibrohistiocytic tumors are a diverse group of neoplasms, primarily composed of fibroblastic and histiocytic cells. Most authorities believe these tumors originate from a multipotential primitive mesenchymal cell that can differentiate fibroblastic and fibrohistiocytic cell lines.[9,16]

Fibrous histiocytoma, the most commonly encountered mesenchymal orbital tumor in adults, may be benign, locally aggressive, or malignant.[17,18]

Although this lesion usually presents with a mixture of fibroblastic and histiocytic cells, it has a broader range of histopathologic appearance. In certain aggressive forms, multinucleated giant cells may be mixed with spindle cells of fibrous histiocytoma. Clinically, the differential diagnosis includes other solid mesenchymal tumors such as leiomyoma, neurilemoma, hemangiopericytoma, and rhabdomyosarcoma.[19,20] Computed tomography (CT) and magnetic resonance (MR) imaging are not very rewarding for distinguishing fibrous masses such as fibrous histiocytoma from orbital tumors of other types.[21,22] As a rule, benign lesions are well delineated and remodel the bone because of chronic compression (Figure 15.4). Malignant fibrous lesions tend to show infiltrating margins like other malignant soft tissue tumors (Figure 15.5). Enhancement patterns of CT and MR im-

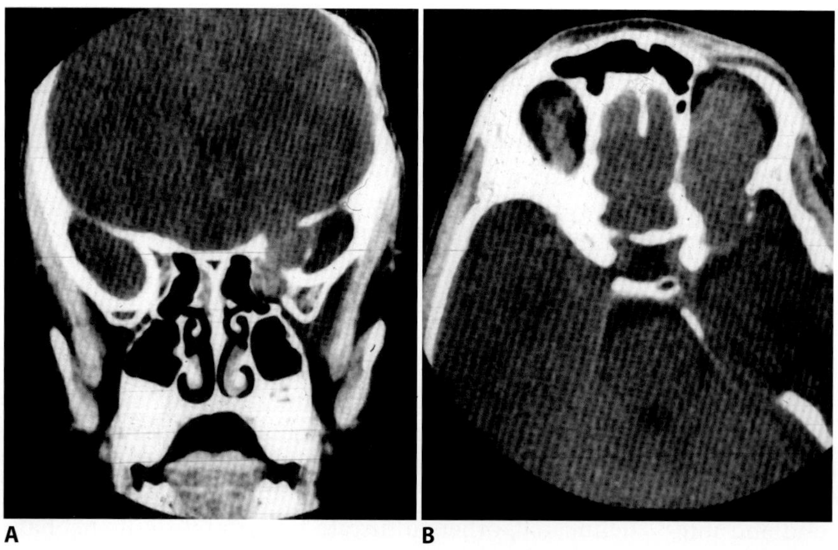

FIGURE 15.2. (A) Coronal and (B) axial CT scans showing the extension of recurrent fibrosarcoma into the brain and paranasal sinuses.

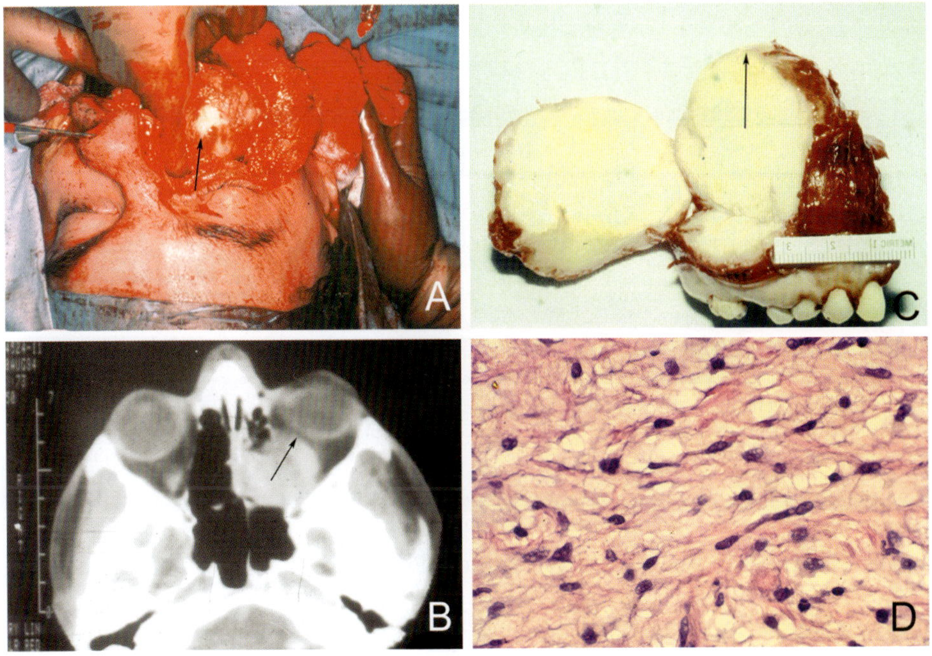

FIGURE 15.3. (A,C) A well-encapsulated maxillary fibromyxoma extending secondarily into the inferior orbit (B); arrows point to the apex of the tumor which was abutting the globe. (D) Histopathologic preparation shows a mixture of elongated fibroblast-like cells mixed with myxomatous matrix.

aging that may vary according to tissue type of the tumor are summarized in Table 15.1.[22]

Fibrous histiocytoma usually presents a heterogeneous, isointense to hyperintense signal with respect to extraocular muscles on T1-weighted studies. Following administration of GDPA enhancement of the tumor is usually heterogeneous. Other soft tissue tumors in the orbit can produce CT and MR features similar to those of fibrohistiocytoma, except for tumors of vascular origin, which enhance markedly and homogeneously.[21] Malignant fibrous histiocytoma has been described as second primary malignancy in children with hereditary retinoblastoma.[23]

Dermatofibrosarcoma protuberans (DFSP) is best known as an aggressive form of fibrous histiocytoma with indeterminate malignant potentials. DFSP con-

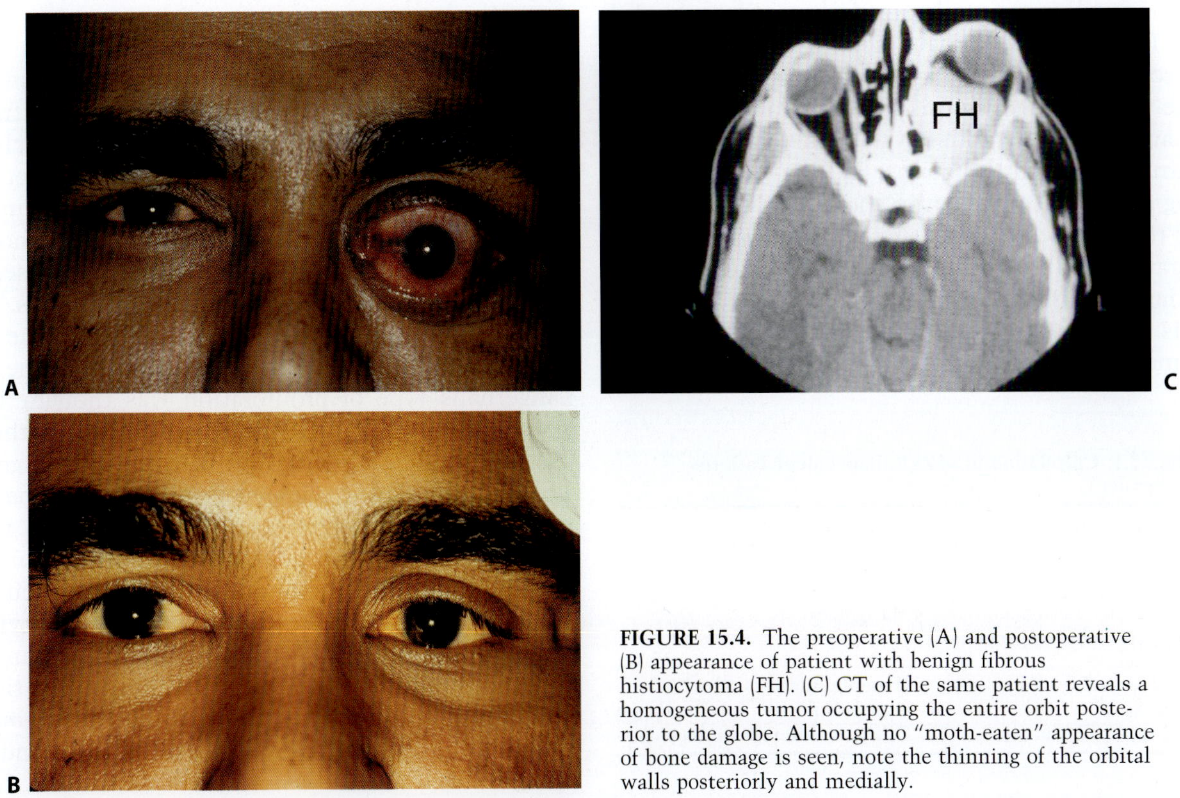

FIGURE 15.4. The preoperative (A) and postoperative (B) appearance of patient with benign fibrous histiocytoma (FH). (C) CT of the same patient reveals a homogeneous tumor occupying the entire orbit posterior to the globe. Although no "moth-eaten" appearance of bone damage is seen, note the thinning of the orbital walls posteriorly and medially.

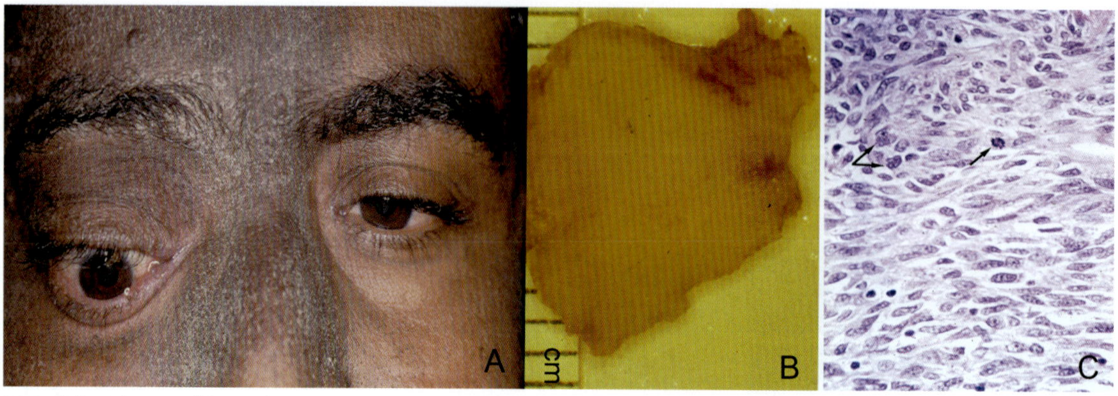

FIGURE 15.5. (A) Malignant fibrous histiocytoma presenting with massive downward proptosis. (B) Gross specimen of the tumor reveals a "firm" appearance of the cut surface. (C) Histopathology also shows the aggressiveness of the tumor with numerous mitotic figures (single arrow) and pleomorphic tumor cells (joined arrows).

sists of fibroblast-like spindle cells. Xanthogranulomatous lesions may present diagnostic problems because of the presence of Touton-type giant cells, particularly when intermingled with a fibroblast-like spindle cell population. Where there is an absence of Langerhans cells, however, these tumors can be definitively differentiated from true histiocytic lesions because of the absence of Langerhans cells.[24,25]

Solitary fibrous tumor is a visceral spindle cell tumor that can also be seen in the orbit.[25] Clinically, it presents as a slowly growing, well-circumscribed intraorbital lesion.[26] Arteriograms have demonstrated these tumors to be very vascular and difficult to differentiate from other well-vascularized orbital lesions such as fibrous histiocytoma, hemangiopericytoma, and paraganglioma. Standardized ultrasonography, CT and MR imaging are not very helpful in differentiating SFT from other solitary vascular lesions. The most accurate way to diagnose this lesion is to perform a biopsy and examine the tissue with hematoxylin–eosin and immunoperoxidase stains; SFT shows diffuse and strong positivity for vimentin and CD34. Occasionally these tumors present with aggressive growth and may infiltrate the orbital bones and recur after excision.[27]

Giant cell fibroblastoma is another fibrous tumor that is histologically benign without potential for distant metastasis, but it may behave clinically as an infiltrative tumor (Figure 15.6), which makes management difficult.[28–30]

TABLE 15.1. Correlation of MRI Enhancement Patterns with Histology.

Enhancement pattern	*Tissue type*
Homogeneous signal Tl, T2 and with Gd DPTA	Benign
Homogeneous T1 signal changing to heterogeneous T2 signal	Malignant
High T2 signal	Hypercellularity, calcification
Low T2 signal	Hypocellularity, more collagen
Intermediate T2 signal	Difficult differential diagnosis

HISTIOCYTOSES

The histiocytoses include both Langerhans cell (Figure 15.7) and non-Langerhans cell proliferations.[29,30] Langerhans cell histiocytosis (formerly known as *histiocytosis X*), is caused by a proliferation of Langerhans cells.[31–33] Although both Langerhans cell histiocytosis and xanthogranuloma (XG) are characterized by the proliferation of histiocytes, significant morphologic and clinical differences exist because their cells of origin are class I and class II histiocytes, respectively.[31]

The light-microscopic features of Langerhans and non-Langerhans cell histiocytoses are quite similar, with a characteristic picture of histiocytic infiltration with lymphocytes, plasma cells, and multinucleated giant cells.[32,33] Histopathologic variability is determinative of the age of the disease; the tumor ultimately scleroses toward the end of the process of pathology. Thus, it has been suggested that histiocytoses are more sensitive to treatment in the early stages.[34]

Both groups of histiocytoses show the same kind of pathology (Figure 15. 8). The landmark of the non-Langerhans type of proliferation was thought to be Touton-type multinucleated giant cells, but the absence of these cells does not rule out the diagnosis. Touton-type multinucleated giant cells may be seen in Langerhans cell histiocytosis as well, and, therefore, their presence or absence is not pathognomonic for either entity. The only certain way to specify the type of histiocytosis is to classify the histiocyte by electron microscopy and/or immunohistochemistry. Histiocytic lesions resulting from the proliferation of Langerhans cells are identified with ultrastructural depiction of intracytoplasmic Birbeck granules and pos-

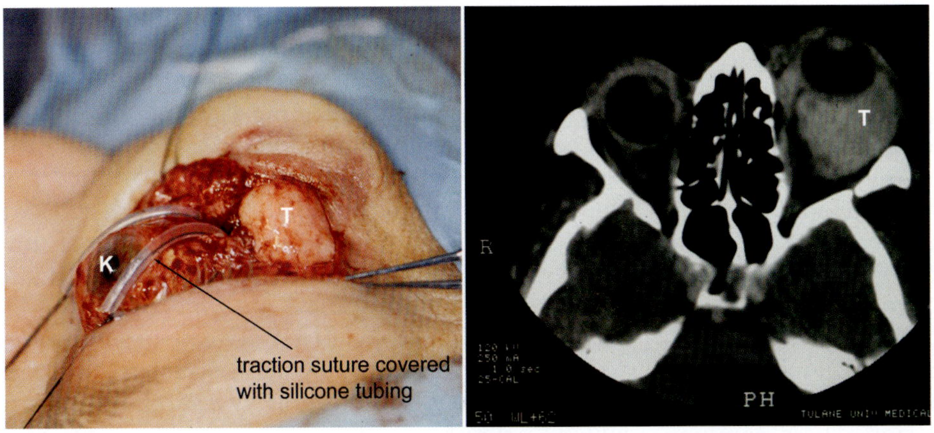

A B

FIGURE 15.6. (A) Intraoperative and (B) CT appearance of a giant cell fibroblastoma. Note the well-delineated but not encapsulated fibrous tumor (T), which offers a very homogeneous appearance on CT because of its hypercellularity. The traction suture through the lateral rectus muscle was pulled medially for easy dissection of the lateral orbital mass; the silk suture was covered with silicone tubing to protect the cornea (K) during traction.

itive reaction to S-100 protein and CD1a. Non-Langerhans cells express other surface markers, including blood clotting transglutaminase factor XIIIa, CD68, Mac387, and vimentin without Birbeck granules.[30] These cell markers have been observed in juvenile xanthogranuloma (JXG), xanthoma disseminatum, and progressive nodular histocytosis.

Patients with Langerhans cell disease are generally younger than those with XG; the majority of these patients present between the ages of 1 and 15 years, with

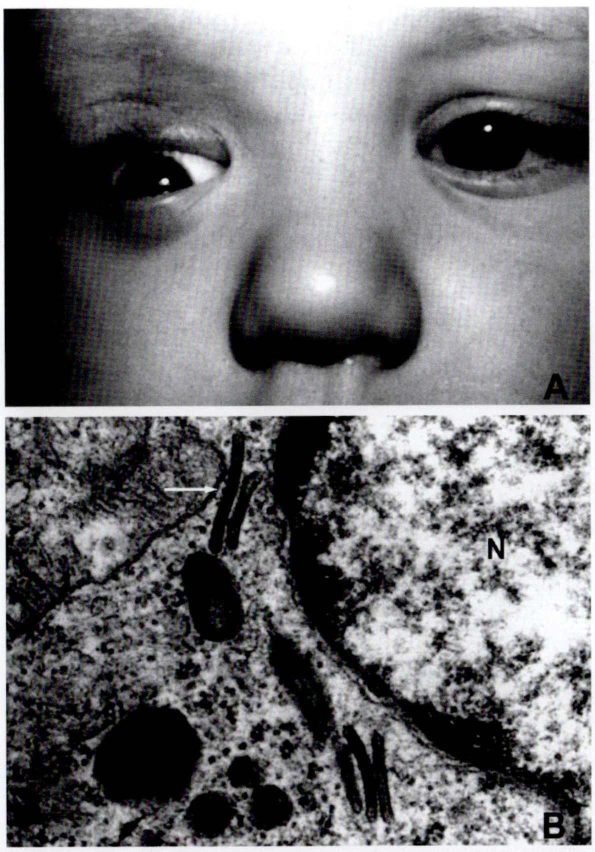

FIGURE 15.7. Langerhans hystiocytosis (eosinophilic granuloma in a young child pushing the right eye inferiorly). (A) Irregular surface of the upper eyelid and superior periorbital skin is due to radiation treatment from which the child benefitted little. (B) Electron microscopic depiction of Langerhans histiocytes with Birbeck granules (white arrow). Identification of these cytoplasmic organelles confirms the tumor cells to be Langerhans histiocytes.

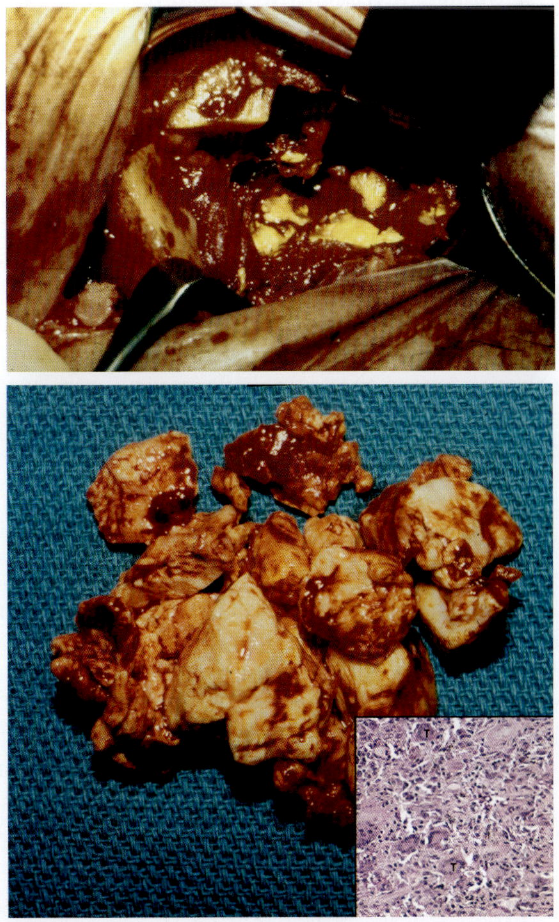

A

B

FIGURE 15.8. (A) Intraoperative appearance of yellowish-orange xanthogranulomatous tumor through lateral orbitotomy. (B) Gross specimen from the same patient showing focally hemorrhagic, yellowish, fatty-looking tissue. *Inset*: Histopathologic appearance of the xanthogranuloma with diffuse infiltration of histiocytic cells and numerous Touton giant cells (T).

the peak ages being 2 to 4 years.[32,35] The three classic forms are eosinophilic granuloma, which primarily affects bone; Hand–Schüller–Christian disease (a triad of exophthalmos, diabetes insipidus, and multiple bone lesions); and Letterer–Siwe disease (a syndrome of multiple soft tissue and bone involvement).[36] It is recommended that a radiographic skeletal survey be obtained when Langerhans-cell histiocytosis is a diagnostic possibility. The lytic bone lesions have a predilection for the flat bones, most often involving the skull.[37] However, radiologic findings in these diseases can be quite varied and include epiphyseal and transepiphyseal lesions, pathologic fractures, and dural extension of vertebral lesions. Less common findings include the involvement of the clavicle and small bones of the hands and feet and, rarely, extracranial "button" sequestra, soft tissue calcification, and neurologic manifestations secondary to spinal disease.[38] When systemic (bone marrow, lung, liver, spleen, central nervous system, etc.) disease occurs, the prognosis of non-Langerhans histiocytosis is much worse.

Although histiocytosis X generally affects young children, rare cases have been observed in adults.[39] These diseases usually present with destructive lesions in orbital and cranial bones associated with secondary soft tissue masses in the orbit.

Orbital involvement is most commonly seen with unifocal Langerhans cell disease (eosinophilic granuloma). A common site for eosinophilic granuloma is the anterior superior orbit. According to Woo and Harris, this is because frontal bone retains active bone marrow, which contains Langerhans cell precursors throughout childhood and adolescence.[39] The same authors propose that osteolysis in eosinophilic granuloma is due to the production of prostaglandin E_2 and interleukin 1 by the abnormal Langerhans cells. Their management recommendations include intralesional corticosteroid injection, which can inhibit the cytokines. The solitary lesions are best managed by debulking of the soft tissue mass with light debridement following an incisional biopsy to confirm the diagnosis. For multifocal, systemic involvement or in recurrent cases, systemic corticosteroids and/or antimetabolites or low-dose external beam radiation therapy (EBRT) are used.[40]

Orbital XG presents as a space-occupying lesion in the orbital and periorbital soft tissues and usually does not affect the orbital bones (Figures 15.9 and 15.10).[41,42] The ocular signs and symptoms depend on the location and the size of the lesion. Generally, orbital XG presents without pain, but pain related to peripheral nerve origin may be the presenting symptom. The clinical differential diagnosis includes space-occupying lesions such as lymphoma, Sjögren's disease, and sarcoidosis, as well as other benign and malignant tumors depending on the age of the patient, laterality, and the location of the lesion (Figure 15.11). In most cases, orbital XG originates from the soft tissues; however, intracerebral XG affecting the orbit secondarily has been reported in both children and adults.[43] The number of MR studies on orbital XG is limited, but this imaging technique usually reveals a destructive lesion with irregular, infiltrating margins of low signal intensity with scattered dark foci (Figure 15.12).[43,44]

CT studies reveal infiltrating, soft tissue masses within the orbit without bone destruction. Enlargement of extraocular muscles away from the lesion site and optic nerve entrapment within lesions have been described with CT examination.[42] Some patients reveal Marcus–Gunn pupils, and others present visual field defects secondary to compressive optic neuropathy.[45] The lacrimal gland may be involved as an extension of infiltrating masses. In our experience, one patient who presented with bilateral lacrimal gland enlargement was falsely diagnosed as having Sjögren's disease because of primary lacrimal gland pathology without other orbital lesions.

Ultrasonography shows irregular soft tissue masses with low-density areas most likely corresponding to necrotic foci, but this is not particularly useful for differential diagnosis. Orbital XG cannot be diagnosed from imaging findings. Rather, diagnosis should be based on histiopathologic, immunohistochemical, and electron microscopic studies. The usefulness of the CT, however, is significant in differential diagnosis of the lesion by allowing one to rule out bone damage and to delineate the extent of the lesion in order to plan surgical and radiation treatments. Furthermore, in some cases, the treatment response may be monitored by imaging studies.[42]

Erdheim–Chester disease (E-Cd) must be ruled out in every case of XG in the eyelids and orbit.[46–48] While the pathogenesis of E-Cd remains unknown, it has recently been reported that the histiocytic element of XG is monoclonal, which suggests that these lesions may be neoplastic. This disease may therefore be con-

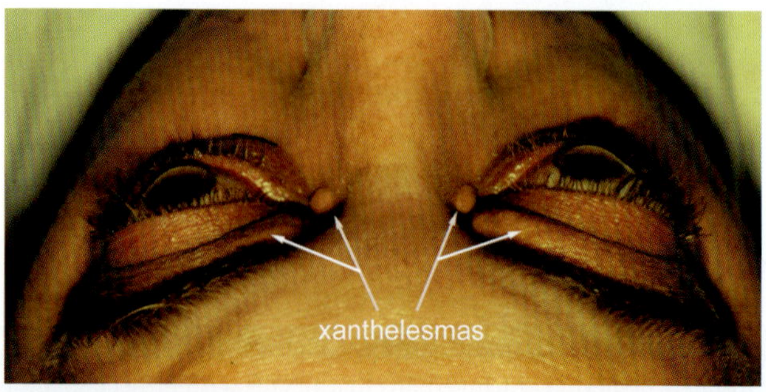

FIGURE 15.9. Bilateral proptosis and xanthalesmas of upper eyelids and medial canthi in a patient with Erdheim–Chester disease.

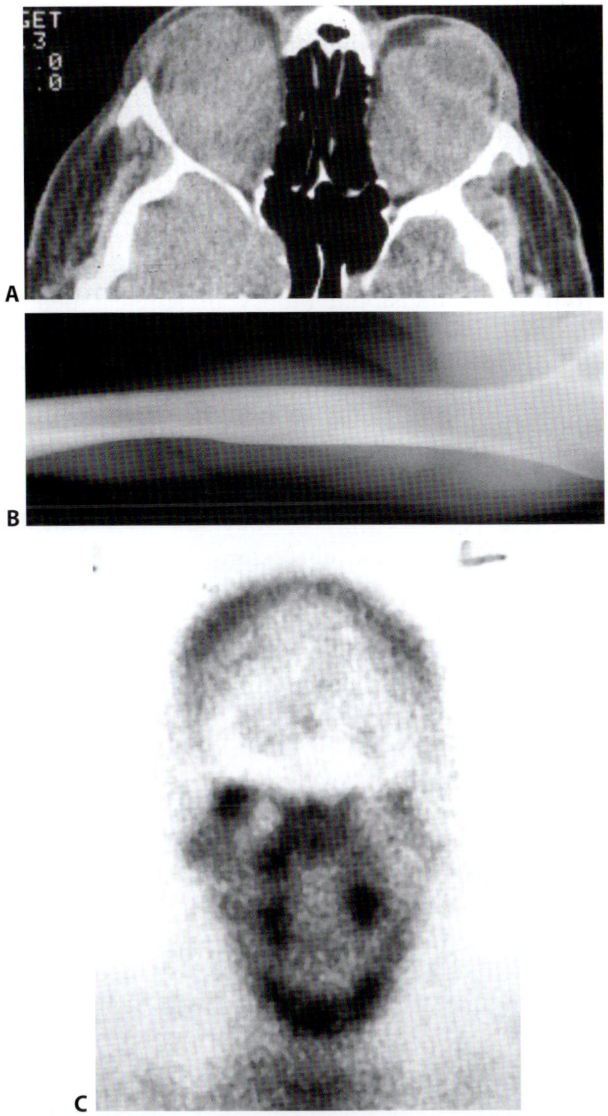

FIGURE 15.10. (A) Axial CT scan showing the homogeneous appearance of xanthogranuloma diffusely involving both orbits. The patient's vision was light perception in both eyes on admission. (B) X-ray of the humerus of the same patient with Erdheim–Chester disease revealing typical lytic and sclerotic changes. (C) Radionucleotide scan of the same patient with increased uptake in orbits.

sidered to be the monocytic counterpart to the dendritic monoclonal expansion of non-Langerhans histiocytosis. The same report suggests that this clonal expansion may also be secondary to an infectious agent, similar to the induction of gastric lymphoma by *Helicobacter pylori*.[47]

E-Cd was first described by Chester in 1930 as an unusual "lipidosis" with distinctive bone changes.[49] Although rarely seen, E-Cd represents the most common form of systemic lipogranulomatosis, predominantly affecting adults, whereas Langerhans histiocytosis is a disease of childhood. E-Cd presents with histiocytic infiltrates involving retroperitoneal soft tissues, long bones, and other viscera including the lungs, heart (conduction network), kidneys, spleen, lymph nodes, and nervous system.[46,50,51] In contrast to the asymmetric, lytic flat bone lesions of Langerhans histiocytosis, patients with E-Cd typically have polyostotic lytic and sclerotic lesions of long bones, with sparing of the appendicular skeleton. X-rays to detect metaphyseal sclerolytic destruction of the long bones, typical for E-Cd, can be easily and inexpensively employed as a screening measure. Systemic involvement should be considered in all cases of orbital XGs, and long bone films should be obtained.

Granulomatous histiocytic infiltrates have been described in the retroperitoneal tissue of E-Cd patients, causing serious renal complications ranging from hydronephrosis to renal failure.[52,53] Although retroperitoneal XG has rarely been reported to regress spontaneously, in many instances it leads to obstructive uropathy, renal failure, and eventual death. The most common treatment measures are surgical excision combined with EBRT and oral steroids, but the prognosis in both local and systemic disease is usually not good.

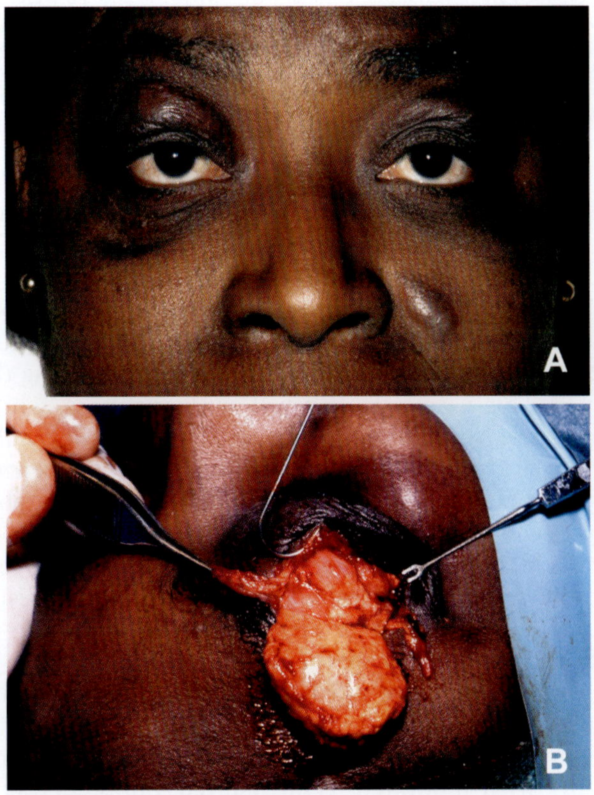

FIGURE 15.11. (A,B) Bilateral xanthogranulomas in superior lateral orbit. The patient later developed multiple skin nodules of the face but no systemic disease. Because of the bilateral superior lateral masses, she was considered to have Sjögren's disease at initial presentation. Later the tissue diagnosis obtained from these lesions revealed the true nature of the pathology. Note the glistening, yellow-orange cut surface of the well-delineated mass from the right superior orbit.

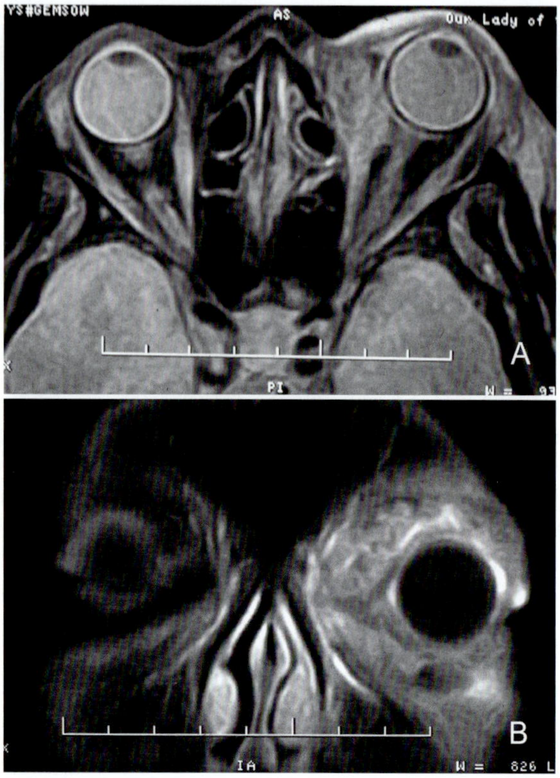

FIGURE 15.12. Axial and coronal MRIs with T1- and T2-weighted images, respectively, showing a mixture of hypo- and hyperintense signals in the superior medial aspect of the globe. One can deduce only that the orbit harbors an infiltrating mass lesion; the appearance is not diagnostic for any specific tumor. Histopathology proved the tumor to be a xanthogranuloma.

Ophthalmologists are most familiar with JXG, a self-limiting disorder of the skin and the iris that may be present at birth, but typically arises during infancy.[54] The lesions consist of several yellow-orange cutaneous nodules on the skin of the head and neck, with the most frequent site of extracutaneous involvement being the uvea. This manifests as a yellowish iris mass, which can cause hyphema and glaucoma. Histopathologically, these are xanthogranulomatous lesions characterized by histiocytic proliferations associated with lymphocytes and Touton giant cells.[32,54] JXG also develops in the orbit as isolated lesions.[55] Whether these cases represent solitary JXG lesions without other manifestations of the disease or are orbital XGs occurring in children is open to speculation.

Another type of xanthogranulomatous disease involving the orbit is necrobiotic xanthogranuloma (Figure 15.13).[56] This rare histiocytic disorder presents with indurated, yellowish-red, nontender skin nodules in the eyelids and periorbital structures. It is a progressive and destructive disease often associated with multiple organ involvement, paraproteinemia, and hematologic and/or lymphoproliferative malignant disorders. The granulomas are made of histiocytes, lymphocytes, and Touton and foreign body giant cells intermixed with focal areas of necrosis. The ocular manifestations are varied and may include eyelid nodules, episcleritis, uveitis, iritis, keratitis, cellulitis, and proptosis.[56] The differential diagnosis of necrobiotic XG includes JXG, granuloma annulare, foreign body granuloma, subcutaneous rheumatoid nodules, xanthoma disseminatum, primary and secondary amyloidosis, and E-Cd.[56] These lesions tend to recur, or there may be an increase in inflammatory activity after incisional biopsy or surgical debulking.[57] Treatment involves chemotherapy with or without radiation and the avoidance of surgery where possible. Lifelong surveillance to detect associated malignancies is advised.

Cutaneous xanthomas may be encountered in patients with solitary orbital XG and in patients with E-Cd. These patients may or may not have elevated serum triglyceride and cholesterol levels. The most common form of cutaneous xanthoma is the xanthelasma palpebrum, also known simply as xanthelasma, which refers specifically to lesions that occur in the eyelids that may present as solitary or diffuse lesions (Table 15.2).[58] Xanthelasmas consist of yellowish placoid skin lesions on the eyelids, usually bilateral, near the inner canthi. The prevalence rate is approximately 2 and 1% in women and men, respectively, increasing with age. Hyperlipidemia, usually Fredrickson hyperlipidemic phenotype IIa, is present in approximately 50% of the patients with xanthelasmas. The histopathology of xanthelasma reveals a great deal of similarity to orbital XG, with aggregates of foamy histiocytes proliferating around the small blood vessels of the superficial dermis and a surrounding lymphocytic reaction with occasional Touton giant cells. The pathogenesis of these lesions is unclear. It is thought that the cholesterol accumulation is derived from the blood, with the low-density lipids leaking through the capillary walls.[59] However, several other factors are likely involved, inasmuch as more than half of hy-

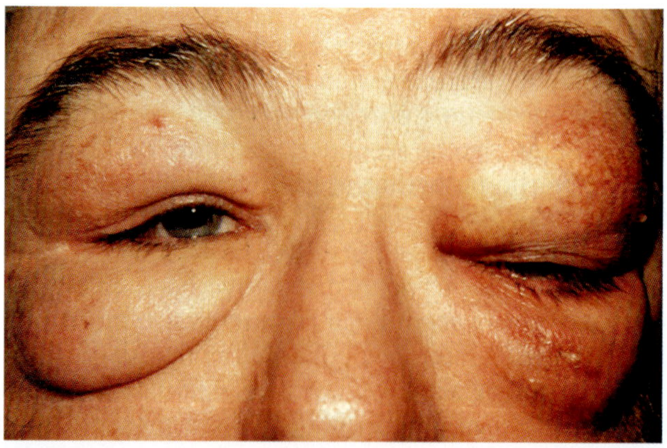

FIGURE 15.13. Yellowish-red skin nodules of the eyelids and periorbital skin in necrobiotic xanthogranuloma.

TABLE 15.2. Clinical and Morphologic Features of Some Xanthomas.

Xanthoma	*Cell of origin*	*Histopathology*	*Ophthalmic manifestations*	*Systemic manifestations*
Xanthogranuloma	Non-Langerhans cell	Foamy histiocytes, Touton GCs, lymphocytes; cholesterol clefts	Solitary or multiple; eyelids, orbit, conjunctiva, optic nerve	Seen in adults; long bones, heart, kidney, retroperitoneal lesions
Juvenile xanthogranuloma (JXG)	Non-Langerhans cell	Foamy histiocytes, lymphocytes, Touton multinucleated GCs	Solitary or multiple iris mass with hyphema, cataract, glaucoma	Seen in infants; skin and scalp lesions
Necrobiotic xanthogranuloma	Non-Langerhans cell?	Foamy histiocytes with Touton and multinucleated GCs; necrosis cholesterol clefts	Periorbital skin lesions, eyelid and orbit mass, keratitis, episcleritis	Multiple violaceous skin nodules on face and trunk
Planar xanthoma (xanthelasma)	Tissue macrophage (non-Langerhans cell?) and lymphocyte	Foamy histiocytes, Touton GCs, lymphocytes	Placoid skin lesions on eyelids	50% Hyperlipidemia
Diffuse planar xanthoma	Tissue macrophage non-Langerhans cell?) and lymphocyte	Foamy histiocytes, Touton GCs, lymphocytes	Placoid skin lesions on eyelids	Confluent xanthelasmas on trunk and face
Progressive nodular histiocytosis	Non-Langerhans cell	Spindly histiocytes, Touton GCs; storiform pattern	Xanthomatous maculopapular lesions on eyelids, ectropion	Yellow, maculopapular skin lesions on face and trunk

Xanthoma	*Associated conditions*	*Workup*	*Laboratory*	*Treatment*	*Prognosis*
Xanthogranuloma	Erdheim–Chester disease, periodontal problems	Long bone films, CT, MRI, radionuclide bone scan	↑ Cholesterol ↑ Triglyceride	Surgery, steroids, EBRT?	Recurrent disease; very poor with E-Cd
Juvenile xanthogranuloma (JXG)	Neurofibromatosis?	Skin biopsy	Normal	Systemic and local steroids; EBRT	Spontaneous regression of systemic disease; poor visual prognosis with hyphema 2° glaucoma
Necrobiotic xanthogranuloma	Multiple myeloma, lymphoma, PC dyscresias	Immune profile	Leukopenia IgG gammopathy Cryoglobulinemia	Chemotherapy, local steroids, minimal surgery	Poor with progressive disease
Planar xanthoma (xanthelasma)	50% Hyperlipidemia, type II	Serum lipid and cholesterol levels	Serum lipid	No surgery, chemotherapy EBRT	50% recurrence after therapy
Diffuse planar xanthoma	40% Multiple myeloma, leukemia, lymphoma, cryoglobulinemia	Serum lipid and cholesterol levels	Serum lipid	Surgery, CO_2 laser, trichloracetic acid	50% recurrence after therapy
Progressive nodular histiocytosis	None	Skin biopsy	High uric acid	Surgery	Spontaneous regression

perlipidemic patients do not develop these lesions, and normolipidemic patients sometimes do. Palpebral and periorbital xanthelasmas were present in three of our cases, including one with E-Cd. Serum cholesterol, lipid, and triglyceride levels were measured in six of our patients but were not helpful as diagnostic tests.

The most commonly used treatment modalities for XG lesions are surgical excision combined with oral corticosteroids and various chemotherapeutic agents, but recurrences are encountered often regardless of the size of the lesion.[41,48,60–62] XG lesions are usually radiation resistant, but some patients are known to respond to EBRT (Figure 15.14). The prognosis in systemic involvement is very poor. According to one report, 22 of 59 E-Cd patients died within a mean of 32 months after diagnosis.[31]

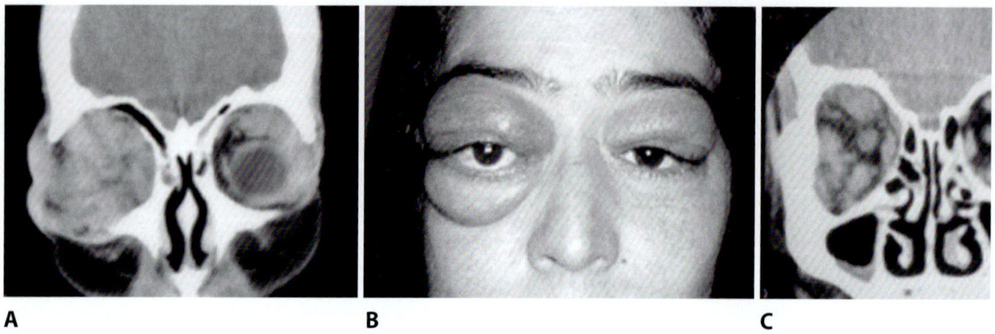

FIGURE 15.14. A patient with bilateral xanthogranulomas before (A,B) and after (C) external beam radiation therapy. She did not have systemic disease and responded quite well to external beam radiation.

References

1. Karcioglu ZA, Carroll G, Nasr AM, Haik BG. Fibrous lesions of the orbit and periorbital tissues. *XXVIII International Congress of Ophthalmology*. Amsterdam; 1998:8.
2. Masson JK, Soule EH. Desmoid tumors of the head and neck. *Am J Surg* 1966;112:6115–6122.
3. Enzinger FM. Fibrous tumors of infancy. In: *Tumors of Bone and Soft Tissue*. Chicago: Year Book Publishers; 1965:375–396.
4. Schreiber MM, Shapiro SI, Sampsel J. Pseudosarcomatous fibromatosis (fasciitis). *Arch Dermatol* 1965;92:661.
5. Schutz JS, Rabkin MD, Schutz S. Fibromatous tumor (desmoid type) of the orbit. *Arch Ophthalmol* 1979;97:703–704.
6. MacKenzie DH. The fibromatoses: a clinicopathological concept. *Br Med J* 1972;4:277–281.
7. Henderson JW. *Orbital Tumors*. Philadelphia: WB Saunders; 1973:209–211.
8. Hidayat AA, Font RL. Juvenile fibromatosis of the periorbital region and eyelid. A clinicopathologic study of six cases. *Arch Ophthalmol* 1980;98:280–285.
9. Allen PW. Nodular fasciitis. *Pathology* 1972;4:9–26.
10. Font RL, Zimmerman LE. Nodular fasciitis of the eye and adnexa. A report of ten cases. *Arch Ophthalmol* 1966;75:475–481.
11. Levitt JM, DeVeer JA, Oguzhan MC. Orbital nodular fasciitis. *Arch Ophthalmol* 1969;81:235–237.
12. Perry RH, Ramani PS, McAllister V, et al. Nodular fasciitis causing unilateral proptosis. *Br J Ophthalmol* 1975;59:404–408.
13. Lattes R. *Tumors of the Soft Tissues. Atlas of Tumor Pathology*. 2nd ser, FI. Washington, DC: Government Printing Office; 1990:123–130.
14. Dymock RB, Allen PW, Stirling JW, et al. Giant cell fibroblastoma. A distinctive, recurrent tumor of childhood. *Am J Surg Pathol* 1987;11:263–271.
15. Karcioglu ZA, Al-Rasheed W, Gray A. Second malignant neoplasms in retinoblastoma. *Middle East J Ophthalmol* 1997; 5:99–104.
16. Jabi M, Jeans T, Dardick I. Ultrastructural heterogeneity in malignant fibrous histiocytoma of soft tissue. *Ultrastruct Pathol* 1987;11:583–592.
17. Char D, Caputo G, Miller T. Orbital fibrous histiocytomas. *Orbit* 2000;19:155–159.
18. Font RL, Hidayat AA. Fibrous histiocytoma of the orbit. A clinicopathologic study of 150 cases. *Hum Pathol* 1982;13: 199–209.
19. Jakobiec FA, Howard GM, Jones IS, Tannenbaum M. Fibrous histiocytomas of the orbit. *Am J Ophthalmol* 1974;77:333–345.
20. Karcioglu ZA, Haik BG, Nasr AM. Orbital hemangiopericytoma. *Am J Ophthalmol* 1997;12:661–672.
21. Mafee MF, Putterman A, Valvassori GE, et al. Orbital space-occupying lesions: role of computed tomography and magnetic resonance imaging. An analysis of 145 cases. *Radiol Clin North Am* 1987;29:529–559.
22. Dalley RW. Fibrous histiocytoma and fibrous tumors of the orbit. *Radiol Clin North Am* 1999;37:185–194.
23. Shields JA, Husson M, Shields CL, et al. Orbital malignant fibrous histiocytoma following irradiation for retinoblastoma. *Ophthalmic Plast Reconstr Surg* 2001;17:58–61.
24. Karcioglu ZA, Nasr AM, Mullaney PB. Xanthogranulomatous lesions in the eye and adnexa. *11th Congress of the European Society of Ophthalmology*. Bologna: Monduzzi, 1997:1273–1276.
25. Kim HY, Lee SY, Kang SJ, et al. Solitary fibrous tumor of the orbit: a poorly recognized orbital lesion. *Acta Ophthalmol Scand* 1999;77:704–708.
26. Lanuza A, Lazaro R, Salvador M, et al. Solitary fibrous tumour of the orbit. Report of a new case. *Int Ophthalmol* 1998; 22:265–268.
27. Polito E, Tosi M, Toti P, et al. Orbital solitary fibrous tumor with aggressive behavior. Three cases and the review of the literature. *Graefes Arch Exp Ophthalmol* 2002;240:570–574.
28. Caroll G, Haik BG, Karcioglu ZA. Orbital giant cell fibroblastoma. *Orbit* 1999;18:25–32.
29. Van Furth R, Cohn ZA, Hirsch JG, et al. The mononuclear phagocyte system: a new classification of macrophages, monocytes and their precursor cells. *Bull World Health Organ* 1972;46:845–855.
30. Chu AC. The confusion state of the histiocytoses. *Br J Dermatol* 2000;143:475–476.
31. Chu AC, Dangio G, Favara D. Histocytosis syndrome in children. *Lancet* 1987;1:208–209.
32. Malone M. The histiocytosis of childhood. *Histopathology* 1991;19:105–119.
33. Dahlmann AH, Simmons I, Picton S, et al. Single–Langerhans cell histiocytosis of the orbit. *Eye* 2000;14:109–110.
34. Gonzalez Ruiz A, Bernal Ruiz A, Aragoneses Fraile H, et al. Progressive nodular histiocytosis accompanied by systemic disorders. *Br J Dermatol* 2000;143:628–631.
35. Koch BL, Myer CM. presentation and disgnosis of unilateral maxillary swelling in children. *Am J Otolaryngol* 1999;20: 106–129.
36. Hidayet AA, Mafee MF, Laver NV, Noujaim S. Langerhans cell histiocytosis and JXG orbit. Clinicopathologic, CT and MRI features. *Radiol Clin North Am* 1998;36:1229–1240.
37. Stull MA, Krandsdorf MJ, Devaney KO. Langerhans cell histiocytosis of the bone. *Radiographics* 1992;12:801–823.
38. Hindman W, Thomas RD, Young LW, Yu L. Langerhans cell histiocytosis: unusual skeletal manifestations observed in thirty-four cases. *Skeletal Radiol* 1998;27:177–181.
39. Woo KI, Harris GJ. Eosinophilic granuloma of the orbit: understanding the paradox of aggressive destruction responsive to minimal intervention. *Ophthalmic Plast Reconstr Surg* 2003;19:429–439.

40. Broadbent V, Gadner H. Current therapy for Langerhans cell histiocytosis. *Hematol Oncol Clin North Am* 1998;12:327–338.
41. Shields JA, Karcioglu ZA, Shields CL, et al. Orbital and eyelid involvement with Erdheim–Chester disease. A report of two cases. *Arch Ophthalmol* 1991;109:850–854.
42. Miszkiel KA, Sohaib SAA, Rose GE. Radiological and clinicopathological features of orbital XG. *Br J Ophthalmol* 2000; 84:251–258.
43. Schultz KD, Petronio J, Nerad J, Hunter SB. Solitary intracerebral juvenile xanthogranuloma. Case report and review of the literature. *Pediatr Neurosurg* 1997;26:315–321.
44. Yamada K, Miura M, Miyayama H, et al. Symptomatic solitary xanthogranuloma occupying the cavernous sinus. *J Neurosurg* 2001;94:322–326.
45. Karcioglu ZA, Sharara N, Boles TL, Nasr AM. Orbital xanthogranuloma; clinical and morphologic features in 8 patients. *Orbital Plast Reconstr Surgery.* 2003;19:372–381.
46. Veyssier-Belot C, Cacoub P, Caparros-Lefebvre D, et al. Erdheim–Chester disease. Clinical and radiologic characteristics of 59 cases. *Medicine (Baltimore)* 1996;75:157–169.
47. Chetritt J, Paradis V, Dargere D, et al. Chester–Erdheim disease: a neoplastic disorder. *Hum Pathol* 1999;30:1093–1096.
48. Alper MG, Zimmerman LE, la Piana FG. Orbital manifestations of Erdheim–Chester disease. *Trans Am Ophthalmol Soc* 1983;81:64–85.
49. Chester W. Über Lipogranulomatose. *Virchows Arch Path Anat* 1930;279:561–602.
50. Molnar CP, Gottschalk R, Gallagher B. Lipid granulomatosis: Erdheim–Chester disease. *Clin Nucl Med* 1988;13:736–741.
51. Egan AJM, Boardman LA, Tazelaar HD, et al. Erdheim–Chester disease. Clinical, radiologic, and histopathologic findings in five patients with interstitial lung disease. *Am J Surg Pathol* 1999;23:17–26.
52. Eble JN, Rosenberg AE, Young RH. Retroperitoneal xanthogranuloma in a patient with Erdheim–Chester disease. *Am J Surg Pathol* 1994;18:843–848.
53. Suzuki K, Miura N, Ueda T, et al. Retroperitoneal xanthogranuloma: a case report. *Acta Urol Japonica* 1992;38: 315–318.
54. Karcioglu ZA, Mullaney PB. Diagnosis and management of iris juvenile xanthogranuloma. *J Pediatr Ophthalmol Strabismus* 1997;34:44–51.
55. Shields CL, Shields JA, Buchanon HW. Solitary orbital involvement with juvenile xanthogranuloma. *Arch Ophthalmol* 1990;108:1587–1589.
56. Ugurlu S, Bartley GB, Gibson LE. Necrobiotic xanthogranuloma: long-term outcome of ocular and systemic involvement. *Am J Ophthalmol* 2000;129:651–657.
57. Robertson DM, Winkelmann RK. Ophthalmic features of necrobiotic xanthogranuloma with paraproteinemia. A review of 22 cases. *Am J Ophthalmol* 1984;97:173–183.
58. Domonkos AN, Arnold HL Jr, Odom RB, eds. *Andrews' Diseases of the Skin: Clinical Dermatology.* 7th ed. Philadelphia: WB Saunders, 1982:658–660.
59. Bergman R. The pathogenesis and clinical significance of xanthelasma palpebrum. *J Am Acad Dermatol* 1994;30(2 pt 1): 236–242.
60. Devouassoux G, Lantuejoul S, Chatelain P, et al. Erdheim–Chester disease. a primary macrophage cell disorder. *Am J Respir Crit Care Med* 1998;157:650–653.
61. Esmaeli B, Ahmadi A, Tang R, et al. Interferon therapy for orbital infiltration secondary to Erdheim–Chester disease. *Am J Ophthalmol* 2001;132:945–947.
62. Jakobson AM, Kreuger A, Hagberg H, Sundstrom C. Treatment of Langerhans cell histiocytosis with alpha-interferon. *Lancet* 1987;2:1520–1521.

16

Fibro-osseous and Cartilaginous Tumors and Tumorlike Conditions

Zeynel A. Karcıoglu

Primary orbital bone and cartilage tumors are rare. More often these lesions develop in neighboring paranasal and nasal bones and involve the orbit secondarily. In most unusual circumstances they originate from the trochlear cartilage and from primitive mesenchymal soft tissues. For the sake of simplicity, in this chapter these lesions are divided into groups of bone and cartilage-forming lesions, fibrous and fibro-osseous lesions, giant-cell-rich lesions, and cystic lesions (Box 16.1).

BONE-FORMING LESIONS

Osteoma

The most common tumor of the orbital bones is the osteoma, which is a benign lesion consisting primarily of mature cancellous bone (Figure 16.1).[1,2] It has not been determined whether osteomas are true neoplasms or the result of an inflammatory reaction. Most of these lesions develop in the fourth to fifth decades of life; they are rare in children.[1] There is evidence that osteoma is more commonly encountered in males.[1,3]

The standard way of labeling the cranial osteomas is to name them according to the bone of origin (e.g., zygomatic osteoma) whereas osteomas of the paranasal sinus are labeled according to which sinus they invade (e.g., frontal osteoma).[3–5] Most osteomas are asymptomatic, but if they grow to sufficient size, they may cause displacement and/or proptosis of the globe and signs of nasolacrimal duct obstruction, particularly by ethmoidal lesions.[6,7] Osteomas usually develop anteriorly; therefore, they do not cause visual disturbances. The exception to this rule is the sphenoid sinus osteoma, which encroaches on the optic foramen and may produce optic nerve damage.[8]

Although these are solitary tumors, multiple lesions occasionally develop, particularly in patients with Gardner syndrome, a hereditary condition in which orbital osteomas can be associated with intestinal polyposis and carcinomatosis.[9,10]

Histopathologically, these tumors are composed of irregular bony trabeculae and fibrovascular tissue (Figure 16.1).[1] Traditionally the osteomas are divided into three types based on histopathologic appearance: eburnated (ivory), fibrous, and mature. The eburnated osteoma is primarily composed of thick bony trabeculae with little fibrous tissue. The fibrous type contains highly vascularized fibroadipose tissue between the bone elements, which may lead to a misdiagnosis of ossifying fibroma or osteogenic sarcoma.[2] Typically, osteomas manifest with well-delineated homogeneous radiodensity in plain films and CTs. On plain skull films, osteomas are identified as well-delineated, dense lesions adjacent to a paranasal sinus.[11]

The differential diagnosis of these lesions should include endochondroma, osteogenesis imperfecta, bone infarction, fibrous dysplasia, low-grade osteogenic sarcoma, ossifying fibroma, and, in unusual cases, calcified meningioma.[12–14]

Only patients with symptomatic osteomas should be treated; when the osteomas are located anteriorly, simple excision will effect a cure, since recurrences are rare. However, when paranasal sinus osteomas invade the orbit posteriorly, particularly with optic canal involvement, the surgery is complex and should be performed by a craniofacial surgical team.

Osteoblastoma

Osteoblastomas are benign bone-forming tumors that account for approximately 10% of all tumors developing in skull bones. However, they are very rarely seen in the orbit.[15]

Osteogenic Sarcoma

Osteogenic sarcoma (osteosarcoma) is the most common primary malignant tumor of bone.[16] It is also the most common malignant tumor of the craniofacial skeleton as well as of the orbit.[17,18] The majority of patients seen are over the age of 40, and the disease more often affects men.[19,20] The clinical presentation depends on the location and size of the tumor and its rate of growth.[16]

BOX 16.1. Fibro-osseous and Cartilaginous Lesions of the Orbit

Bone-forming lesions	Osteoma Osteoblastoma Osteogenic sarcoma Parosteal osteogenic sarcoma
Cartilage-forming lesions	Chondroma Chondrosarcoma Mesenchymal chondrosarcoma Multiple endochondromatoses
Fibro-osseus lesions	Fibrous dysplasia Ossifying fibroma
Fibrous lesions	
Giant-cell-rich lesions	Giant cell reparative granuloma Osteitis fibrosa cystica (brown tumor) Giant cell tumor
Cystic lesions	Simple bone cyst Aneurysmal bone cyst Epidermal cyst

Radiologic studies show a poorly defined infiltrating lesion that can be sclerotic, lytic, or mixed sclerotic and lytic. Early changes discernible on computed tomography (CT) include increased bone marrow attenuation and calcification (Figure 16.2).[21] The tumor is densely sclerotic in approximately 50% of cases. In the other 50% of cases, osteogenic sarcoma has an ossifying, destructive appearance, or it may present as a pure osteolytic lesion. The classic "sunburst" pattern produced as a result of periosteal new bone formation is not a helpful feature in skull tumors. Contrast-enhanced CT can determine the vascularity and the distribution of the blood vessels within the soft tissue component. Radionuclide bone scan is more sensitive for early changes than plain films and CT, whereas MRI is the most sensitive method of imaging.[22] MRI defines the extent of the tumor much more accurately than CT. High or low signal intensity can occur on T2-weighted images owing to cellularity and osteosclerosis, respectively. The relationship of the tumor to the compartments of the cranium is best assessed with magnetic resonance imaging (MRI). Magnetic resonance angiography (MRA) may also prove to be useful to demarcate tumor vessels.

Clinical manifestations depend on the location of the tumor, its size, and rate of growth. Most patients present with swelling of the orbit, proptosis, and pain, particularly at night.[23,24] Osteosarcomas originating from ethmoid and frontal bones present as palpable and often visible masses, whereas tumors originating posteriorly, particularly from the sphenoid bone, produce proptosis without a palpable mass. Serum alkaline phosphatase levels are often elevated in osteogenic sarcoma.

Osteogenic sarcomas are composed of pleomorphic spindle cells containing hyperchromatic nuclei and numerous mitotic figures intermixed with neoplastic bone formations. Depending on the matrix of the tumor, they are subgrouped as chondroblastic or fibromatoid types.

It is known that cranio-orbital osteosarcomas are more often seen with Paget's disease, with fibrous dysplasia, and after radiation treatment with or without retinoblastoma.[25–27] The incidence of osteogenic sar-

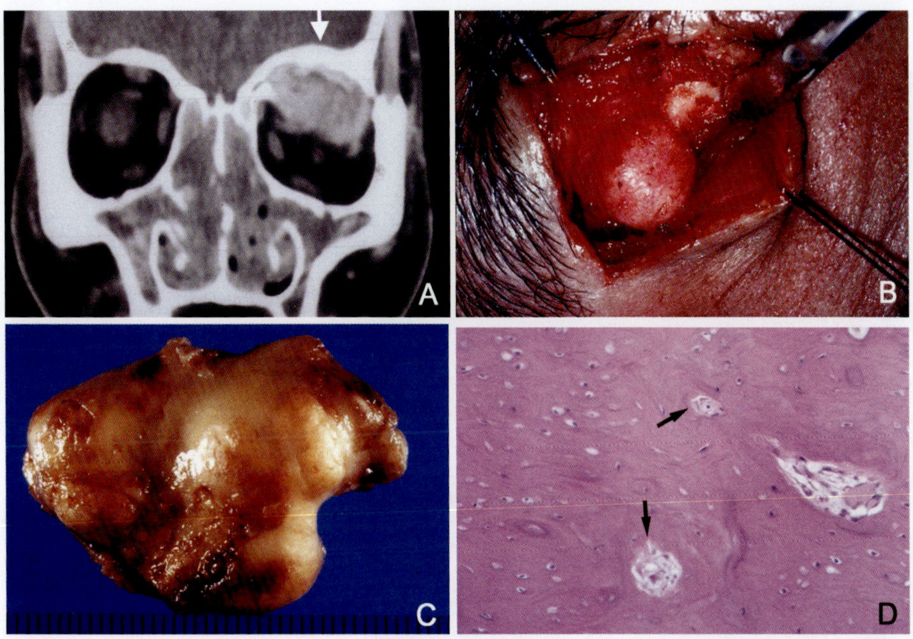

FIGURE 16.1. (A) Coronal CT image showing a densely sclerotic osteoma of the frontal bone. Note the thickening of the superior orbital rim (white arrow). (B) The intraoperative picture of another case of superior orbital rim osteoma. (C) Gross photograph of the same tumor with bosselated, well-circumscribed appearance. (D) Histopathology of the same osteoma reveals dense cortical-type bone with haversian systems (black arrows) of varying size and shapes.

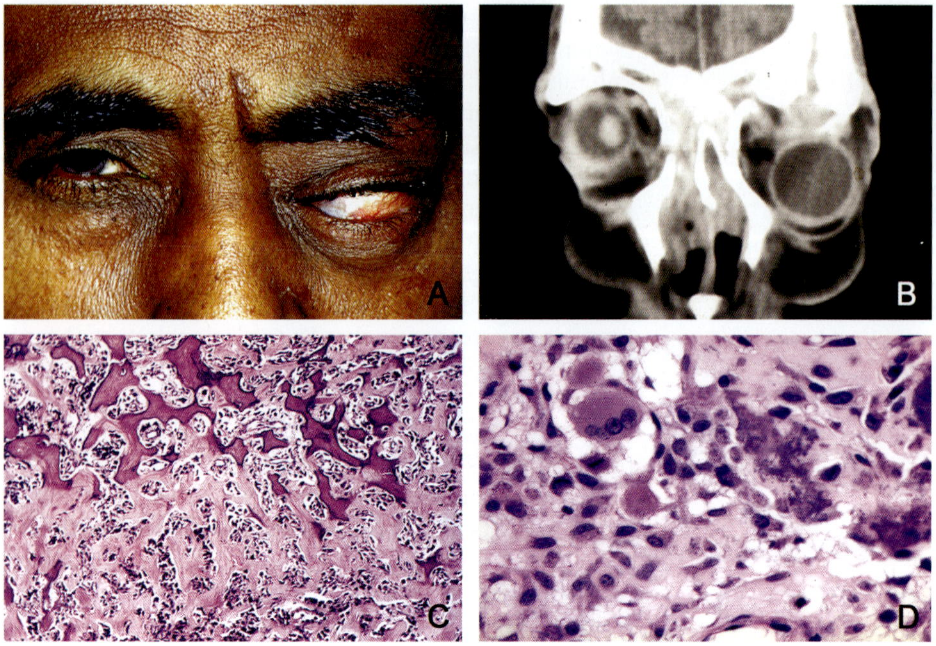

FIGURE 16.2. (A) Proptosis and inferior displacement of the left eye secondary to osteogenic sarcoma of the superior orbit. (B) Coronal CT image shows a poorly defined, infiltrating lesion with alternating areas of sclerosis and lysis pushing the globe inferiorly. (C) The histopathology consists of clusters of fusiform, atypical connective tissue cells surrounding deposits of neoplastic bone. (D) Atypical osteoblastic proliferation.

coma developing as a second primary tumor in survivors of retinoblastoma is high (see Chapter 5).[16,17,28]

Treatment of osteogenic sarcoma is surgical, but clear margins in the craniofacial cases may be difficult to obtain because frozen section of the bone cannot be done during excision. CT and MRI are the best means of determining the bone and soft tissue extent of the tumor.[29] Preoperative chemotherapy has been reported to increase the survival.[30]

Parosteal Osteogenic Sarcoma (Low-Grade Osteogenic Sarcoma)

Parosteal osteosarcoma rarely involves the orbit; its craniofacial involvement is usually limited to the jaw bones (Figure 16.3).[31–34] It originates in the periosteum or from the immediate parosteal connective tissue and is a rare type of osteogenic sarcoma, representing about 5% of all tumors.

Accurate diagnosis and subclassification of parosteal osteosarcoma is important because although the tumor is fairly rare (approximately 16% of cases), dedifferentiation is associated with a worse prognosis. Parosteal osteosarcoma may dedifferentiate into a higher grade sarcoma, such as liposarcoma, rhabdomyosarcoma, or malignant fibrous histiocytoma.[31]

Because surrounding tissue is frequently invaded by parosteal osteosarcoma, local recurrence is common. One study found as high as 46% soft tissue involvement adjacent to tumor, and 22% had adjacent

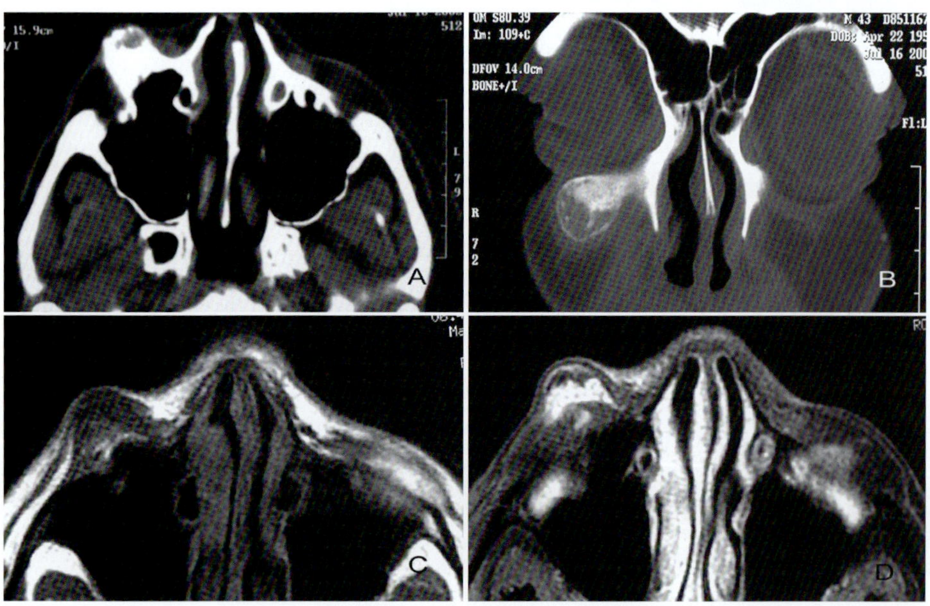

FIGURE 16.3. (A,C,D) Axial CT and MR images of focally sclerotic, well-delineated tumor of the inferior orbital rim. (B) Bone window study shows well-delineated tumor with intralesional deposits of young bone.

neurovascular bundle involvement.[33] Therefore, wide excision is advocated (Figure 16.4). Along with appropriate surgical management, continued monitoring is important. Craniofacial parosteal osteosarcomas are detected early, and prognosis for these tumors, when fully excised, is better than for the conventional osteogenic sarcoma.

CARTILAGE-FORMING LESIONS

Chondroma

Benign cartilaginous tumors of the orbit are rare, but they are known to occur in the region of the trochlea, the only cartilaginous structure in the orbit.[35] Orbital chondroma presents as a slowly enlarging, well-delineated mass in the superior nasal quadrant of the orbit. Microscopically, it is composed of lobulated hyaline cartilage that may occasionally show mild atypia.[36] Since the orbital chondroma is a benign tumor with no capacity to malignant transformation, it responds well to surgical excision.

Chondrosarcoma

Chondrosarcoma is a commonly encountered tumor of the skeleton. However, in the cranium it is uncommon, and its occurrence in the orbit and periorbital sinus is exceptionally rare.[37,38] These tumors originate mainly from the nasal cavity; nasopharynx and orbital invasion may occur secondarily.[39] Most chondrosarcomas are made of pleomorphic hyaline cartilage cells scattered throughout a myxoid matrix (Figure 16.5). The clinical findings depend on the location and the size of the tumor, which may compress and/or infiltrate orbital structures.[40] Chondrosarcoma infrequently metastasizes, and, therefore, local control is the goal of treatment. Chondrosarcomas of the craniofacial skeleton are difficult to excise totally short of major procedures including exenteration. Radiation therapy is an important adjunct that should be used whenever total excision cannot be accomplished.[41]

Mesenchymal Chondrosarcoma

Mesenchymal chondrosarcoma is a rare, more aggressive subtype of chondrosarcoma; however, it is encountered in and around the orbit more often than the conventional chondrosarcoma.[42–44] It may rarely be multicentric.[44] Radiologically, mesenchymal chondrosarcoma leads to haphazard infiltration of the bone and, therefore, presents with ill-defined margins. Dense irregular calcifications are frequently found within these tumors.[45–47] Mesenchymal chondrosarcoma is treated with extensive surgery with adjunct chemotherapy and radiation therapy; the survival rate for these patients is poor.[45]

Multiple Enchondromatoses

Multiple enchondromatosis syndromes (Ollier disease and Maffucci syndrome) are congenital disorders that

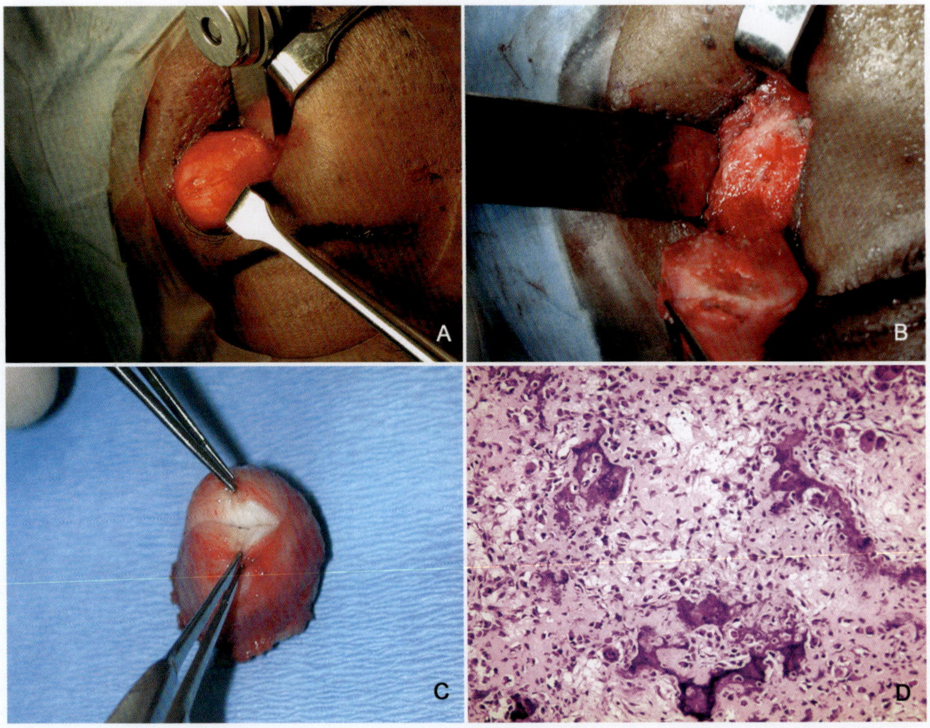

FIGURE 16.4. (A,B) Excision of a parosteal osteogenic sarcoma with the use of oscillating saw. (C) The gross specimen, showing the cut surface of the fibrous cap of the lesion. (D) Histopathology reveals proliferation of spindle cells and irregular deposits of malignant bone surrounded by extensive osteoblastic activity.

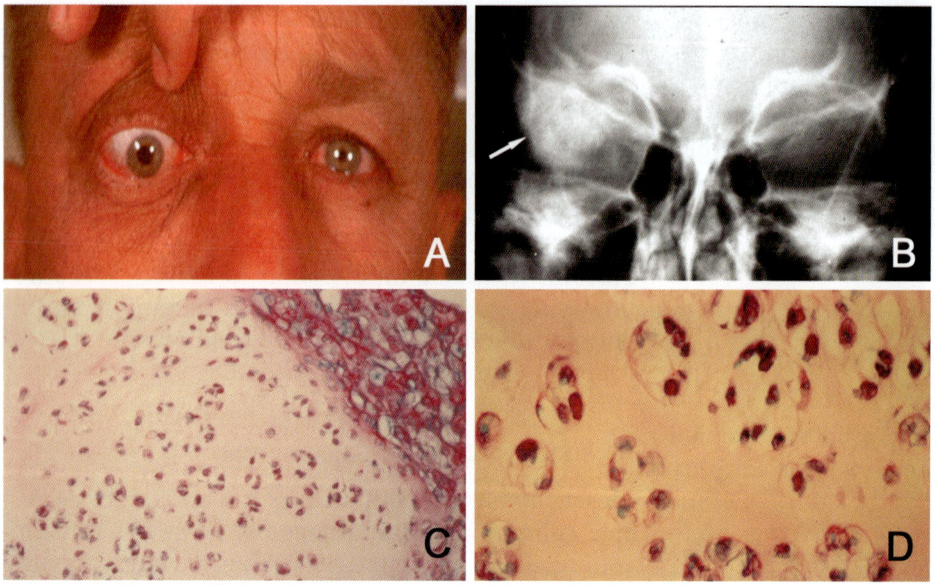

FIGURE 16.5. (A) Right axial proptosis secondary to orbital chondrosarcoma. (B) Plain film showing moderately sclerotic, lobulated orbital mass (arrow). (C,D) Hypercellular hyaline cartilage composed of atypical chondrocytes clustered within lacunae. The atypical nature of the chondrocytes is better seen in (C). (Courtesy of Dr. James Allen, New Orleans, Louisiana.)

are considered to be in the spectrum of mesodermal dysplasias.

Maffucci syndrome is a nonfamilial disease that presents with multiple enchondromas and subcutaneous hemangiomas.[48,49] Ollier disease most often presents with multiple cartilaginous masses in long bones of the extremities, but hemangiomatous masses are missing. Ollier disease rarely develops in paranasal sinuses and may secondarily involve the orbit.[50] Radionuclide studies may be of help to diagnose Ollier disease.[51]

The mesodermal dysplasia syndromes are also known to develop other benign and malignant tumors including skull chondrosarcomas, low grade astrocytomas, pituitary adenomas, and carcinomas of the genitourinary and gastrointestinal tracts.[52–54] In addition, orbital hemangiomas have been reported in Maffucci disease (Figure 16.6).[55] These intracranial and orbital tumors may present with a number of ocular and orbital symptoms including proptosis, diplopia, visual loss, and cranial nerve palsies.[56] Periodic orbital and neuro-ophthalmologic examinations and imaging studies are appropriate for the patients with Ollier disease and Maffucci syndrome. The treatment of these lesions includes surgery and radiotherapy.

FIBRO-OSSEOUS LESIONS

Fibro-osseous lesions, a mixture of bone and fibrous tissue, occur commonly in the craniofacial bones. At one end of the spectrum is fibrous dysplasia, which is dominated by the fibrous element. At the other end is ossifying fibroma, in which the lamellar bone formation defines the lesion.

Fibrous Dysplasia

Fibrous dysplasia is a benign developmental disorder of the bone that results from the arrest in the maturation of primitive woven bone into mature lamellar bone containing osteoblasts.[57] It can be considered to be a hamartomatous disorder. In fibrous dysplasia osteoblastic activity is arrested and the mature lamellar bone is not formed.[57] The anomaly is considered to be the result of a specific mutation of the Gs alpha gene.[58] In approximately 75% of cases, the disease involves only one bone (monostotic), and in 25% of cases, multiple bones (polyostotic) are involved. Polyostatic fibrous dysplasia develops at an earlier age than the single bone involvement and is rarely found as a part of Albright (McCune–Albright) syndrome, a rare endocrine dysfunction consisting of precocious puberty, hyperthyroidism, and cutaneous hyperpigmentation.[58,59] The most frequently affected sites of the skull are frontal, ethmoidal, sphenoidal, and temporal bones.[60,61] Orbital fibrous dysplasia is usually not associated with Albright syndrome, but, a few cases of Albright syndrome with orbital involvement have been described.[62]

Fibrous dysplasia is usually diagnosed coincidentally, but if it becomes symptomatic, the signs and symptoms correlate well with the primary bone involved and the extent of the involvement.[63] The globe is usually displaced inferiorly with or without proptosis because of the common involvement of the frontal bone (Figure 16.7). The most feared ocular manifestation is the compressive optic neuropathy secondary to sphenoid bone disease, which may present as an acute or chronic loss of visual acuity and fields.[64,65] In advanced cases, the facial asymmetry may lead to serious distortion of the orbit, causing sig-

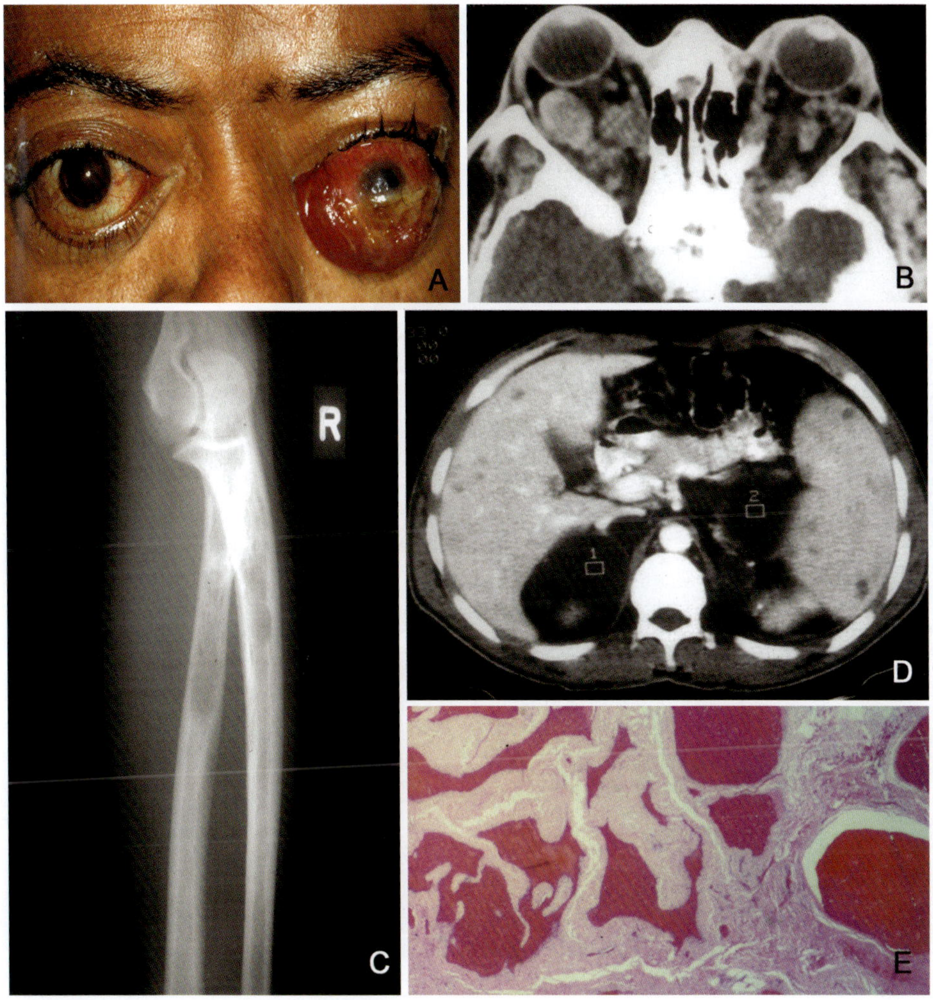

FIGURE 16.6. (A,B) Bilateral proptosis of a patient with Maffucci syndrome, secondary to bilateral orbital cavernous hemangioma. (C) Plain x-ray of the arm displays multiple radiolucent areas consistent with enchondromas of the proximal radius and ulna. (D) CT scan of the abdomen shows multiple hypodense areas in the liver and spleen. (E) Histopathology of the hemangioma shown in (A). (Courtesy of Dr. Thomas E. Johnson, Miami, Florida.)

nificant proptosis, ptosis, and lacrimal drainage system obstruction.[66,67]

CT is the imaging method of choice for initial diagnosis as well as for monitoring the disease during its course and postoperatively, particularly with three-dimensional re-formations. The imaging features, which vary depending on the stage of the disease and the extent of the fibrous stromal replacement, present with Pagetoid, cystic, and sclerotic patterns.[68] MRI patterns of fibrous dysplasia consists of nonhomogeneous low intensity with a sharp margin on T1-weighted images. Signal enhancement may be seen with contrast studies, but this simply offers information regarding the vascularity of the lesion rather than its fibrocellular activity.[69,70]

The diagnosis should be confirmed by means of a biopsy specimen; however, if the radiologic features are typical for fibrous dysplasia in a patient without symptoms, the biopsy may be delayed. Particularly when the involvement is within the posterior orbit, the task of obtaining a biopsy sample may require rather extensive surgery. Therefore, the biopsy may be postponed until the symptomatology justifies surgical excision of bone (Figure 16.8). Fibrous dysplasia compromising the optic foramen is best operated through a transcranial approach to unroof the optic canal and excise tissue from the involved bone as much as possible.[71] In most cases, surgical intervention is delayed until optic nerve compression is imminent or severe asymmetry of the face becomes a serious cosmetic issue.[71]

The histopathology consists of irregularly shaped osteoid deposits and immature, irregular bone originating from the fibrovascular stroma that creates bizarre geometric patterns resembling Chinese letters (Figure 16.7). The metaplastic bone deposits are seen without osteoblastic activity, which is helpful to differentiate fibrous dysplasia from other bone pathologies particularly from ossifying fibroma, which usually contains osteoblasts. The size of the biopsy should be as large as possible, since the histopathologic differential diagnosis may be difficult, particularly when there is malignant transformation of fibrous dysplasia into osteogenic sarcoma and fibrosarcoma.[72]

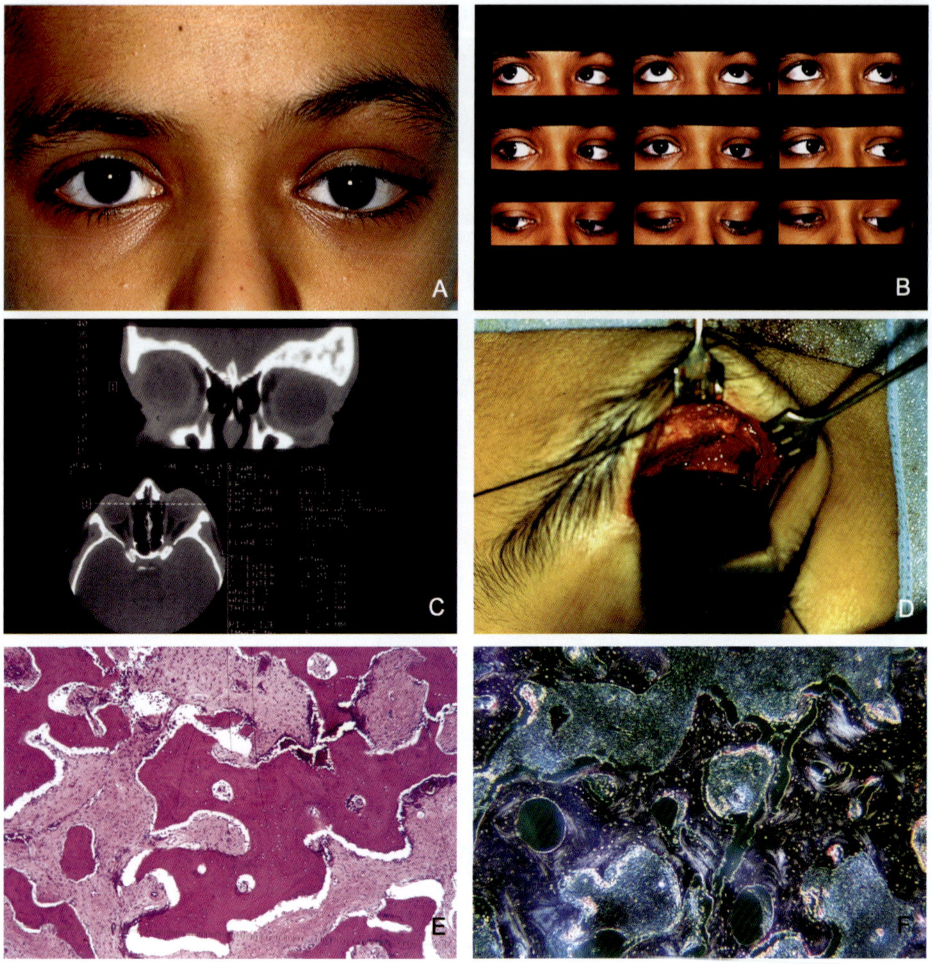

FIGURE 16.7. (A, B) A 9-year-old patient with fibrous dysplasia showing elevation of the left eyebrow and inferior displacement of the left globe that are most apparent in straight and right upper gaze photographs. (C) Coronal CT image shows the irregular sclerosis of the frontal bone including the internal and external trabulae. (D) Intraoperative photograph reveals the knotty thickening of the superior orbital rim. (E) Histopathology reveals a mixture of fibrous tissue composed of uniform spindle cells and irregular discontinuous trabeculae of bone without osteoblastic activity. (F) The birefringence of young deposits of lamellar bone formation is seen through a polarizing lens.

Ossifying Fibroma

Ossifying fibroma, otherwise known as juvenile ossifying fibroma or psammomatoid ossifying fibroma, is a fibro-osseous lesion less commonly seen than fibrous dysplasia (Figure 16.9).[73–76] This is another hamartomatous, indolent fibro-osseous lesion that commonly involves the cranial bones and in almost all cases presents as a monostotic disease. Histopathology of the ossifying fibroma reveals irregular bony spicules surrounded by extensive osteoblastic activity. As opposed to fibrous dysplasia, it is more common in females and in an age group involving adolescents and young adults. Displacement of the globe, optic nerve, and lacrimal drainage system may be seen, depending on the location of the tumor.[76]

On CT, ossifying fibroma presents as a well-delineated sclerosing mass with osseous trabeculae.[77] Maxillary and mandibular involvement are common.[78] The ossifying fibromas usually reveal intermediate signal intensity on T1-weighted MR images and a hypointense signal on T2-weighted images; however, MRI is not very helpful in classifying these lesions.

The best management of ossifying fibroma is early surgical removal; in most instances the surgery is performed by a craniomaxillary team.

FIBROUS LESIONS

Fibrous lesions, which rarely develop in the craniofacial skeleton, include desmoplastic fibroma, myofibroma, and infantile myofibromatosis. These lesions represent locally aggressive tumors with a high rate of recurrence without distant metastasis.[79,80]

GIANT CELL-RICH LESIONS

Giant Cell Reparative Granuloma

Giant cell granuloma (GCG), or giant cell reparative granuloma, is a reactive, nonneoplastic process that occasionally affects the bones of the skull and orbit.[81–84]

The majority of GCGs occur within the first two decades of life and are approximately twice as common

A

B

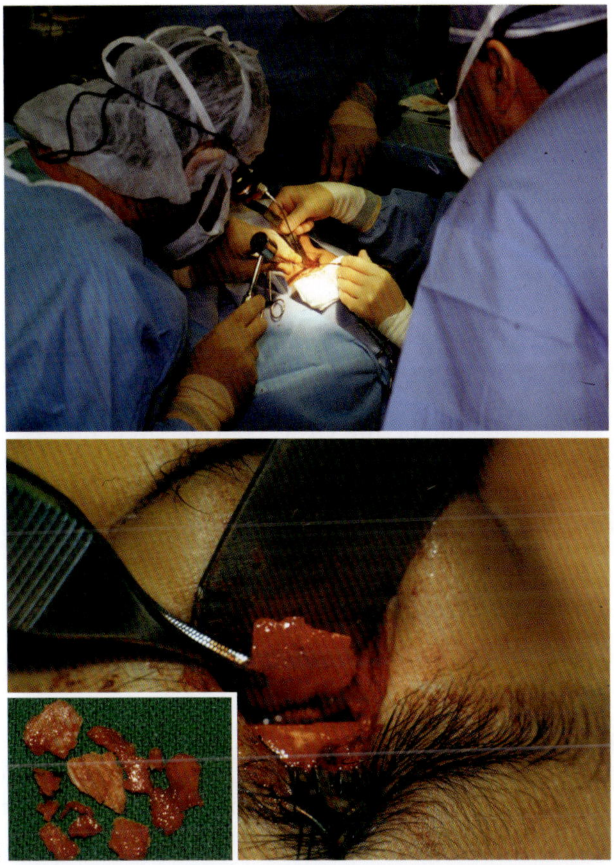

FIGURE 16.8. Intraoperative photographs show the use of the mallet and the osteotome to debulk the thickened dysplastic bone of the orbital roof in a lamellar fashion. *Inset*: Gross photograph of the resected, thin bone chips from dysplastic bone of the orbital roof.

in girls as in boys.[85] These lesions have a hemorrhagic appearance on gross inspection and microscopically consist of groups of spindle-shaped fibroblasts that are mixed with collagen and numerous, multinucleated osteoclast-like giant cells. Additionally, extensive hemorrhages, hemosiderin deposits and reactive woven bone are identified.[86] The histopathologic differential diagnosis includes brown tumor of hyperparathyroidism and giant cell tumor of bone. Histopathologically, the lesion is identical to brown tumor. Only the absence of biochemical findings of hyperparathyroidism would differentiate these two lesions.

The clinical presentation is associated with painful proptosis and encroachment onto orbital structures, depending on the location of the lesion. Radiographically, central GCG forms a well-demarcated, radiolucent, multiloculated lesion.[87] The treatment of choice is aggressive surgical curettage, after which the lesion usually heals and becomes ossified.[86]

Osteitis Fibrosa Cystica

Osteitis fibrosa cystica, otherwise known as brown tumor, is a reactive destructive process that occurs in patients with hyperparathyroidism. In histology it is very similar if not identical to giant cell reparative granuloma and aneurysmal bone cysts; however, the latter lesions are not associated with endocrine abnormality. Brown tumor is rarely seen in the orbital region.[88] CT scans and plain x-rays reveal irregular osteolytic lesions involving the bones that may resemble the radiologic appearance of other fibro-osseous conditions (Figure 16.10).[89] Once a lesion has been established as being composed of fibrous proliferation with scattered giant cells and irregular spicules of bone, appropriate endocrine studies should be done to rule out hyperparathyroidism.

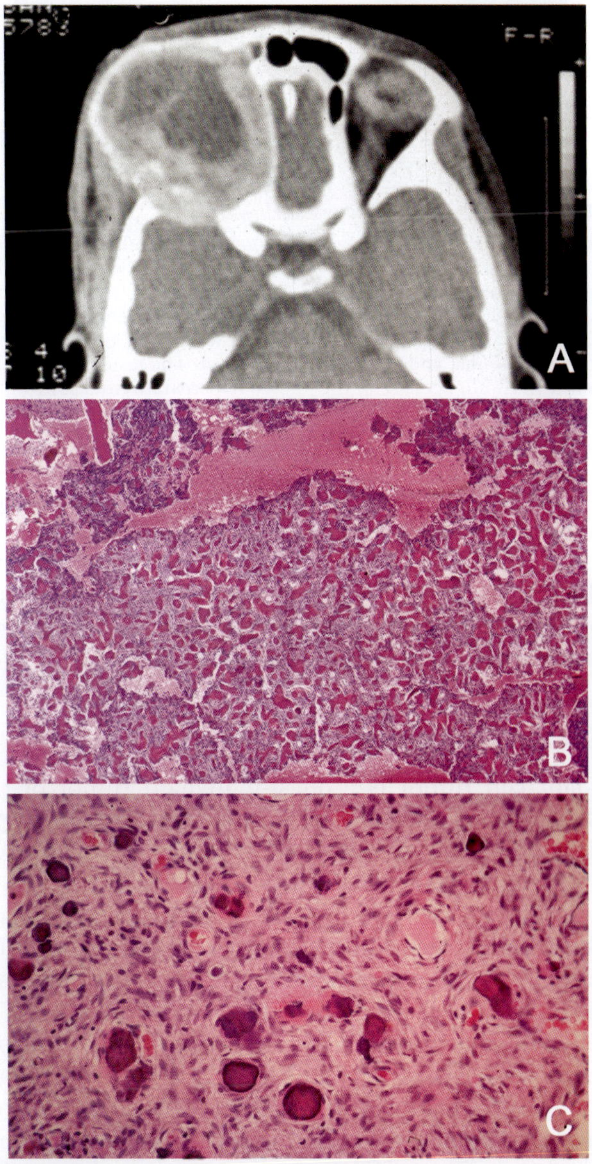

FIGURE 16.9. (A) Axial CT scan showing a variably demineralized, well-delineated ossifying fibroma of the superior orbit and frontal sinus. (B,C) Histopathologically, the lesion is composed of an admixture of woven bony trabeculae and cellular fibrous tissue containing numerous psammoma bodies. (Courtesy of Dr. Curtis Margo, Tampa, Florida.)

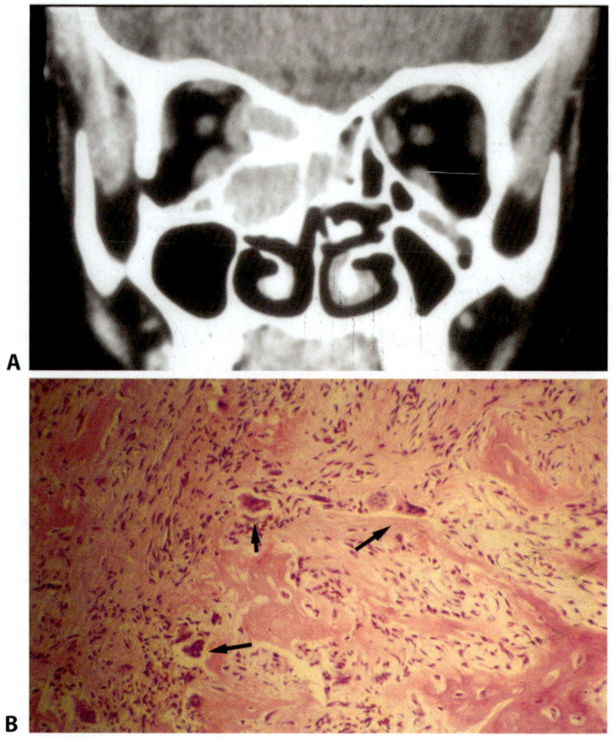

FIGURE 16.10. (A) Coronal CT showing a multiloculated, destructive lesion of the ethmoidal sinus extending into the medial orbit. (B) The histopathology revealed numerous multinucleated giant cells (arrows) scattered within the fibrous tissue matrix with new bone formation, consistent with brown tumor, giant cell reparative granuloma, and aneurysmal bone cyst. The lesion was labeled as brown tumor because of the known hyperparathyroid state of the patient.

The treatment of this lesion is surgical curettage, to which the lesion responds well. However, if the destructive process produces optic nerve compression, the visual prognosis may be poor. Systemic prognosis, on the other hand, depends on the effective management of the hyperparathyroidism.

Giant Cell Tumor

Giant cell tumor is a quasi-malignant tumor of the skeletal connective tissue commonly occurring in patients between the ages of 20 and 40 years.[81,90] Approximately 20% behave in a malignant fashion; however, it is not possible to predict the malignant behavior of these tumors histopathologically or clinically.[91,92] The classic appearance is a round, expansile, radiolucent lesion with light trabeculation. CT is valuable to define the soft tissue component; with contrast enhancement it provides useful information about the tumor's vascularity, which may be similar to that of aneurysmal bone cyst.[93] MRI is superior to plain films and CT in defining the extent of the lesion. T1-weighted images show diminished signal intensity; T2-weighted images show isointense or hyperintense signal intensity of the tumor.[94] Radionuclide bone scans are unreliable in GCT.

Craniofacial lesions represent approximately 2% of all giant cell tumors of bone, and GCT very rarely affects the orbit and paranasal sinuses.[95] The true incidence of giant cell tumor in the craniofacial skeleton is difficult to estimate, since it is believed that many lesions that had been reported as GCT probably represent giant cell reparative granulomas.[96–98]

Clinical features depend on the location and range from displacement of the globe and decreased visual acuity and field.[98] Plain films and CT images usually show destructive radiolucent and poorly defined lesions often associated with a soft tissue mass (Figure 16.11).[97]

The treatment for GCT is wide excision, as extensive as exenteration in some cases.[99] Tumor-free margins should be obtained whenever possible because malignant transformation of these tumors has been reported.[98]

CYSTIC LESIONS

Simple Bone Cyst

Simple bone cyst is a unilocular, fluid-filled cyst lined by a fibrous wall. Although it affects mostly the long bones, occasionally it is seen in the craniofacial area.[100]

Aneurysmal Bone Cyst

Aneurysmal bone cyst is an expansile, cystic lesion that develops within the bone from a preexisting pathology or de novo of unknown etiology.[101,102] Although these lesions are most often seen in long bones, about 5% occur within the craniofacial skeleton, and a small minority is seen in the orbital region.[103] Orbital aneurysmal bone cysts usually develop without any other bony pathology.[104] Most of these lesions affect the orbital roof and produce gradually developing proptosis. In occasional cases, the proptosis develops rapidly, raising the clinical suspicion of malignancy.[105] If the location of the aneurysmal bone cyst is sufficiently posterior, it may compress the optic nerve.[106]

Histopathologically, an aneurysmal bone cyst consists of blood-filled cystic spaces that are lined not by endothelial cells but with plump, fibroblast-like cells (Figure 16.12). Between the cystic places, a fibrovascular stroma containing osteoclast-type giant cells is present. Sometimes there are so many giant cells that the aneurysmal bone cyst is difficult to distinguish from a giant cell lesion of bone. These lesions also contain woven bone and partially calcified, cartilage-like matrix adjacent to cystic places.[107,108] In plain films and CT findings, an aneurysmal bone cyst appears as a mildly enhancing loculated partially cystic mass.

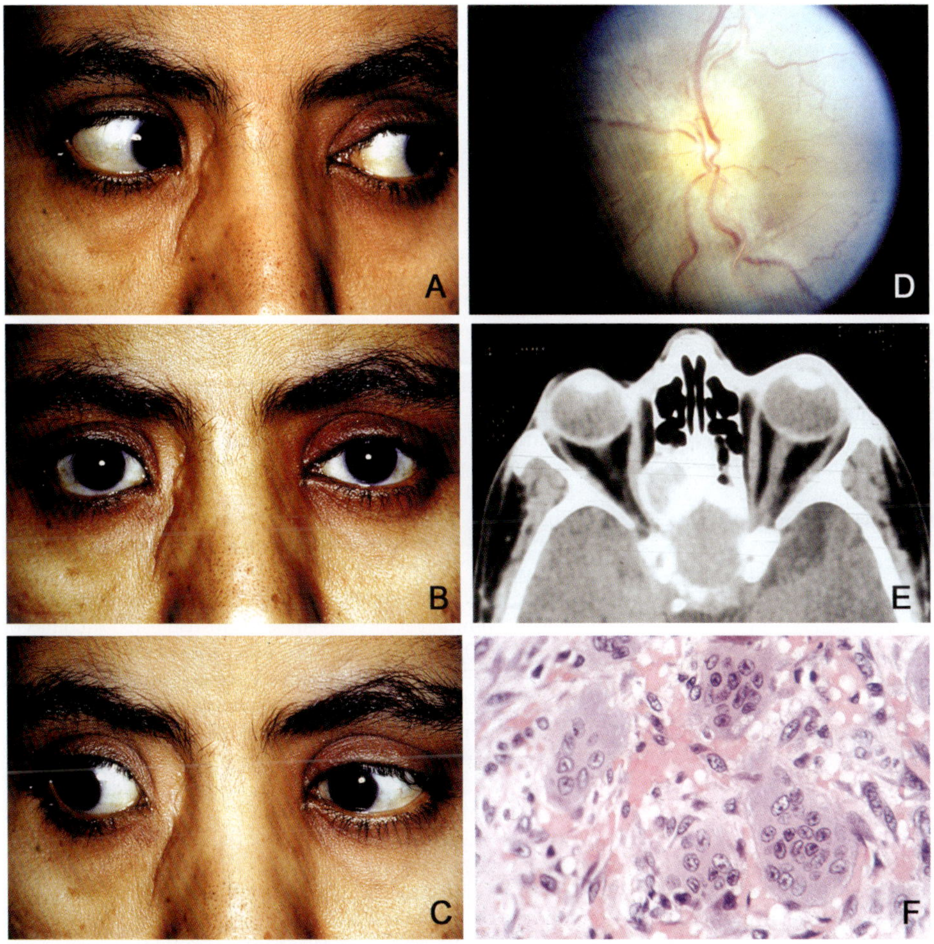

FIGURE 16.11. (A–C) Mild axial proptosis and lateral gaze limitation of the right eye. (D) Disk edema secondary to optic nerve compression by the giant cell tumor. (E) Axial CT scan shows poorly defined, partially cystic and partially sclerotic tumor originating from the sphenoid bone with extension into the posterior orbit. (F) Histopathology shows multinucleated tumor giant cells with innumerable nuclei.

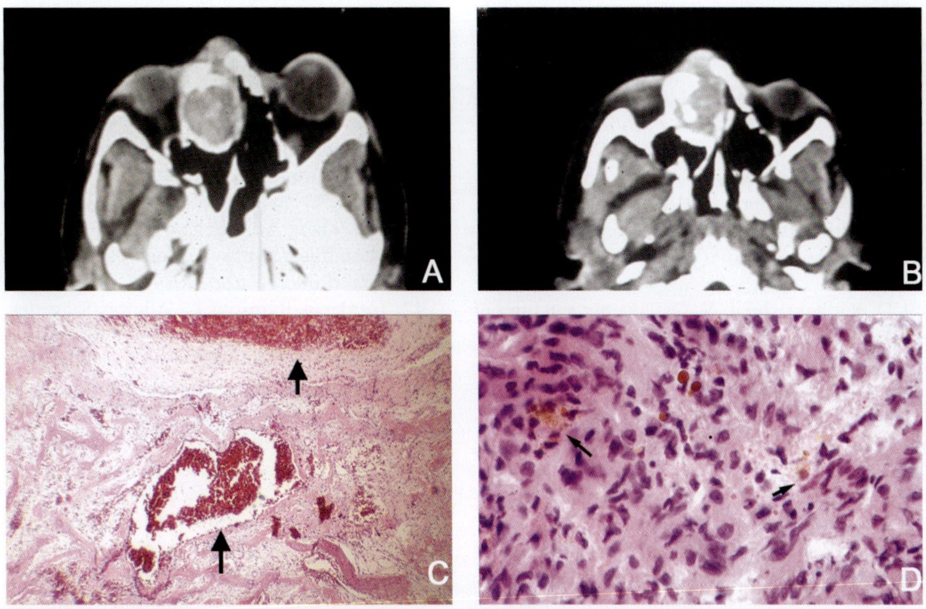

FIGURE 16.12. (A,B) Axial CT images reveal a cystic lesion surrounded by a bony re-formation consistent with a very small bone cyst. There are numerous intralesional densities. (C,D) Microscopic blood-filled cystic spaces lined by spindle-shaped cells containing blood are identified. Clusters of plump, spindle-shaped fibroblasts are scattered among the pseudocystic spaces. Focal deposits of hemosiderin (arrows), indicating old hemorrhages, are also present.

Management of aneurysmal bone cysts is by surgical excision, which is usually done with curettage; the extent of the lesion should be determined carefully during surgery, particularly in superior orbital lesions.

References

1. Fechner RE, Mills SE. *Tumors of the Bone and Joints*. Washington DC: Armed Forces Institute of Pathology; 1993.
2. Jakobiec FA, Jones IS. Mesenchymal and fibro-osseous tumors. In: Jones IS, Jakobiec FA, eds. *Diseases of the Orbit*. New York: Harper & Row; 1979:461–502.
3. Earwaker J. Paranasal sinus osteomas: a review of 46 cases. *Skeletal Radiol* 1993;22:417–423.
4. Boysen M. Osteomas of the paranasal sinuses. *J Otolaryngol* 1978;7:366–370.
5. Smith ME, Calcaterra TC. Frontal sinus osteoma. *Ann Otol Rhinol Laryngol* 1989;98:896–900.
6. Miller NR, Gray J, Sni PR. Giant mushroom-shaped osteoma of the orbit originating from the maxillary sinus. *Am J Ophthalmol* 1977;83:587–591.
7. Sternberg I, Levine MR. Ethmoidal sinus osteoma: a primary cause of nasolacrimal obstruction and dacryocystorhinostomy failure. *Ophthalmic Surg* 1984;15:295–297.
8. Thakur V, Nema HV. Osteoma of the lesser wing of the sphenoid. *Eye Ear Nose Throat Mon* 1969;48:619–621.
9. VanGehuchten DV, Lemagne J-M, Weber S, et al. A case of exophthalmos—an early symptom of Gardner's syndrome. *Orbit* 1982;1:61–69.
10. Whitson WE, Orcutt JC, Walkinshaw MD. Orbital osteoma in Gardner's syndrome. *Am J Ophthalmol* 1986;101:236–241.
11. Wilbur AC, Dobben GD, Linder B. Paraorbital tumors and tumor-like conditions: role of CT and MRI. *Radiol Clin North Am* 1987;25:631–646.
12. Smith GD, Chalmers J, et al. Osteosarcoma arising in relation to an endochondroma. *J Bone Joint Surg Am* 1986;68:315–319.
13. Heater K, Collins PA. Osteosarcoma in association with infarction of bone. *J Bone Joint Surg Am* 1987;69:300–302.
14. Resnik CS, Aisner SC, Young JWR, et al. Case report 767. *Skeletal Radiol* 1993;22:58–61.
15. Lucas DR, Unni KK, McLeod RA, et al. Osteoblastoma: clinicopathologic study of 306 cases. *Hum Pathol* 1994;25:117–134.
16. Huvos AG. *Bone Tumors: Diagnosis, Treatment and Prognosis*. Philadelphia: WB Saunders; 1991:179–200.
17. Nora FE, Unni KK, Pritchard DJ, et al. Osteosarcoma of extragnathic craniofacial bones. *Mayo Clin Proc* 1983;58:268–272.
18. Rao VRK, Rout D, Radhakrishnan V. Osteogenic sarcoma of the skull. *Neuroradiology* 1983;25:51–53.
19. Bertoni F, Dallera P, Bacchini P, et al. The Istituto Rizzoli–Beretta experience with osteosarcoma of the jaw. *Cancer* 1991;68:1555–1563.
20. Clark JL, Unni KK, Dablin DC, et al. Osteosarcoma of the jaw. *Cancer* 1983;51:2311–2316.
21. de Santos LA, Edeiken BS. Subtle early osteosarcoma. *Skeletal Radiol* 1985;13:44–48.
22. Cofre C, Vanel D, et al. Problems and pitfalls in the use of computed tomography for the local evaluation of long bone osteosarcoma: Report on 30 cases. *Skeletal Radiol* 1985;13:147–153.
23. Henderson JW, Farrow GM. *Orbital Tumors*. 2nd ed. New York: BC Decker (Thieme-Stratton); 1980:198–247.
24. Nora FE, Unni KK, Pritchard DJ, et al. Osteosarcoma of extragnathic craniofacial bones. *Mayo Clin Proc* 1983;58:268–272.
25. Moore TE, King AR, Kathol MH, et al. Sarcoma in Paget disease of bone: clinical, radiologic, and pathologic features in 22 cases. *Am J Radiol* 1991;156:1199–1203.
26. Epley KD, Lasky JB, Karesh JW. Osteosarcoma of the orbit associated with Paget disease. *Ophthalmic Plast Reconstr Surg* 1998;14:62–66.
27. Abramson DH, Lee TC, Driscoll C. Osteogenic sarcoma in a survivor of metastatic germline retinoblastoma: the possible influence of human growth hormone. *J Pediatr Ophthalmol Strabismus* 2002;39:347–348.
28. Aung L, Gorlock RG, Shi W, et al. Second malignant neoplasms in long-term survivors of osteosarcoma: Memorial Sloan-Kettering Cancer Center Experience. *Cancer* 2002;95:1728–1734.
29. Smith J, Heelan RT, Huvos AG. Radiographic changes in primary osteogenic sarcoma following intensive chemotherapy. *Radiology* 1982;143:355–360.
30. Chuang VP, Benjamin R, Jaffe N, et al. Radiographic and angiographic changes in osteosarcoma after intraarterial chemotherapy. *Am J Radiol* 1982;139:1065–1069.
31. Parmar DN, Luthert PJ, Cree IA, et al. Two unusual osteogenic orbital tumors: presumed parosteal osteosarcomas of the orbit. *Ophthalmology* 2001;108:1452–1456.
32. Edeiken J, Farrel C, Ackerman LV, et al. Parosteal sarcoma. *AJR Am J Roentgenol* 1971;111:579–583.
33. Okada K, Frassica FJ, Sim FH, et al. Parosteal osteosarcoma: a clinicopathological study. *J Bone Joint Surg Am* 1994;76:366–378.
34. Kumar R, Moser RP, Madewell JE, et al. Parosteal osteogenic sarcoma arising in cranial bones. Clinical and radiologic features in eight patients. *Am J Radiol* 1990;155:113–117.
35. Jepson CN, Wetzig PC. Pure chondroma of the trochlea. A case report. *Surv Ophthalmol* 1966;11:656–659.
36. Henderson JW, Farrow GM. *Orbital Tumors*. 2nd ed. New York: BC Decker (Thieme-Stratton); 1980:198–247.
37. Cianfriglia F, Pompili A, Occhipinti E. Intracranial malignant cartilaginous tumors. Report of two cases and review of literature. *Acta Neurochir* 1978;45:163–175.
38. Saito K, Unni KK, Wollan PC, et al. Chondrosarcoma of the jaw and facial bones. *Cancer* 1995;76:1550–1558.
39. Fu YS, Perzin KH. Non-epithelial tumors of the nasal cavity, apranasal sinuses, and nasopharynx: a clinicopathologic study. III. Cartilaginous tumors (chondroma, chondrosarcoma). *Cancer* 1974;34:453–463.
40. Holland MG, Allen JH, Ichinose H. Chondrosarcoma of the orbit. *Trans Am Acad Ophthalmol Otolaryngol* 1961;65:898–905.
41. Rosenberg AE, Nielsen GP, Efrid JT, et al. Base of the skull chondrosarcomas. a clinicopathologic study of 130 cases [abstract]. *Mod Pathol* 1997;9:12.
42. Cardenas-Ramirez L, Albores-Saavedra J, de Buen S. Mesenchymal chondrosarcoma of the orbit. Report of the first case in orbital location. *Arch Ophthalmol* 1971;86:410–413.
43. Sevel D. Mesenchymal chondrosarcoma of the orbit. *Br J Ophthalmol* 1974;58:882–887.
44. Pepe AJ, Kuhlmann RF, Miller DB. Mesenchymal chondrosarcoma: a case report. *J Bone Joint Surg Am* 1977;59:256–258.
45. Huvos AG, Rosen G, Dabska M, et al. Mesenchymal chondrosarcoma. A clinicopathologic analysis of 35 patients with emphasis on treatment. *Cancer* 1983;51:1230–1237.
46. Nakashima Y, Unni KK, Shives TC, et al. Mesenchymal chondrosarcoma of bone and soft tissue. A review of 111 cases. *Cancer* 1986;57:2444–2453.
47. Vencio EF, Reeve CM, Unni KK, et al. Mesenchymal chondrosarcoma of the jaw bones: clinicopathologic study of 19 cases. *Cancer* 1998;82:2350–2355.

48. Kaplan RP, Wang JT, Amron DM, et al. Maffucci's syndrome: two case reports with a literature review. *J Am Acad Dermatol* 1993;29:894–899.
49. Ramina R, Neto MC, Meneses MS, et al. Maffucci's syndrome associated with a cranial base chondrosarcoma: case report and literature review. *Neurosurgery* 1997;41:269–272.
50. Delaey JJ, DeSchryver A, Kluyskens P, et al. Orbital involvement in Ollier's disease (multiple enchondromatosis). *Int Ophthalmol* 1982;5:149–154.
51. Trikha V, Gupta V, Kumar R. Ollier's disease: characteristic Tc-99m MDP scan features. *Clin Nucl Med* 2003;28:56–57.
52. Clifton AG, Kendall BE, Crockard HA, et al. Intracranial chondrosarcoma in a patient with Ollier's disease. *Br J Radiol* 1991; 64:633–636.
53. Traflet RF, Barbaria AR, Barolat G, et al. Intracranial chondroma in a patient with Ollier's disease. *J Neurosurg* 1989;70: 274–276.
54. Albregts AE, Rapini RP. Malignancy in Maffucci's syndrome. *Dermatol Clin* 1995;13:73–78.
55. Johnson TE, Nasr AM, Nalbandian RM, et al. Enchondromatosis and hemangioma (Maffucci's syndrome) with orbital involvement. *Am J Ophthalmol* 1990;110:153–159.
56. Balcer LJ, Galetta SL, Cornblath WT, et al. Neuro-ophthalmic manifestations of Maffucci syndrome and Ollier disease. *J Neuro-Ophthalmol* 1999;19:62–66.
57. Jaffe T, Castillo M, Naidich TP, et al. Facies to remember: fibrous dysplasia. *Int J Neuro-Radiol* 1997;4:112–120.
58. Marie PJ, Pollack C, de Chanson P, et al. Increased proliferation of osteoblastic cells expressing the activating Gs alpha mutation in monostotic and polyostotic fibrous dysplasia. *Am J Pathol* 1997;150:1059–1069.
59. Albright F, Butler AM, Hampton AO, et al. Syndrome characterized by osteitis fibrosa disseminata, areas of pigmentation and endocrine dysfunction with precocious puberty in females. *N Engl J Med* 1937;216:727.
60. Daffner RH, Kirks DR, Gehweiler JA Jr, et al. Computed tomography of fibrous dysplasia. *Am J Radiol* 1983;139:943–948.
61. Mohammadi-Araghi H, Haery C. Fibro-osseous lesions of craniofacial bones: the role of imaging. *Radiol Clin North Amer* 1993;31:121–134.
62. Moore AT, Buncic JR, Munro IR. Fibrous dysplasia of the orbit in childhood. Clinical features and management. *Ophthalmology* 1985;92:12–20.
63. Katz BJ, Nerad JA. Ophthalmic manifestations of fibrous dysplasia: a disease of children and adults. *Ophthalmology* 1998;105:2207–2215.
64. Melen O, Weinberg PE, Kim KS, et al. Fibrous dysplasia of bone with acute visual loss. *Ann Ophthalmol* 1980;12:734–739.
65. Ronner HJ, Trokel SL, Hilal SK. Acute blindness in a patient with fibrous dysplasia. *Orbit* 1982;1:231–234.
66. Horgan MA, Delashaw JB, Dailey RA. Bilateral proptosis: an unusual presentation of fibrous dysplasia. *Br J Neurosurg* 1999;13:335–337.
67. Moore RT. Fibrous dysplasia of the orbit. *Surv Ophthalmol* 1969;13:321–334.
68. Sharma RR, Mahapatra AK, Pawar SJ, et al. Symptomatic cranial fibrous dysplasias: clinicoradiological analysis in a series of eight operative cases with follow-up results. *J Clin Neurosci* 2002;9:381–390.
69. Faul S, Link J, Behrendt S, et al. MRI features of craniofacial fibrous dysplasia. *Orbit* 1998;17:125–132.
70. Casselman JE, Dejonge T, Neyt L, et al. MRI in craniofacial fibrous dysplasia. *Neuroradiology* 1993;35:234–237.
71. Ricalde P, Horswell BB. Craniofacial fibrous dysplasia of the fronto-orbital region: a case series and literature review. *J Oral Maxillofac Surg* 2001;59:157–167.
72. Liakos GM, Walker CB, Carruth JAS. Ocular complications in craniofacial fibrous dysplasia. *Br J Ophthalmol* 1979;63: 611–616.
73. Margo CE, Ragsdale BD, Perman KI, et al. Psammomatoid (juvenile) ossifying fibroma of the orbit. *Ophthalmology* 1985; 92:150–159.
74. Vandekerchkove K, van den Abeele K, van den Broecke C, et al. Psammamatoid ossifying fibroma of the ethmoid. *Bull Soc Belge Ophtalmol* 2003;287:9–14.
75. Shields JA, Nelson LB, Brown JF, et al. Clinical, computed tomographic, and histopathologic characteristics of juvenile ossifying fibroma with orbital involvement. *Am J Ophthalmol* 1983;96:650–653.
76. Shields JA, Peyster RG, Handler SD, et al. Massive juvenile ossifying fibroma of maxillary sinus with orbital involvement. *Br J Ophthalmol* 1985;69:392–395.
77. Shand JM, Heggie AA, Radden BG, et al. Juvenile ossifying fibroma of the midface. *J Craniofac Surg* 1999;10:442–446.
78. Mavel JB, Marsh MA, Catlin FI. Ossifying fibroma of the midface and paranasal sinuses: diagnostic and therapeutic considerations. *Otolaryngol Head Neck Surg* 1991;104:803–808.
79. Pensak ML, Nestok BR, Van Loveren H, et al. Desmoplastic fibroma of the temporal bone. *Am J Otol* 1997;18:627–631.
80. Selfa-Morena S, Arana-Fernandez E, Fernandez-Latorre F, et al. Desmoplastic fibroma of the skull. Case report. *J Neurosurg* 1995;82:119–120.
81. Bertoni F, Unni KK, Beabout JW. Giant cell tumor of the skull. *Cancer* 1992;70:1124–1132.
82. Watkins LD, Uttley D, Archer DJ, et al. Giant cell tumors of the sphenoid bone. *Neurosurgery* 1992;30:576–581.
83. Wolfe JT 3rd, Scheithauer BW, Dahlin DC. Giant-cell tumor of the sphenoid bone. Review of 10 cases. *J Neurosurg* 1983;59:322–327.
84. Hoopes FC, Anderson RL, Blodi FC. Giant cell (reparative) granuloma of the orbit. *Ophthalmology* 1981;88:1361–1366.
85. Waldron CA, Shafer WG. The central giant cell reparative granuloma of the jaws. An analysis of 38 cases. *Am J Clin Pathol* 1966;45:437–447.
86. Hirschl S, Katz A. Giant cell reparative granuloma outside the jaw bone. Diagnostic criteria and review of the literature with the first case described in the temporal bone. *Hum Pathol* 1974;5:171–181.
87. Som PM, Lawson W, Cohen BA. Giant-cell lesions of the facial bones. *Radiology* 1983;147:129–134.
88. Naiman J, Green WR, d'Heurle D, et al. Brown tumor of the orbit associated with primary hyperparathyroidism. *Am J Ophthalmol* 1980;90:565–571.
89. Scully RE, Mark EJ, McNeely BU. Case records of the Massachusetts General Hospital. Weekly clinicopathologic exercises. Case 10-1984. *N Engl J Med* 1984;310:642–648.
90. Dahlin DC. Giant cell tumor of bone: highlights of 407 cases. *AJR Am J Roentgenol* 1985;144:955–960.
91. Rock MG, Pritchard DJ, Unni KK. Metastases from histologically benign giant-cell tumor of bone. *J Bone Joint Surg Am* 1984;66:269–274.
92. Tubbs WS, Brown LR, Beabut JW, et al. Benign giant-cell tumor of bone with pulmonary metastases: Clinical findings and radiologic appearance of metastases in 13 cases. *AJR Am J Roentgenol* 1992;158:331–334.
93. deSantos LA, Murray JA. Evaluation of giant-cell tumor by computerized tomography. *Skeletal Radiol* 1978;2:205–212); Yaghamai I. *Angiography of Bone and Soft Tissue Lesions.* New York: Springer-Verlag; 1979.
94. Herman SC, Mesgarzadeh M, Bonafdarpour A, et al. The role of magnetic resonance imaging in giant cell tumor of bone. *Skeletal Radiol* 1987;16:635–643.
95. Vernet O, Ducrey N, Deruaz JP, et al. Giant cell tumor of the orbit. *Neurosurgery* 1993;32:848–851.

96. Hoopes PC, Anderson RL, Blodi FC. Giant cell (reparative) granuloma of the orbit. *Ophthalmology* 1981;88:1361–1366.
97. Schajowica F. Bone-forming tumors. In: *Tumors and Tumor-like Lesions of Bone. Pathology, Radiology and Treatment.* New York: Springer-Verlag, 1994:30–35
98. Fu YS, Perzin KH. Non-epithelial tumors of the nasal cavity, paranasal sinuses, and nasopharynx. A clinicopathologic study. II. Osseous and fibro-osseous lesions, including osteoma, fibrous dysplasia, ossifying fibroma, osteoblastoma, giant cell tumor, and osteosarcoma. *Cancer* 1974;33:1289–1305.
99. Abdalla MI, Hosni F. Osteoblastoma of the orbit. *Br J Ophthalmol* 1966;50:95–98.
100. Matsumura S, Murakami S, Kakimoto N, et al. Histopathologic and radiographic findings of the simple bone cyst. *Oral Surg Oral Med Oral Pathol Oral Radiol Endosc* 1998;85:619–625.
101. Kransdorf MJ, Sweet DE. Aneurysmal bone cyst: concept, controversy, clinical presentation and imaging. *Am J Radiol* 1995;164:573–580.
102. Vergel De Dios AM, Bond JR, Shives TC, et al. Aneurysmal bone cyst. A clinicopathologic study of 238 cases. *Cancer* 1992;69:2921–2931.
103. Ronner HJ, Jones IS. Aneurysmal bone cyst of the orbit: a review. *Ann Ophthalmol* 1983;15:626–629.
104. Hunter JV, Yokoyama C, Moseley IF, et al. Aneurysmal bone cyst of the sphenoid with orbital involvement [review]. *Br J Ophthalmol* 1990;74:505–508.
105. Fite JD, Schwartz JF, Calhoun FP. Aneurysmal bone cyst of the orbit. A clinicopathologic case report. *Trans Am Acad Ophthalmol Otolaryngol* 1968;72:614–618.
106. Yee RD, Cogan DG, Thorp R, et al. Optic nerve compression due to aneurysmal bone cyst. *Arch Ophthalmol* 1977;95:2176–2179.
107. Bertoni F, Bacchini P, Capanna R, et al. Solid variant of aneurysmal bone cyst. *Cancer* 1993;71:729–734.
108. Dehner LP, Sibley RK, Sauk JJ Jr, et al. Malignant melanotic neuroectodermal tumor of infancy: a clinical, pathologic ultrastructural and tissue culture study. *Cancer* 1979;43:1389–1410.

17

Peripheral Nerve Tumors

Kaan Gündüz

Peripheral nerve tumors of the orbit arise from cranial nerves III, IV, V, and VI and the ciliary ganglion. These peripheral nerves, in contrast to the optic nerve, are ensheathed by Schwann cells. Some of these tumors may originate from neural or neuroganglionic tissues in the orbit as well. The peripheral nerve tumors covered in this chapter are schwannoma, neurofibroma, malignant peripheral nerve sheath tumor (MPNST), granular cell tumor, alveolar soft part sarcoma (ASPS), paraganglioma, amputation neuroma, melanotic neuroectodermal tumor of infancy, primary orbital neuroblastoma, and primary orbital carcinoid.

Table 17.1 shows the frequencies of various orbital peripheral nerve tumors cited in five major reviews on histopathologically proven orbital tumors from different geographical locations.[1–5] Peripheral nerve tumors of the orbit are rare, accounting for 1.4 to 5.3% of all orbital tumors (Table 17.1). The most common peripheral nerve tumors of the orbit are schwannoma and neurofibroma. Since these tumors have an association with neurofibromatosis, this phakomatosis is also discussed at the end of the chapter.

SCHWANNOMA (NEURILEMOMA)

Schwannoma (neurilemoma) is a benign peripheral nerve tumor of the orbit. It accounts for 0.7 to 2.3% of all histopathologically proven orbital tumors (Table 17.1).[1–5] Since it has been recognized that the tumor consists primarily of Schwann cells, *schwannoma* has been the preferred term. Schwannoma generally occurs as an isolated tumor. However, in 2 to 18% of the cases, it is associated with neurofibromatosis.[6]

Clinical Features

Orbital schwannoma usually arises from the sensory branches of the ophthalmic division of the trigeminal nerve. The supraorbital and supratrochlear nerves are more commonly affected than the infraorbital nerve. Less commonly, schwannoma may develop from one of the motor nerves including the oculomotor and ciliary nerves.[7,8]

Orbital schwannoma generally occurs in young to middle-aged adults. It presents as a well-circumscribed mass located in an intraconal or extraconal position, sometimes producing proptosis (Figures 17.1A, 17.2A, 17.3A).[9–11] When schwannoma develops from the supraorbital and supratrochlear nerves, it may produce downward displacement of the globe.[9–11] When the tumor arises from the infraorbital nerve, it may produce upward displacement of the globe. The patient may complain of pain.[9–11]

Orbital schwannoma can demonstrate invasion into the cavernous sinus through the superior orbital fissure.[12] Conversely, schwannoma arising from the cavernous sinus may show invasion into the orbit through the superior orbital fissure, simulating a primary orbital tumor.[10] Rarely, orbital schwannoma can present as an intramuscular[13] or epibulbar tumor.[14]

Radiologic Features

Orbital schwannomas display low internal reflectivity and acoustic hollowness on A- and B-scan orbital ultrasonography, respectively.[15] On computed tomography (CT), orbital schwannoma is seen as a round to oval well-circumscribed mass.[16] Schwannoma usually occurs in the superior orbit and does not involve the orbital apex.[7,16] However, 24% of orbital schwannomas demonstrate enlargement of the superior orbital fissure and invasion into the cavernous sinus on CT.[8,16]

Magnetic resonance imaging (MRI) shows that schwannoma is isointense with respect to the extraocular muscle and cerebral gray matter on T1-weighted images (Figures 17.1B, 17.2B, 17.3B), is hyperintense on T2-weighted images (Figures 17.1D, 17.2D, 17.3C), and shows moderate contrast enhancement (Figure 17.2C).[9,17,17a] The tumor may display heterogeneous signal changes on T2-weighted images corresponding to the myxoid changes in the tumor (Figure 17.2D). The myxoid regions of the tumor (Antoni B pattern) with their greater water content demonstrate a higher signal intensity on T2-weighted images than the more cellular (Antoni A pattern) regions of the tumor.[17a] The myxoid regions of the tumor demonstrate greater contrast enhancement than the cellular regions.[9] Schwannoma can undergo necrosis and present with a cavitary appearance on MRI (Figure 17.1C). Under these circumstances, cavitary schwannoma can be confused with a cystic

TABLE 17.1. Frequency of Various Peripheral Nerve Tumors of the Orbit.

Author	*No. of cases*	*Schwannoma*	*Neurofibroma*	*MPNST*	*Granular cell tumor*	*Amputation neuroma*	*ASPS*	*Paraganglioma*
Shields et al.[1]	645	5 (0.8%)	5 (0.8%)	—	—	3 (0.5%)	1 (0.2%)	—
Sen[5]	266	6 (2.3%)	8 (3.0%)	—	—	—	—	—
Günalp and Gündüz[3]	1092	8 (0.7%)	4 (0.4%)	2 (0.2%)	—	1 (0.1%)	—	1 (0.1%)
Henderson et al.[2]	1376	15 (1.1%)	35 (2.5%)	2 (0.1%)	—	—	—	—
Seregard and Sohlin[4]	300	5 (1.7%)	4 (1.3%)		1 (0.3%)			

orbital tumor.[17a,18,19] Other orbital tumors that exhibit cavitary appearance on MRI include inflammatory lesions, adenoid cystic carcinoma, cavernous hemangioma, lymphangioma, and rhabdomyosarcoma.[20]

Morphologic Features

Grossly, schwannoma is yellow-gray, with a well-circumscribed appearance (Figure 17.3D). The nerve of origin is identifiable in about 32[8] to 47%[7] of orbital schwannomas. Results of the histopathologic examination show that the encapsulated tumors are composed of cells with eosinophilic cytoplasm having indistinct cellular borders and oval nuclei.[7,11] The nuclei either form solid structures (Antoni A pattern) or are arranged in a loose myxomatous background (Antoni B pattern) (Figures 17.1E, 17.2E, 17.3E). In the Antoni A pattern, the nuclei form palisading and occasional tangles of fibrillary processes called Verocay bodies (Figure 17.3E).[7,11] The demonstration of Verocay bodies is important in the diagnosis of schwannoma.

Schwannoma shows positive immunoreactivity with S-100.[14] This immunohistochemical staining is not specific for schwannoma; neurofibroma also demonstrates positive but weaker immunoreactivity for S-100. Transmission electron microscopy performed on fresh tumor tissue reveals extracellular long-spacing collagen (Luse bodies) in schwannoma.[7,12]

Rarely, a schwannoma demonstrates increased cellularity, nuclear pleomorphism and hyperchromatism

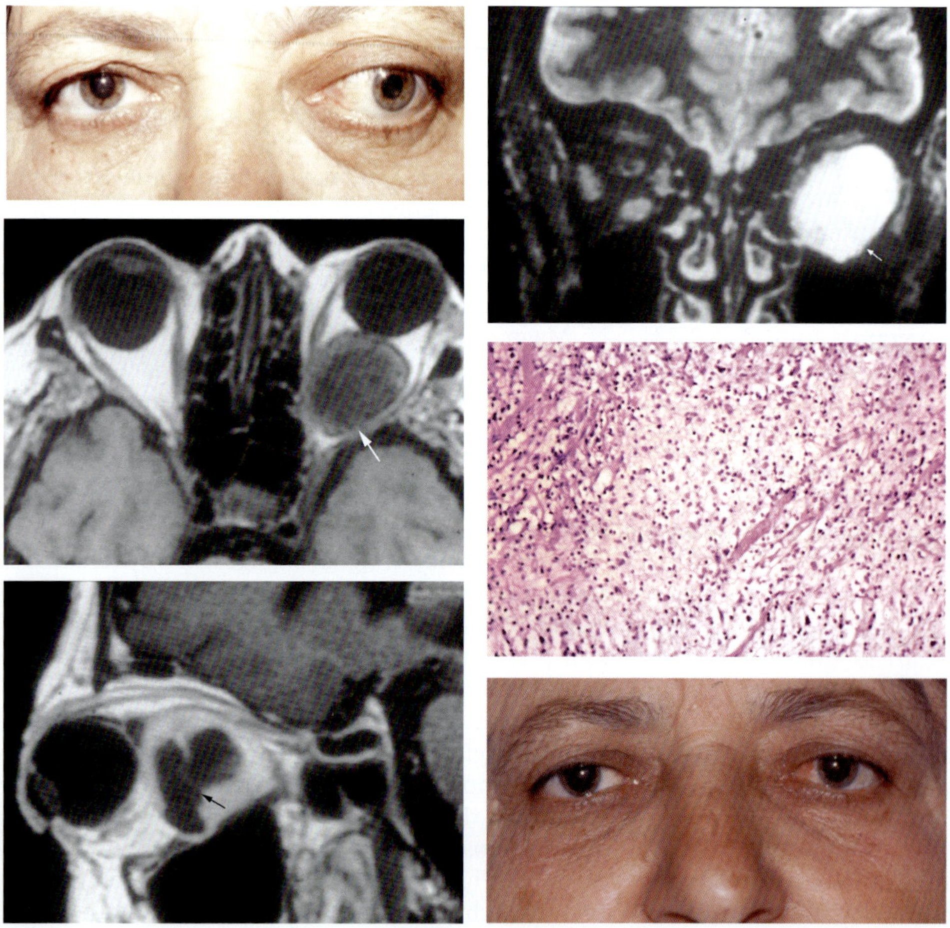

A B C D E F

FIGURE 17.1. A 56-year-old woman with left orbital schwannoma. (A) Preoperative facial photograph showing left proptosis with inferotemporal displacement of the globe. (B) T1-weighted axial MR image showing the oval intraconal schwannoma isointense to the extraocular muscle and cerebral gray matter (arrow). (C) T1-weighted sagittal MRI demonstrating the intraconal schwannoma with central cavitary changes (arrow). (D) T2-weighted coronal MR image demonstrating the intraconal schwannoma hyperintense to the extraocular muscle and cerebral gray matter (arrow). (E) Histopathologic examination shows that the tumor is composed predominantly of Antoni B pattern with some Antoni A areas [hematoxylin–eosin (H&E), original magnification ×200). (F) Postoperative facial photograph 2 years after anterior orbitotomy with inferotemporal orbital rim approach. There is no proptosis of the left eye.

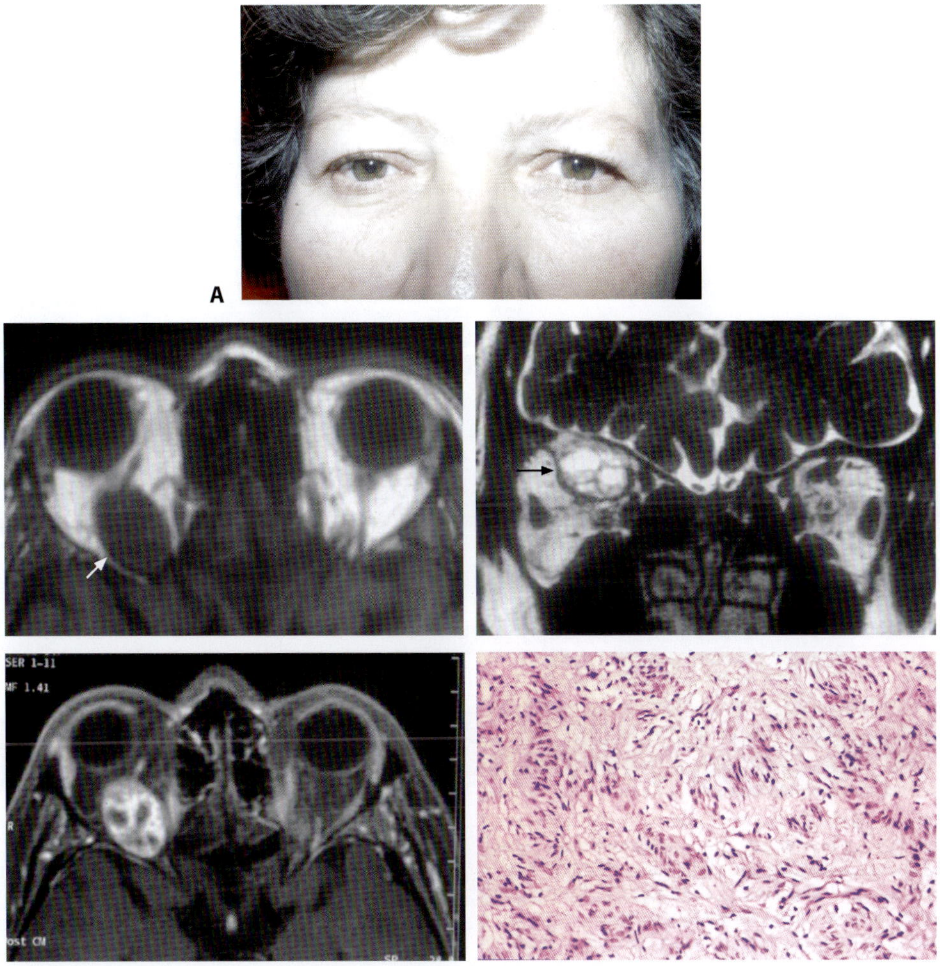

FIGURE 17.2. A 43-year-old woman with right orbital schwannoma. (A) Preoperative facial photograph of the patient with 2 mm proptosis of the right eye. (B) T1-weighted axial MR image showing the fusiform schwannoma isointense to the extraocular muscle and cerebral gray matter (arrow). (C) T2-weighted axial MR image showing the schwannoma hyperintense to the extraocular muscle and cerebral gray matter. Antoni B portions demonstrate a higher signal intensity due to increased water content (arrow). (D) T1-weighted coronal MR image demonstrating the superiorly located schwannoma with marked enhancement after contrast injection (arrow). (E) Histopathologic examination demonstrates that the tumor is composed of Antoni A and B patterns (H&E, original magnification ×200).

in the absence of mitotic figures, creating confusion because of resemblance to a malignant tumor. Such tumors have been pathologically designated as ancient schwannoma.[21]

Management and Prognosis

The treatment of orbital schwannoma is total excision. Most of the tumors are managed surgically by means of either an anterior or superolateral orbitotomy (Figures 17.1A, F). A Krönlein orbitotomy may be necessary in selected intraconal and superiorly located tumors to ensure total removal of thc tumor. In the series of Rose and Wright, complete tumor excision was achieved in 72% of the patients with orbital schwannoma.[8] Postoperatively, a sensory deficit in the skin occurs in 32% of patients with orbital schwannoma.[8]

Although orbital schwannoma is benign, total excision is advised to prevent recurrence and the rare malignant transformation. In the series of Rose and Wright, no recurrence was noted after incomplete excision of six orbital schwannomas at a median follow-up of 2.8 years.[8] Rootman and associates similarly reported no recurrence after incomplete excision of orbital schwannomas.[7] However, long-term follow-up is necessary. Late recurrence and malignant transformation of an incompletely excised benign schwannoma generally occur in the presence of neurofibromatosis.[6]

NEUROFIBROMA

Neurofibroma is probably the most frequent peripheral nerve tumor of the orbit. It accounts for 0.8 to 3.0% of all histopathologically proven orbital lesions (Table 17.1).[1–5] Orbital neurofibroma is classified into three subsets: plexiform, diffuse, and localized. In the

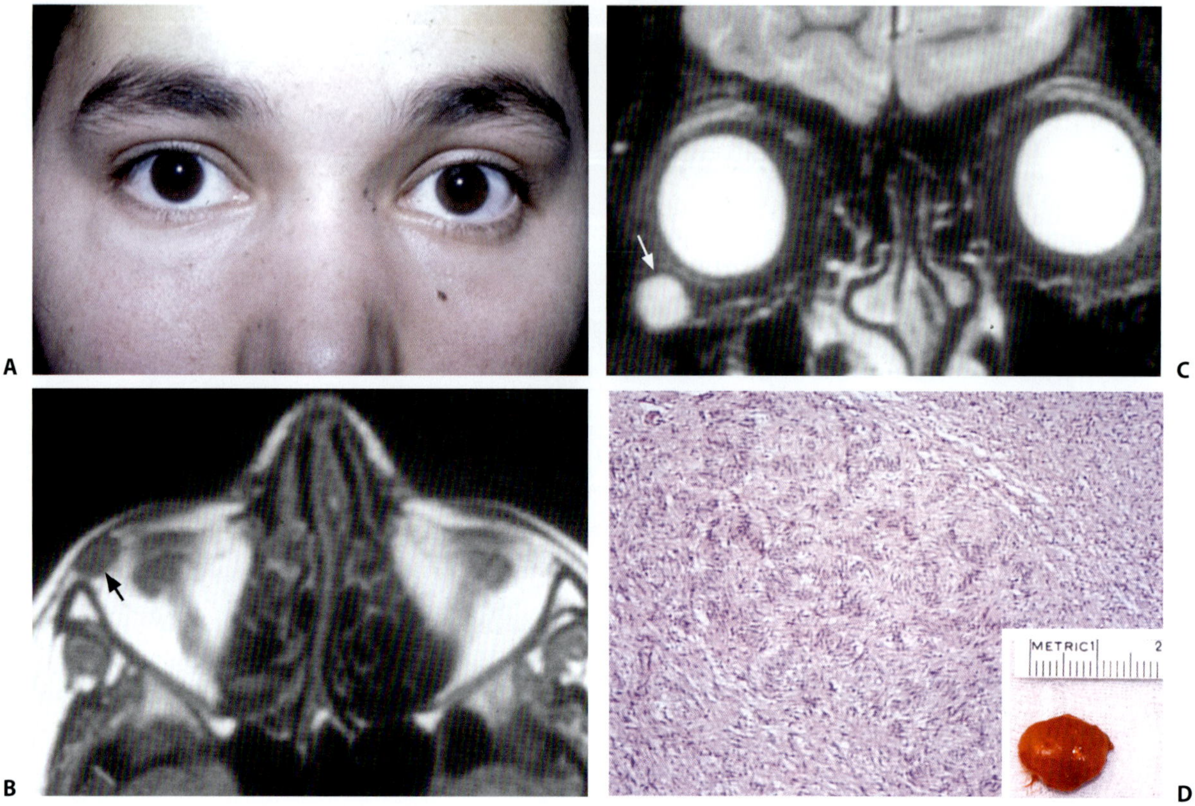

FIGURE 17.3. An 18-year-old woman with right orbital schwannoma. (A) Preoperative facial photograph showing the orbital mass producing swelling of the eyelid along the right inferotemporal orbital rim. (B) T1-weighted axial MR image showing the round extraconal schwannoma isointense to the cerebral gray matter (arrow). (C) T2-weighted coronal MR image showing the extraconal schwannoma hyperintense to the cerebral gray matter (arrow). (D) Histopathologic examination shows that the tumor is composed primarily of Antoni A pattern with palisading of the nuclei (H&E, original magnification, ×40). *Inset*: Gross photograph of the excised tumor showing a gray-colored well-circumscribed mass.

periorbital region, the diffuse type is less common than the plexiform and localized types. The characteristics of plexiform and diffuse neurofibromas are similar.

The plexiform neurofibroma is considered to be pathognomonic of neurofibromatosis.[22,23] Virtually all patients with plexiform neurofibroma have neurofibromatosis. However, only 5% of the patients with neurofibromatosis develop plexiform orbital neurofibroma.[22] The diffuse type has a more variable association with neurofibromatosis than the plexiform type. The localized type is only seldom associated with neurofibromatosis.[11]

Clinical Features

The clinical features vary with the type of neurofibroma (i.e., whether it is plexiform, localized, or diffuse). The plexiform neurofibroma generally becomes clinically apparent in the first decade of life in a patient who characteristically has signs of neurofibromatosis (Figure 17.4A, C).[24] Involvement of the eyelids is seen in approximately 66% of the patients with plexiform neurofibroma.[25] The plexiform neurofibroma generally begins as an eyelid mass. As the tumor grows, the hypertrophy of the eyelid becomes more localized to its lateral third, giving the eyelid an S-shaped appearance (Figure 17.4A). In time, the tumor extends into the orbit, leading to proptosis.[25]

The localized orbital neurofibroma behaves like many other solitary well-circumscribed soft tissue tumors in the orbit.[26,27] The localized orbital neurofibroma presents at a later age than the plexiform type. The typical patient is a young or middle-aged adult (Figure 17.5A).[26,27] Clinical features include proptosis and downward displacement of the globe owing to the preferential location of the tumor in the superior orbit (Figure 17.5B).[26] The inferior orbit can also be affected.[27] Isolated neurofibroma can occur in the lacrimal gland region, simulating a lacrimal gland tumor.[28] It can also develop in an extraocular muscle.[17] Long-standing orbital neurofibroma can also demonstrate bone destruction and invasion into the adjacent sinus.[27]

There have been several reports demonstrating the occurrence of multiple isolated neurofibromas in patients with and without clinical signs of neurofibromatosis.[28] The presence of multiple well-circumscribed orbital tumors, especially in association with pain, should raise the suspicion for the diagnosis of neurofibroma in a patient.[28]

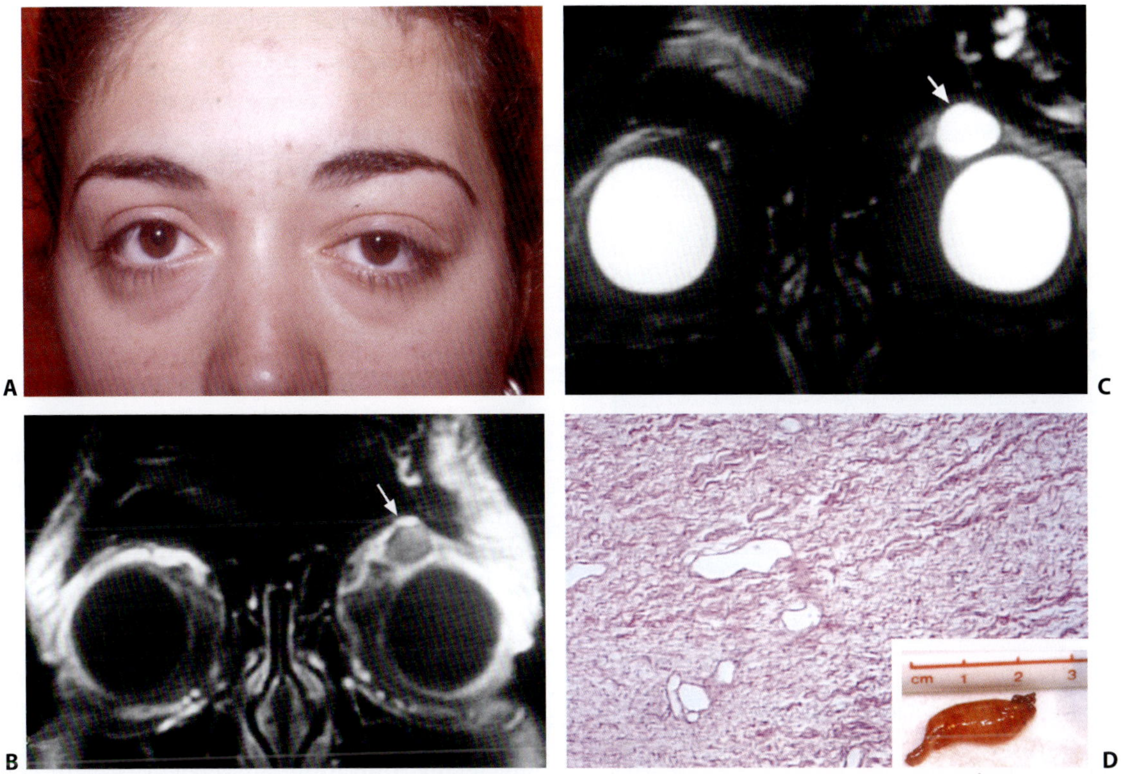

FIGURE 17.4. A 21-year-old woman with left isolated neurofibroma in the left orbit. (A) Preoperative facial photograph demonstrating 1 mm of upper eyelid ptosis and edema. (B) Coronal T1-weighted MRI demonstrating superiorly located isolated neurofibroma isointense to the extraocular muscle and cerebral gray matter (white arrow). (C) Coronal T2-weighted MRI showing the isolated neurofibroma hyperintense the extraocular muscle and cerebral gray matter (arrow). (D) Histopathologic examination demonstrates that the isolated neurofibroma is composed of interwoven bundles of axons, Schwann cells, and endoneural fibroblasts within a mucoid matrix (H&E, original magnification ×200). *Inset*: Gross photograph of the excised lesion demonstrating the isolated neurofibroma and the peripheral nerve from which it originated.

The diffuse orbital neurofibroma seems to represent a lesion closely simulating the plexiform type. Age at onset parallels that of the plexiform variety. The affected patient generally presents with unilateral proptosis with or without involvement of the eyelids.

Radiologic Features

In localized neurofibromas, orbital CT reveals a well-circumscribed ovoid mass generally in the superior orbit and less commonly in the inferior orbit. The tumor generally occupies an extraconal position and does not involve the orbital apex. Localized neurofibroma can demonstrate extension into the superior orbital fissure in 33% of the cases.[8] Magnetic resonance imaging demonstrates that the tumor is isointense with respect to the extraocular muscle and cerebral gray matter on T1-weighted images (Figure 17.5B) and hyperintense on T2-weighted images (Figure 17.5C). The tumor shows moderate contrast enhancement.

In plexiform and diffuse orbital neurofibromas, orbital CT and MRI demonstrate an ill-defined oblong or diffuse soft tissue mass, sometimes filling the entire orbit. The MRI features with respect to internal features are similar to those of the isolated neurofibroma (Figure 17.4B).

Morphologic Features

On gross examination, the localized orbital neurofibroma appears as a well-defined yellow or white lesion (Figure 17.5D). The lesion usually has a capsule. The surgical specimen of an isolated orbital neurofibroma often includes a piece of the nerve from which the tumor arises (inset, Figure 17.5D). In the series of Rose and Wright, the nerve of origin was evident in 63% of neurofibromas.[8] The diffuse or plexiform neurofibromas appear ill-defined on gross examination.

Microscopically, localized neurofibromas are composed of interwoven bundles of axons, Schwann cells, and endoneural fibroblasts within a mucoid matrix (Figure 17.5D).[25] The plexiform orbital neurofibroma is characterized additionally by the presence of a well-demarcated cellular perineurium defining individual tumor cords or fascicles (Figure 17.4D). Diffuse orbital neurofibroma differs from plexiform orbital neurofibroma in its extension beyond the confines of the perineurium.[25]

Immunohistochemical stains for S-100 protein may be positive. However, neurofibroma stains less intensely with S-100 protein than to schwannoma.[25]

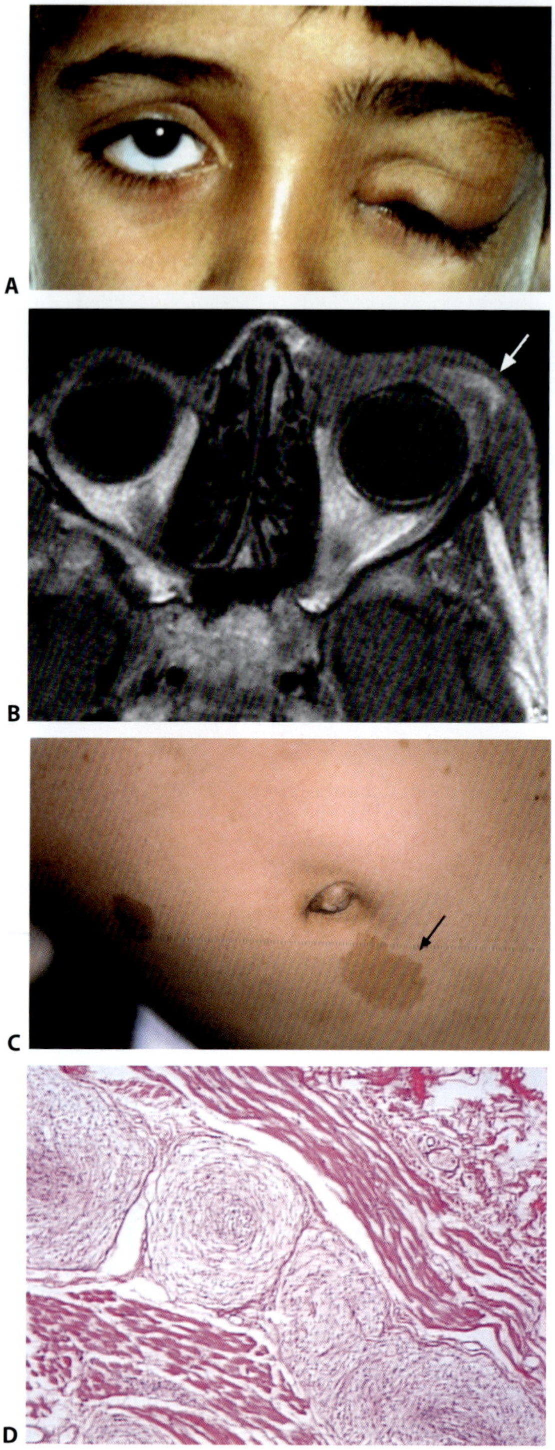

FIGURE 17.5. A 6-year-old girl with neurofibromatosis having plexiform neurofibroma of the left upper eyelid. (A) Facial photograph demonstrating the S-shaped ptosis of the left upper eyelid. (B) Axial T1-weighted MR image demonstrating plexiform neurofibroma isointense to the extraocular muscle and cerebral gray matter (arrow). (C) Café-au-lait spot in the umbilical area of the patient (arrow). (D) Histopathologic examination of the tumor shows intertwining bundles of enlarged nerves in a connective tissue mass. The perineurium separates individual tumor cords or fascicles (H&E, original magnification ×40).

Management and Prognosis

The management of localized orbital neurofibroma consists of total excision. Postoperatively, a sensory skin deficit was present in 72% of the patients with an isolated orbital neurofibroma.[8] These tumors can usually be dissected free from the surrounding orbital contents. In the series of Rose and Wright, complete tumor excision was possible in 46% of the patients with isolated orbital neurofibroma.[8] Incompletely excised tumors are not at particular risk for recurrence. No recurrence has been reported at a median follow-up of 6 years after incomplete excision of 11 cases of isolated orbital neurofibroma.[8]

The management of plexiform and diffuse orbital neurofibroma presents a much more complex problem. Eyelid sparing orbital exenteration and orbital reconstruction may be the best treatment approach in the presence of total eyelid ptosis and severe visual loss.[29] The diffuse infiltrating nature of this tumor makes complete surgical removal difficult. Surgical removal of large tumors with intracranial invasion and the management of associated sphenoidal, orbital, and facial bone dysplasia requires a team approach of physicians from different specialties.[25] In contrast to the isolated neurofibroma, the plexiform and diffuse tumors may show recurrence after incomplete excision. Recurrent tumors may develop invasion into the cranial cavity, causing death. In patients with neurofibromatosis, malignant transformation of the cutaneous neurofibroma into neurofibrosarcoma occurs in about 10 to 29% of the cases.[29] The incidence of malignant transformation in orbital neurofibroma is probably lower. Recurrence and malignant transformation may complicate the course of an incompletely excised orbital plexiform neurofibroma. Therefore, these patients should be followed closely.

MALIGNANT PERIPHERAL NERVE SHEATH TUMOR

Malignant peripheral nerve sheath tumor is a very rare tumor in the orbit. The frequency in different histopathologically proven orbital tumor series ranges from 0 to 0.2% (Table 17.1).[1–5] MPNST usually arises de novo in the orbit, although it may also arise from a neurofibroma or schwannoma. Schwann cell origin has not been demonstrated in all cases of MPNST; therefore, the term *malignant peripheral nerve sheath tumor* is preferred over *malignant schwannoma*, used earlier.

Clinical Features

MPNST usually occurs in adults.[30,31] However, it can occur rarely in children.[32] MPNST usually presents with rapidly progressive proptosis and displacement of the globe. The mass usually occurs in the superior orbit because of the tendency of this tumor to arise from the supraorbital and supratrochlear nerve.[30,31] However, MPNST can occur in other orbital locations (Figure 17.6A, B).[31] Unlike benign orbital peripheral nerve tumors, they are more likely to be accompanied by pain, ptosis, and signs of optic nerve compression, which reflect the rapidly progressive nature of this tumor.[30,31]

MPNST has a tendency to develop perineural spread, resulting in orbital recurrence and intracranial invasion. Orbital recurrence is usually associated with metastasis. Metastasis from orbital MPNST usually occurs to the regional lymph nodes and the lung.[30,31] Metastasis usually develops within the first 2 years after diagnosis.[30]

Malignant triton tumor is a sarcomatous variant of the MPNST showing areas of skeletal muscle differentiation. It can occur in the orbit. Triton tumor has a strong association with neurofibromatosis, is very aggressive in growth and has a high rate of metastasis.[33]

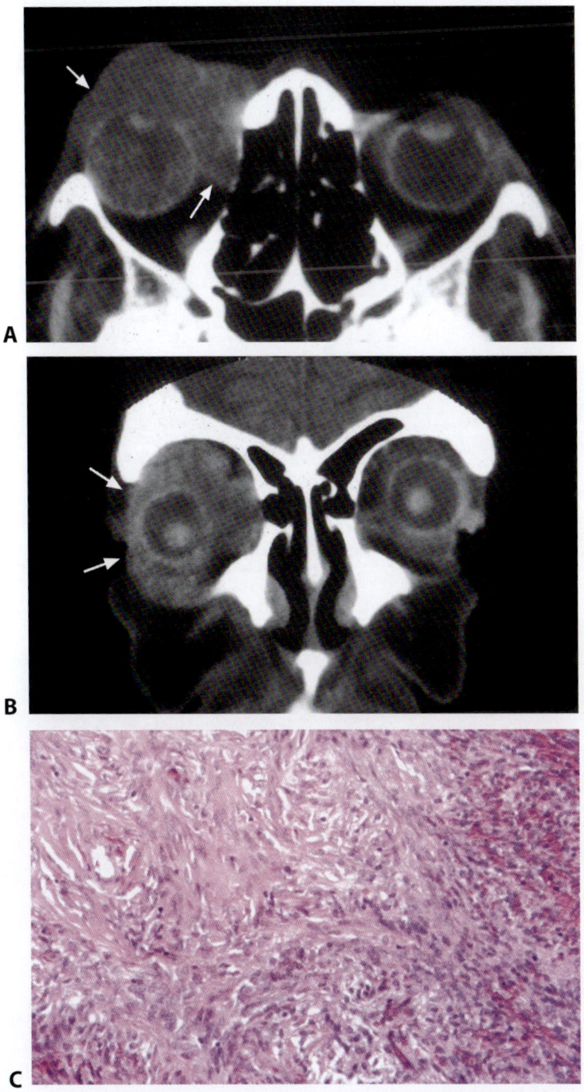

FIGURE 17.6. Malignant schwannoma in a 67-year-old patient. (A) Axial CT shows that the tumor occupies the anterior and middle orbit (arrows). (B) Coronal CT demonstrates that the malignant schwannoma occupies the superior and inferior orbit (arrows). (C) Histopathologic examination shows that malignant peripheral nerve sheath tumor is a highly cellular tumor composed of spindle cells with nuclear pleomorphism and hyperchromatism (H&E, original magnification ×200).

Radiologic Features

On CT, malignant peripheral nerve sheath tumors generally have ill-defined irregular borders. There may be adjacent bone invasion.[30,31]

Morphologic Features

Grossly, the MPNST is an ill-defined gray-white lesion with a nodular configuration. Pathologically, there is usually no capsule,[31] although in rare instances the tumor appears to be encapsulated.[32] The tumor is composed of spindle-shaped cells with nuclear pleomorphism, hyperchromatism, and mitotic figures (Figure 17.6C). Occasionally, epithelioid cells and multinucleated giant cells are present.[30,31] The nerve of origin in MPNST is evident in 50% of the cases.[8]

With S-100, MPNST shows positive immunoreactivity that is less uniform and focal than in schwannoma. Transmission electron microscopy demonstrates prominent nucleoli suggesting a malignant tumor. The presence of long-spacing extracellular collagen (Luse bodies) suggesting a Schwann cell origin has not been convincingly demonstrated in all MPNSTs.[30,31]

Management and Prognosis

Treatment of MPNST consists of total excision of the soft tissue tumor. Adjacent bone should be removed if there is bone invasion. The risk of metastasis increases if the patient develops orbital recurrence. Therefore, it is important to obtain clear margins at the time of initial surgery to reduce the risk of metastasis. If this is not possible or documentable, some authors have suggested an aggressive approach consisting of exenteration and radiotherapy (50–60 Gy).[30,31] Others recommend continued observation with serial neuroimaging studies after complete excision of the orbital tumor.[32] Chemotherapy has been used in patients with distant metastasis, but there is no substantial evidence that it is effective.[30,31]

The prognosis for survival in patients with MPNST of the orbit appears to be poor. In one series, 9 of 13 patients with orbital MPNST were deceased within 5 years after diagnosis.[31]

GRANULAR CELL TUMOR

Granular cell tumor commonly occurs in the skin, tongue, chest wall, and arms.[34] (In this chapter, the lesion is designated GCT, the acronym used elsewhere for giant cell tumor.) Rarely, the orbit can also be primarily affected by a GCT (Table 17.1).[35–38] Although 10 to 15% of patients with GCT may have lesions at multiple sites, orbital GCT usually occurs as a solitary lesion.[34] Orbital GCT can also be a metastatic deposit originating from a primary tumor elsewhere in the body.[39] Because GCT was presumed to be associated with striated muscle, it was referred to as *granular cell myoblastoma* in the older literature.[40]

The pathogenesis of GCT is still obscure. Possible cells of origin for this tumor include myoblast, histiocyte, astrocyte, or the Schwann cell. Based on the unequivocal staining with the S-100 protein, the most likely origin for the GCT is the Schwann cell.[36] It is possible that orbital GCT originates from branches of small peripheral nerves supplying the extraocular muscles.[41]

Clinical Features

Orbital GCT usually occurs in adult patients, although it can also occur in children.[36,41] The age range of the patients with orbital GCT at the time of diagnosis is between 3[41] and 74[36] years. However, the majority of the patients are 40 to 60 years old. There is no distinguishing feature for periorbital GCT. Most patients present with a slowly growing orbital or eyelid tumor resulting in proptosis, ptosis, or diplopia (Figure 17.7A).[35–38,42] The tumor is attached to the orbicularis or rectus muscle in about 25% of the cases.[36] Orbital GCT can lead to dilation of the epibulbar vessels in the quadrant(s) where the tumor is located.

A malignant variant of GCT with metastatic potential has been reported.[39] Primary malignant GCT is rare in the orbit. However, histopathologically benign orbital GCT can demonstrate invasion into the adjacent tissues.[37]

Radiologic Features

Computed tomography shows that orbital GCT can present as a well-circumscribed orbital mass (Figure 17.7B),[35,36,38] or as an ill-defined mass infiltrating the posterior orbit.[37] The tumor may be attached to an extraocular muscle. As such, orbital GCT is indistinguishable from other well-circumscribed or ill-defined orbital tumors in neuroimaging studies.[35–39]

Morphologic Features

The excised orbital GCT can be well circumscribed or ill defined. It is yellow-gray in color. The well-

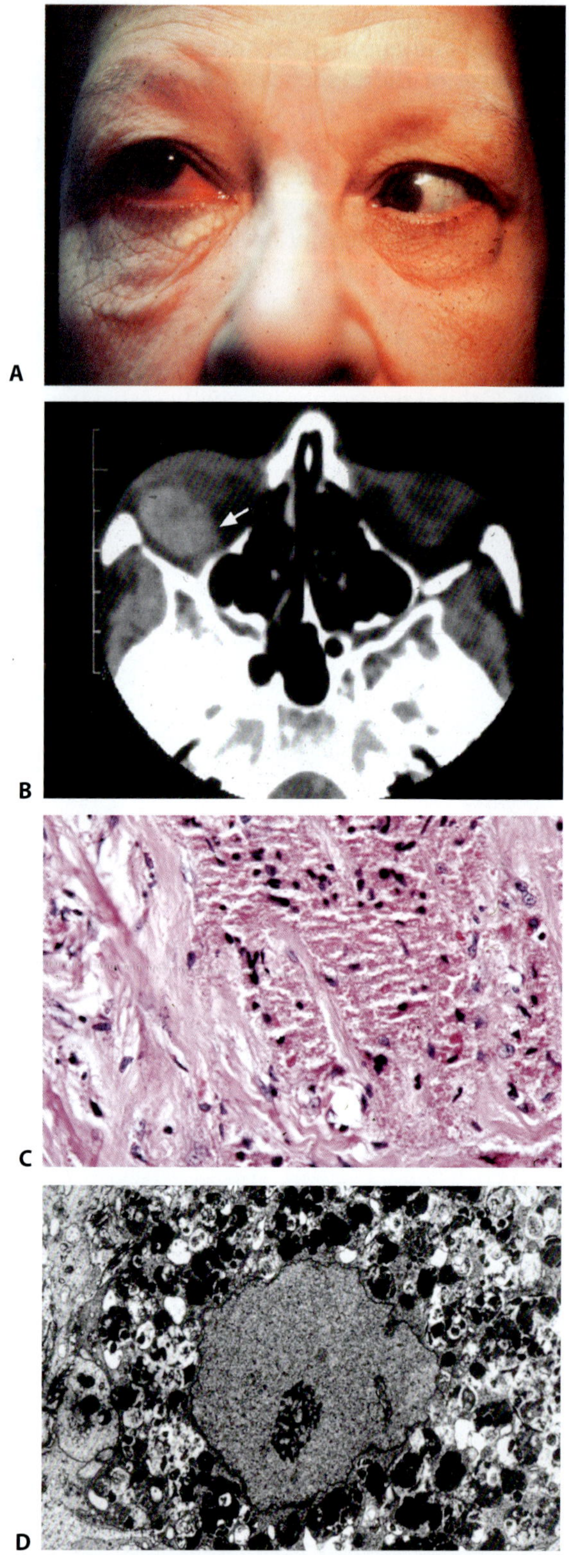

FIGURE 17.7. A 65-year-old woman with orbital granular cell tumor. (A) Facial photograph showing the motility restriction of the right eye in right gaze owing to the location of the tumor in the temporal orbit. (B) Axial CT showing the extraconally located orbital granular cell tumor in close association with the lateral rectus muscle (arrow). (C) Histopathologic examination demonstrates that the tumor is composed of round cells with granular eosinophilic cytoplasm and small nuclei. The tumor cells lie in a collagenous tissue stroma (H&E, original magnification ×400). (D) Transmission electron micrograph shows that the cytoplasm of tumor cells are filled with several membrane-bound inclusions.

circumscribed tumor appears to have a capsule.[35] Microscopically, the tumor is composed of lobules of round or oval cells with a granular eosinophilic cytoplasm and small nuclei.[35–37,42] The tumor cells are arranged in clusters or fascicles between strands of collagenous tissue or skeletal muscle cells (Figure 17.7C). With immunostaining, the tumor is positive for neural markers including S-100 protein, neuron-specific enolase (NSE), and various myelin proteins.[35–37,39,42] The positive immunoreactivity with S-100 protein provides support for the Schwann cell origin of this tumor.[36]

Transmission electron microscopy shows that the cytoplasm of tumor cells are filled by numerous membrane-bound cytoplasmic inclusions that are the ultrastructural counterpart of granularity noted histopathologically (Figure 17.7D). These inclusions contain cellular debris including mitochondria, myelin figures, rough endoplasmic reticulum, and residual axons.[36,37]

Management and Prognosis

The best treatment for orbital GCT is surgical excision.[35,36] For infiltrative tumors, complete surgical excision may be difficult.[37] Orbital GCT is radioresistant.[42] Exenteration probably should be employed only in recurrent tumors.[41] The visual and systemic prognosis for patients with orbital GCT is good if the tumor is completely excised.[41]

ALVEOLAR SOFT PART SARCOMA

Alveolar soft part sarcoma (ASPS) is a malignant tumor of the soft tissues in which the cells are arranged in an alveolar pattern, from which the name of the tumor is derived. It most often develops in the buttocks and thighs, being closely related to skeletal muscles.[43] ASPS can rarely occur in the orbit (Table 17.1).[44–49] There is considerable overlap between orbital granular cell tumor, alveolar soft part sarcoma, and paragangliomas reported in the earlier literature. Many cases reported as granular cell tumor or paraganglioma have been shown after careful pathologic examinations, to be ASPS.

Clinical Features

The ages of the patients reported in the literature range from 11 months to 69 years, with a median of approximately 18 years.[44] Females are affected more often than males. Most patients present with rapidly progressive proptosis. In some instances the tumor presents with eyelid swelling and in others as an epibulbar mass. When the tumor is located anteriorly in the orbit, dilated epibulbar blood vessels in the quadrant(s) of the tumor may be evident.[44,47] ASPS may secondarily involve the orbital bone and soft tissues from the nasal cavity and paranasal sinuses.

ASPS has a tendency to metastasize to the lungs, bone, and brain.[44] Prognosis is variable depending on the completeness of surgical excision and tumor histopathology. Patients with completely resected tumors appear to have a better prognosis than those whose tumors have been incompletely resected.

Radiologic Features

CT images reveal that the tumor is usually well circumscribed.[45,47] The tumor generally occupies an anterior position in the orbit where it is attached to one of the extraocular muscles. In some cases, it may be located deep in the orbit and appears ill defined on neuroimaging studies.

Morphologic Features

On gross examination, the tumor is pink or red, generally well circumscribed, but in some cases ill defined. In some cases, the tumor appears to be encapsulated.[44] The tumor cells are arranged in an alveolar pattern similar to metastatic renal cell carcinoma. The tumor cells are polygonal or rounded and have a large cytoplasm with eccentrically placed nuclei and prominent nucleolus.[44,45] An important finding of ASPS is the presence in the cytoplasm of tumor cells of diastase-resistant crystalline structures that elicit a positive reaction to the periodic acid–Schiff (PAS) stain. These crystals have never been demonstrated in any other neoplasm. Therefore, their presence is considered to be highly characteristic and virtually diagnostic of ASPS.[44] In contrast to most peripheral nerve tumors of the orbit, the tumor stains negative for S-100 protein.[45]

Management and Prognosis

Wide surgical excision is the treatment of choice for ASPS. Tumors located anteriorly in the orbit in close association to an extraocular muscle can be completely excised.[45,47,49] Tumors located deep in the orbit that cannot be excised completely are treated with exenteration. Supplemental external beam radiation therapy (50–60 Gy) has been used in patients with incompletely resected tumors or recurrences.[44,47]

Based on the limited literature data, orbital ASPS seems to have better systemic prognosis than nonorbital lesions. In a report of 17 patients with orbital ASPS, 11 were alive at follow-ups ranging from 4 to 16 years.[44] Two patients died from tumor metastasis at intervals of 14 and 21 years after treatment. Two patients died from causes unrelated to the tumor, and 2 patients were lost to follow-up.

PARAGANGLIOMA

Paraganglioma, also known as *chemodectoma,* is a benign and uncommon tumor of paraganglion cells (glomus bodies). Paraganglion cells are of neural crest origin. This tumor usually occurs in the head and neck region but can also occur in the thorax and abdomen. The most common site of origin is the carotid body, followed by jugulotympanic and vagal paragangliomas.[50] In the orbit, paraganglioma is a rare tumor (Table 17.1). Orbital paraganglioma is believed to arise from the ciliary ganglion, ciliary nerve, or related neural tissue.[50] Multiple paragangliomas can occur in 10 to 20% of the patients. Paragangliomas may occur simultaneously in the orbit and carotid body.[51]

It has been speculated that the development of carotid body paragangliomas may be related to higher altitudes (>2000 m) and accompanying hypoxia.[52] All paragangliomas contain neurosecretory granules in their cytoplasm. However, only 1 to 3% of paragangliomas are clinically functional and secrete norepinephrine. Functional paragangliomas are usually located in the adrenal glands. Paragangliomas at other locations including the orbit are usually nonfunctional and do not secrete norepinephrine.[50]

Clinical Features

In 13 cases that have been reported in the literature by Archer and associates, the ages of the patients ranged between 3 and 68 years.[51] The patient with orbital paraganglioma most frequently develops proptosis.[51] The tumor is generally attached to an extraocular muscle, causing motility restriction. Tumors located in the anterior orbit may lead to dilation of episcleral blood vessels.[52] In the differential diagnosis of dilated episcleral blood vessels, orbital tumors including granular cell tumor, alveolar soft part sarcoma, and paraganglioma should be considered. Paraganglioma may also occur deep in the orbit in the region of the ciliary ganglion.[51,53] In such cases, the tumor may present with diplopia, papilledema, and decreased vision.[51,53]

About 5 to 10% of all paragangliomas are malignant. Malignant paragangliomas can demonstrate local invasion and metastasis. Metastasis usually occurs to distant organs or to regional lymph nodes.[50]

Radiologic Features

Orbital CT and MR images demonstrate a well-circumscribed tumor that may be attached to a rectus muscle.[53] In some cases, the tumor may appear ill-defined, occupying the posterior orbit.[51] In most cases, there is no orbital bone involvement. However, rarely a malignant orbital paraganglioma can demonstrate orbital bone destruction.[51] Malignant paragangliomas of the nasal cavity and paranasal sinuses can also secondarily invade the orbit through the medial orbital wall.

Morphologic Features

Grossly, the paraganglioma is usually well circumscribed. Rarely, it can also be ill defined. The lesion is pink. Histopathologically, there is no true capsule. The tumor is composed of clusters of cells sometimes called *zellballen,* which are separated from one another by delicate septae that contain blood vessels. The cells are polygonal, with round to oval nuclei. Mitosis is uncommon.[52,53]

The PAS reaction is useful in the differentiation of paraganglioma from ASPS because ASPS contains PAS-positive cytoplasmic crystalline inclusions; however, paraganglioma is PAS negative. In ASPS, immunostaining is positive for neuron-specific enolase (NSE).[52,53] Transmission electron microscopy reveals membrane-bound neurosecretory granules.[53]

Management and Prognosis

The best treatment of orbital paraganglioma is total surgical excision. Tumors located anteriorly in the orbit may be amenable to total excision. However, those located deeper in the orbit in the region of the ciliary ganglion may be treated with incisional biopsy followed by external beam radiation therapy (50 Gy).[51] Orbital paraganglioma is generally radiosensitive,[51,55] although in rare instances it does not respond to external beam radiation therapy.[54] Radical orbital surgery such as exenteration should be withheld until definite signs of orbital recurrence or malignant transformation are noted.

Metastasis can develop at follow-up periods ranging from a few months to as long as 42 years.[55] Therefore, given the long interval between the primary tumor and metastases, these patients require extended follow-up.

AMPUTATION NEUROMA

Orbital amputation neuroma is a rare tumor (Table 17.1). Amputation (traumatic) neuroma occurs at the proximal stump of severed peripheral nerves in the orbit. Amputation neuroma develops after orbital surgery, usually enucleation,[56,57] but it can also develop after strabismus surgery[58] and orbital bone fractures.[59] Following transection of a peripheral nerve, axonal sprouting characterized by proliferating Schwann cells, fibroblasts, and axons starts at the proximal stump. This proliferative activity represents an attempt of the proximal nerve to establish continuity with its distal counterpart. If there is a large defect that cannot be bridged, or if the distal segment has been removed, an amputation neuroma results. Orbital amputation neuromas are not known to arise from the optic nerve.

Clinical Features

The amputation neuroma usually manifests as a painless orbital mass, many months after orbital surgical procedures or trauma.[56–59] If the enucleation was performed for a malignant intraocular tumor, the possibility of orbital recurrence is usually the first diagnostic consideration.

Although a higher frequency of amputation neuromas following orbital surgery or trauma may be expected, these tumors have rarely been reported in the literature. Many neuromas arising from the small severed peripheral nerves do not reach a large enough size to be clinically detectable. The amputation neuroma rarely causes pain, hence is usually asymptomatic.

Radiologic Features

Orbital CT shows a well-circumscribed mass in an anophthalmic socket.[57,59] Amputation neuroma may occur in association with a conjunctival implantation cyst.[57] The cysts seen on CT in two cases were confirmed histopathologically to be adjacent conjunctival implantation cysts. Their relationship to the amputation neuroma is unclear, but they are probably coincidental.[57]

Morphologic Features

Grossly, the amputation neuroma presents as a circumscribed white-gray mass. There is no capsule. Microscopically, the mass is composed of proliferated axons, Schwann cells, and fibroblasts.[57] The presence of distinct perineurium helps to differentiate this lesion from a plexiform neurofibroma. The typical clinical history and the absence of neurofibromatosis also are helpful in making this distinction.

Management and Prognosis

The recommended management of orbital amputation neuroma is surgical excision of the mass and orbital reconstruction if necessary. A dermis fat graft or a mucous membrane graft may be required for orbital reconstruction.[57] Since the tumor is benign with no malignant potential, the systemic prognosis of the patient with an orbital amputation neuroma is excellent.

MELANOTIC NEUROECTODERMAL TUMOR OF INFANCY

The melanotic neuroectodermal tumor of infancy, or retinal anlage tumor, is a benign pigmented lesion that frequently involves the head and neck region.[60,61] The tumor usually originates in the anterior portion of the maxillary bone, but it rarely arises from the zygomatic bone, producing orbital manifestations.[60–62] This tumor generally occurs in infants under 1 year of age. Melanotic neuroectodermal tumor is probably of neural crest origin.[61,63]

Clinical Features

The child with melanotic neuroectodermal tumor in the zygomatic bone develops a mass on the face with medial displacement of the eye. Since the mass is related to the bone, it is usually hard and immobile to palpation.[64] There is no pain or eyelid ecchymosis, features that would help to differentiate it from a metastatic neuroblastoma. Elevated serum vanilmandelic acid level has been reported in patients with melanotic neuroectodermal tumor. Other laboratory studies are normal.[60,61]

In nonorbital locations, local recurrence develops in 10 to 45% of the patients and metastasis is about 3%.[60,61] Periorbital tumors appear to have a better prognosis. In a report of six cases, recurrence was noted in one patient (16%). None of the patients developed malignant transformation and metastasis.[62]

Radiologic Features

Orbital CT imaging reveals a lytic lesion in the lateral orbital wall with sclerosis of the adjacent bone.

Morphologic Features

On gross examination, the tumor is ill-defined and is gray to blue-black, depending on the melanin content. Light microscopy reveals two cell types: small poorly differentiated cells and larger pigmented cells. The small poorly differentiated cells are probably of neuroblastic origin. The pigmented cells bear a striking similarity to the retinal pigment epithelium in the eye. Immunohistochemical staining is positive for epithelial, melanocytic, and neural markers. Transmission electron microscopy demonstrates electron-dense granules in the cytoplasm of the pigmented cells.[61,63]

Management and Prognosis

The management consists of total excision. The prognosis of the patient with melanotic neuroectodermal tumor is generally good provided the tumor is adequately resected.[60–62] The patient should be followed closely, however, for signs of possible recurrence and metastasis.

PRIMARY ORBITAL NEUROBLASTOMA

Primary orbital neuroblastoma is very rare. Orbital involvement in neuroblastoma is usually secondary or metastatic. Secondary orbital neuroblastoma develops from orbital invasion of olfactory neuroblastoma (esthesioneuroblastoma). Metastatic orbital neuroblastoma originates from the adrenal medulla, retroperitoneum, and mediastinal and cervical sympathetic ganglia and spreads hematogenously to the orbit.[64] There has been only one well-documented case of primary orbital neuroblastoma, diagnosed in a 49-year-old woman in whom no other primary lesion could be found.[65] Over 12 years, the patient underwent five local excisions, external beam radiation therapy to the orbit, and finally orbital exenteration. Computed tomography performed before orbital exenteration demonstrated an ill-defined mass filling the entire orbit.[65]

Histopathologic examination of the tumor in this case showed spindle cells with benign cytologic features, no mitotic activity, palisading of the nuclei, and Homer–Wright rosettes. Immunohistochemical staining was positive for NSE but negative for glial fibrillary acidic protein (GFAP). Transmission electron microscopy demonstrated the presence of electron dense neurosecretory granules in the cytoplasm.[65]

Primary orbital neuroblastoma is unlikely to be diagnosed clinically or radiologically. It is difficult to make any treatment recommendations based on this single case in the literature. It is best to remove the orbital tumor totally. If this is not possible, external beam radiation therapy or exenteration can be employed for the residual tumor.

PRIMARY ORBITAL CARCINOID TUMOR

Carcinoid tumors arise from the enterochromaffin system (Kultschitzsky cells). They usually occur in the appendix, ileum, and bronchi. Carcinoid tumors of gastrointestinal origin are more likely to metastasize to the orbit, whereas bronchial carcinoids are more likely to metastasize to the uvea.[66]

Although the majority of orbital carcinoid tumors represent metastatic foci, the following reported case is believed to be a true primary orbital carcinoid tumor. A 71-year-old woman presented with a slowly progressive proptosis of 11 years' duration.[67] The affected eye had been blind for 4 years at the time of presentation. Orbital CT disclosed an infiltrative tumor with ill-defined borders. The orbit was exenterated. Histopathologic examination showed that the tumor was composed of small cells with round or oval hyperchromatic nuclei arranged in solid lobules and rosettelike configuration in some areas. Cytoplasmic neurosecretory granules were demonstrated by transmission electron microscopy. These findings were found to be consistent with the diagnosis of carcinoid tumor. Urinary level of 5-hydroxyindolacetic acid was normal. No primary tumor was found. There was no orbital recurrence or metastasis 15 years after orbital exenteration according to the latest follow-up data.[11]

Primary orbital carcinoid tumor is unlikely to be diagnosed clinically and by imaging studies. An attempt should be made to excise the orbital tumor completely. After the diagnosis of orbital carcinoid is made, it is appropriate to make a systemic evaluation looking for a primary site. If the results of the systemic evaluation are negative, the residual orbital tumor should be treated with external beam radiation therapy. The radiation dose for metastatic orbital carcinoid tumor is around 40 Gy, so a similar dose may also be appropriate for primary orbital carcinoid tumor.[64]

NEUROFIBROMATOSIS

Neurofibromatosis, an oculoneurocutaneous syndrome characterized by multisystem involvement, can lead to a wide variety of clinical symptoms and signs.[68] There are two distinct subtypes of neurofibromatosis. Neurofibromatosis type 1 (NF1) affects about 1 in 4000 individuals, and neurofibromatosis type 2 (NF2) affects about 1 in 50,000.[69]

NF1 is also known as *peripheral neurofibromatosis* or *von Recklinghausen's syndrome*. It is characterized by many peripheral cutaneous manifestations and is recognized to occur from an abnormality of chromosome 17.[68] The gene responsible for the development of this disorder is called *NF1*. NF2 is called *central* or *bilateral acoustic neurofibromatosis*. It is characterized by central neural tumors and early onset of posterior subcapsular cataract and is recognized to be related to an abnormality in chromosome 22.[69] The gene for this disorder is called *NF2*. Both forms of neurofibromatosis are transmitted by an autosomal dominant mode of inheritence.

Although the penetrance of both *NF1* and *NF2* is greater than 95%, the expressivity of the disease is highly variable.[68,70] Some patients have only a mild form of the disease and others a severe form of the disease.[68] The gene for NF1 encodes a protein termed *neurofibromin*, and the gene for NF2 encodes a protein termed *merlin* or *schwannomin*. Both proteins have tumor suppressor activity, downregulating the activity of proto-oncogenes.[70–72]

Although there is considerable overlap between NF1 and NF2, the ophthalmic manifestations are discussed separately. The diagnostic criteria for NF1 and NF2 are given in Boxes 17.1 and 17.2. Strict criteria should be met before the diagnosis of neurofibromatosis is made.

Ophthalmic Manifestations of Neurofibromatosis Type 1

Ophthalmic involvement in NF1 include abnormalities in the uveal tract (80%), eyelid (25%), cornea (25%), optic nerve (12%), retina (9%), and conjunctiva (4%).[73]

BOX 17.1. Diagnostic Criteria for Neurofibromatosis Type 1

Presence of two or more of the following criteria:
- Café-au-lait macules, six or more (>5 mm in diameter in prepubertal individuals and >15 mm in postpubertal individuals)
- Neurofibromas, two or more of any type, or one plexiform neurofibroma
- Freckling in the axillary or inguinal regions
- Optic gliomas
- Lisch nodules, two or more
- Distinctive osseous lesion (sphenoid dysplasia or thinning of long bone cortex with or without pseudoarthrosis)
- First-degree relative with neurofibromatosis type 1 by the foregoing criteria

Eyelids

Patients with NF1 may develop café-au-lait spots, fibroma molluscum (dermal neurofibromas), and plexiform neurofibroma in the eyelids. The first two conditions may not produce visual problems, but plexiform neurofibroma results in the typical S-shaped curvature of the upper eyelid, a finding that is believed to be highly characteristic of neurofibromatosis. In about 25% of the patients with eyelid plexiform neurofibroma, the tumor extends to involve the orbit.[73] The eyelid plexiform neurofibroma is treated by surgical debulking, and frontalis suspension procedures are necessary to reduce ptosis.

Orbit

Proptosis may be observed in NF1 and may occur from a variety of reasons: optic nerve glioma or rarely meningioma, orbital tumors including neurofibroma or schwannoma, and bony defects in the greater wing of the sphenoid.[68] Bony defects in the greater wing of the sphenoid enable the pulsations of brain to be transmitted to the orbit, resulting in proptosis. The tumor that is most characteristic of NF1 is optic nerve glioma. Other tumors are more rarely seen than optic nerve glioma.

The optic nerve can be involved with pilocytic astrocytoma (glioma) or meningioma. In patients with pilocytic astrocytoma, the reported incidence of neurofibromatosis has ranged from 9 to 30%.[22] Juvenile pilocytic astrocytoma of the optic nerve is a slowly progressive lesion that can lead to proptosis (Figure 17.8A), optic disk edema (Figure 17.8C), retinal venous obstruction, optic atrophy, and visual loss. Optociliary (or retinochoroidal) shunt vessels, a characteristic finding in optic nerve sheath meningioma, occur rarely with optic glioma (Figure 17.8C).

Gliomas may either involve the intraorbital portion of the optic nerve or the chiasm and optic tracts. In the majority of cases, optic nerve gliomas are self-limited or grow very slowly. Tumors located to the optic nerve at the time of diagnosis infrequently extend into the chiasm subsequently.[74,75] Some studies indicate that optic nerve gliomas associated with NF1 carry a more benign prognosis than those unassociated with NF1[76]; other studies failed to disclose such a relationship.[74]

Diagnosis of optic nerve glioma is usually based on orbital imaging. In CT and MR images, optic nerve glioma appears as oval or fusiform enlargements of the optic nerve (Figure 17.8D). Increased length of the intraorbital nerve segment results in kinking of the optic nerve. Optic nerve meningioma, in contrast, tends to produce a "railroad track" appearance. MRI is generally considered to be superior to CT for demonstrating the optic nerve features and showing the extent of intracranial disease. In patients with NF1, optic nerve glioma may rupture through the pia surrounding the optic nerve and proliferate in the subarachnoid space. This manifests on MRI as arachnoidal hyperplasia surrounding the optic nerve (Figure 17.8D, inset).

Observation is generally recommended if there is no clinical or radiographic evidence of progression of an optic nerve glioma.[75] If the patient has chiasmal involvement that threatens to extend into surrounding structures resulting in progressive visual loss, hydrocephalus, or other serious complications, surgical excision or radiotherapy can be employed.[77] Complete surgical excision may not be possible in many extrachiasmal cases. External beam radiation therapy (40–50 Gy) is used either alone or after incomplete excision in such cases.[77]

Extraocular Muscles

Congenital absence of the superior oblique tendon and inferior rectus muscle have been reported in patients with NF1.[78,79]

BOX 17.2. Diagnostic Criteria for Neurofibromatosis Type 2

Bilateral eighth nerve masses (acoustic neuromas)
or
First-degree relative with neurofibromatosis type 2 and
- Unilateral eighth nerve mass
- or
- Two of the following: neurofibroma, schwannoma, glioma, meningioma, juvenile posterior subcapsular cataract

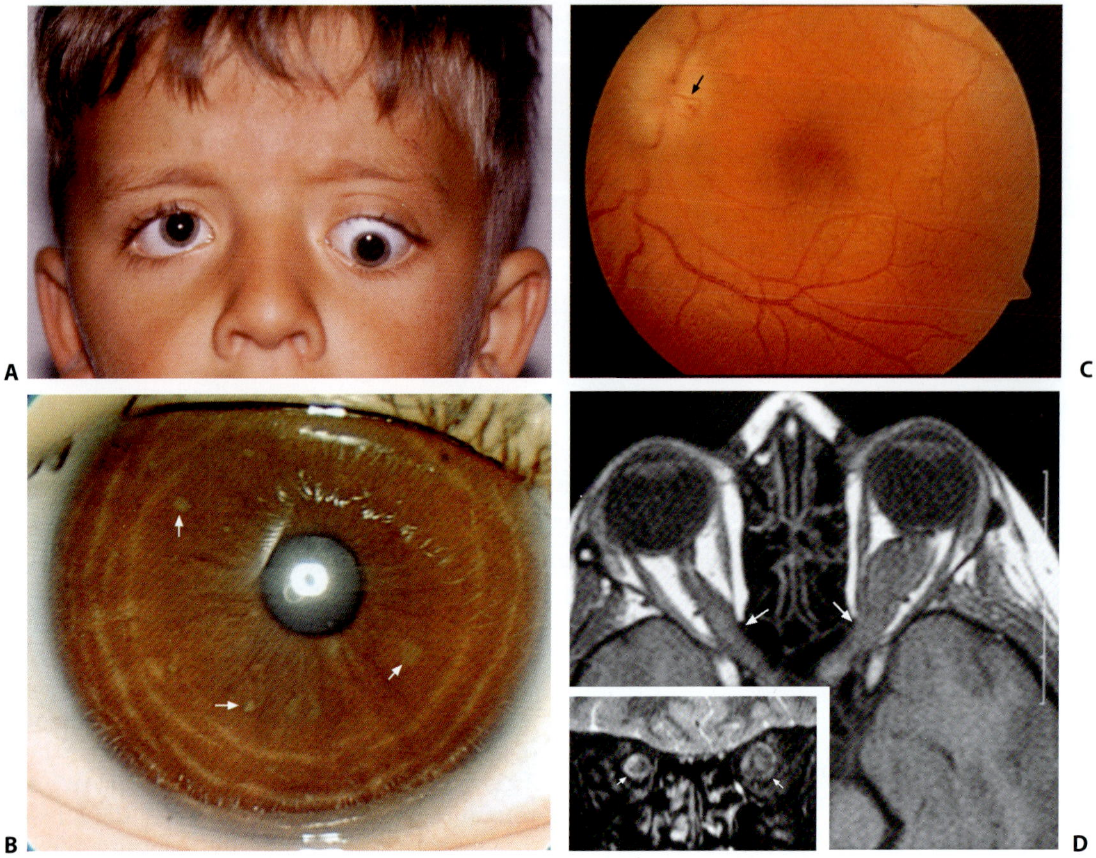

FIGURE 17.8. A 5-year-old boy with NF1 and bilateral optic nerve gliomas. (A) Facial photograph demonstrating downward proptosis of the left eye. (B) Anterior segment photograph showing multiple Lisch nodules located on the anterior iris surface (arrows). (C) Fundus photograph of the left eye showing optic disk edema and optociliary shunt vessel (arrow). (D) Axial orbital T1-weighted MR image showing bilateral optic nerve gliomas isointense to the extraocular muscle and cerebral gray matter (arrows). *Inset*: Coronal orbital T1-weighted MR image demonstrating bilateral arachnoidal hyperplasia surrounding the optic nerve gliomas (arrows).

Conjunctiva

The conjunctiva may rarely be involved by neurofibromas in a patient with NF1.[73]

Anterior Segment

Iris melanocytic hamartoma, known as Lisch nodules, is the most common uveal abnormality, occurring in nearly 80% of the patients with NF1.[73] Lisch nodules are small, sharply demarcated, dome-shaped, lightly pigmented lesions on the anterior surface of the iris (Figure 17.8B). The finding of two or more Lisch nodules is a diagnostic criterion for NF1, but often dozens of them are present. They usually become apparent around age 5 years. Unlike iris nevi, the nodules are raised and have a gelatinous appearance. Histologically, Lisch nodules are focal aggregates of melanocytes and glial cells on the anterior border layer of the iris. Another anterior segment finding in NF1 is the presence of enlarged corneal nerves.[73]

Glaucoma

Unilateral congenital glaucoma appears to occur more commonly in patients who have neurofibromatous involvement of the eyelids. The most important cause of glaucoma is the obstruction of aqueous outflow by diffuse neurofibromatous thickening of the trabecular meshwork.[80] Glaucoma may also develop from maldevelopment of the anterior chamber angle, angle closure due to forward displacement of the iris by a ciliary body tumor, or iris neovascularization.[80] Medical treatment of this type of glaucoma is uniformly unsuccessful. Surgical options include goniotomy, filtering procedures, cyclocryotherapy, and cyclophotocoagulation. However, the long-term prognosis is quite poor.

Retina and Choroid

Hamartomas similar to those that occur in the iris can also occur in the choroid of patients with neurofibromatosis. The choroidal lesion is similar histopathologically to the iris lesion and probably represents a nevus.[73]

Other patients with neurofibromatosis have a diffuse thickening of the uveal tract, which can be difficult to recognize on clinical examination. This uveal thickening probably results from the proliferation of neurofibromatous (Schwann cells and in some cases ganglions) and melanocytic elements.[81] Other choroidal tumors that can occur in patients with neurofibromatosis are choroidal melanoma and neurilemoma (schwannoma).[82,83] Choroidal melanoma and neurilemoma are managed with one of several methods including enucleation, local resection, plaque radiotherapy, and transpupillary thermotherapy.

Retinal manifestations in NF1 that require no treatment include retinal astrocytic hamartoma, myelinated nerve fibers, multifocal congenital hypertrophy of the retinal pigment epithelium, retinal hamartoma (i.e., phakomatosis) similar to the combined pigment epithelial and retinal hamartoma, and retinal vascular occlusions (retinal vein and arterial occlusions).[73,84] The vascular occlusions probably develop from the proliferating Schwann cells in the vascular walls occluding the vessels.

Ophthalmic Manifestations of NF2

The three major ocular manifestations of NF2 are juvenile posterior subcapsular or cortical cataracts (69%), retinal hamartomas (22%), and ocular motor abnormalities (12%). The subcapsular and cortical cataract in patients with NF2 usually develops before age 30 years. Ocular motor palsies are due either to the presence of a tumor or to increased intracranial pressure.[85]

In another report focusing on the posterior segment findings of NF2, the most frequent retinal finding was an epiretinal membrane observed in 80% of the patients.[86] Additionally, a lesion similar to the combined pigment epithelial and retinal hamartoma was observed in 7% of the patients.[86] Epiretinal membranes, which do not generally develop in patients with NF1, are observed in patients with NF2.[86] The retinal hamartoma resembles the combined pigment epithelial and retinal hamartoma in some respects. However, the retinal hamartoma may also represent an atypical lesion consisting of an epiretinal membrane associated with a retinal glial hamartoma similar to the one seen in tuberous sclerosis. If the retinal glial hamartoma is too small initially to be detectable on funduscopy the lesion may be observed as an epiretinal membrane.[86] It is speculated that cells of neural crest origin at the vitreoretinal juncture and in the retina proliferate or develop abnormalities resulting in epiretinal membrane and retinal hamartoma. Similar changes occurring in the ectodermal cells of the lens result in cataract.[86]

Other rare ophthalmic manifestations of NF2 include Lisch nodules,[85] pseudopapilledema caused by epiretinal membrane extending onto the optic disk,[87] papilledema from increased intracranial pressure,[88] optic nerve glioma and optic nerve sheath meningioma,[85] and morning glory disk abnormality.[89]

Systemic Features of Neurofibromatosis

The most common cutaneous manifestations of neurofibromatosis include pigmented macules (café-au-lait spots), axillary and inguinal freckling, benign nerve sheath tumors (most commonly neurofibroma but also schwannoma), and nevi.[68] Most of these skin lesions become clinically apparent at puberty, although some instances have been noted at birth. Café-au-lait spots are highly characteristic of neurofibromatosis seen in 94 to 100% of patients with NF1.[68] Axillary and inguinal freckling is seen in approximately 67% of the patients.[68] The benign cutaneous and subcutaneous nerve sheath tumors (neurofibromas and schwannomas) are particularly pronounced in the facial area.

The pigmented macule (café-au-lait spot) is characterized as a patch of light brown pigmentation with fairly well-defined borders. It can occur anywhere on the skin and can assume a variety of size and configurations. Approximately 25% of the normal population can have one to three café-au-lait spots. However, patients with neurofibromatosis have more and larger café-au-lait spots.[68]

The central nervous system manifestations of neurofibromatosis vary with the size and the extent of the associated tumors. Acoustic neuromas, particularly if bilateral, are considered to be pathognomonic of NF2. Other associated tumors include gliomas in the region of the third ventricle, pituitary tumors, and spinal cord meningiomas.[68,81]

Some patients with NF1 develop seizure disorder and mild intellectual impairment. Bright lesions seen on T2-weighted MRI may represent brain dysplasia or heterotopias. The significance of these bright lesions in relation to seizure disorder and intelligence problems is not known.[68]

Skeletal abnormalities are common in patients with NF1. Vertebral defects and scoliosis can occur. An uncommon problem is the development of pseudoarthroses (false joints). Pseudoarthroses result from thinning of long bones, fractures, and abnormal callus formation.[68]

Other benign and malignant systemic tumors that have been associated with neurofibromatosis include neurofibrosarcoma, pheochromocytoma, breast carcinoma, genitourinary tumors, gastrointestinal tumors, and cutaneous melanoma. Patients with neurofibromatosis are recognized to have a slightly higher incidence of pheochromocytoma.[68,81]

References

1. Shields JA, Bakewell B, Augsburger JJ, Flanagan JC. Classification and incidence of space-occupying lesions of the orbit. *Arch Ophthalmol* 1984;102:1606–1611.
2. Henderson JW, Campbell RJ, Farrow GM, Garrity JA. *Orbital Tumors.* New York: Raven Press; 1994:43–52.

3. Günalp I, Gündüz K. Biopsy-proven orbital lesions in Turkey. A survey of 1092 cases over 30 years. *Orbit* 1994;13:67–79.
4. Seregard S, Sahlin S. Panorama of orbital space-occupying lesions. The 24-year experience of a referral center. *Acta Ophthalmol Scand* 1999;77:91–98.
5. Sen DK. Aetiological pattern of orbital tumors in India and their clinical presentations. A 20-year retrospective study. *Orbit* 1990;9:299–302.
6. Schatz H. Benign orbital neurilemmoma: sarcomatous transformation in von Recklinghausen's disease. *Arch Ophthalmol* 1971;86:268–273.
7. Rootman J, Goldberg C, Robertson W. Primary orbital schwannomas. *Br J Ophthalmol* 1982;66:194–204.
8. Rose GE, Wright JE. Isolated peripheral nerve sheath tumours of the orbit. *Eye* 1991;5:668–673.
9. Carroll GS, Haik BG, Fleming JC, et al. Peripheral nerve tumors of the orbit. *Radiol Clin North Am* 1999;37:195–202.
10. Shen WC, Yang DY, Ho WL, et al. Neurilemoma of the oculomotor nerve presenting as an orbital mass: MR findings. *AJNR Am J Neuroradiol* 1993;14:1253–1254.
11. Shields JA. *Diagnosis and Management of Orbital Tumors.* Philadelphia: WB Saunders; 1989:149–169.
12. Shields JA, Kapustiak J, Arbizo V, Augsburger JJ, Schnitzer RE. Orbital neurilemoma with extension through the superior orbital fissure. *Arch Ophthalmol* 1986;104:871–873.
13. Capps DH, Brodsky MC, Rice CD, Mrak RE, Glasier CM, Brown HH. Orbital intramuscular schwannoma. *Am J Ophthalmol* 1990;110:535–539.
14. Marc'hadour FL, Romanet JP, Fdili A, Peoc'h M, Pinel N. Schwannoma of the bulbar conjunctiva. *Arch Ophthalmol* 1996;114:1258–1260.
15. Byrne BM, van Heuven WAJ, Lawton AW. Echographic characteristics of benign orbital schwannomas (neurilemomas). *Am J Ophthalmol* 1988;106:194–198.
16. Dervin JE, Beaconsfield M, Wright JE, Moseley IF. CT findings in orbital tumors of nerve sheath origin. *Clin Radiol* 1989;40:475–479.
17. Abe T, Kawamura N, Homma H, et al. MRI of orbital schwannomas. *Head Neck Radiol* 2000;42:466–468.
17a. Gündüz K, Shields CL, Günalp I, Shields JA, Erden E. Orbital schwannoma: correlation of magnetic resonance imaging and pathologic findings. *Graefes Arch Clin Exp Ophthalmol* 2003;241:593–597. Erratum in: *Graefes Arch Clin Exp Ophthalmol* 2004;242:188.
18. Tsuzuki N, Katoh H, Ohnuki A, et al. Cystic schwannoma of the orbit: case report. *Surg Neurol* 2000;54:385–387.
19. Lam DSC, Ng JSK, To TAF, et al. Cystic schwannoma of the orbit. *Eye* 1997;11:798–800.
20. Fetkenhour DR, Shields CL, Chao AN, et al. Orbital cavitary rhabdomyosarcoma masquerading as lymphangioma. *Arch Ophthalmol* 2001;119:1208–1210.
21. Khwarg SI, Lucarelli MJ, Lemke BN, et al. Ancient schwannoma of the orbit. *Arch Ophthalmol* 1999;117:262–264.
22. Lewis RA, Gerson LP, Axelson KA, et al. Von Recklinghausen neurofibromatosis. II. Incidence of optic gliomata. *Ophthalmology* 1984;91:929–935.
23. Kobrin JL, Blodi FC, Weingeist TA. Ocular and orbital manifestations of neurofibromatosis. *Surv Ophthalmol* 1979;24:45–51.
24. Mamalis N, Apple DJ, Williams RD, et al. Surgical removal of an "inoperable" neurofibroma. *Ophthalmic Surg* 1988;19:37–41.
25. Henderson JW, Campbell RJ, Farrow GM, Garrity JA. *Orbital Tumors.* New York: Raven Press; 1994:221–237.
26. Krohel GB, Rosenberg PN, Wright JE, Smith RS. Localized orbital neurofibromas. *Am J Ophthalmol* 1985;100:458–464.
27. Rocca RCD, Roen J, Labay GR, Bedrossian E. Isolated neurofibroma of the orbit. *Ophthalmic Surg* 1985;16:634–638.
28. McDonald P, Jakobiec FA, Hornblass A, Iwamoto T. Benign peripheral nerve sheath tumors (neurofibromas) of the lacrimal gland. *Ophthalmology* 1983;90:1403–1413.
29. Jackson IT, Laws ER Jr, Martin RD. The surgical management of orbital neurofibromatosis. *Plast Reconstr Surg* 1983;71:751–758.
30. Jakobiec FA, Font RL, Zimmerman LE. Malignant peripheral nerve sheath tumors of the orbit: a clinicopathologic study of eight cases. *Trans Am Ophthalmol Soc* 1985;83:332–366.
31. Lyons CJ, McNab AA, Garner A, Wright JE. Orbital malignant peripheral nerve sheath tumors. *Br J Ophthalmol* 1989;73:731–738.
32. Eviatar JA, Hornblass A, Herschorn B, Jakobiec FA. Malignant peripheral nerve sheath tumor of the orbit in a 15-month-old child. *Ophthalmology* 1992;99:1595–1599.
33. Brooks JSJ, Freeman M, Enterline HT. Malignant "triton" tumor. Natural history and immunohistochemistry of nine new cases with review of the literature. *Cancer* 1985;55:2543–2549.
34. Enzinger FM, Weiss SW. *Soft Tissue Tumors.* St. Louis: CV Mosby-Year Book; 1995:821–888.
35. Allaire GS, Laflamme P, Bourgouin P. Granular cell tumour of the orbit. *Can J Ophthalmol* 1995;30:151–153.
36. Jaeger MJ, Green WR, Miller NR, Harris GJ. Granular cell tumor of the orbit and ocular adnexae. *Surv Ophthalmol* 1987;31:417–423.
37. Dolman PJ, Rootman J, Dolman CL. Infiltrating orbital granular cell tumour: a case report and literature review. *Br J Ophthalmol* 1987;71:47–53.
38. Moseley I. Granular cell tumour of the orbit: radiological findings. *Neuroradiology* 1991;33:399–402.
39. Callejo SA, Kronish JW, Decker SJ, et al. Malignant granular cell tumor metastatic to the orbit. *Ophthalmology* 2000;107:550–554.
40. Obayashi K, Yamada Y, Kozaki M. Granular cell myoblastoma of the orbit. *Jpn J Ophthalmol* 1969;20:566–574.
41. Henderson JW, Campbell RJ, Farrow GM, Garrity JA. *Orbital Tumors.* New York: Raven Press; 1994:239–268.
42. Karcioglu ZA, Hemphill GL, Wool BM. Granular cell tumor of the orbit. Case report and review of the literature. *Ophthalmic Surg* 1983;14:125–129.
43. Lieberman PH, Foote WH Jr, Steward WH, Berg JW. Alveolar soft part sarcoma. *JAMA* 1966;198:1047–1051.
44. Font RL, Jurco S, Zimmerman LE. Alveolar soft-part sarcoma of the orbit: a clinicopathologic analysis of seventeen cases and review of the literature. *Hum Pathol* 1982;13:569–579.
45. Coupland SE, Heimann H, Hoffmeister B, et al. Immunohistochemical examination of an alveolar soft part sarcoma. *Graefes Arch Clin Exp Ophthalmol* 1999;237:266–272.
46. Bunt AH. Alveolar soft part sarcoma of the orbit. *Ophthalmology* 1981;88:1339–1346.
47. Grant GD, Shields JA, Flanagan JC, Horowitz P. The ultrasonographic and radiologic features of a histologically proven case of alveolar soft-part sarcoma of the orbit. *Am J Ophthalmol* 1979;87:773–777.
48. Jordan DR, MacDonald H, Noel L, Carpenter B, Brownstein S, Munro S. Alveolar soft part sarcoma of the orbit. *Ophthalmic Surg* 1995;26:269–270.
49. Litricin O. Alveolar soft-part sarcoma. *Am J Ophthalmol* 1982;94:554–555.
50. Myssiorek D. Head and neck paragangliomas. An overview. *Otolaryngol Clin North Am* 2001;34:829–836.
51. Archer KF, Hurwitz JJ, Balogh JM, Fernandes BJ. Orbital nonchromaffin paraganglioma. A case report and review of the literature. *Ophthalmology* 1989;96:1659–1666.
52. Rodriguez-Cuevas S, Lopez-Garza J, Labastida-Almendaro S. Carotid body tumors in inhabitants of altitudes higher than 2000 meters above sea level. *Head Neck Surg* 1998;20:374–378.

53. Bednar MM, Trainer TD, Aitken PA, et al. Orbital paraganglioma: case report and review of the literature. *Br J Ophthalmol* 1992;76:183–185.
54. Ahmed A, Dodge OG, Kirk RS. Chemodectoma of the orbit. *J Clin Pathol* 1969;22:584–588.
55. Rosenwasser H. Current management of glomus jugulare tumors. *Ann Otol Rhinol Laryngol* 1967;76:603–610.
56. Blodi FC. Amputation neuroma in the orbit. *Am J Ophthalmol* 1949;32:929–932.
57. Messmer EP, Camara J, Boniuk M, Font RL. Amputation neuroma of the orbit. Report of two cases and review of the literature. *Ophthalmology* 1984;91:1420–1423.
58. Wolter JR, Benz CA. Bilateral amputation neuromas of eye muscles. *Am J Ophthalmol* 1964;57:287–289.
59. Okuba K, Asai T, Sera Y, Okada S. A case of amputation neuroma presenting proptosis. *Ophthalmologica* 1987;194:5–8.
60. Kapadia SB, Frisman DM, Hitchcock CL, Ellis GL, Popek EJ. Melanotic neuroectodermal tumor of infancy. Clinicopathological, immunohistochemical and flow cytometric study. *Am J Surg Pathol* 1993;17:566–573.
61. Cutler LS, Chaudhry AP, Topazian R. Melanotic, neuroectodermal tumor of infancy: an ultrastructural study, literature review, and reevaluation. *Cancer* 1981;48:257–270.
62. Lamping KA, Albert DM, Lack E, et al. Melanotic neuroectodermal tumor of infancy (retinal anlage tumor). *Ophthalmology* 1985;92:143–149.
63. Navas Palacios JJ. Malignant melanotic neuroectodermal tumor; light and electron microscopic study. *Cancer* 1980;46:529–536.
64. Shields JA. *Diagnosis and Management of Orbital Tumors.* Philadelphia: WB Saunders; 1989:291–315.
65. Jakobiec FA, Klepach GL, Crissman JD, Spoor TC. Primary differentiated neuroblastoma of the orbit. *Ophthalmology* 1987;94:255–266.
66. Shetlar DJ, Font RL, Ordonez N, et al. A clinicopathologic study of three carcinoid tumors metastatic to the orbit. Immunohistochemical, ultrastructural, and DNA flow cytometric studies. *Ophthalmology* 1990;97:257–264.
67. Zimmerman LE, Stangl R, Riddle PJ. Primary carcinoid tumor of the orbit. A clinicopathologic study with histochemical and electron microscopic observations. *Arch Ophthalmol* 1983;101:1395–1398.
68. Sippel KC. Ocular findings in neurofibromatosis type 1. *Int Ophthalmol Clin* 2001;41:25–40.
69. The National Institutes of Health Consensus Development Conference. Neurofibromatosis. *Arch Neurol* 1988;45:575–578.
70. Rettele GA, Brodsky MC, Merin LM, et al. Blindness, deafness, quadriparesis and a retinal malformation: The ravages of neurofibromatosis 2. *Surv Ophthalmol* 1996;41:135–141.
71. Gutmann DH, Collins FS. The neurofibromatosis type 1 gene and its protein product, neurofibromin. *Neuron* 1993;10:335–343.
72. Basu TN, Gutmann DH, Fletcher JA, et al. Aberrant regulation of Ras proteins in malignant tumour cells from type 1 neurofibromatosis patients. *Nature* 1992;356:713–715.
73. Lewis RA, Riccardi VM. Von Recklinghausen neurofibromatosis. Incidence of iris hamartoma. *Ophthalmology* 1981;88:348–354.
74. Hoyt WF, Baghdassarian SA. Optic glioma of childhood: natural history and rationale for conservative management. *Br J Ophthalmol* 1969;53:793–798.
75. Imes RK, Hoyt WF. Childhood chiasmal gliomas: update on the fate of patients in the 1969 San Francisco study. *Br J Ophthalmol* 1986;70:179–182.
76. Listernick R, Darling C, Greenwald M, et al. Optic pathway tumors in children: the effect of neurofibromatosis on clinical manifestations and natural history. *J Pediatr* 1995;127:718–722.
77. Kovalic JJ, Grigsby PW, Shepard MJ, et al. Radiation therapy for gliomas of the nerve and chiasm. *Int J Radiat Oncol Biol Phys* 1990;18:927–932.
78. Newman RM, Cogen MS. Congenital absence of the superior oblique tendon in a patient with neurofibromatosis. *J Pediatr Ophthalmol Strabismus* 1997;34:192–194.
79. Majid MA, Ah-Fat FG, Wilson R, Marsh IB. Congenital absence of the inferior rectus muscle in a patient with neurofibromatosis. *Eye* 2001;15:795–796.
80. Grant WM, Walton DS. Distinctive gonioscopic findings in glaucoma due to neurofibromatosis. *Arch Ophthalmol* 1968;79:127–134.
81. Shields JA, Shields CL. Systemic hamartomatoses ("phakomatoses"). In: Shields JA, Shields CL, eds. *Intraocular Tumors. A Text and Atlas.* Philadelphia: WB Saunders; 1992;513–539.
82. Wiznia RA, Freedman JE, Mancini AD, Shields JA. Malignant melanoma of the choroid in neurofibromatosis. *Am J Ophthalmol* 1978;86:684–687.
83. Freedman SF, Elner VM, Donev I, et al. Intraocular neurilemoma arising from the posterior ciliary nerve in neurofibromatosis. *Ophthalmology* 1988;95:1559–1564.
84. Mori F, Kawai M, Sato E, et al. Branch retinal vein occlusion in a Japanese patient with neurofibromatosis 1. *Jpn J Ophthalmol* 2001;45:634–635.
85. Ragge NK, Baser ME, Klein J, et al. Ocular abnormalities in neurofibromatosis type 2. *Am J Ophthalmol* 1995;120:634–641.
86. Meyers SM, Gutman FA, Kaye LD, Rothner AD. Retinal changes associated with neurofibromatosis 2. *Trans Am Ophthalmol Soc* 1995;93:245–252; discussion, 252–257.
87. Lueder GT, Doll JT. Pseudopapilledema in neurofibromatosis type 2. *Am J Ophthalmol* 2000;129:405–407.
88. Thomas DA, Trobe JD, Cornblath WT. Visual loss secondary to increased intracranial pressure in neurofibromatosis type 2. *Arch Ophthalmol* 1999;117:1650–1653.
89. Brodsky MC, Landau K, Wilson RS, Boltshauser E. Morning glory disc anomaly in neurofibromatosis type 2. *Arch Ophthalmol* 1999;117:839–841.

18

Lacrimal Gland Tumors

Yoon-Duck Kim

Lacrimal gland tumors typically present with upper eyelid fullness, alteration of the upper eyelid contour, and downward and nasal displacement of the globe. Lacrimal fossa masses consist of inflammatory, neoplastic, and structural disorders. In managing lacrimal tumors appropriately, it is imperative to differentiate benign mixed tumors of the lacrimal gland with diagnostic accuracy so that the initial management is complete extirpation without preceding incisional biopsy.

Traditionally it has been said that about 50% of lacrimal masses are epithelial and 50% are nonepithelial.[1] More recent data indicate that inflammatory lesions and lymphoid tumors of the lacrimal gland are two to three times more common than epithelial tumors.[2,3] In reported series on epithelial tumors of larger size, the relative frequency is approximately 50% benign mixed tumors and 50% carcinomas. About half of the malignancies are adenoid cystic carcinoma (Table 18.1).[4–8] The incidence of epithelial tumors of the lacrimal gland ranges from 5 to 8% of orbital neoplasia.[1,6,9]

In managing lacrimal fossa mass lesions, preoperative characterization of a particular lesion is highly desirable. This recommendation is based on the duration of symptoms, the presence of pain, and radiologic findings.[10,11] Acute onset of swelling, periorbital pain, chemosis, or an erythematous indurated lid indicate an inflammatory process of either idiopathic or of bacterial or viral etiology (Figure 18.1). A computed tomography (CT) scan will reveal a diffuse lacrimal enlargement with irregular margins, frequently demonstrating contrast enhancement and no bony change. Most cases of bacterial dacryoadenitis resolves rapidly with appropriate systemic antibiotics. Idiopathic acute inflammation can be treated with a short course of corticosteroids (Figure 18.2). Failure to resolve over a few weeks should lead to incisional biopsy, since acute inflammatory episodes may be related to an underlying carcinoma.[10]

Orbital lymphoproliferative lesions are another common cause of lacrimal gland swelling (see Chapter 13). They are characterized by insidious and painless onset in a slightly older population and can often be bilateral. CT scans show that all lymphoid tumors mold themselves around the existing orbital structures, such as the globe and the bony orbit, without eroding bone or enlarging the orbit (Figure 18.3).[12]

When painless swelling in the upper lid without inflammatory symptoms and signs presents for more than 12 months, benign mixed tumor (pleomorphic adenoma) should be suspected. On CT scans pleomorphic adenomas usually show round to oval, well-circumscribed mass and enlargement of the lacrimal fossa without invasion of overlying bone. Such a tumor should be excised intact through a lateral orbitotomy.[10,13] When biopsy is done before excision, the 5-year recurrence rate is estimated to be 32%, and many of these recurrences undergo malignant transformation.[4] Biopsy of pleomorphic adenoma should be avoided. It is advisable to completely remove all encapsulated or well-circumscribed masses without incisional biopsy.

Most patients with malignant epithelial tumors present with painful swelling in the upper eyelid that developed within one year.[14] High-resolution CT reveals more elongated mass extending along the lateral orbital wall with expansion of the lacrimal fossa with bone invasion. Calcifications are more commonly seen in malignant tumors. A biopsy through a transseptal incision should be performed without delay in all these patients.

Dermoid cysts are not true lacrimal gland tumors; rather, they originate from epithelial rests located in the orbit, particularly in the superolateral quadrant. Deep dermoids in the lacrimal fossa most often present as painless proptosis in a younger age group. Bony change in the superolateral wall is common. When a tumor extends through the suture line, it may appear on both sides of the bone (the "dumbbell" dermoid). Rarely, these patients present inflammatory reaction when the cyst ruptures. Dermoid cysts can be diagnosed easily by typical findings on CT or magnetic resonance (MR) images of a lesion of fatty density with no or only faint enhancement and smoothly outlined osseous changes. It appears as an image of low intensity on T1-weighted and high intensity on T2-weighted MR images (Figure 18.4).[15]

TABLE 18.1. Incidence of Primary Epithelial Neoplasms of the Lacrimal Gland.

Authors	*Number of cases*	*Benign mixed*	*Malignant mixed*	*Adenoid Cystic*	*Other carcinoma*
Font and Gamel[4]	265	136 (51%)	34 (13%)	70 (27%)	25 (9%)
Ni et al.[5]	160	90 (56%)	10 (6%)	46 (29%)	14 (9%)
Henderson[6]	66	25 (38%)	10 (15%)	22 (34%)	9 (13%)
Wright[7]	54	30 (56%)	3 (6%)	11 (20%)	10 (18%)
Ashton[8]	54	30 (55%)	2 (4%)	13 (24%)	9 (17%)
Total	599	311 (52%)	59 (10%)	162 (27%)	67 (11%)

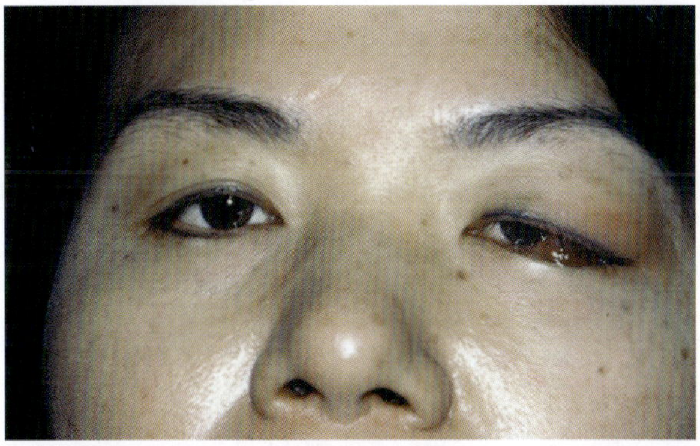

FIGURE 18.1. Acute dacryoadenitis in a 39-year-old woman with a 1-week history of pain and swelling over the left lacrimal gland with marked chemosis.

DACRYOPS (LACRIMAL DUCTAL CYSTS)

The ducts of the lacrimal gland may become obstructed, leading to a cystic mass in the lacrimal region. The palpebral lobe is affected far more commonly than the orbital lobe. The typical findings of dacryops are bluish transilluminating cystic swellings visible through the conjunctiva (Figure 18.5A). Imaging usually reveals a cyst without any bone changes (Figure 18.5B). On histopathologic examination they are typically composed of two layers: an inner cuboidal or columnar layer and an outer flattened myoepithelial layer (Figure 18.5C).[16] The treatment is

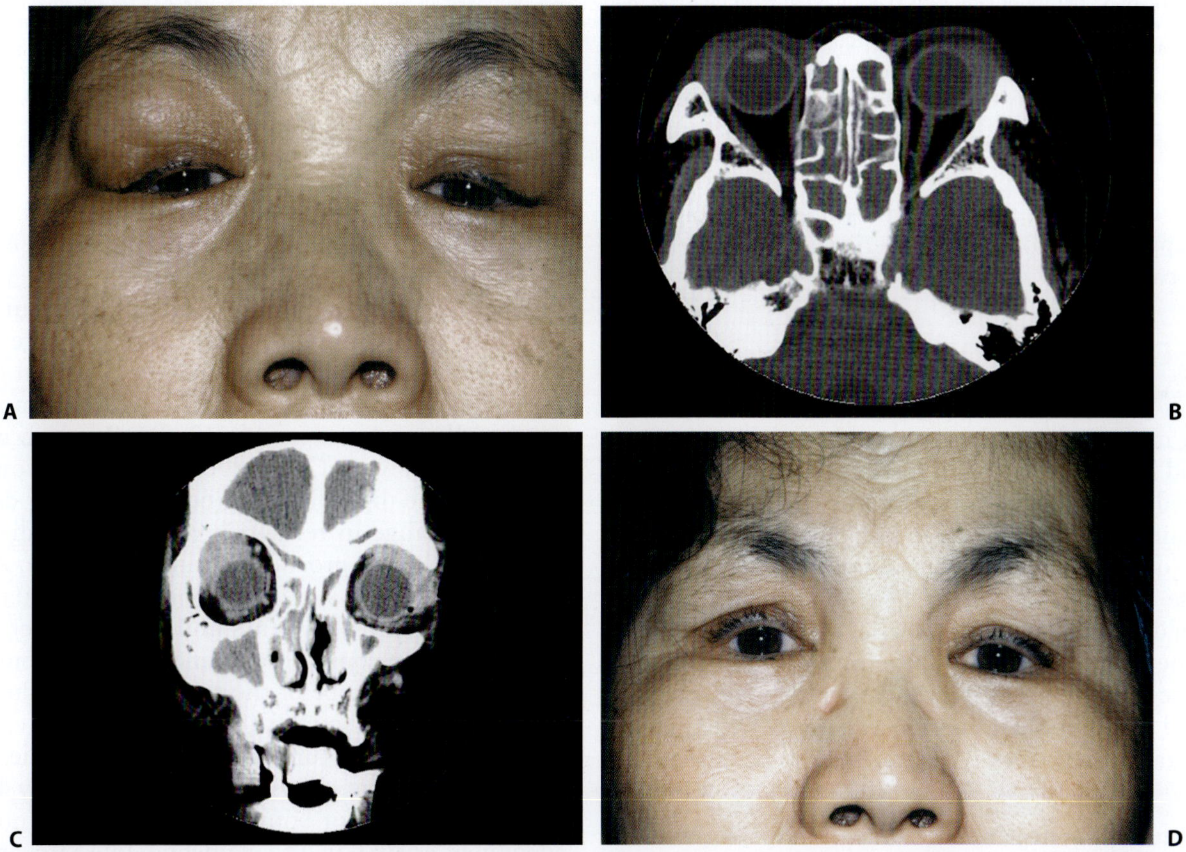

FIGURE 18.2. Idiopathic inflammatory pseudotumor in a 63-year-old woman with bilateral, nontender masses in the lacrimal gland region for 3 months (A). The S-shaped eyelid is typical for lacrimal gland enlargement. (B) Axial and (C) coronal CT images demonstrate bilateral enlargement of the lacrimal glands. (D) The patient 2 months after systemic steroid therapy.

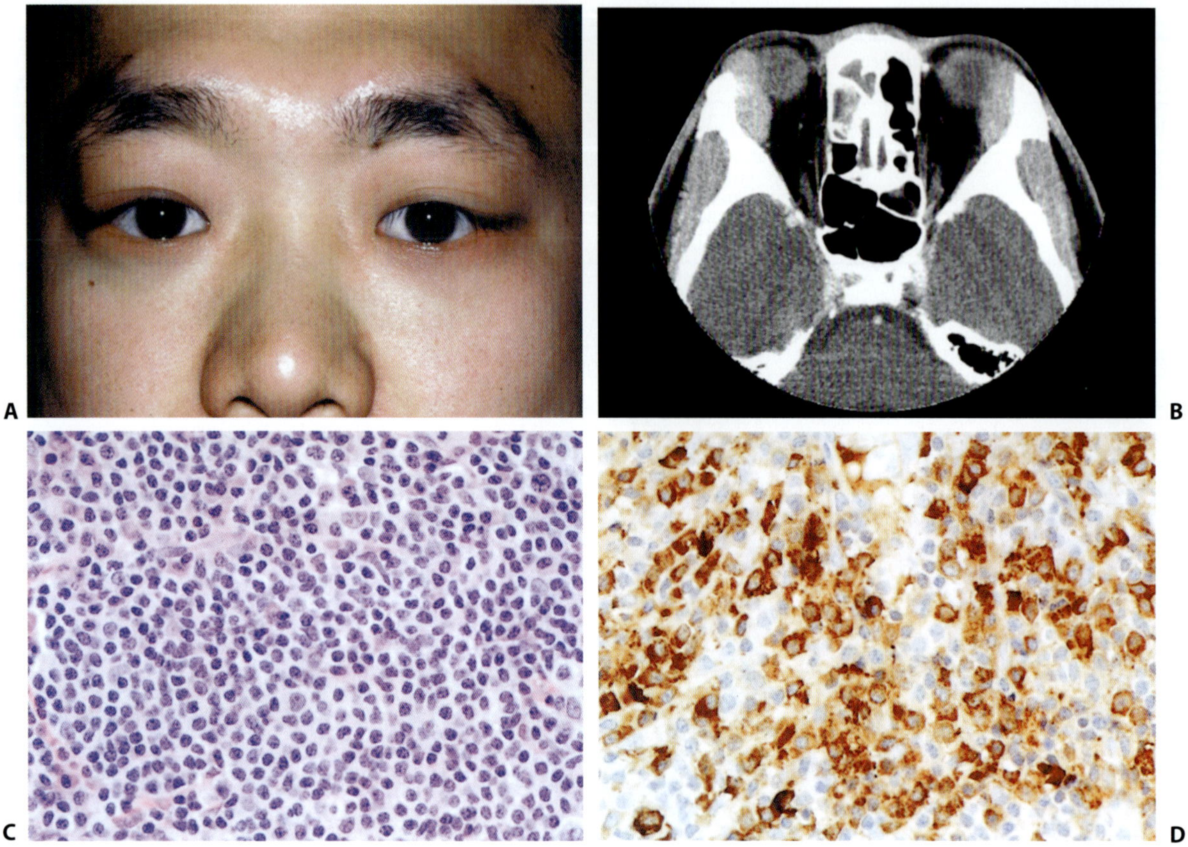

FIGURE 18.3. Lymphoma in a 26-year-old man with bilateral, nontender enlargement of the lacrimal glands. (A) Facial photograph. (B) Axial CT image shows diffuse enlargement of the lacrimal glands that is smooth in outline, of homogeneous density, and molds around the eyeball. (C) Low-grade, marginal zone B-cell lymphoma is composed of small lymphocytes [H&E, original magnification ×400]. (D) Immunohistochemical stain shows monoclonality of tumor cells for kappa light chain (original magnification ×400).

meticulous and complete removal of the intact cyst. An approach through the superior cul-de-sac with lateral cantholysis is adequate (Figure 18.5D).

PLEOMORPHIC ADENOMA (BENIGN MIXED TUMOR)

The most common benign neoplasm of the lacrimal gland is the pleomorphic adenoma. The term "benign mixed tumor" came from an earlier hypothesis, which remains popular, that these tumors derive from a mixture of epithelial and mesodermal elements. In fact, these tumors are epithelial in origin. Ductal epithelium develops into the epithelial component, and cells in the stroma and myoepithelium develop into cells in the stroma.[17] The World Health Organization proposed the name *pleomorphic adenoma*, which more accurately describes the nature of the neoplasm.

Clinical Features

Pleomorphic adenomas usually occur in the fourth and fifth decade of life, and incidence is equal for both genders.[13] However the age range is wide, and the tumor has been reported in children as young as 6 years old.[18]

Pleomorphic adenomas commonly present with symptoms of painless, unilateral progressive proptosis and downward and inward displacement of the globe (Figures 18.6A and 18.7A). These symptoms are usually present for over 12 months with no inflammatory signs. Other presenting symptoms or signs include diplopia or an ocular motility disturbance, a change in refractive error, orbital discomfort, lacrimation, ptosis, and choroidal folds. A palpable mass in the superotemporal orbital quadrant is present in most patients and is not tender.[13]

Although pleomorphic adenomas commonly involve the orbital lobe of the lacrimal gland, they can involve the palpebral lobe in about 10% of cases.[13] The palpebral lobe tumors are freely movable, nontender, and present for a shorter duration. They do not produce proptosis or bony changes.[19,20] Pleomorphic adenomas arising in the palpebral lobe are excised with some normal lacrimal gland tissue through a lid crease incision.[19]

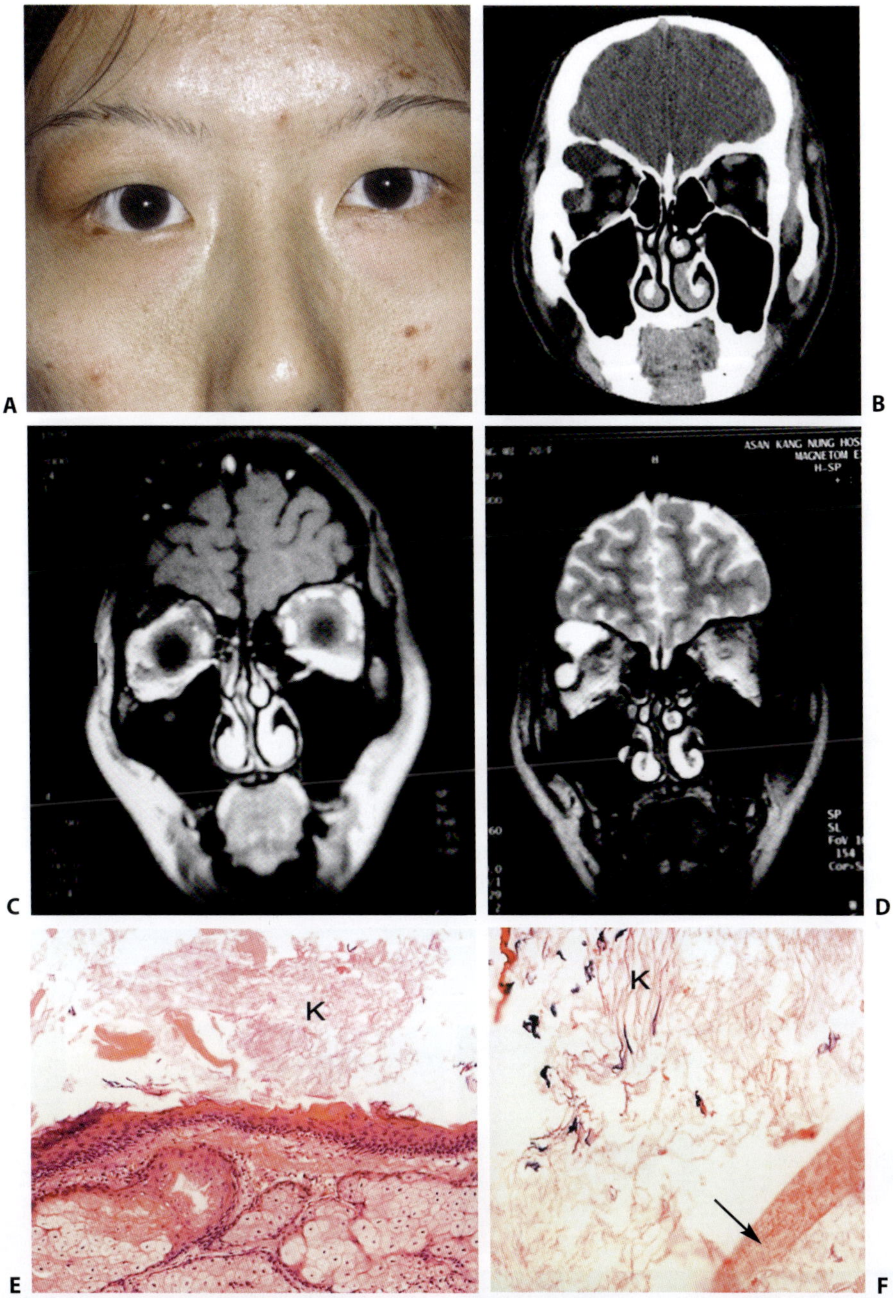

FIGURE 18.4. (A) Dermoid cyst in a 21-year-old woman who had experienced slowly progressive proptosis of the right eye for several years. (A) Facial photograph. (B) Coronal CT image shows a large cystic mass that erodes the superior and lateral walls of the orbit. (C) T1-weighted MR image shows a low-intensity mass with no enhancement. (D) The mass shows high intensity on a T2-weighted MR image. (E) The cyst wall is lined by well-differentiated epidermal and dermal tissues containing all the skin appendages (H&E, original magnification ×100). (F) The cystic lumen is filled with keratin materials (K), sebum and hairs (arrow) (H&E, original magnification ×200).

Radiologic Features

CT images show round to oval, well-defined lesions that are smooth in outline, displacing and deforming the globe (Figure 18.6B,C). The contrast enhancement is moderate to marked. Some long-standing large tumors show lobulations and radiolucent areas of cystic degeneration. In the bone window, the lacrimal fossa is prominent owing to pressure erosion. This condition can progress to a defect in the orbital roof with contact of tumor and dura.[21]

On MRI the tumor is of low signal intensity on the T1-weighted image and of high signal intensity on the T2-weighted image, frequently of heterogeneous distribution. The contrast enhancement is intense (Figure 18.7B). Large tumors can show liquefied portions centrally (Figure 18.8). The pseudocapsule may appear

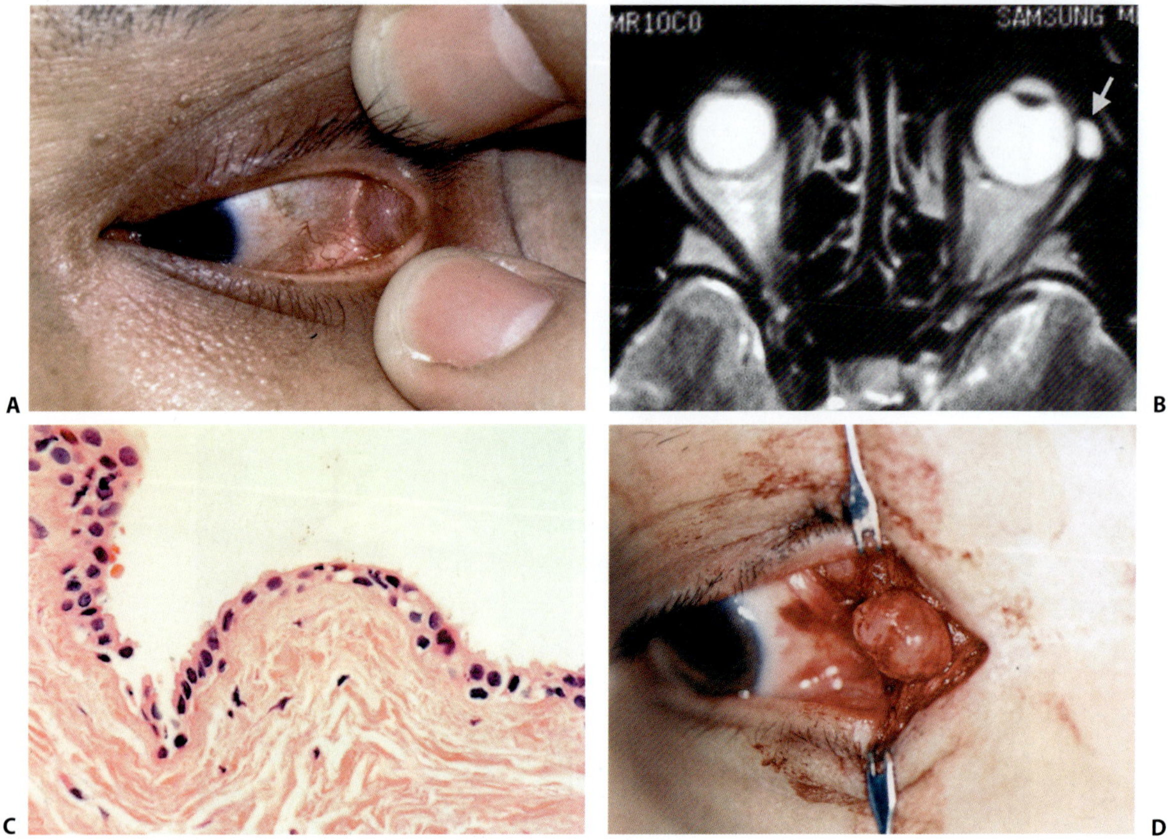

FIGURE 18.5. Dacryops. (A) The transilluminating, cystic mass is visible through the conjunctiva. (B) T2-weighted MR image showing a cystic mass. (C) Histopathologically, the cyst wall is lined by two layers of epithelial cells (H&E, original magnification ×400). (D) The mass is excised by lateral cantholysis.

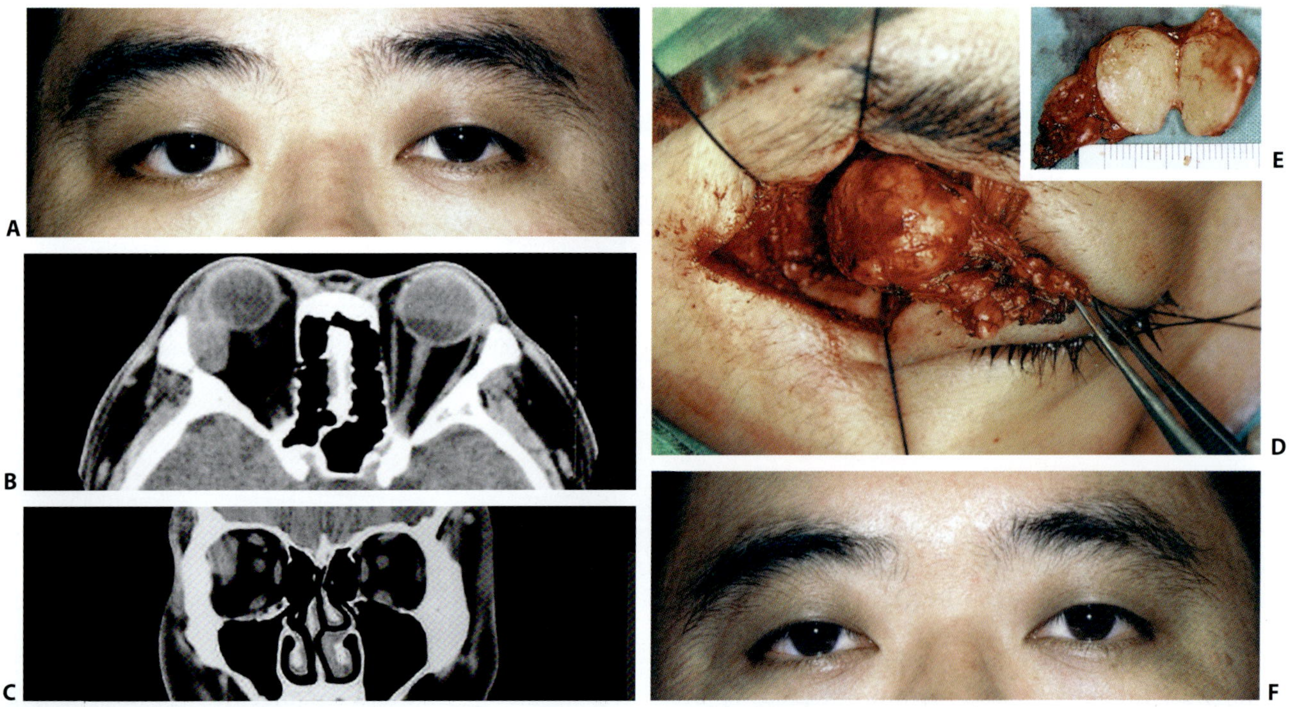

FIGURE 18.6. Pleomorphic adenoma in a 33-year-old man who had experienced progressive proptosis and inferior dystopia of right eye for 1 year. (A) Facial photograph. (B) Axial and (C) coronal CT images show well-defined oval mass with smooth excavation of the adjacent orbital bone. (D) The tumor, inside its pseudocapsule, is removed along with surrounding lacrimal gland. (E) The cut surface shows hyalinized appearance. (F) The patient one year after operation; there had been no recurrences.

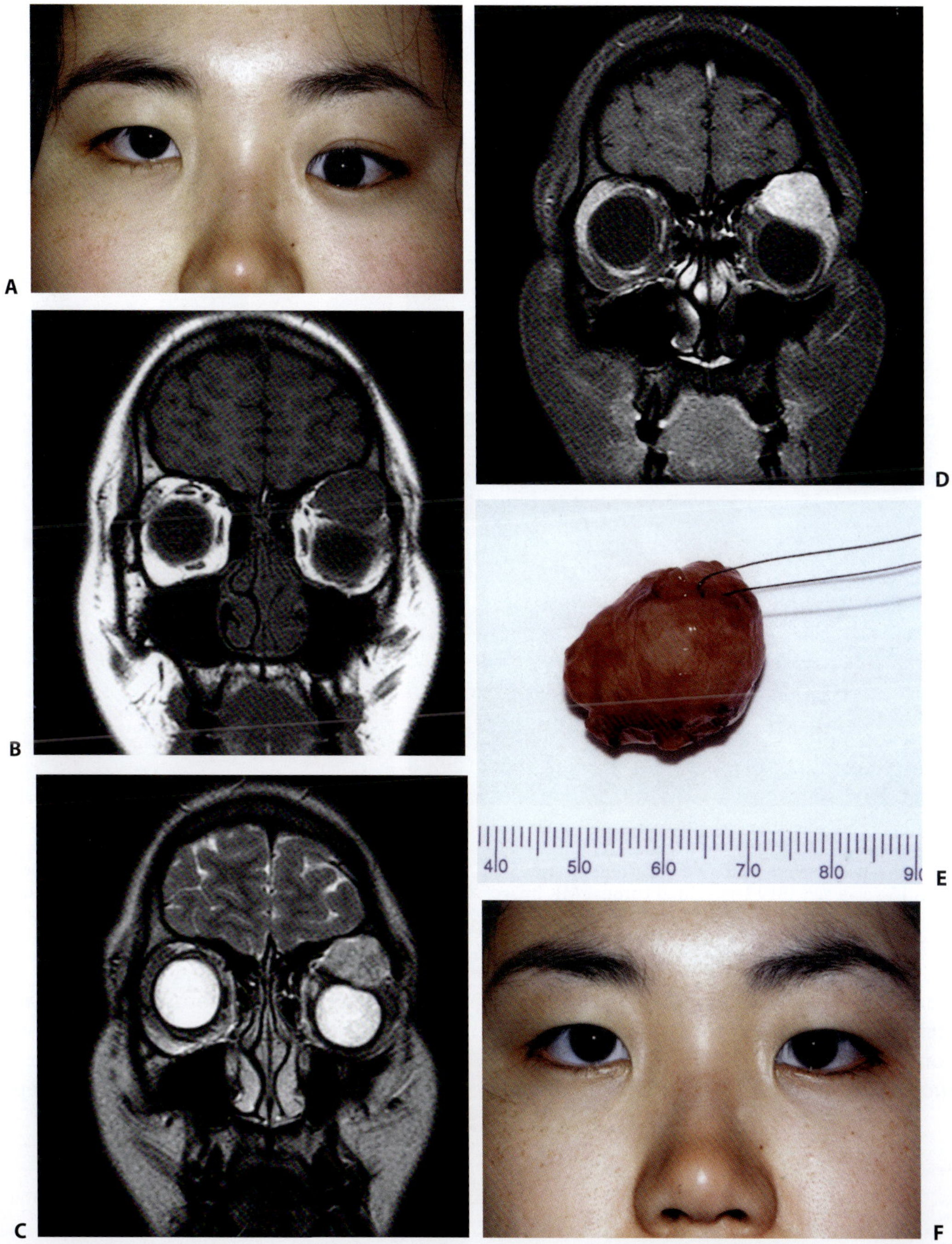

FIGURE 18.7. Pleomorphic adenoma in a 19-year-old woman who presented with slowly progressive proptosis and had experienced downward displacement of the left eye for 3 years. (A) Facial photograph. (B) T1-weighted coronal image shows well-demarcated lacrimal gland mass of low signal intensity with pressure erosion of the superior orbital wall. (C) T2-weighted coronal image shows mass of high signal intensity; the globe is deformed by the mass. (D) After gadolinium DTPA enhancement, visibility of details of the mass is markedly improved. (E) The tumor is excised with its capsule intact. (F) Photograph taken 2 years after the operation demonstrating no tumor recurrence.

as a linear rim of low signal intensity on T1- and T2-weighted images.[21]

Pathology

Grossly, the tumor is grayish white, bosselated, solitary, and well circumscribed by a thin pseudocapsule formed by compressed adjacent tissue and reactive fibrosis. Small tumor cell nests may be seen outside the pseudocapsule; these cause a high incidence of recurrence when a margin of normal tissue is not removed with the tumor. Their cut surfaces show soft mucinous areas alternating with tough fibrous areas.

Histopathologic examination shows the mixture of epithelial and mesenchymal elements that led to the term "benign mixed tumor." As noted earlier, how-

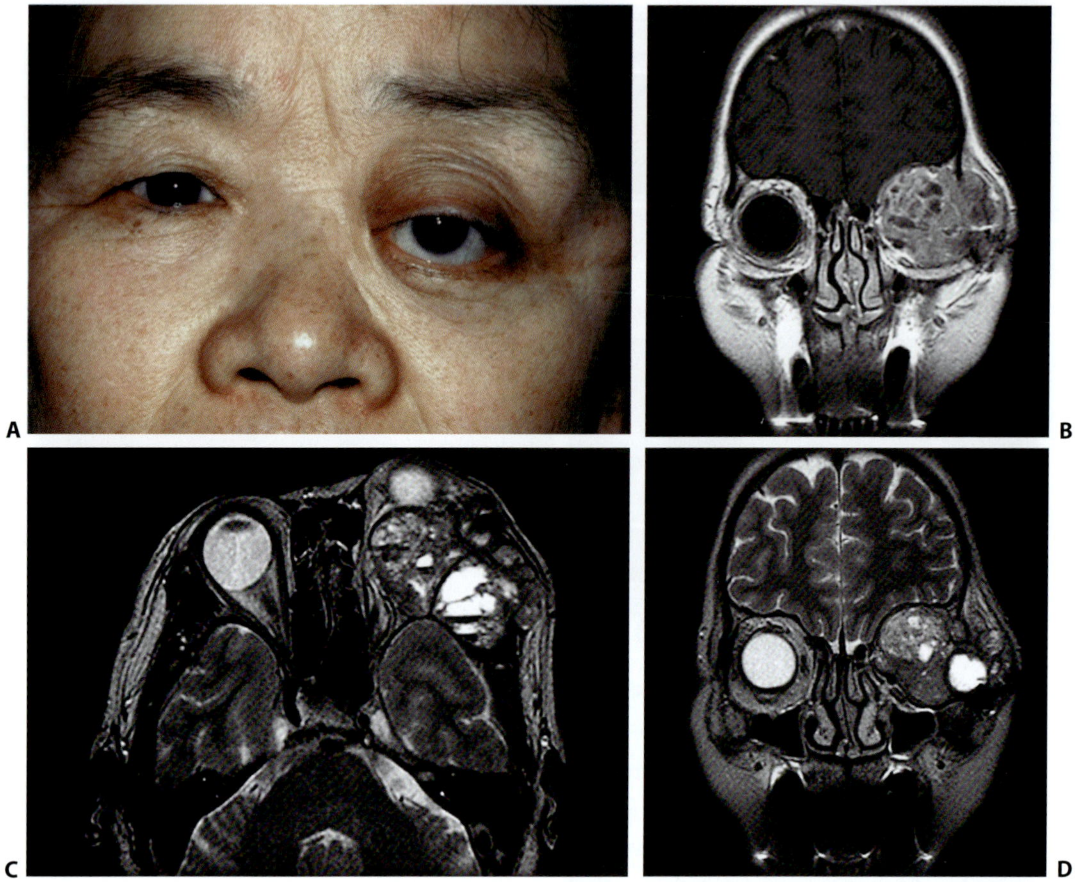

FIGURE 18.8. Pleomorphic adenoma. (A) A 68-year-old woman had had long-standing proptosis and downward displacement of the left eye for 30 years. She had experienced two recurrences after incomplete removal 15 years ago. (B) T1-weighted coronal MR image shows the huge mass of heterogeneous intensity filling the entire orbital cavity and extending into the temporal fossa. The focal area of low-signal intensity in the tumor mass demonstrates the area of cystic degeneration. T2-weighted axial (C) and coronal (D) MR images demonstrate a huge mass with focal areas of high signal intensity and fluid–fluid level of cystic degeneration.

ever, immunohistochemical studies support the hypothesis that this tumor arises from pleomorphism of epithelial components rather than a mixed origin.[17] Thus *pleomorphic adenoma* is the more preferable term. The epithelial components are variably sized ducts containing an inner cuboidal to columnar epithelium and an outer flattened, spindle-shaped myoepithelial layer (Figure 18.9A). The myoepithelial cells

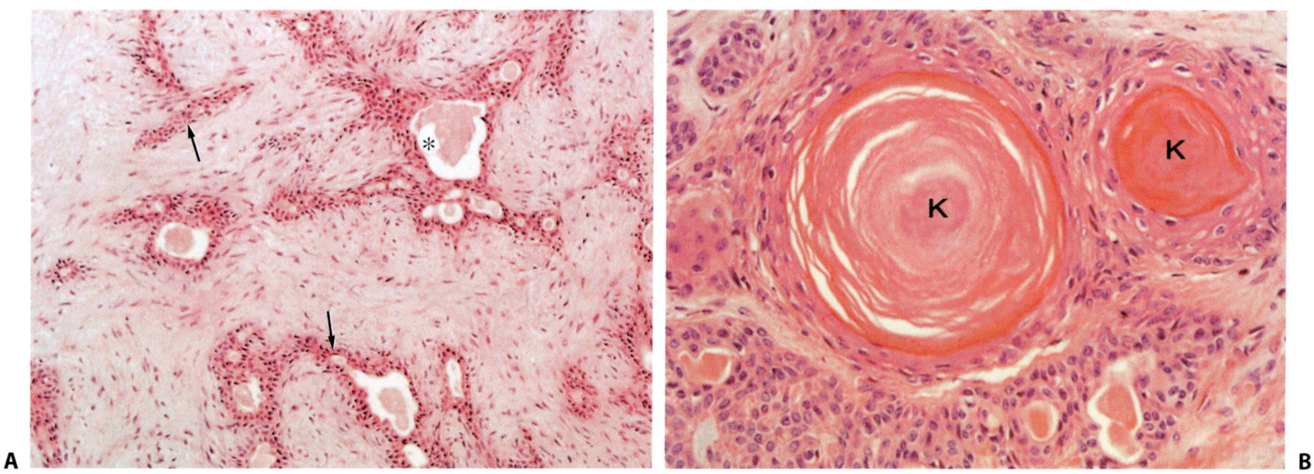

FIGURE 18.9. Pleomorphic adenoma. (A) Histopathologic appearance of the tumor shows the myxomatous matrix and cords of epithelial cells. Duct formation is apparent, with ducts lined with a double layer of cuboidal cells, surrounded by myoepithelial cells (arrows). Secreted eosinophilic material (asterisk) is present in the lumen of the duct (*) (H&E, original magnification ×100). (B) Focal area of squamous metaplasia with keratin formation (K) (H&E, original magnification ×200).

undergo metaplasia to form myxoid tissue, cartilage, and bone. Focal squamous metaplasia and keratin production may be observed (Figure 18.9B).[6,22]

Management and Prognosis

The best management is complete excision of the tumor within its pseudocapsule via a lateral orbitotomy (Figures 18.6D and 18.7E). To minimize any tumor seeding from microscopic extensions through the pseudocapsule, an adequate margin of the surrounding lacrimal gland and the adjacent periorbita should be removed in the extirpation.[6,13] In some cases, small satellite nodules of pleomorphic adenoma may be left behind even after careful in toto excision of the main mass. Therefore, it is good practice to inspect the surgical bed and ensure that no residual tumor nodules remain. When properly handled, the prognosis of pleomorphic adenomas is excellent (Figures 18.6F and 18.7F). Some advocate additional removal of the palpebral lobe of the lacrimal gland with excretory ductules to reduce the recurrence rate.[9] However, preservation of the palpebral lobe greatly reduces the incidence of postoperative dry eye and the need for topical lubricants.[13]

Font and Gamel[4] have emphasized the high recurrence rate following incomplete excision or incisional biopsy. The 5-year recurrence rate was 3% for completely excised lesions and 32% for incompletely excised tumors. Recurrent pleomorphic adenoma can undergo malignant change. Font and Gamel[4] estimated that about 10% of adenomas undergo malignant change by 20 years after first treatment and 20% by 30 years. Because biopsy of pleomorphic adenomas can have disastrous consequences, these tumors should be diagnosed before surgery so that biopsy can be avoided. For patients with pleomorphic adenoma who have had a biopsy, the biopsy track and skin scar are excised in continuity with a total removal of lacrimal gland.[13]

MALIGNANT MIXED TUMOR

The reported incidence of the malignant mixed tumor has ranged from 4 to 15% of the epithelial tumors of the lacrimal gland.[2,4,6,8,23] A malignant mixed tumor represents a pleomorphic adenoma that has undergone malignant degeneration. Patients with malignant mixed tumors tend to be older than those with pleomorphic adenoma. Font and Gamel[4] described different sex ratios for subtypes of these tumors. Men are more often affected by an adenocarcinoma arising from pleomorphic adenoma, whereas women are more often affected by an adenoid cystic carcinoma arising from pleomorphic adenoma.

Clinical Features

Malignant mixed tumors usually present in three clinical ways. First, the patient whose benign mixed tumor was not removed totally may develop a sudden recurrence several years later (Figure 18.10A). Second, the patient with indolent long-standing lacrimal tumor history presents with sudden expansion of the mass, as well as pain and swelling of the upper eyelid. Third, the patient has rapidly developing symptoms of pain and bone destruction, and the tumor is diagnosed as malignant at the first presentation. The third presentation could be considered to be de novo.[6,23,24]

Radiologic Features

On CT, an enlarged lacrimal fossa surrounded by bone destruction means malignant tumors. The bone window shows the osseous changes best. Contrast enhancement helps to reveal involvement of the dura and intracranial extension. It is not possible to differentiate malignant mixed tumor from other carcinomas of the lacrimal gland on CT.[15,21] At times, carcinoma in pleomorphic adenoma may have a smooth contour and no bony changes (Figure 18.10B,C).

Pathology

Malignant mixed tumors have the histologic features of a benign mixed tumor with areas of malignant change. In most cases the malignant elements are poorly differentiated adenocarcinoma (Figure 18.10D, E). The other malignant elements are adenoid cystic carcinoma, squamous cell carcinoma, and, rarely, spindle cell sarcoma.[4,23,24]

Management and Prognosis

When preoperative evaluation indicates a malignant tumor, the recommended therapy is transseptal biopsy followed by complete removal of the tumor. Henderson and Neault[25] proposed a one-stage procedure for the surgical removal of the tumor and adjacent adnexa: an en bloc resection of the neoplasm, its periorbital base, and surrounding bone. A radical orbitectomy with regional and cervical lymph node dissection has been advised because an adenocarcinoma arising in a benign mixed tumor may disseminate early via lymphatics. Postoperative radiotherapy may also be recommended.[22,26] If metastases have occurred, treatment is often limited to surgical debulking followed by postoperative radiotherapy.

Even with extensive surgery, patient mortality remains high. Font and Gamel[4] reported that 30% of their patients had died of a tumor at 5 years, 45% at 11 years, and 50% by 12 years. Henderson[6] described 8 of the 9 patients who died during the mean follow-

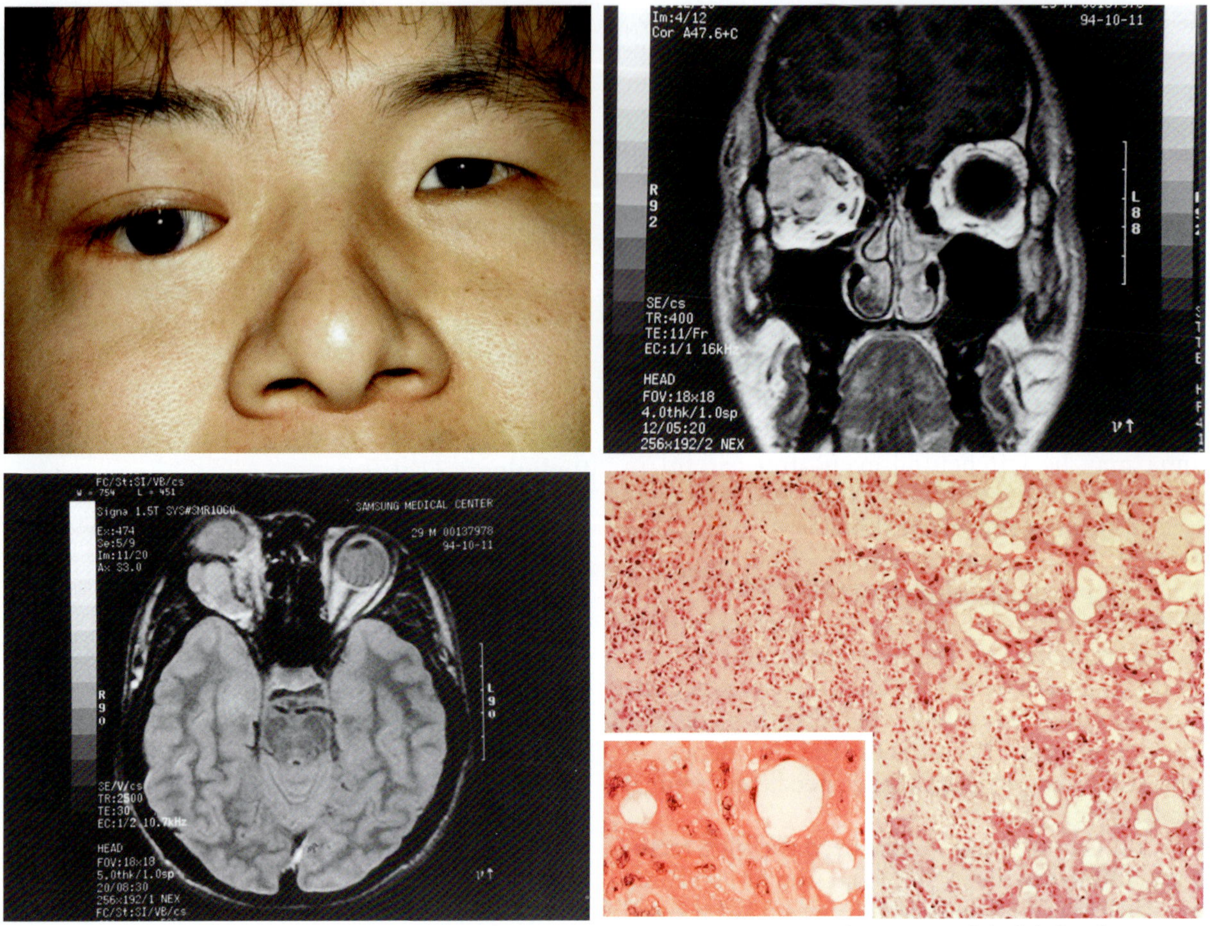

FIGURE 18.10. Malignant mixed tumor. (A) A 28-year-old male presented with a 12-year history of proptosis and downward displacement of the right eye. He experienced multiple recurrences of incompletely excised pleomorphic adenomas for 10 years. The globe was 11 mm proptosed and became frozen in all directions over a 6-month period. (B) Proton-density axial MR image shows a large, lobulated soft tissue mass extends backward along the lateral wall of the right orbit. (C) Coronal enhanced T1-weighted image demonstrates homogeneous enhancement of the lobulated mass. Note erosion of the superolateral bony wall. (D) Histopathologic examination of the tumor shows adjacent area of a benign mixed tumor on the left with solid epithelial tubules on the right indicating malignant transformation (H&E, original magnification ×100). *Inset*: The epithelial component showing the features of the adenocarcinoma (H&E, original magnification ×400).

up period of 14.1 years. The longest survival was 30 years in a patient whose original tumor was benign. Henderson introduced the concept that patients whose original tumor was benign will live longer (mean 19.2 years) than patients with tumors of the de novo type (mean 7.7 years). The cause of death is intracranial extension of the tumor and distant metastases to lung, chest wall, or bone.

ADENOID CYSTIC CARCINOMA

Adenoid cystic carcinoma is the second most common epithelial tumor of the lacrimal gland and the most common malignant epithelial tumor of the lacrimal gland. It accounts for about 1.6% of all orbital tumors and 3.8% of all primary orbital tumors.[6] It occurs in both sexes. Patients are about 40 years of age at presentation, with a range of 6.5 to 79 years.[14,27] Wright and associates suggested a bimodal peak in the fourth and sixth decades.[14] Because this tumor may present at an earlier age, a high clinical suspicion is indicated for any unilateral mass in the upper temporal quadrant, even in teenagers and children, where these tumors might be mistaken for dermoids.[27–29]

Clinical Features

A patient with adenoid cystic carcinoma presents mass effect with a more rapid temporal sequence usually under 1 year (Figures 18.11A, 18.12A, and 18.13A). The presenting symptoms are pain, globe displacement, mass or swelling, numbness, diplopia, visual change, lacrimation, and ptosis. Because this tumor invades perineurally and into adjacent bone, there may be pain and, more rarely, numbness. The reported in-

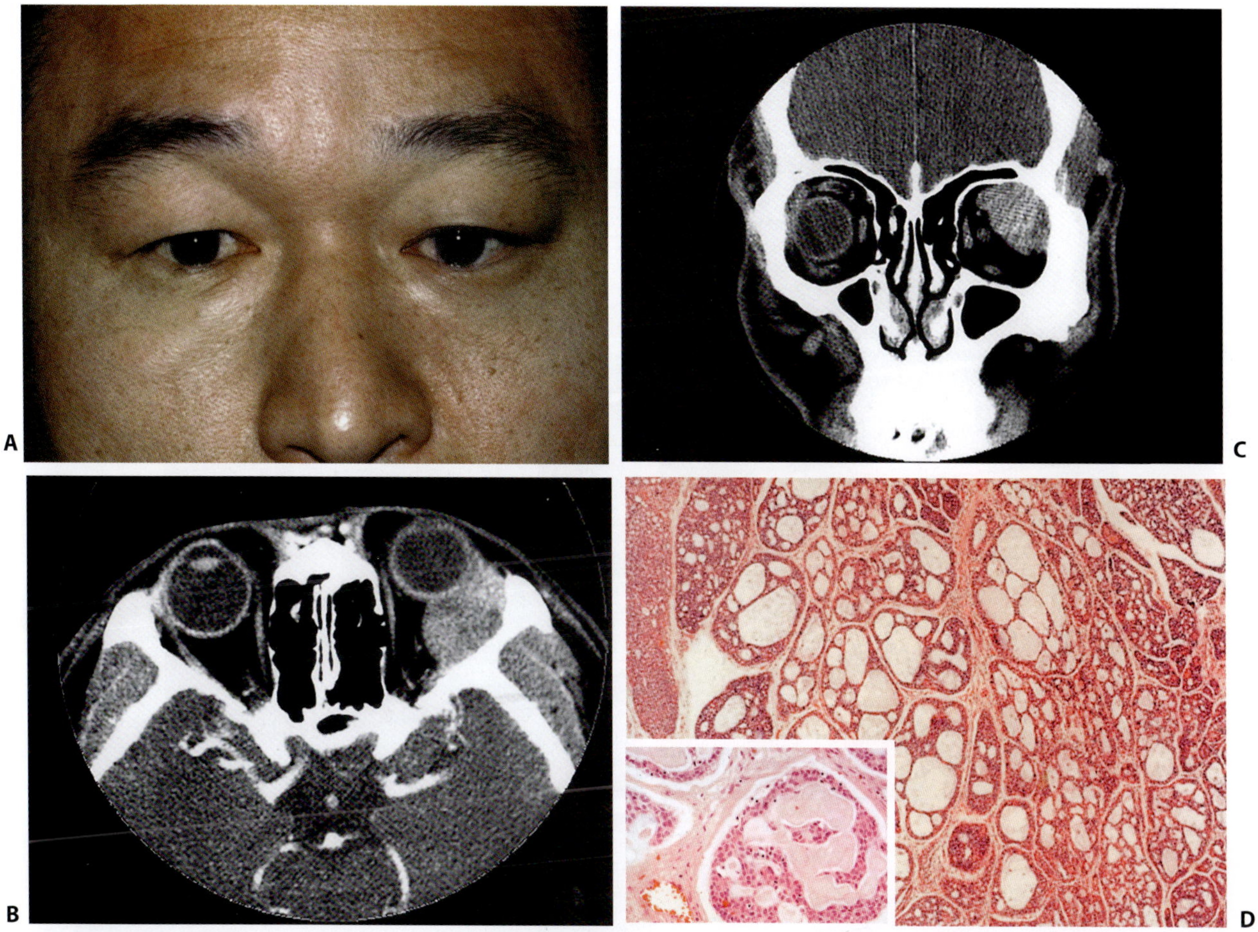

FIGURE 18.11. Adenoid cystic carcinoma. (A) A 40-year-old man presenting proptosis of the left eye for 5 months. (B) Axial and (C) coronal CT images show well-defined oval mass with pressure erosion of the adjacent orbital bone. (D) Histopathologically, the tumor proved to be an adenoid cystic carcinoma with a typical cribriform (Swiss cheese) pattern (H&E, original magnification ×40). *Inset*: Glandlike spaces (pseudocysts) are filled with eosinophilic basal lamina materials (H&E, original magnification ×200).

cidence of pain is variable, between 37.5 and 79%.[6,14,30]

Radiologic Features

High-resolution CT shows more elongated mass extending along the lateral orbital wall, with expansion of the lacrimal fossa with bone invasion.[15,31] This tumor can be globular or round and usually reveals more irregular and serrated borders than those seen in pleomorphic adenoma (Figures 18.11B,C, 18.12B, and 18.13B). In the series of Wright and colleagues', CT abnormalities consisted of bone erosion (75%), bone destruction (34%), and soft tissue calcification (22%).[14] High-resolution CT with bone windows is recommended. Contrast enhancement helps to reveal involvement of the dura and intracranial extension.

MRI with enhancement is best for assessing the invasion of the tumor into the cavernous sinus, brain, and bone marrow (Figures 18.12C and 18.13C). The tumor is hypointense on the T1-weighted image and hyperintense on the T2-weighted image with contrast enhancement.

Pathology

The gross appearance of adenoid cystic carcinoma is grayish-white, firm, nodular, and deceivingly circumscribed. The tumor is more difficult to dissect during surgery than a pleomorphic adenoma.

Microscopically, five histologic patterns have been described: cribriform ("Swiss cheese") (Figure 18.11D), solid (basaloid), sclerosing, comedocarcinomatous, and tubular (ductal), in order of frequency.[32] All or several of these patterns may be present in one tumor, but one pattern usually predominates. In Gamel and Font's series of 54 adenoid cystic carcinomas, patients with a basaloid pattern in their tumor had a 5-year survival rate of 21% and a median survival of 3 years, whereas patients whose tumor contained no trace of a basaloid component had a 5-year survival rate of 71% and a median survival of 8 years.[32] In a study of

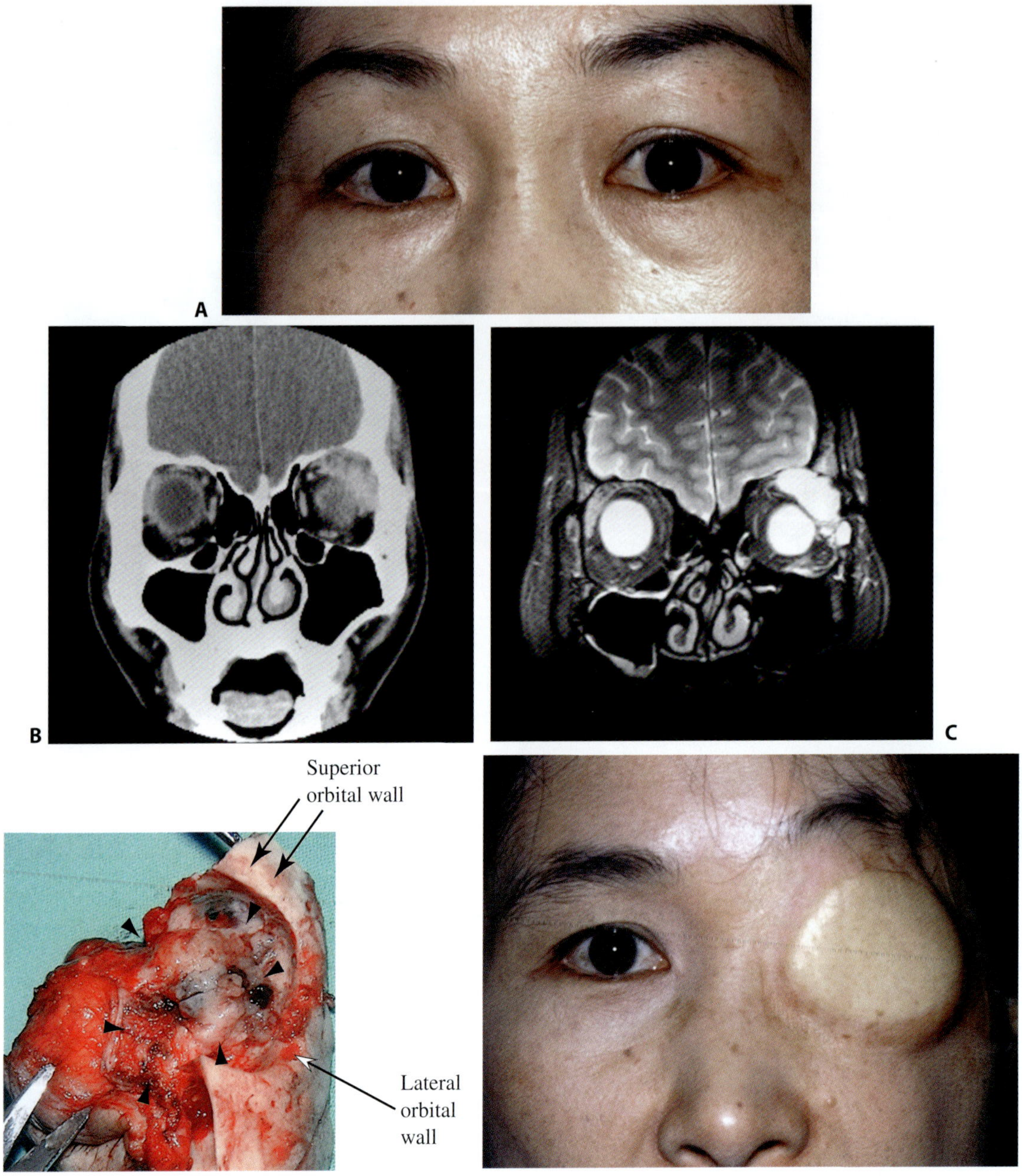

FIGURE 18.12. Adenoid cystic carcinoma. (A) A 39-year-old woman developed painful swelling of left eyelid and headache from several months ago. She had undergone lateral orbitotomy 13 years earlier to remove an unknown benign tumor of the left lacrimal gland. There is 2 mm of proptosis in her left eye. Firm, tender mass is palpable in the left lacrimal gland area. (B) Coronal CT scan of the orbit shows heterogeneously enhancing mass in superolateral portion of the left orbit with excavation of adjacent bone. (C) T2-weighted coronal MR image shows well-defined mass lesion, which, from the superotemporal portion of the left orbit, invades the bony cortex of the superior and lateral wall of the orbit. (D) An orbitozygomatic approach was used to perform radical orbital exenteration with removal of superior and lateral orbital wall. Solid arrows indicate the tumor. (E) The orbital defect was reconstructed with calvarian bone graft and rectus abdominis free flap. This photograph was taken 6 months after the operation.

26 orbital adenoid cystic carcinomas by Lee et al., the "Swiss cheese" pattern was associated with longer survival and the basaloid pattern was not.[30] The basaloid pattern may occur more frequently in patients older than 40 years and is associated with a reduction in estimated disease-free survival.[14]

Perineural invasion is frequently observed in exenteration specimens, accounting for the symptoms of pain and numbness. Tumor cells tend to infiltrate the contiguous bone of the lacrimal fossa to produce the bony changes observed in radiologic studies.

Management and Prognosis

The optimal treatment for patients with adenoid cystic carcinoma has yet to be determined. Tumor removal and postoperative radiotherapy comprise the most common treatment. The surgical techniques of

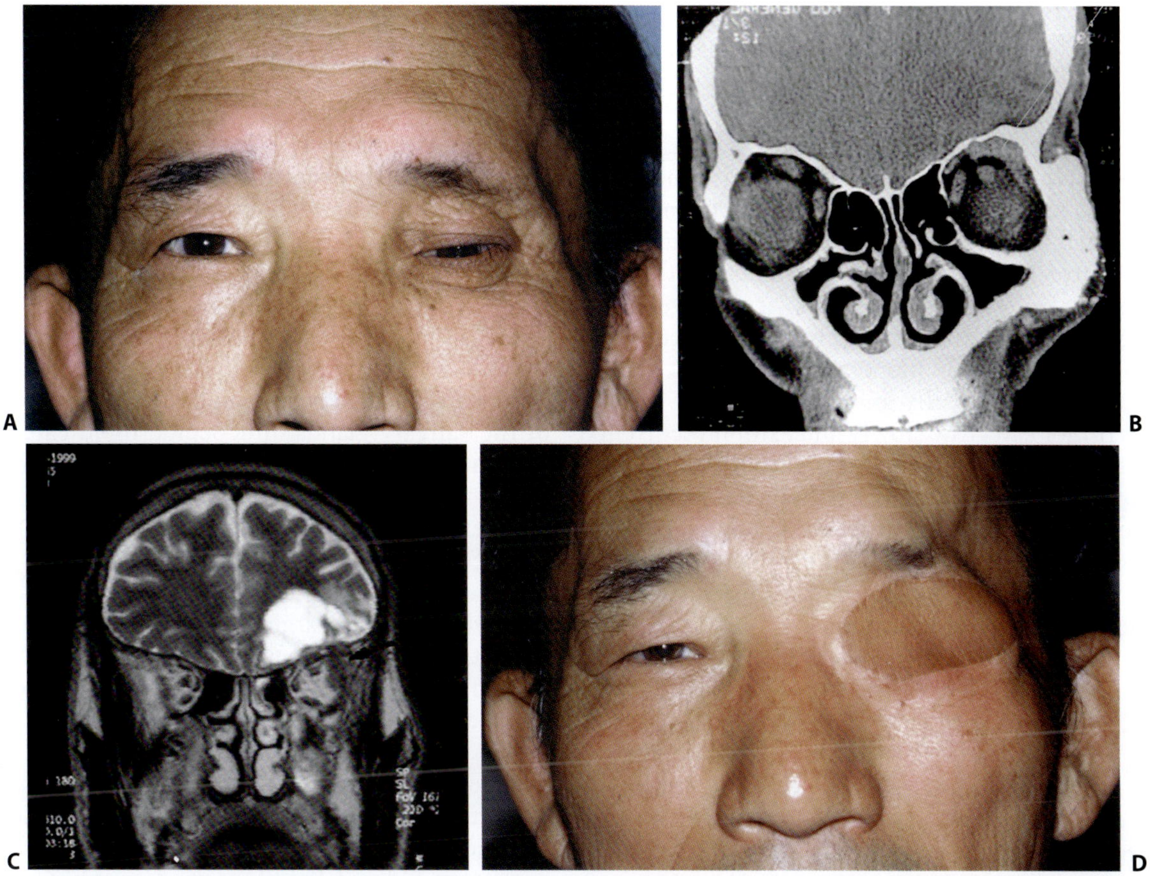

FIGURE 18.13. Adenoid cystic carcinoma. (A) A 57-year-old man had undergone tumor removal by lateral orbitotomy 12 years earlier for adenoid cystic carcinoma of the left lacrimal gland. There were perineural and adjacent bony invasion at that time. He received radiation therapy right after the operation. Upon developing motor aphasia, he visited our clinic. There is 2 mm of proptosis in his left eye. The left upper eyelid is ptotic and hard mass is palpable in the upper lid. The upward movement of the eye is restricted. (B) Coronal CT scan of the orbit shows tubular mass in superolateral portion of the left orbit with excavation of adjacent bone. (C) T2-weighted coronal MR image shows a well-defined 3.5 cm cystic lesion in the left basal frontal lobe from previous radiation necrosis and a tubular mass lesion in superotemporal portion of the left orbit that is isosignal with muscle. (D) Incisional biopsy of the orbital mass revealed recurrence of adenoid cystic carcinoma. Radical orbital exenteration with removal of surrounding orbital wall was performed through orbitozygomatic approach. The intracranial cyst was removed and dura was sutured. The orbital defect was reconstructed with splitted calvarian bone graft and rectus abdominis free flap. There has been no recurrence after 5 years.

tumor removal include local resection, en bloc removal, exenteration, and radical exenteration (radical orbitectomy).[25,33–37] Radical exenteration with removal of the orbital roof, the lateral wall, and the anterior portion of the temporalis muscle where the zygomaticofrontal and zygomaticotemporal nerves extend has been recommended (Figures 18.12D,E and 18.13D). Even with this radical approach, the survival rate has been 20% at 10 years, and the median survival was 5 years.[32] Patients usually die of intracranial spread as a result of perineural invasion and pulmonary metastasis. In one series, cranio-orbital resection did not reduce the incidence of recurrence but might lead to improved survival.[14]

Radiation therapy in the dose of 50 to 60 Gy after local resection of adenoid cystic carcinoma significantly delays the onset of tumor recurrence and prolongs survival. It might be as effective as cranio-orbital resection with radiotherapy.[14] Our experience also shows that good tumor control can be obtained in lesions that have local disease and contiguous spread. We have treated 5 patients with adenoid cystic carcinoma who refused radical exenteration with local resection and adjuvant radiation therapy, and the results were good during a 13- to 17-year follow-up. This is, however, too short a follow-up period to permit us to draw final conclusions. One interesting surviving patient in our series had undergone tumor removal by lateral orbitotomy and radiation therapy for adenoid cystic carcinoma of the left lacrimal gland, 17 years earlier, at which time there were perineural and adjacent bony invasions. Twelve years later motor aphasia from radiation necrosis of the frontal lobe developed. A recurrent tumor was diagnosed by radiologic studies and managed by radical orbital exenteration with removal of surrounding orbital wall. There has been no recurrence or metastasis to date (5-year follow-up, Figure 18.13). This case is noteworthy because the patient was able to avoid destructive surgery for 12 years.

Implanted sources of radiation (brachytherapy) have been tried on 7 patients with adenoid cystic carcinoma and have yielded good results in 6 patients with an average follow-up period of 3.2 years.[38] However the long-term results are unknown.

Intra-arterial chemotherapy has recently been advocated for supplemental management. Intracarotid cisplatin and intravenous doxorubicin were used before and after exenteration and radiation with long-term survival of 9.5 and 7.5 years, respectively.[39,40] The sample size is small, but this modality could be tried for patients with inoperable tumors to shrink them to a more surgically amenable size.

This tumor can grow slowly and exhibit recurrence and metastasis years after the initial treatment. Long-term follow-up of treatment methods has been difficult to obtain. Some patients die early; others may live asymptomatically for years. A long follow-up, perhaps up to 15 years, is needed before meaningful conclusions regarding a cure can be made.

ADENOCARCINOMA

Adenocarcinoma is more common in males and tends to occur in an older population ranging from 18 to 80 years (median age 56 years).[4,6,22,41] This tumor constitutes 7% of epithelial neoplasms of the lacrimal gland.[4,6]

Adenocarcinoma metastasizes earlier and is associated with a shorter patient survival time than adenoid cystic carcinoma. It often manifests as a rapidly growing mass, exceeding the limits of adequate surgical excision at the time of presentation. The most common symptom at presentation is a palpable mass. Other symptoms included proptosis, pain, globe displacement, visual loss, diplopia, and ptosis (Figure 18.14A–C).[14,41]

Histopathologic examination shows pleomorphic cells with many mitotic figures arranged in sheets and cords, and lumen formation with mucin production (Figure 18.14D,E). The mucin content of the adenocarcinoma may be demonstrated with mucicarmine and alcian blue stains. The undifferentiated type does not show mucin production.

Management and Prognosis

In the Mayo Clinic series, adenocarcinoma showed great malignancy. Four of the 5 patients died of the tumor, with a mean survival of only 1.5 years from initial presentation. The shorter survival of the patients with adenocarcinoma probably is related to early lymphatic dissemination to regional lymph nodes and pulmonary metastasis. Henderson recommended a monobloc craniofacial orbitectomy combined with a regional lymph node dissection for longer survival.[6]

In a retrospective study of 13 patients with adenocarcinoma, 4 of 7 patients who received exenteration followed by radiation therapy were alive without recurrence.[41] The authors recommend treatment of primary adenocarcinoma of the lacrimal gland with exenteration and radiation therapy as soon as a diagnosis has been confirmed pathologically.

MUCOEPIDERMOID CARCINOMA

Although it is the most common primary carcinoma of the salivary glands, mucoepidermoid carcinoma is rare in the lacrimal gland. The age range of mucoepidermoid carcinoma patients is 12 to 81 years,[6,42] with an average of 49 years; there is a slight (3:2) preponderance of males over females.[43]

Mucoepidermoid carcinoma usually presents as a painless, slowly enlarging mass of the lacrimal gland fossa that is sometimes mistaken preoperatively for benign mixed tumor.[6,42] Pain, proptosis, diplopia, and globe displacement may occur.

Histologically, these tumors comprise various numbers of mucus-secreting cells interspersed with epidermoid and basal cells. Mucus-secreting cells can assume a signet ring appearance and stain positively with periodic acid–Schiff stain, Alcian blue, and mucicarmine dyes. It is classified as either low or high grade depending on the degree of differentiation and the number of mucin-producing cells. Grade 1(low-grade) tumors have large, well-differentiated cells with abundant cytoplasm, a relative paucity of the epidermoid cells, and no mitotic figures. Grade 3 (high-grade) tumors have smaller cells with hyperchromatism and frequent mitotic figures predominated by epidermoid elements. Grade 2 tumors are intermediate in histologic activity.[43]

Management and Prognosis

The clinical behavior and prognosis parallel the histologic grading. Eviatar and Hornblass[43] reviewed a series of 25 cases of mucoepidermoid carcinoma. Seven of 8 patients with low-grade tumors survived, and 1 of 8 patients with high-grade tumors has remained tumor-free. The authors recommended exenteration, radiation, and resection of involved orbital bone for patients with high-grade tumors. Patients with low-grade tumors can be expected to do well with extirpation with or without adjuvant radiation.

OTHER TUMORS

The following lacrimal gland tumors are rarely encountered even in busy ocular oncology practices.

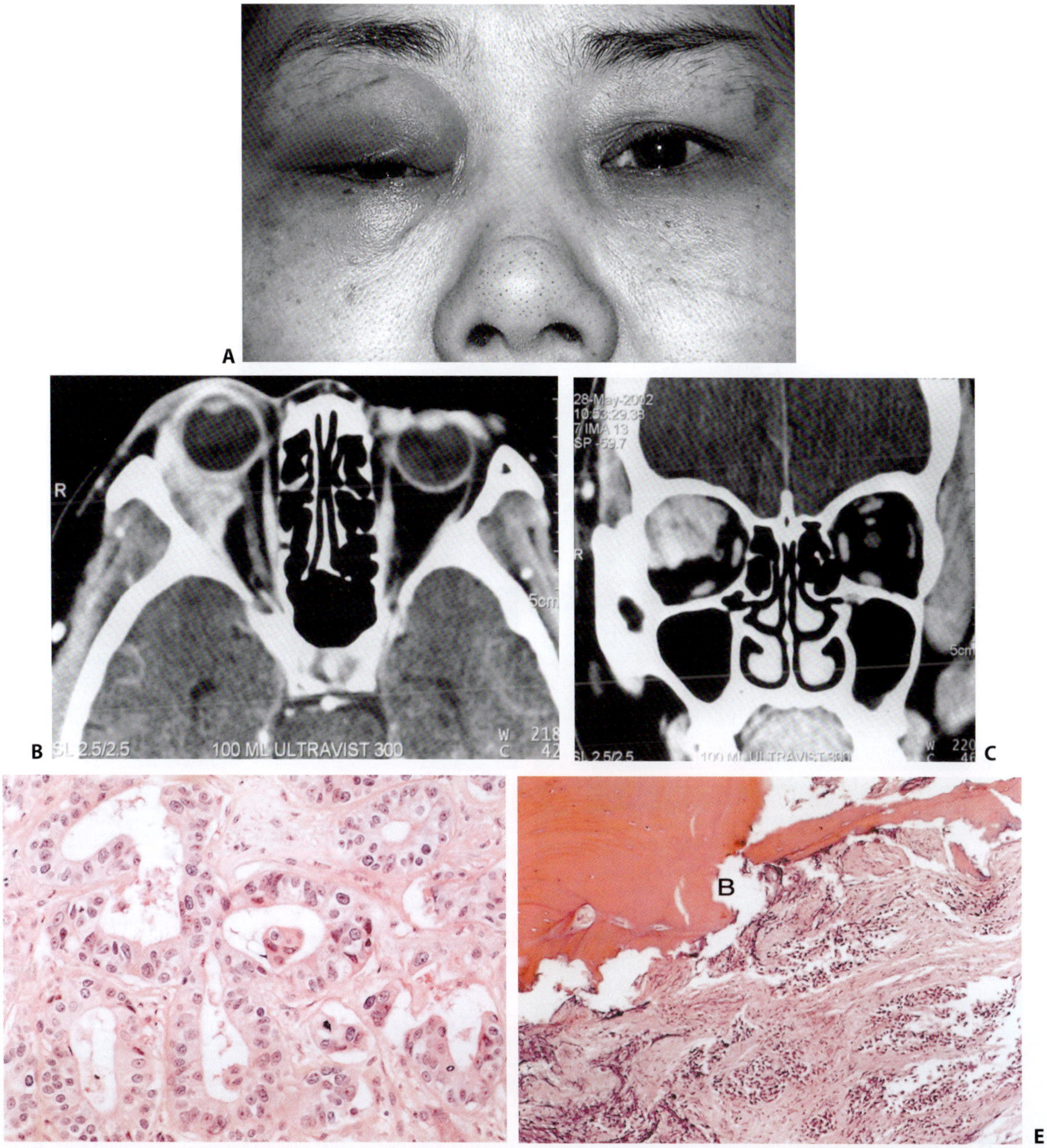

FIGURE 18.14. Adenocarcinoma. (A) A 51-year-old woman was referred with a 3-month history of right upper eyelid swelling and proptosis. She complained of deep orbital pain. Her eyelid was swollen and ptotic; there was limitation of upgaze. (B) Axial CT demonstrating an enhancing mass in the right orbit extending posteriorly in the area of the lacrimal gland. (C) Coronal CT demonstrating an enhancing mass in superolateral portion of the right orbit with excavation of adjacent bone and involvement of superior and lateral rectus muscles. (D) Histopathologic examination shows well-formed glandular or ductal structures composed of malignant epithelial cells with prominent nuclei and dark-staining cytoplasm (H&E, original magnification ×200). (E) The bone (B) is invaded by the tumor (H&E, original magnification ×100).

However, they are briefly reviewed here for the sake of completeness.

Acinic Cell Carcinoma

Acinic cell carcinoma is an uncommon tumor of salivary gland origin that comprises 2 to 4% of primary parotid gland neoplasms. There is a female preponderancc and a peak incidence in the sixth decade. Only a few cases in the lacrimal gland were reported in patients from 18 to 56 years of age.[44–46] This cancer manifests as a painless, slow-growing mass but can invade intracranially in a more aggressive manner.

Microscopically, there are four growth patterns: solid, microcystic, papillary cystic, and follicular. The solid and microcystic patterns are considered to be the most common. The reported cases were treated by tumor excision, exenteration, and exenteration with cranial bone resection, with no tumor recurrences during follow-up periods of 2.5 to 4.5 years.[44–46]

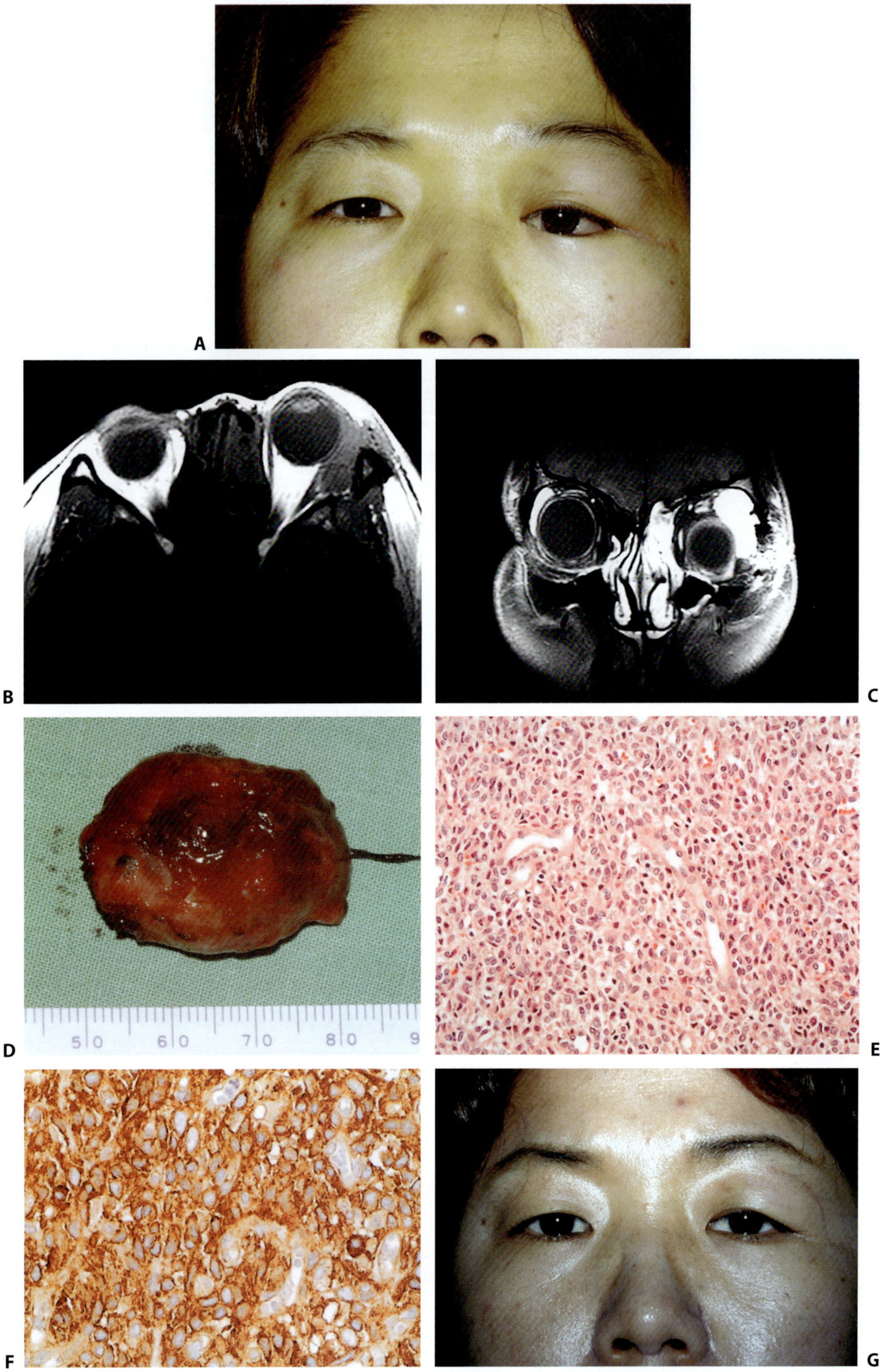

FIGURE 18.15. Solitary fibrous tumor. (A) A 27-year-old woman had had eyelid swelling, chemosis, proptosis, and inferior displacement of left eyeball for 9 months. Three months before referral, she had undergone incomplete tumor removal via lateral orbitotomy. (B) T1-weighted axial image shows well-demarcated oblongated lacrimal gland mass of low signal intensity. Lateral orbital wall is deformed from previous orbitotomy. (C) T1-weighted enhanced coronal image shows marked enhancement of the mass. (D) Complete excision of the tumor was performed via lateral orbitotomy. (E) Histopathologically, the proliferation of mesenchymal spindle cells in a collagenous stroma shows "patternless pattern." The prominent vascularity is noted (H&E original magnification ×100). (F) The tumor cells are strongly stained with antibodies to CD34 (original magnification ×400). (G) Six months after operation, there was no recurrence of tumor.

Oncocytoma (Oxyphil Cell Adenoma)

Because of their eosinophilic cytoplasm, oncocytes are also called *oxyphil cells*. These large cells with acidophilic staining properties may be found in mucous membranes such as the caruncle, conjunctiva, lacrimal sac, and lacrimal glands and seem to increase in number with age. Benign and malignant oncocytomas have been reported in the lacrimal gland. The tumors are usually benign and sometimes cystic. Malignant oncocytoma could show intracranial extension. The tumor tends to occur in older patients and is rare in children.[6,47]

Spindle Cell Myoepithelioma

Myoepithelioma is a monomorphic adenoma with a pure proliferation of myoepithelial cells. Myoepithelioma is defined as a tumor composed of myoepithelial cells with up to 10% ductal elements. The more common pleomorphic adenoma has a proliferation of both epithelial and myoepithelial elements in various combinations.[48–50]

CT scan reveals a well-circumscribed mass in superotemporal orbit. The tumor usually presents as a well-encapsulated mass and should be removed intact through a lateral orbitotomy. Most epitheliomas are benign and exhibit biological behavior similar to that of pleomorphic adenoma.[50]

Sebaceous Carcinoma

Primary sebaceous carcinoma of the lacrimal gland, possibly arising from heterotopic sebaceous tissue, is very rare. It must be differentiated from secondary invasion of the orbit by an eyelid tumor or metastatic spread. The tumor is highly malignant. Orbital exenteration, regional lymph node dissection, and postoperative radiotherapy should be considered in the management.[51,52]

Solitary Fibrous Tumor

Solitary fibrous tumor is a rare spindle cell neoplasm that most frequently develops in the pleura. This tumor usually presents with a painless unilateral proptosis with gradual onset.[53,54] CT scan shows mild remodeling of the bony orbit without calcification. Thus the clinical presentation is similar to that of pleomorphic adenoma. The management is en bloc excision via lateral orbitotomy (Figure 18.15). Generally, the aggressiveness of this tumor is associated with large tumor size, high cellularity, numerous mitoses, pleomorphism, and the presence of necrosis.[54] Solitary fibrous tumors of pleura and mediastinum demonstrated aggressive clinical behavior, such as adjacent tissue invasion, local recurrence, and distant metastases. Careful and continued follow-up is needed for this tumor because there may be recurrence after several years.

Malignant Rhabdoid Tumor

Malignant rhabdoid tumor is a rare and highly aggressive renal tumor of infants. Niffenegger et al.[55] described this tumor in a 50-year-old man. It manifested as a rapidly growing mass in the area of the right lacrimal gland. Because of the highly malignant nature of the tumor, the patient was treated with radical surgery and adjunctive radiotherapy and chemotherapy; he showed no recurrences during a 15-month follow-up period.

Hemangioma

Cavernous hemangioma, hemangioendothelioma, and epithelioid hemangioma have been reported to occur in the lacrimal gland.[56] Simple excision to preserve the lacrimal gland is sufficient treatment if the tumor is limited to the gland.[57]

Warthin Tumor

Warthin tumor frequently occurs in the parotid gland; the extraparotid localization is very rare. Bonavolonta et al.,[58] who described Warthin tumor in a 62-year-old woman, treated the patient with complete excision via lateral orbitotomy.

References

1. Reese AB. Expanding lesions of the orbit (Bowman lecture). *Trans Ophthalmol Soc U K* 1971;91:85–104.
2. Shields CL, Shields JA, Eagle RC, et al. Clinicopathologic review of 142 cases of lacrimal gland lesions. *Ophthalmology* 1989;96:431–435.
3. Font RL, Smith SL, Bryan RG.. Malignant epithelial tumors of the lacrimal gland. A clinicopathologic study of 21 cases. *Arch Ophthalmol* 1998;116:613–616.
4. Font RL, Gamel JW. Epithelial tumors of the lacrimal gland: an analysis of 265 cases. In: Jacobiec FA, ed. *Ocular and Adnexal Tumors*. Birmingham, AL: Aesculapius Publishing; 1978:787–805.
5. Ni C, Cheng SC, Dryja TP, et al. Lacrimal gland tumors: a clinicopathologic analysis of 160 cases. *Int Ophthalmol Clin* 1982;22:99–120.
6. Henderson JW. *Orbital Tumors*. 3rd ed. New York: Raven Press; 1994:323–342.
7. Wright JE. Factors affecting the survival of patients with lacrimal gland tumors. *Can J Ophthalmol* 1982;17:3–9.
8. Ashton N. Epithelial tumors of the lacrimal gland. *Mod Probl Ophthalmol* 1975;14:306–323.
9. Rootman JA. *Diseases of the Orbit: A Multidisciplinary Approach*. Philadelphia: JB Lippincott, 1988:384–405.
10. Wright JE, Stewart WB, Krohel GB. Clinical presentation and management of lacrimal gland tumours. *Br J Ophthalmol* 1979;63:600–606.
11. Jakobiec RA, Yeo JH, Trokel SL, et al. Combined clinical and computed tomographic diagnosis of primary lacrimal fossa lesions. *Am J Ophthalmol* 1982;94:785–807.

12. Som PM, Curtin HD. *Head and Neck Imaging*. St Louis: Mosby; 1996;1119–1125.
13. Rose GE, Wright JE. Pleomorphic adenoma of the lacrimal gland. *Br J Ophthalmol* 1992;76:395–400.
14. Wright JE, Rose GE, Garner A. Primary malignant neoplasms of the lacrimal gland. *Br J Ophthalmol* 1992;76:401–407.
15. Mafee MF, Edward D, Koeller KK, et al. Lacrimal gland tumors and simulating lesions. Clinicopathologic and MR imaging features. *Radiol Clin North Am* 1999;37:219–239.
16. Bullock JD, Fleishman JA, Rosset JS. Lacrimal duct cysts. *Ophthalmology* 1986;93:1355–1360.
17. Grossniklaus HE, Abbuhl MF, McLean IW. Immunohistologic properties of benign and malignant mixed tumor of the lacrimal gland. *Am J Ophthalmol* 1990;110:540–549.
18. Faktorovich EG, Crawford JB, Char DH, et al. Benign mixed tumor (pleomorphic adenoma) of the lacrimal gland in a 6-year-old boy. *Am J Ophthalmol* 1996;122:446–447.
19. Parks SL, Glover AT. Benign mixed tumors arising in the palpebral lobe of the lacrimal gland. *Ophthalmology* 1990;97:526–530.
20. Vangveeravong S, Katz SE, Rootman J, et al. Tumors arising in the palpebral lobe of the lacrimal gland. *Ophthalmology* 1996;103:1606–1612.
21. Hosten N, Bornfeld N. *Imaging of the Globe and Orbit. A Guide to Differential Diagnosis*. Stuttgart-New York: Thieme; 1998:110–122.
22. Jakobiec FA, Bilyk JR, Font RL. Lacrimal gland tumors. In: Spencer WH, ed. *Ophthalmic Pathology. An Atlas and Textbook*. 4th ed. Philadelphia: WB Saunders; 1996:2485–2525.
23. Perzin KH, Jakobiec FA, Lovolsi VA, et al. Lacrimal gland malignant mixed tumors (carcinomas arising in benign mixed tumors): a clinicopathologic study. *Cancer* 1980;45:2593–2606.
24. Henderson JW, Farrow GM. Primary malignant mixed tumors of the lacrimal gland. Report of 10 cases. *Ophthalmology* 1980;87:466–475.
25. Henderson JW, Neault RW. En bloc removal of intrinsic neoplasms of the lacrimal gland. *Am J Ophthalmol* 1976;82:905–909.
26. Jakobiec FA. In discussion of Ref 24. *Ophthalmology* 1980;87:466–475.
27. Tellad MV, McLean, Specht CS, et al. Adenoid cystic carcinomas of the lacrimal gland in childhood and adolescence. *Ophthalmology* 1997;104:1622–1625.
28. Shields JA, Shields CL, Eagle RC, et al. Adenoid cystic carcinoma of the lacrimal gland simulating a dermoid cyst in a 9-year-old boy. *Arch Ophthalmol* 1998;116:1673–1676.
29. Dagher G, Anderson RL, Ossoinig KC, et al. Adenoid cystic carcinoma of the lacrimal gland in a child. *Arch Ophthalmol* 1980;98:1098–1100.
30. Lee DA, Campbell RJ, Waller RR, et al. A clinicopathologic study of primary adenoid cystic carcinoma of the lacrimal gland. *Ophthalmology* 1985;92:128–134.
31. Lloyd GAS. Lacrimal gland tumours: the role of CT and conventional radiology. *Br J Radiol* 1981;54:1034–1038.
32. Gamel JW, Font RL. Adenoid cystic carcinoma of the lacrimal gland: the clinical significance of a basaloid histologic pattern. *Hum Pathol* 1982;13:219–225.
33. Byers RM, Berkeley RG, Luna M, et al. Combined therapeutic approach to malignant lacrimal gland tumors. *Am J Ophthalmol* 1975;79:53–55.
34. Forrest AW. Pathologic criteria for effective management of epithelial lacrimal gland tumors. *Am J Ophthalmlol* 1971;71:178–192.
35. Marsh JL, Wise DM, Smith M, et al. Lacrimal gland adenoid cystic carcinoma: intracranial and extracranial en bloc resection. *Plast Reconstr Surg* 1981;68:577–585.
36. Henderson JW. Past, present, and future surgical management of malignant epithelial neoplasia of the lacrimal gland. *Br J Ophthalmol* 1986;70:727–731.
37. Janecka I, Housepian E, Trokel S, et al. Surgical management of malignant tumors of the lacrimal gland. *Am J Surg* 1984;148:539–541.
38. Tyl JWM, Blank LECM, Koornneef L. Brachytherapy in orbital tumors. *Ophthalmology* 1997;104:1475–1479.
39. Meldrum ML, Tse DT, Benedetto P. Neoadjuvant intracarotid chemotherapy for treatment of advanced adenocystic carcinoma of the lacrimal gland. *Arch Ophthalmol* 1998;116:315–321.
40. Goldberg RA. Intra-arterial chemotherapy. A welcome new idea for the management of adenocystic carcinoma of the lacrimal gland. *Arch Ophthalmol* 1998;116:372–373.
41. Heaps RS, Miller NR, Albert DM, et al. Primary adenocarcinoma of the lacrimal gland. A retrospective study. *Ophthalmology* 1993;100:1856–1860.
42. Sofinski SJ, Brown BZ, Rao N, et al. Mucoepidermoid carcinoma of the lacrimal gland. Case report and review of the literature. *Ophthalmic Plast Reconstr Surg* 1986;2:147–151.
43. Eviatar JA, Hornblass A. Mucoepidermoid carcinoma of the lacrimal gland: 25 cases and a review and update of the literature. *Ophthalmic Plast Reconstr Surg* 1993;9:170–181.
44. DeRosa G, Zeppa P, Tranta F, et al. Acinic cell carcinoma in a lacrimal gland: first case report. *Cancer* 1986;57:1988–1991.
45. Rosenbaum PS, Mahadevia PS, Goodman LA, et al. Acinic cell carcinoma of the lacrimal gland. *Arch Ophthalmol* 1995;113:781–785.
46. Jang J, Kie JH, Lee SY, et al. Acinic cell carcinoma of the lacrimal gland with intracranial extension. *Ophthalmic Plast Reconstr Surg* 2001;17:454–457.
47. Biggs SL, Font RL. Oncocytic lesions of the caruncle and other ocular adnexa. *Arch Ophthalmol* 1977;95:474–478.
48. Heathcote JG, Hurwitz JJ, Dardick I. A spindle-cell myoepithelioma of the lacrimal gland. *Arch Ophthalmol* 1990;108:1135–1139.
49. Font RL, Garner A. Myoepithelioma of the lacrimal gland: report of a case with spindle cell morphology. *Br J Ophthalmol* 1992;76:634–636.
50. Grossniklaus HE, Wojno TH, Wilson MW, et al. Myoepithelioma of the lacrimal gland. *Arch Ophthalmol* 1997;115:1588–1590.
51. Harvey PA, Parsons MA, Rennie IG. Primary sebaceous carcinoma of lacrimal gland: a previously unreported primary neoplasm. *Eye* 1994;8:592–595.
52. Briscoe D, Mahmood S, Bonshek R, et al. Primary sebaceous carcinoma of the lacrimal gland. *Br J Ophthalmol* 2001;85:625–626.
53. Scott IU, Tanenbaum M, Rubin D, et al. Solitary fibrous tumor of the lacrimal gland fossa. *Ophthalmology* 1996;103:1613–1618.
54. Woo KI, Suh YL, Kim YD. Solitary fibrous tumor of the lacrimal sac. *Ophthalmic Plast Reconstr Surg* 1999;15:450–453.
55. Niffenegger JH, Jakobiec FA, Shore JW, et al. Adult extrarenal rhabdoid tumor of the lacrimal gland. *Ophthalmology* 1992;99:567–574.
56. Kargi S, Ozdal P, Kargi E, et al. Hemangioma of the lacrimal gland. *Plast Reconstr Surg* 2001;108:1829–1830.
57. Seiff SR, McFarland JE, Shorr N, et al. Cavernous hemangioma of the lacrimal fossa. *Ophthalmic Plast Reconstr Surg* 1986;2:21–24.
58. Bonavolonta G, Staibano S, Di Matteo G, et al. Warthin tumor of the lacrimal gland. *Am J Ophthalmol* 1997;124:857–858.

19

Tumors of the Lacrimal Drainage System

Jeffrey J. Hurwitz

The nasolacrimal sac is situated at a crossroad in the face. It is in intimate relation with the nose and ethmoid sinuses and has a close proximity to the maxillary antrum, the globe and orbit, and to the cribriform plate and ultimately to the cranial cavity. The rich blood supply and substantial lymphatic vessels in the area allow distant spread of neoplastic cells. Whereas most swellings in the nasolacrimal sac are not due to tumors, one must be aware that a tumor may exist in an occult fashion and give rise to a potentially life-threatening situation.

DIFFERENTIAL DIAGNOSIS OF MASSES IN THE LACRIMAL SAC FOSSA REGION[1]

Swellings arising in the lacrimal sac fossa region along the medial side of the nose may have two etiologies:

1. Lacrimal sac disease
2. Other diseases arising from surrounding structures

The most common lacrimal sac swelling is a lacrimal sac mucocele in which there is a blockage at the lacrimal sac–duct junction and a buildup of mucus within the sac.[2] The mucoceles may be regurgitating or nonregurgitating. The regurgitating type allows for egress of fluid, mucus, or pus through the puncta when one presses over the sac. In a nonregurgitating mucocele, there is a fluctuant swelling of the sac but no egress of fluid through the puncta. This may be due to obstruction of the puncta and/or canaliculi, a common canalicular–lacrimal sac membrane, or most frequently a kinking of the common canaliculus due to swelling of the sac that proceeds in a lateral direction. If the swelling is big enough, it may transilluminate.

Lacrimal sac stones[3] may develop within the lacrimal sac either primarily or secondary to a blockage of the sac–duct junction. These stones may be palpable through the skin overlying the lacrimal sac, but more often they lodge more deeply within the sac and/or within the nasolacrimal bony canal (Figure 19.1).

Lesions that are within the lacrimal sac fossa but not arising from the lacrimal sac may be arising from the soft tissues in the lacrimal sac fossa region, such as skin, subcutaneous glands, blood vessels, nerves, or lymphatics.[4] As well, swellings from the ethmoid sinuses, antrum, nose, or cranial cavity (meningocele and encephalocele) may produce swelling in this region.[5–8] Epistaxis, cerebrospinal fluid (CSF) leak, loss of smell, nasal stuffiness, and olfactory anesthesia are all signs that the swelling may be of ear–nose–throat origin, not primarily from the lacrimal sac.

LACRIMAL SAC TUMOR PRESENTATION

There are three presentations of lacrimal sac tumors (Table 19.1):

1. Unsuspected sac tumors
2. Suspected sac tumors
3. Known sac tumors

Unsuspected Sac Tumors

An unsuspected sac tumor may occur during a routine dacryocystorhinostomy (DCR) when the surgeon notices a hard or irregular mass within the lacrimal sac or an abnormality in the color and/or consistency of the sac mucosa. Excessive bleeding from the mucosa may also suggest a tumor.

Suspected Sac Tumors

A patient with a suspected sac tumor will present with a mass in the lacrimal sac fossa. There will be no regurgitation of the mass with pressure over it. Because the tumor arises from the mucosa and grows toward the lumen of the sac, the sac is often patent to syringing. The mass itself is nonfluctuant. Bloodstained tears are suggestive of a tumor. If there is suspicion of

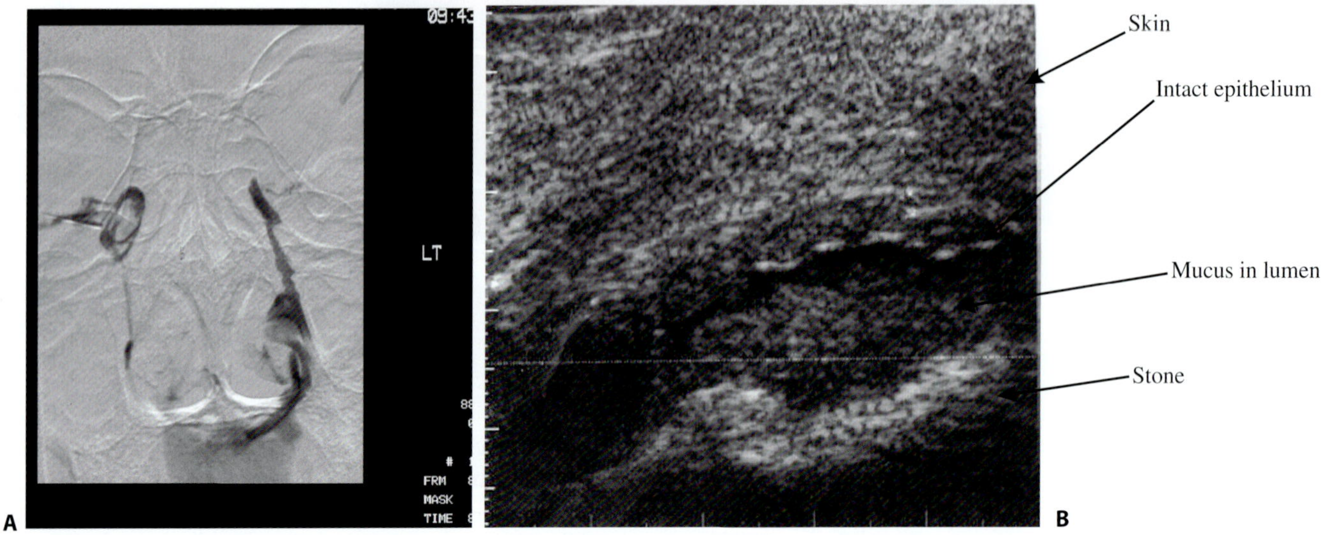

FIGURE 19.1. (A) Dacryocystogram showing large filling defects in large lacrimal sac suggestive of stones. (B) Ultrasound biomicroscopy (UBM) showing stone within sac. Epithelium is well demarcated.

a tumor, a dacryocystogram is extremely helpful diagnostically.

Known Sac Tumor

If a patient has had a biopsy of a mass in the lacrimal sac that proved to be positive for malignancy, one must determine whether the tumor is primary or has spread to the sac from elsewhere. It is also important to determine whether the tumor has spread from the sac to the surrounding tissues such as the sinus, nose, or orbit. Signs of nasosinus extension are nosebleeds, CSF leak, numbness around the roof or the nose, loss of smell, nasal stuffiness (Box 19.1). If the tumor has spread to the orbits, one might expect to find displacement and/or proptosis of the globe, motility restriction with diplopia, or optic neuropathy (Box 19.2).

INVESTIGATION

Symptoms of a sac tumor are a painless mass, often accompanied by bloody tears or bloody discharge (Table 19.2). The patient may not be tearing because the lumen is still patent. There is a nontender, nonregurgitating, nonfluctuant mass. There may be orbital, nasal, or sinus signs.

Nasal endoscopy is mandatory in assessing these patients.[9] It must be determined whether the sac tumor has eroded through the ethmoids and/or into the nose because such erosion would make management much more complex. It is also important to view the inferior meatus to determine whether any tumor has grown down the bony nasolacrimal canal and is projecting through into the nose. Such growth also would make tumor resection much more extensive.

Dacryocystography is extremely useful.[10] A dacryocystogram that shows irregular filling defects in a patent system is suggestive of a tumor. These irregular filling defects are present in all projections, which tends to rule out the presence of a stone or air. Ultrasonography is extremely useful in demonstrating whether there is fluid in the sac and in assessing the thickness of the sac and the walls, as well as the potential for extension outside the sac.[11] Ultrasound biomicroscopy (UAM) gives a very accurate appreciation of the thickness of the lacrimal sac mucosa.[12–14] Computed tomography (CT) scanning is extremely useful

TABLE 19.1. Lacrimal Sac Tumors: Three Presentations.

Unsuspected sac tumor	At routine dacryocystorhinostomy, a hard or irregular mass
Suspected sac tumor	Bloodstained tears
	Nonfluctuant mass in fossa
	Mass nontender, nonregurgitating
	Patency to syringing
	Dacryocystogram suspicion
Known sac tumor	Previous positive biopsy
	Spread of malignancy from elsewhere to sac
	Spread from sac to surrounding structures (nose, sinus, orbit)

BOX 19.1. Lacrimal Sac Tumor: Signs of Nasosinus Extension

Nosebleed
CSF leak
Numbness around roof of nose
Loss of smell
Nasal stuffiness

BOX 19.2. Lacrimal Sac Tumors: Signs of Orbital Extension

Displacement and/or proptosis of globe
Motility restriction with diplopia
Hypesthesia
Optic neuropathy
  Relative afferent pupillary defect
  Color vision defect
  Visual field abnormality
  Visual loss

to see the extent of the tumor and the bony involvement.[15,16] Magnetic resonance imaging (MRI) is useful to determine the interface between the sac and the tumor.[17,18]

Biopsy

If a sac tumor is suspected, it is useful to perform a biopsy of the lesion and obtain paraffin sections as well as frozen sections so that appropriate management can be undertaken. This can be done under local anesthesia. We prefer an open biopsy rather than a needle biopsy to obtain more tissue to facilitate the diagnostic potential for the pathologist.

Pathology of Lacrimal Sac Tumors[19]

Lacrimal sac tumors may be divided into epithelial and nonepithelial lesions (Table 19.3). Most lacrimal sac tumors are squamous and may be papillomas, transitional papillomas (carcinomas), or frank carcinomas.

Papillomas[20–22]

Papillomas may grow in two main patterns: exophytic and endophytic (Figure 19.2). There may also be a mixed variety. The amount of dysplasia will vary from mild (atypical cells in the lower third of epithelium) to moderate (atypical cells in the middle third) to severe (atypical cells throughout the whole thickness) to carcinoma in situ (full thickness plus epithelium polarity loss and surface cells maturation loss) (Table 19.4). If at surgery an abnormal epithelium of the sac is discovered, and the frozen section suggests a papilloma, it is advised not to proceed with the DCR until the paraffin sections have been obtained. This will minimize the chance of spreading malignant cells through into the nose. The sac tumor itself can be excised, and if paraffin sections suggest that the lesion is benign, a canaliculo-DCR can be performed at a later sitting.

Inverted papilloma (Schneiderian papilloma) is a special type of epithelial growth in lacrimal passages that may be encountered by the ophthalmologists as a primary lesion in the lacrimal system or as a secondary extension into the orbit from nasal and paranasal cavities. Most of these lesions are benign, but they tend to recur after treatment. In nasal Schneiderian papillomas, the incidence of malignancy ranges from less than 5% to 15%.[23–25]

The exact frequency of carcinomatous changes associated with the lacrimal sac papillomas is not known. The actual histologic documentation of the transformation of a papilloma to carcinoma is difficult to demonstrate in many cases but seems to occur more often in the lacrimal sac region than the nasal cavity and sinuses. Ryan and Font reported nine papillomas showing pure or partial (mixed) inverted patterns, three of which had been documented to contain a transition zone from benign to malignant proliferation.[22] This is certainly higher than any reported incidence of malignancy associated with nasal Schneiderian papillomas. Furthermore, one should keep in mind that the overall incidence of malignant epithe-

TABLE 19.2. Lacrimal Sac Tumors: Investigation.

Symptoms	Painless mass
	Not tearing
	Bloody tears or discharge
Signs	Nontender, nonregurgitating, nonfluctuant mass
	Patency to syringing
	Orbital, nasal, or sinus signs
Imaging	Dacryocystograph: irregular filling defect, patency
	Ultrasonography: no fluid in sac, thickened walls, extrasac extension
	Computed tomography: Bone involvement
	Sac–tumor interface

TABLE 19.3. Pathology of Lacrimal Sac Tumors.

Epithelial	Squamous
	Papilloma
	Inverted papilloma
	Carcinoma
	Transitional carcinoma
	Adenocarcinoma
	Mucoepidermoid carcinoma
	Adenoid cystic carcinoma
	Oncocytoma
Nonepithelial	Stromal
	Fibrous tissue: histiocytoma
	Skeletal muscle: rhabdomyosarcoma
	Peripheral nerve: neurilemmoma; neurofibroma
	Hematopoetic
	Lymphoma
	Plasmocytoma
	Leukemia
	Sarcoma
	Neuroectoderm
	Melanoma
	Neuroendocrine
	Secondary oat-cell carcinoma

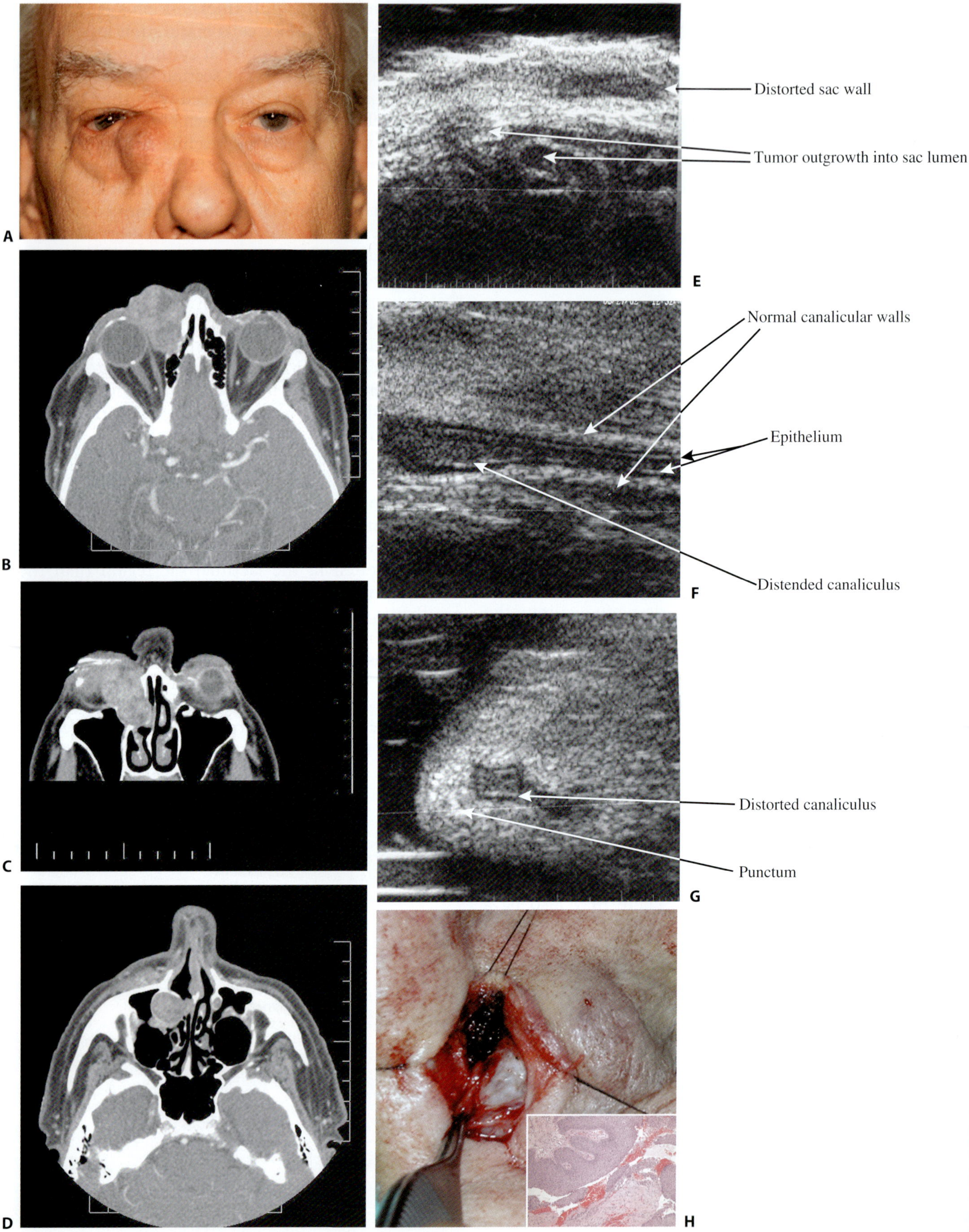
A
B
C
D
E
F
G
H
Distorted sac wall
Tumor outgrowth into sac lumen
Normal canalicular walls
Epithelium
Distended canaliculus
Distorted canaliculus
Punctum

TABLE 19.4. Epithelial Tumors—Papilloma.

Growth patterns	*Exophytic, endophytic, or mixed*
Degree of dysplasia	Mild: atypical cells lower third of epithelium Moderate: atypical cells into middle third Severe: atypical cells through whole thickness Carcinoma in situ: full thickness, plus epithelium polarity loss and surface cell maturation loss

lial tumors of lacrimal drainage system is approximately 60%, which is 20% more common than their benign counterparts. Radiation therapy and chronic inflammation have been suggested as causes of malignant transformation.[26]

Patients with primary papillomas of the lacrimal drainage system usually present with epiphora and a slowly growing mass in the inner canthus. These masses are usually firm and nonfixed when they do not harbor foci of infiltrating carcinoma. Tenderness, hyperemia, and warmth of the overlying skin are commonly absent in neoplastic lesions. Tumors of this area may mimic acute and/or chronic dacryostenosis. Inflammatory lesions, however, present with discrete symptomatology and a rather abrupt onset. In acute cases, tenderness, erythema, and warmth of the overlying skin are the usual findings. In chronic dacryocystitis, symptoms are recurrent, and the mass is usually compressible. Bloody discharge is not a regular finding with the inflammatory lesions but may be seen with tumors on occasion.

Clinical evaluation of the lacrimal drainage system in epiphora with a space-occupying lesion in the inner canthal area should include probing and irrigation. In many reported cases of inverted papilloma, the system could be easily probed and sometimes successfully irrigated. This is probably secondary to the intraluminal nature of the early mass, which allows the passage of a probe or fluid between the tumor and the wall. Therefore, the patency of the lacrimal drainage system to probing or irrigation should not rule out the presence of a papilloma.

Carcinomas of the lacrimal sac, on the other hand, usually show complete occlusion because of their infiltrative growth pattern into neighboring structures. Flanagan et al. stressed the importance of the location of the inner canthal mass in relation to the medial canthal tendon. In their experience, a mass above the medial canthal tendon almost always signifies a neoplastic process, and below the medial canthal tendon, inflammation.[27] Proptosis is almost always absent in primary lacrimal drainage system papillomas at the time of initial presentation but not necessarily on recurrence. Proptosis should indicate the presence of recurrence or of a secondary extension of the papilloma eroding the orbital wall to displace the orbital structures.[28]

Less common complaints such as postnasal discharge, diplopia, and nasal speech are observed in cases with secondary extension into the orbit.[29] Dacryocystography is a helpful tool in evaluating cases with multiple components. This radiographic procedure may be helpful in differential diagnosis of inflammatory versus neoplastic lesions. Dacryocystitis commonly reveals a dilated sac in the film, or dacryocystogram. The dacryocystogram of a benign tumor initially presents a discrete mass protruding toward the lumen of the lacrimal sac, whereas malignant tumors usually show a complete obstruction of the system.

The importance of CT and MRI as diagnostic aids should also be adequately emphasized. The initial choice of treatment for both primary and secondary papillomas with or without carcinoma is surgery with wide excision. Considering the recurrent nature of these tumors, the surgery should be performed under frozen section control, and every effort should be made not to leave any residual elements of the tumor. The surgical excision margins should be as wide as possible. In papillomas with malignant component, the excision may include the surrounding soft tissues and the orbital bony wall.

Squamous Carcinomas[30]

Squamous carcinomas are graded according to the differentiation of the cells as mild, moderate, or poorly differentiated (Table 19.5). Certain cytologic features suggest malignancy; if present, these require further investigation into the possibility of dissemination and the role of wider surgery and/or radiation (Table 19.6).

At the time of surgery, a frozen section should be done. Certain lesions that occur in the lacrimal sac may present diagnostic difficulty on frozen section (Table 19.7). With malignant melanomas (Figure

TABLE 19.5. Epithelial Tumors: Squamous Carcinoma.

Histology	Desmosomes (intercellular bridges) Keratin (on electron microscopy or immunohistochemical)
Differentiation	Mild Moderate Poor

←

FIGURE 19.2. Papilloma. (A) Large swelling in lacrimal sac region. Blocked sac, hard mass, some mucus regurgitating. A lacrimal sac tumor was suspected. CT images showing (B) large tumor in lacrimal sac fossa, (C) extension into ethmoids, and (D) growth into an expanded bony nasolacrimal canal. (E) UBM showing tumor in sac with fingerlike extensions. The epithelium is distorted. (F) Longitudinal UBM of lower canaliculus shows normal epithelium and walls with some distension and mucus in channel (confirmed surgically). (G) Cross section UBM of lower punctum showing canaliculus distorted by tumor. (H) Intraoperative photograph of the tumor at the time of biopsy. *Inset*: Histopathologic appearance of inverted papilloma.

TABLE 19.6. Cytological Features Suggesting Malignancy.

Nucleus	Nuclear pleomorphism Increased ratio of nuclear to cytoplasmic cells (enlarged nucleus) Irregular nuclear contours (angulation) Hyperchromasia (increased staining due to DNA synthesis) Nuclear molding (nuclear compression, fragile membranes)
Cytoplasm	Smaller surface area (more immature cell, larger nucleus)

TABLE 19.7. Tumors Presenting Diagnostic Difficulty on Frozen Section.

Malignant melanoma	Difficult to assess spread because cells are distorted on frozen section
Lymphoma	Need immunohistochemical test
Epithelial lesions	Papillomas: squamous, transitional Easier diagnosis if invasive

19.3),[31] it is difficult to assess the spread because the cells are distorted on frozen section. With lymphomas, immunohistochemical tests are needed to differentiate between a true lymphoma and a pseudotumor. With papillomas, it is difficult to determine on the basis of frozen section whether the lesion is a squamous or transitional papilloma.

MANAGEMENT OF LACRIMAL SAC TUMORS (Table 19.8)

Unsuspected Sac Tumor

At DCR, if the sac appears abnormal, it is wise to do a frozen section biopsy. If a confirmed tumor is present, dacryocystectomy should be performed. If a round-cell infiltrate is present that cannot be identified with certainty as lymphoma or pseudotumor, the sac should not be removed. With a tumor present, it is best not to open into the nose until the final pathology results are available. There is always the fear of spreading a tumor into the nose with a DCR, or even by an intubation.

Suspected Sac Tumor

A dacryocystectomy is the treatment of choice for suspected sac tumor. The procedure may be done under

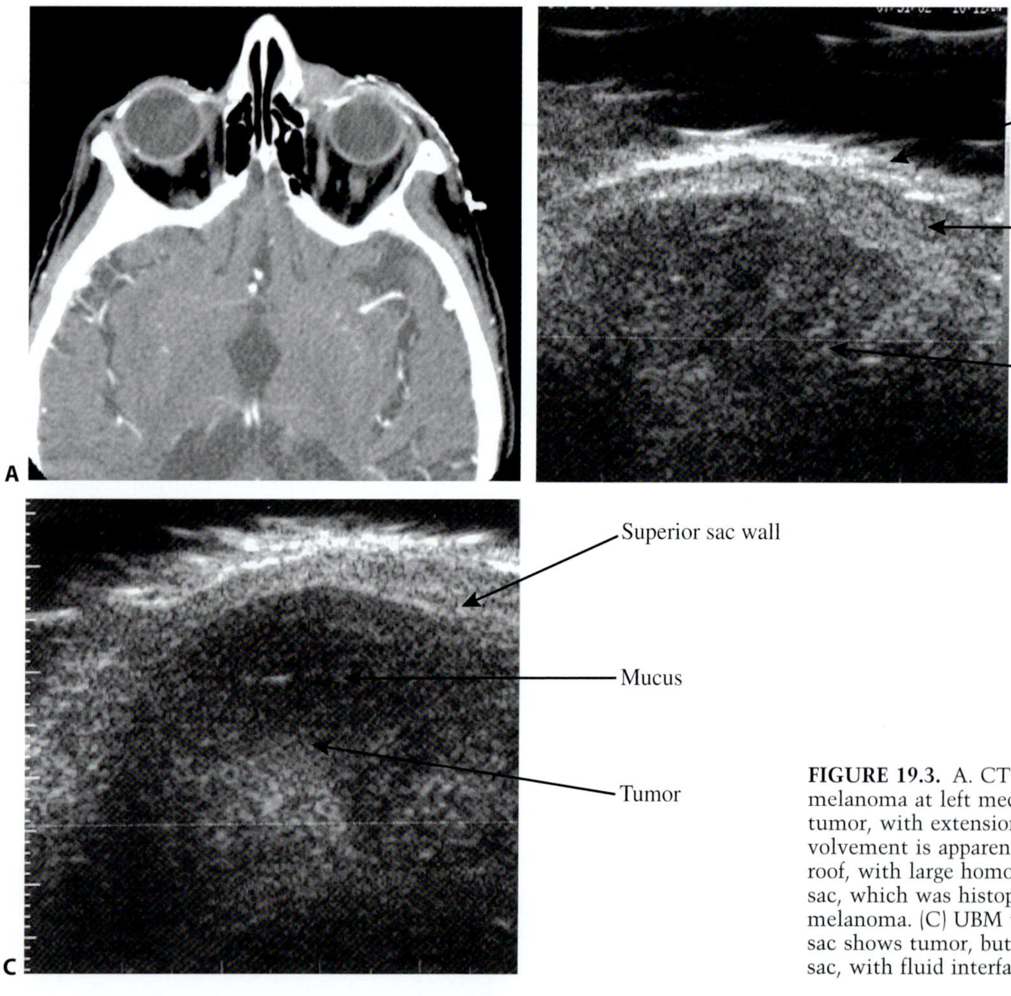

FIGURE 19.3. A. CT image of patient with large melanoma at left medial canthus. The sac is full of tumor, with extension into soft tissues. No bony involvement is apparent. (B) UBM shows distended sac roof, with large homogeneous tumor filling up the sac, which was histopathologically proven to be a melanoma. (C) UBM through section higher up in sac shows tumor, but not extending to wall of sac, with fluid interface (confirmed surgically).

TABLE 19.8. Lacrimal Sac Tumors: Management.

Unsuspected sac tumor	Biopsy–frozen section If malignant: Dacryocystectomy If benign: If inflammatory, proceed with DCR If definitely benign, remove mass and perform DCR If questionable Lymphoma: close after biopsy with or without tubes (preradiation) at later date Transitional papilloma: dacryocystectomy; then close and wait for permanent section
Suspected sac tumor	Biopsy for confirmation Dacryocystectomy Cryoprobe freezing to prevent spillage of cells
Known tumor	En bloc excision, especially if extension beyond sac Possibly postoperative radiation Later reconstruction and/or prosthesis

local anesthesia or general anesthesia. If the tumor is isolated to the sac, a dacryocystectomy alone should suffice. A cryoprobe may be used to seal the site of the biopsy and prevent spillage of cells, and then the sac can be removed as one mass. If there is any question about the diagnosis on frozen section, one should err on the side of conservatism, remove the sac, and realize that a canaliculo-DCR can be performed later. If malignant tissue is observed around the sac, a wider excision, often with an en bloc bone removal, may be necessary.

Known Tumor with Extension

A known tumor with extension requires a larger en bloc excision, which must be planned preoperatively. Radiation is often of use in these patients postoperatively.[32] If tearing occurs postoperatively, when one can be assured that there is no recurrence of tumor, a tear duct reconstruction procedure can be performed later.

Dacryocystectomy[33]

Dacryocystectomy is the basic operation for the management of a malignant sac tumor with no extension (Box 19.3) (Figure 19.4). The operation may be performed under local or general anesthesia. The patient must be warned that there may be tearing postoperatively, depending on the amount of tear secretion, and that a tear duct reconstructive procedure may be required later. An incision is made on the side of the nose, as with a standard DCR incision. The section is carried down to bone. The sac should be mobilized laterally, with care being taken not to penetrate the thin lacrimal bone or ethmoids. Once the sac has been mobilized, a biopsy can be performed. When a tumor is confirmed, there is a good tissue plane between the periosteum and the surrounding bone in which dissection and sac mobilization can be performed. The common canaliculus should be amputated as laterally as possible, and the nasolacrimal membranous duct should be amputated as inferiorly as possible within the canal. One may use tissue forceps to extract remnants of nasolacrimal duct mucosa from the bony lacrimal canal. Absorbable cellulose packs may be used for hemostasis. The skin incision is closed and a pressure dressing placed on the surgical site.

CONCLUSIONS

Suspicion is the key to the diagnosis of lacrimal sac tumors. A firm mass in the lacrimal sac fossa with suspicious signs and symptoms necessitates more elaborate investigation. Appropriate extirpative surgery helps to remove the tumor and prevent dissemination. Lacrimal reconstructive procedures such as DCR or canaliculorhinostomy can always be performed at a later date if epiphora is a problem (Figures 19.5 and 19.6).

BOX 19.3. Dacryocystectomy: Key Points

- Anesthesia: local with sedation.
- Skin incision as in DCR.
- No bone removal; avoid entering ethmoid processes.
- Sac mobilized, then biopsy performed.
- Amputate common canaliculus.
- Amputate nasolacrimal duct as deep in canal as possible.
- Remove tissue from within body of nasolacrimal canal.
- Use absorbable cellulose packs for hemostasis.
- Close and apply pressure dressing to surgical site.

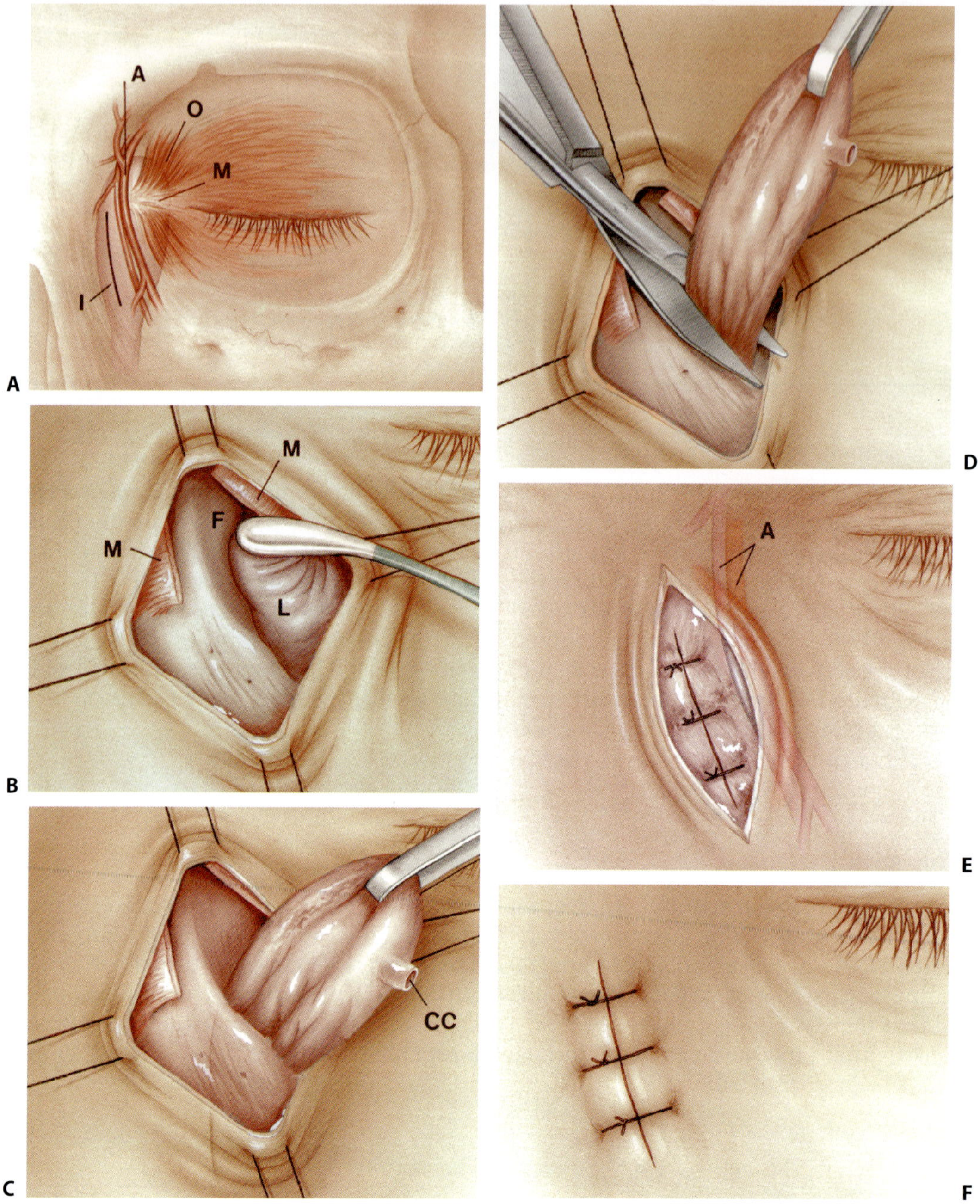

FIGURE 19.4. Six stages of dacryocystectomy. (A) Incision I, showing angular vein A, orbicularis muscle O, and medial canthal tendon M. (B) The lacrimal sac L is separated from the lacrimal fossa F. (C) The sac is elevated from the fossa. The common canaliculus (CC) has been transected. The sac is transected as low as possible into nasolacrimal canal. (E) The subcutaneous tissues sutured. (F) The skin is sutured (Reprinted with permission from Hurwitz, JJ, Tumours of the nasolacrimal system. Courtesy of Benjamin F. Boyd, MD, FACS, Editor-in-Chief, *World Atlas Series of Ophthalmic Surgery, Highlights of Ophthalmology*, English ed., Vol IV, 1999.)

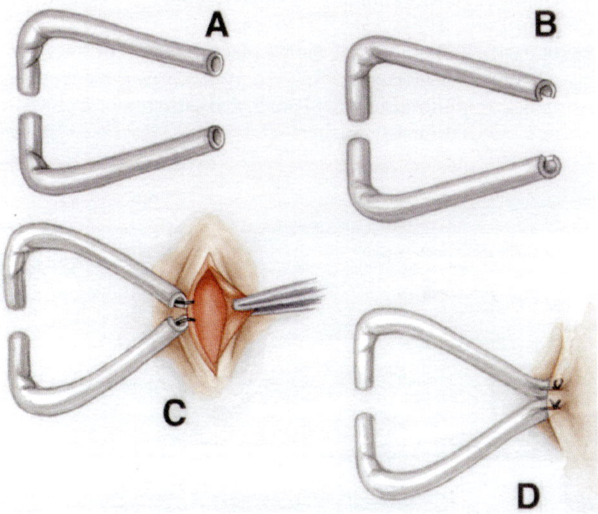

FIGURE 19.5. Canaliculorhinostomy. (A) Medial ends of canaliculi identified. (B) Slits in canaliculi to make "funnels." (C) Posterior flaps sutured to posterior nasal mucosa flap. (D) Anterior flaps sutured to anterior nasal mucosa flap. (Reprinted with permission from Hurwitz, JJ, Tumours of the nasolacrimal system. Courtesy of Benjamin F. Boyd, MD, FACS, Editor-in-Chief, *World Atlas Series of Ophthalmic Surgery, Highlights of Ophthalmology*, English ed., Vol IV, 1999.)

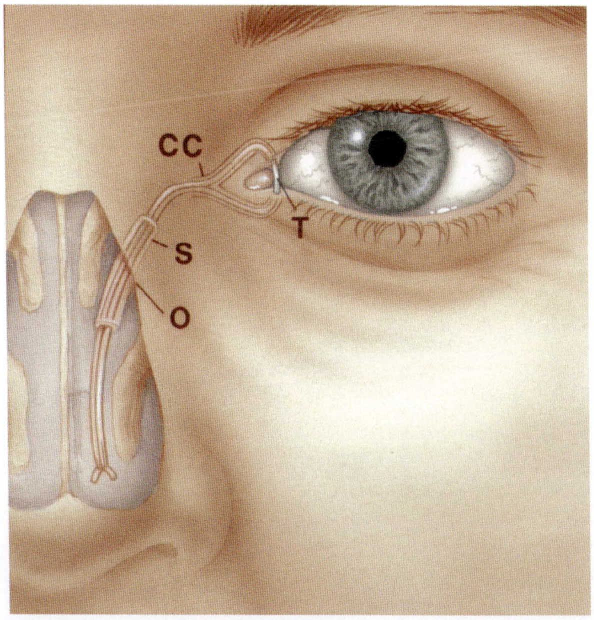

FIGURE 19.6. Intubation after common canaliculorhinostomy: T, tube; CC, common canaliculus; S, sleeve; O, opening in bone. (Reprinted with permission from Hurwitz, JJ, Tumours of the nasolacrimal system. Courtesy of Benjamin F. Boyd, MD, FACS, Editor-in-Chief, *World Atlas Series of Ophthalmic Surgery, Highlights of Ophthalmology*, English ed., Vol IV, 1999.)

Acknowledgments The author thanks Dr. Charles J. Pavlin for the ultrasound biomicroscopy photographs, Dr. David Howarth for the pathology photographs, Dr. Edward Kassel for the radiology photographs, and Ms. Rosemary Williams for preparing the manuscript.

References

1. Hurwitz JJ. Lacrimal sac tumours. In: Hurwitz JJ, ed. *The Lacrimal System*, Philadelphia: Lippincott-Raven, 1996: chap 28.
2. Jones LT, Linn M. The diagnosis and treatment of epiphora. *Am J Ophthalmol* 1969;67:75.
3. Herzig S, Hurwitz JJ. Lacrimal sac calculi. *Can J Ophthalmol* 1979;14:17.
4. Nolan J. Granuloma of lacrimal sac: simulating a neoplasm. *Am J Ophthalmol* 1966;62:156.
5. Rice DH. Chronic frontal sinus disease. *Otol Clin North Am* 1993;26:4.
6. Bordley JE, Bosley WR. Mucocele of the frontal sinus: causes and treatment. *Ann Otol Rhino Laryngol* 1973;82:696.
7. Conley JJ. Sinus tumors invading the orbit. *Trans Am Acad Ophthalmol Otol* 1966;70:615.
8. Wilbur AC, Dobben GD, Linder B. Paraorbital tumors and tumor-like conditions: role of CT and MRI. *Radiol Clin North Am* 1987;25:631.
9. Metson R. Endoscopic surgery for lacrimal obstruction. *Otol Head Neck Surg* 1991;104:473.
10. Lloyd GAS, Welham RAN. Subtraction macrodacryocystography. *Br J Radiol* 1974;47:379.
11. Dutton JJ. Standard echography in the diagnosis of lacrimal drainage dysfunction. *Arch Ophthalmol* 1989;107:1010.
12. Pavlin CJ, Sherar MD, Foster FS. Subsurface ultrasound microscopic imaging of the intact eye. *Ophthalmology* 1990;97:244.
13. Pavlin CJ, Sherar MD, Harasiewicz K, Foster FS. Clinical use of ultrasound biomicroscopy. *Ophthalmology* 1991;98:287.
14. Pavlin CJ, Hurwitz JJ. Ultrasound biomicroscopy. In: Hurwitz JJ, ed. *The Lacrimal System.* Philadelphia: Lippincott-Raven Press: 1995 Chap 16.
15. Ashenhurst ME, Jaffer N, Hurwitz JJ, Corin SM. Combined computerized tomography and dacryocystography for complex lacrimal obstruction. *Can J Ophthalmol* 1991;26:278.
16. Char DH, Norman D. The use of computerized tomography and ultrasonography in the evaluation of orbital masses. *Surv Ophthalmol* 1982;27:49.
17. Edelstein WA, Schenck JP, Hart HR. Surface cell magnetic resonance imaging. *JAMA* 1985;253:828.
18. Zimmerman RA, Bilaniuk LT, Yanoff M, et al. Orbital magnetic resonance imaging. *Am J Ophthalmol* 1985;100:312.
19. Howarth JC, Hurwitz JJ. Lacrimal sac tumours. Pathology. In: Hurwitz JJ, ed. *The Lacrimal System*. Philadelphia: Lippincott-Raven; 1996: Chap 27.
20. Harry J, Ashton N. The pathology of tumours of the lacrimal sac. *Trans Ophthalmol Soc UK* 1969;88:19.
21. Jones IS. Tumours of the lacrimal sac. *Am J Ophthalmol* 1956;42:561.
22. Ryan SJ, Font RL. Primary epithelial neoplasms of the lacrimal sac. The exact frequency of carcinomatous changes associated. *Am J Ophthalmol* 1973;76:73.
23. Hyams VJ. Papillomas of the nasal cavity and paranasal sinuses a clinicopathological study of 315 cases. *Ann Otol Rhino Laryngol* 1971;80:192–196.
24. Trible WM. Inverting papilloma of the nose and para-nasal sinuses. Report of 30 cases. *Laryngoscope* 1971;81:663–668.
25. Batsakis JG. Nasal Schneiderian papillomas. *Ann Otol Rhinol Laryngol* 1981;90:190–191.
26. Spaeth EB. Carcinoma in the region of the lacrimal sac. *Arch Ophthalmol* 1957;57:689–693.
27. Flanagan JC, Strokes DP. Lacrimal sac tumors. *Ophthalmology* 1978;85:1282–1287.
28. Karcioglu ZA, et al. Proptosis and pseudocyst formation from inverted papilloma. *Ann Ophthalmol* 1982;14:443–448.
29. Vrabec DP. The inverted Schneiderian papilloma: a clinical and pathological study. *Laryngoscope* 1975;85:186–220.

30. Ashton N, Choyce DP, Fison LC. Carcinoma of the lacrimal sac. *Br J Ophthalmol* 1951;35:366.
31. Yamade S, Kitagawa A. Malignant melanoma of the lacrimal sac. *Ophthalmologica* 1978;177:30.
32. Sternberg I, Levine M. Radiation therapy for carcinoma of the lacrimal sac. In: Bosniuk SL, Smith BC, eds. *Advances in Ophthalmic, Plastic, and Reconstructive Surgery*. Oxford: Pergamon Press; 1984.
33. Hurwitz JJ. Tumours of the nasolacrimal system. In: Boyd BF, ed. *World Atlas Series of Ophthalmic Surgery*. Vol IV. *Highlights of Ophthalmology*. Panama: Highlights of Ophthalmology International Publishers; 284.

PART FOUR

Secondary Tumors of the Adult Orbit

20

Eyelid and Periocular Skin Tumors

Georgina Kourt and Peter Martin

Skin cancers commonly affect the eyelids and periocular region. Orbital invasion is a serious and potentially fatal complication of cutaneous neoplasia. The most frequent skin cancers resulting in orbital invasion are basal cell carcinoma, squamous cell carcinoma, sebaceous gland carcinoma, and malignant melanomas. Orbital invasion from eyelid tumors usually results from a delayed presentation, incomplete excision with subsequent recurrences, and highly aggressive invasive tumors.

Basal cell carcinomas represent 90% of periocular tumours with orbital invasion and occur predominantly from the medial and lateral canthal regions by direct extension. Medial canthal basal cell carcinomas that invade the orbit via contiguous spread often have minimal external changes and are known as an *iceberg type*. Squamous cell carcinomas may invade the orbit by direct extension, by metastatic spread, or by perineural spread.

The most important external cause of basal cell carcinomas, squamous cell carcinomas, and malignant melanomas is exposure of fair-skinned people to sunlight, in particular, to wavelengths in the ultraviolet B (UV-B) range. The amount of UV-B in sunlight increases with increasing proximity to the equator, posing a particular risk for nonindigenous populations who migrate from temperate to tropical and subtropical zones. Ultraviolet irradiation damages DNA in the skin either by direct absorption or via damage to chemical mechanisms.[1] Australia has the highest incidence of skin cancers in the world, ranging from 650 to 1560 cases per 100,000 persons compared with 300 cases per 100,000 persons in Texas and Arizona. In the United States, basal cell carcinomas and squamous cell carcinomas are classified as non-melanoma skin cancers; their incidence decreases with increasing latitude. The high incidence of skin cancers in Australia has been partly attributed to holes in the ozone layer.[2]

The morbidity and mortality of patients with nonmelanoma skin cancers is significant, particularly in patients with a late presentation. Patients with basal cell carcinoma rarely die from the disease, but morbidity increases with advanced cases, particularly those with orbital invasion. Metastases from squamous cell carcinoma occur in 2 to 6% of cases.

BASAL CELL CARCINOMA

Basal cell carcinoma (BCC) is the most common skin malignancy involving the eyelids. It accounts for over 90% of malignant eyelid tumors. It rarely metastasizes but can cause significant morbity and mortality by invading contiguous structures in the head and neck. The mortality rate from BCC has been reported at levels ranging from 1 to 11%.[3] Intracranial extension is usually fatal and is associated with significant delay in diagnosis and inadequate initial treatment.[4]

Clinical Features

There are four main types of BCC, each with a different clinicopathologic pattern and with distinct biological behavior: nodular ulcerative BCC, sclerosing (also known as morpheaform type), superficial multifocal, and basosquamous.

The *localized nodular–ulcerative* subtype is the most common form of basal cell carcinoma, accounting for 75% of all tumors.The tumor begins as a small translucent papule. As it grows there is central ulceration and necrosis as the tumor outstrips its blood supply. It is often referred to as a rodent ulcer and is characterized by a raised pearly margin, central ulceration, and telangiectatic vessels coursing over the surface (Figure 20.1).

Orbital invasion can occur with the nodular–ulcerative type of BCC, although it is more common in the diffuse morpheaform type. In their study of 13 cases of orbital invasion of cutaneous malignancy, Howard et al. found eight morpheaform basal cell carcinomas, two basosquamous cell carcinomas, two squamous cell carcinomas, and one nodular–ulcerative BCC.[5]

The *morpheaform or sclerosing* subtype accounts for 15% of all BCCs and is responsible for the majority of tumors invading the orbit.[5] It may be difficult to diagnose, since the margins are clinically indistinct. The lesion may present as a depressed plaque of indurated tissue with loss of the sharp posterior lid margin and loss of lashes. Morpheaform BCCs are characterized by deep invasion into the dermis and deeper tissues.

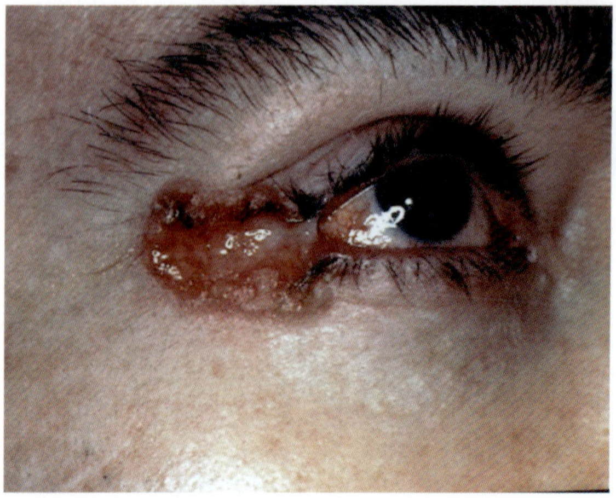

FIGURE 20.1. A 45-year-old Caucasian male with an ulcerated lesion at the lateral canthus of more than 12 months' duration. There was evidence of orbital invasion at presentation.

BOX 20.1. Clinical Features Suggestive of Orbital Invasion

Involvement of canthal angles (Figure 20.2)
Tethering to the conjunctiva or to periosteum
Palpation of a deeper mass
Involvement of the facial or trigeminal nerves
Diplopia
Ophthalmoplegia
Proptosis
Limitation of movement

The *superficial or multifocal* subtype of BCC may appear as a scaly area that resembles chronic dermatitis.

The *basosquamous* subtype of BCC shows squamous differentiation. It may be clinically indistinguishable from the nodular type. However, biologically, it behaves in a more aggressive manner with perineural invasion and distant metastatic potential.

Three syndromes are associated with BCCs:

1. The basal cell nevus syndrome of Gorlin–Goltz[6]
2. The linear unilateral basal cell nevus[7]
3. The Bazex syndrome[8]

Orbital Invasion

Although it is unusual BCC may invade the orbit in four ways:

1. Contiguous spread grows slowly and relentlessly, invading tissue and destroying adjacent tissue.
2. Periosteal spread travels along the periosteum without actually invading bone.
3. Perineural spread grows along peripheral nerves and gains access to the orbit and deeper structures without contiguous spread. Perineural spread may be asymptomatic, or it may be heralded by pain, parasthesias, or motor paresis.
4. Intracranial spread travels along cranial nerves through the superior orbital fissure and cranial foramina.

Risk Factors for Orbital Invasion

Delay in diagnosis is the critical factor in the development of orbital invasion.[9] This factor becomes even more critical for patients in rural regions away from tertiary referral centers. Risk also increases when the initial lesion has been incompletely excised and is therefore prone to recurrences.

Radiotherapy is associated with a high recurrence rate[9,10] and should be avoided. Recurrent tumors behave in a more biologically aggressive manner following radiotherapy.

The most common sites for BCCs on the eyelids are, in order, the lower lid, the medial canthus, the lateral canthus, and the upper lid.

The typical patient is a middle-aged or older person who has been exposed to actinic radiation.There is also evidence that immunologic factors may play a role in the development of BCCs, for example in younger patients with acquired immune deficiency syndrome.[3]

Suspicion of Orbital Invasion

The clinician should suspect orbital invasion in recurrent lesions of the morpheaform type, particularly in the medial and lateral canthal regions (Box 20.1).[9–11] Most of the patients in the Howard series presented with an orbital mass and incomitant strabismus at the initial examination.[5]

Perineural spread should be suspected if the patient complains of intermittent or constant pain, altered sensation such as formication (the sensation of insects

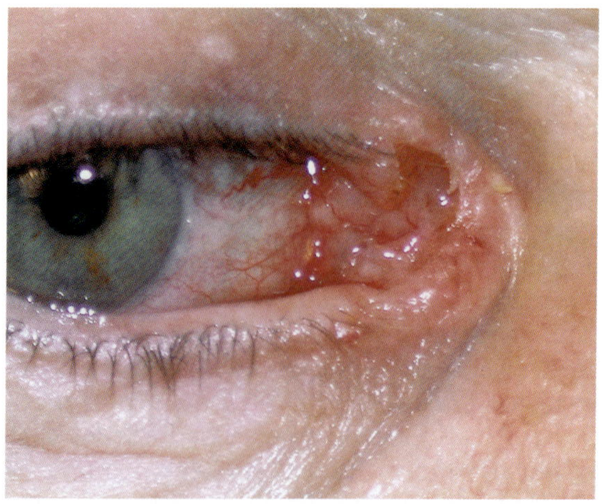

FIGURE 20.2. A 62-year-old Caucasian male with diplopia and a mass in the medial orbit. He had a medial canthal basal cell carcinoma that extended into the caruncular region and invaded the orbit.

crawling on the skin), numbness, and intermittent tingling.

As the tumor continues to spread, the pain may become more severe and may be described as burning, shooting, or stinging. Motor abnormalities may also appear, including ptosis, ophthalmoplegia, or general facial weakness.

The *iceberg type BCC* described and coined by Dr Peter Rogers at the Sydney Eye Hospital in the 1970s, often has minimal external signs of tumor, the bulk lying deep in the orbit (Figures 20.3A and B). This clinical subtype of BCC is found in tumors from the medial and lateral canthal regions. The clinician should palpate for deep extension and note any distortion of the canthal angles. Imaging is essential to establish the extent of the tumor. A history of radiotherapy is associated with recurrent lesions. The biological activity of the tumor may change to a more aggressive pattern after radiotherapy.

Signs of invasion from the lateral canthus include loss of canthal angle, loss of lashes, loss of the posterior margin, irregularity of the lid, increasing scleral show as the lid is tethered down, invasion of local structures such as muscle and lacrimal gland, and adherence to the periosteum and invasion of bone.

Differential Diagnosis

The differential diagnosis includes squamous cell carcinoma (SCC), melanoma, sebaceous gland carcinoma (SGC), and other skin appendage tumors. Pigmented BCCs in particular should be differentiated from melanoma. It may be impossible, however, to clinically distinguish between a pigmented BCC and a melanoma.[12] Likewise, without histopathological examination, an amelanotic melanoma may be mistaken for a BCC. Pigmented BCCs tends to occur in pigmented individuals. It is often difficult to distinguish between an SGC and a BCC with sebaceous cell differentiation. Histopathologic examination with an oil-red-0 stain may be helpful.

Trichoepithelioma is a benign adnexal tumor that may histologically resemble BCC. A desmoplastic trichoepithelioma is a variant of trichoepithelioma that should be considered in any child diagnosed with a morpheaform BCC.[13]

Metastatic carcinomas may also resemble morpheaform BCC. In breast carcinoma metastatic to skin, the cells are usually arranged in single file and display pleomorphic nuclei. In morpheaform BCC, the cells are usually more than one layer thick and are less pleomorphic.

A

B

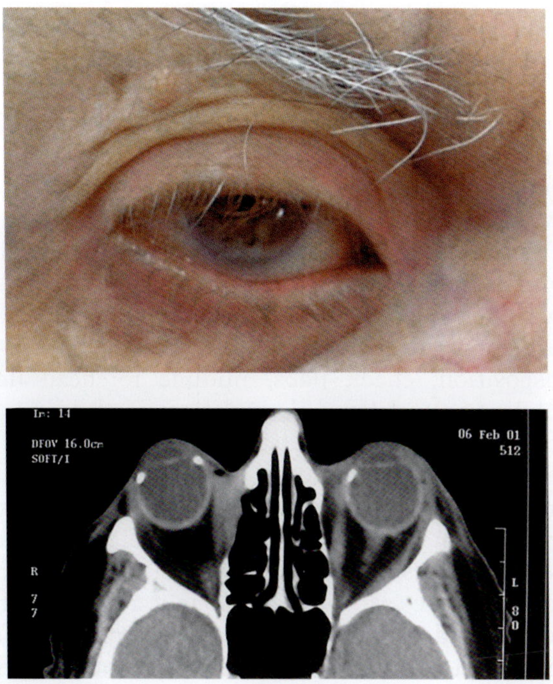

FIGURE 20.3. (A) A 72-year-old Caucasian male whose medial canthal basal cell carcinoma had been treated with radiotherapy 10 years earlier. The patient re-presented with limitation of movement and a mass in the medial orbit. (B) The CT scan of the patient shows the mass extending down the medial orbital wall.

Investigation

Imaging remains the mainstay of investigations in the management of orbital invasion of skin malignancy. Computerized tomography (CT) may show an orbital mass originating from the eyelid region and extending into the orbit (Figure 20.3B). Bone window settings may be useful in determining bony involvement There may be bony involvement in the presence of a normal CT scan.[11] Always guided by the clinical picture, the surgeon should not be deterred from removing clinically abnormal bone and submitting it for histopathology.

Magnetic resonance imaging (MRI) may be useful in determining the extent of orbital and neural invasion prior to surgery. MRI features of the orbital mass are a low signal intensity on T1-weighted images (T1W) and a low to high signal intensity on T2-weighted (T2W) images with respect to orbital fat. Primary eyelid carcinoma shows marked enhancement after the administration of gadolinium diethylenetriamine pentaacetic acid (Gd-DTPA). Fat suppression techniques may be extremely useful in establishing the extent of orbital involvement from the eyelid tumor.[14]

The preferred mode of imaging when perineural spread is suspected in MRI, which provides better soft tissue definition. CT is used to complement MRI data by defining foramina destruction and enlargement at the base of the skull. Radiologic findings suggestive of perineural spread include nerve enlargement and enhancement, foraminal enlargement/destruction, and obliteration of fat planes and convexity of the lateral cavernous sinus wall.[15]

Histopathology

BCC is characterized by a proliferation of cells with oval nuclei and scant cytoplasms. The cells are uniform in appearance and rarely appear anaplastic. Two main histologic types correlate with the clinical types.

In the *nodular* type, nests of cells resembling basal cells show peripheral palisading (Figure 20.4). Cells within the nests may be pleomorphic and atypical and may contain mitotic figures. The cells are continuous with the basal layer of the surface epithelium. There may also be areas of necrosis that correspond to surface ulceration clinically, areas of glandular formation, and squamous and sebaceous differentiation. Surrounding tissues often contain many fibroblasts, which may be large, numerous, and often bizarre in morphology.

The *morpheaform or fibrosing* type is characterized by elongated strands of infiltrating tumor cells. The fingerlike projections of tumor cells may be several layers thick and may extend below otherwise normal epithelium. This correlates well clinically as the clinical margin may be difficult to detect. There is an absence of typical palisading, and the stroma contains abundant collagen and a variable number of fibroblasts (Figure 20.5). The morpheaform type of growth pattern has been consistently correlated with deep invasion.[4,5,16]

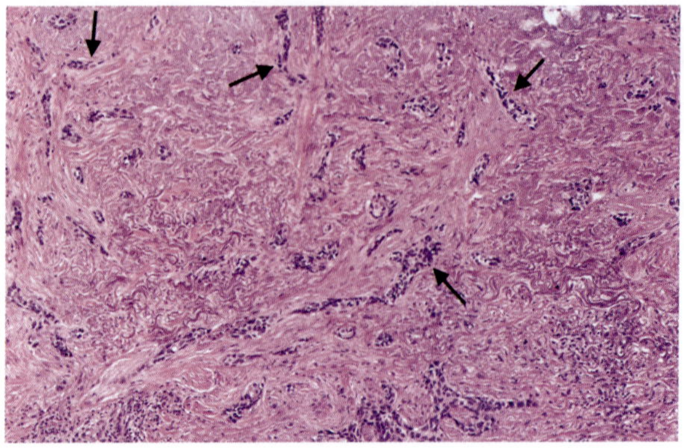

FIGURE 20.5. An infiltrative basal cell carcinoma invading the orbit of the patient shown in Figure 20.3. There are infiltrating cords of basal cell carcinoma (arrows) in a dense fibrous stroma. This pattern is known as morpheaform histology.

Management

Surgical management of BCC with evidence of orbital invasion is managed by two surgical techniques: en bloc excision and the Mohs micrographic surgical technique. En bloc surgical exision is performed with clear margins under frozen section control and confirmed by paraffin section by an experienced ocular pathologist.

Mohs micrographic surgery is employed when the tumor is excised close to the clinical margin and processed with frozen sections. This technique allows any residual tumor to be identified and reexcised. The process is time-consuming and involves a series of frozen section examinations and reexcisions until clear margins are reached. It is a labor-intensive method designed to minimize the removal of normal tissue. In many cases of orbital invasion, cure is possible only with exenteration.

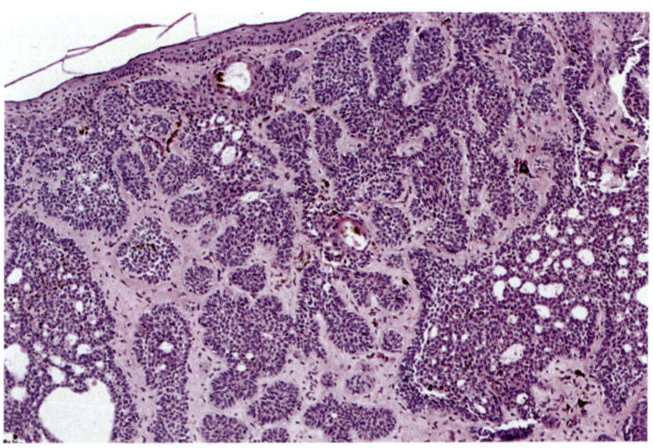

FIGURE 20.4. Nodular type basal cell carcinoma with nests of tumor cells with peripheral palisading. Note that some of the tumor cells contain melanin pigment which on occasion may cause pigmentation of the tumor to be confused with melanoma. (Courtesy of Dr. Alun Wang of New Orleans, Louisiana.)

The patient with orbital invasion is best managed by using a multidisciplinary approach incorporating the expertise of ocular pathologists, head and neck surgeons, oncologists, radiation oncologists, Mohs micrographic surgeons, and oculoplastic reconstructive surgeons to attempt cure in this potentially fatal disease.

Exenteration

Orbital exenteration is performed in cases of advanced neoplastic spread to the orbit in an attempt to prolong life. It may be a complete exenteration, subtotal exenteration, or an exenteration including the resection of additional tissue. Eyelid-sparing techniques are generally not indicated when there is extensive involvement of the lids.[17]

The bare orbital cavity may be allowed to heal by granulation and epithelialization. Alternatively, it may be lined by full-thickness or split skin grafts. Various flaps may be used, such as temporalis muscle transposition, cheek flaps, midline forehead flaps, frontal periosteal flaps, dermal flaps, and dermis fat grafts or vascular pedicle flaps.

The authors' preferred option, supported by Putterman, Bartley, and others,[17–19] is to allow spontaneous granulation or epithelialization. The main advantage of this technique is that it is relatively simple, and recurrences are more easily detected than if a flap or graft is used. The end result is a smooth cavity lined with skin of good color match. The main disadvantage is that dressings are required over several weeks, or even months, before epithelialization is complete. Exenteration is a radical but important surgical procedure that should be used in the cases described earlier prior to metastatic spread. Patients with basal cell carcinomas invading the orbit tend to do well following exenteration if the tumor is completely removed, since the lesion has little metastatic potential.[20] An exenteration may be necessary to totally eradicate the tumor and preserve life. An excellent cosmetic result is possible with a skillfully crafted, spectacle-mounted prosthesis.

Potential Complications

The mortality rate for exenterated BCCs in the series of Günalp et al. was 8%.[19]

The clinician must determine whether there is bony or periosteal involvement in all cases of orbital invasion by eyelid malignancies; if present, radiotherapy is generally inadvisable as primary treatment.[11] When bone involvement has occurred, the bone and periorbita must be surgically removed adjacent to the bone to achieve clearance. An exenteration may be necessary to totally eradicate the tumor and preserve life (Figure 20.6).

The potential complications of bone removal include cerebrospinal fluid (CSF) leak, sinus fistulas, meningitis, brain abscess, and osteomyelitis. The orbital surgeon should be prepared to manage the potential complications in collaboration with an otolarygologist and/or a neurosurgeon. It is therefore important to establish good working relationships within those disciplines.[11]

Other treatment modalities may be offered to patients who refuse exenteration. Radiotherapy is a useful palliative measure, although it is not to be recommended as an effective treatment because of the significant recurrence rate.

Perineural spread, although more commonly reported with squamous cell carcinoma, can also occur in BCC. It appears to be more common in men with recurrent tumors. Hanke[21] recommends the Mohs technique as being the most likely to identify perineural involvement because of horizontally cut frozen sections that may be missed in vertically cut sections.[21] Treatment of BCC with perineural spread is difficult.

Prognosis and Follow-up

The surgeon should be alert to the possibility of perineural spread. The patient may complain of symptoms prior to the onset of any visible recurrent lesion. Lifelong follow-up should be maintained to detect recurrences. Prognosis depends on the individual case, the pathology, the clearance of the tumor and the extent of the disease. The chances of a successful outcome depend strongly on an early diagnosis.

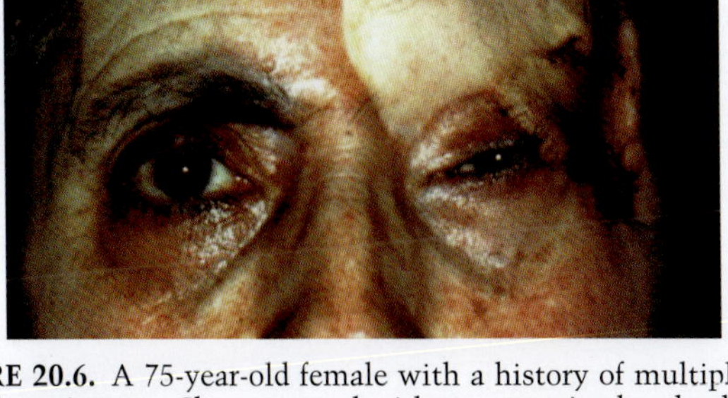

FIGURE 20.6. A 75-year-old female with a history of multiple basal cell carcinomas. She presented with an extensive basal cell carcinoma adherent to periosteum at the lateral canthal region. Treatment consisted of exenteration with removal of bone.

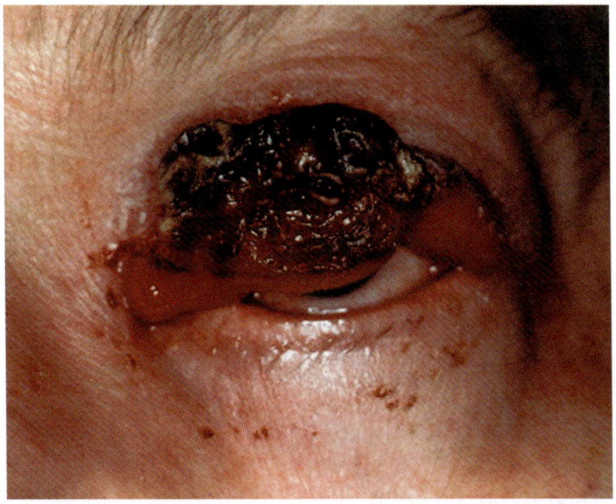

FIGURE 20.7. An 84-year-old Caucasian male with a squamous cell carcinoma of the upper lid that has invaded the orbit.

SQUAMOUS CELL CARCINOMA

Squamous cell carcinoma is the second most common form of skin cancer. It represents approximately 9% of all eyelid tumors but less than 2% of all eyelid malignancies.[22,23] It tends to occur in fair-skinned individuals with a history of exposure to sunlight. The incidence of SCC has risen over the past 30 years. The annual incidence in the United States is approximately 105 cases per 100,000 persons. Australia has the highest incidence of SCC in the world, with an annual incidence of approximately 166 per 100,000. The mechanism of UV-induced photocarcinogenesis appears to involve the inactivation of the tumor suppressor gene *p53*. It is a potentially fatal neoplasm that can metastasize to regional lymph nodes and also exhibit aggressive local spread. Other predisposing factors for the development of SCC are Bowen's disease, solar keratosis, keratoses resulting from arsenic, tar, or irradiation,[23] xeroderma pigmentosum, therapeutic ultraviolet light treatments [e.g., psoralen ultraviolet A range (PUVA)], fair skin, immunosuppression, and chronic inflammation. SCC may arise from a precancerous condition or de novo.

Clinical Features

SCC usually presents as an ulcerated lesion on an encrusted erythematous indurated and elevated base (Figure 20.7). The tumor spreads locally into the dermis and then invades deeper connective tissue, the periorbita, and lacrimal passages. The tumor may spread via the lymphatic glands to the submandibular nodes and submaxillary nodes from the lower lid and medial canthus and to the preauricular nodes if the tumor is in the lateral canthus or upper lid.

SCC tends to have a more rapid course than BCC. According to Duke-Elder, "left unattended, the entire orbital region and major portion of the face are destroyed in a fetid-smelling, ulcerating, fungating crater which may eventually reach the cranial cavity."[24] SCC has the potential for perineural spread and may gain access to the orbit via this modality.[25]

Differential Diagnosis

The differential diagnosis of SCC includes BCC, keratoacanthoma, sebaceous gland carcinoma, amelanotic malignant melanoma, and metastases to the lid and orbit.

Investigation

The same investigations are required as for BCC. Because SCC tends to metastasize, a careful examination of the appropriate lymph nodes should be performed and a systemic examination carried out. Perineural spread from SCC can be seen radiologically as an increase in the size of the nerve or as a widening of neural foramina.

Histopathology

SCC may begin as actinic keratosis where there is subtotal replacement of the epidermis by atypical cells. However, the general stratification from basal cells to the superficial epidermal layers is maintained.

SCC in situ, or intraepidermal SCC (e.g., Bowen's disease), occurs when the entire epidermis is replaced by atypical and disorganized cells. This lesion may arise from a preexisting precancerous lesion or de novo and may lead to invasive SCC. The hallmark of invasive SCC is invasion of the dermis.

Squamous cell carcinoma may be graded by the number of differentiating cells, the degree of atypicality of the cells, the depth of invasion, and the degree of acantholysis. Extensive acantholysis is associated with a more favorable prognosis.[26]

Orbital Invasion

SCC may invade the dermis at different levels and by traveling along various tissue planes—the periosteum, embryonic fusion planes, nerve sheaths, lymphatic vessels, and blood vessels—gain entry to the orbit.[27] SCC has the potential to metastasize to regional lymph nodes.[16,24,28,29]

SCC is responsible for approximately 10% of carcinomas involving the orbit,[25] mainly as a result of direct spread from surrounding tissues. Like orbital invasion by BCC, invasion by SCC tends to result from a delayed diagnosis, inadequate prior treatment with incomplete surgical excision, previous irradiation, and frequent recurrences. SCC may invade the orbit via contiguity with eyelid tumors, the paranasal sinuses, the conjunctiva, or the lacrimal sac (Figure 20.7). SCC may also be metastatic.[30]

Orbital invasion may also be associated with involvement of the orbital nerves, branches of the trigeminal and facial nerves, and cranial nerves.[15,31] Indeed, perineural spread and involvement may be the presenting feature of orbital involvement. Patients may present with pain, parasthesias, decreased or altered sensation such as formication, complete ptosis, and ophthalmoplegia prior to any proptosis, facial weakness, diplopia, or progressive cranial nerve palsies.[31]

Pain, complete ptosis, and ophthalmoplegia (i.e., the orbital apex syndrome, or superior orbital fissure syndrome) indicate that the disease process has reached an advanced state of spread into the orbital apex and cavernous sinus.

Perineural Spread

Pathologists disagree about the precise definition of perineural spread, but Veness and Biankin recommend the following criteria: unequivocal tumor cells must exist within the perineurium; as long as tumor cells are present, they need not encircle the nerve.[15] The location of the nerve in relation to the tumor is not relevant.

Perineural invasion of orbital nerves may also provide a route for intracranial extension. Numbness in the distribution of the nerve is thought to be pathognomonic of perineural involvement; sensory symptoms may precede the clinical recognition of the tumor, particularly in recurrent tumors.[32]

Perineural spread is an important mode of entry of tumor cells into the orbit. Orbital invasion occurs via direct spread, through hematologic and lymphatic routes and via perineural invasion (Figure 20.8). Perineural spread represents a form of metastatic spread in an aggressive tumor. It occurs commonly in SCC (Figure 20.8) but may also occur in BCC, sebaceous gland carcinoma, and malignant melanoma. When it occurs, it should be interpreted as a poor prognostic sign, and the clinician should strongly consider adjuvant therapy in addition to aggressive surgery. It mostly involves superficial branches of the trigeminal and facial nerves. The involvement of cranial nerves may provide access to the cranial cavity.

Spread is usually antegrade (i.e., toward the central nervous system) but may also be retrograde upon reaching a junction point such as the trigeminal gan-

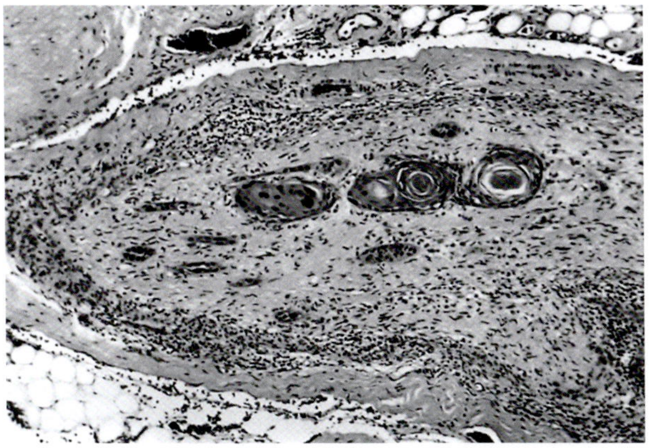

FIGURE 20.8. A 64-year-old Caucasian male had a squamous cell carcinoma with orbital invasion. The patient, who presented with a complete ptosis and orbital mass and pain in the distribution of the supratrochlear nerve, required an exenteration. Image shows intraneural spread in the supratrochlear nerve at some distance from the tumor mass (H&E, original magnification ×122).

glion.[32] In a review of the literature, the incidence of perineural spread in SCCs was reported to vary between 3.7 and 24%.[15] In cases of perineural invasion by SCC, Cottel reported the presence of skip areas of involvement. These are areas in the nerve that appear to be free of tumor, but microscopic analysis using the Mohs technique reveals tumor present in the proximal part of the nerve.[33] There may be an associated inflammatory response around the nerve; such areas should be resected until normal tissue is found.[21,33]

Management

Complete surgical excision under frozen section control remains the recommended treatment for SCC of the eyelids invading the orbit. Mohs surgery has been advocated by some as adequate treatment if the disease is in the early stages, but this technique may miss "skip lesions" occurring at significant distances from the presenting SCC. Some surgeons who use the Mohs technique use adjuvant radiotherapy even if the margins are clear.

When perineural spread has extended to the base of the skull, the orbital apex, or the cavernous sinus, the prognosis is extremely guarded. Radical surgery should be attempted only after consultation with the patient and clinicians from other disciplines and then only if negative margins are possible with an acceptable outcome. Radiotherapy plays a role when the margins are not clear in cases of advanced disease: doses greater than 50 Gy to the involved orbit and cavernous sinus should be given.[34]

Potential Complications

SCC has the potential to metastasize and exhibit perineural spread. It is the most common secondary epithelial malignancy in the orbit.[23]

Prognosis and Follow-up

The mortality rate of SCC of the eyelid is up to 40% in some series.[19,29] Metastases from SCC occur in 2 to 6% of cases. Approximately 2500 patients with SCC die annually in the United States. Most patients with SCC invading the orbit require exenteration. Perineural spread is associated with a poor prognosis,[20,25] depending upon such factors as histological grade of malignancy, delayed diagnosis, previous radiotherapy, previous incomplete excision, and recurrences.

Follow-up for all patients is lifelong.

A delayed presentation and inadequate initial treatment are probably the most important factors contributing to orbital invasion by periocular tumors.[19]

SEBACEOUS GLAND CARCINOMA

Sebaceous gland carcinoma is a relatively rare eyelid tumor that arises from the meibomian glands, the glands of Zeis, or from sebaceous glands in the eyebrow or caruncle.

In Caucasian populations, SGC accounts for up to 6% of all malignant eyelid tumors.[35] It mainly affects patients in the sixth to seventh decades. SGC is more common in the upper lid than the lower lid, probably because there are more meibomian glands in the upper lid.[36]

Known as a masquerader, SGC may mimic apparently benign conditions such as chronic blepharoconjunctivitis or chalazion and be misdiagnosed for months, or even years, resulting in a delay in diagnosis and treatment (Figure 20.9). SGC should be considered in any unilateral chronic inflammatory condition of the eyelids. Patients who present with a chronic inflammatory condition masking SGC often exhibit pagetoid spread or conjunctival intraepithelial

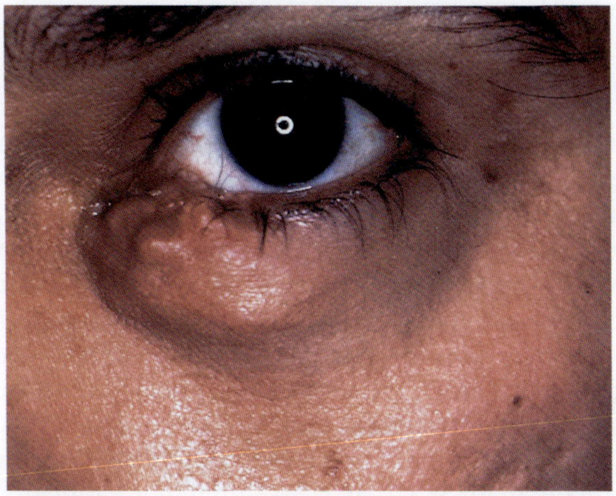

FIGURE 20.9. A 46-year-old male with a sebaceous gland carcinoma invading the medial orbit. He had been treated for recurrent chalazia for more than 2 years.

invasion.[37] Bonuik and Zimmerman studied 88 patients with SGC: 15 exhibited orbital invasion, mainly due to a delay in diagnosis.[38] Direct orbital invasion occurred in 19% of cases reported from the Armed Forces Institute of Pathology.[39]

Clinical Features

SGC may present as an enlarging mass in the eyelid or lid margin or as an orbital mass.[38] It may mimic chronic inflammatory conditions such as blepharoconjunctivitis or a chronic chalazion. In some cases, it may present with a diffuse or nodular thickening of the eyelids associated with loss of lashes, resulting from neoplastic involvement of the hair follicles. Unilateral papillary hypertrophy of the conjunctiva and cicatricial changes in the conjunctiva may also be a sign of SGC.

It may be impossible to determine the exact site of origin of the SGC. Some tumors may appear to originate from both meibomian glands and the glands of Zeis. Those originating from the glands of Zeis tend to have a more favorable prognosis.

Risk Factors for Orbital Invasion

SGC tends toward orbital invasion and a poor prognosis under any of the following conditions:

- Location in the upper lid or involving both lids
- Presence for longer than 6 months
- Multicentric origin
- Infiltrative histological pattern
- Moderate to poor sebaceous differentiation
- Evidence of intraepithelial carcinomatous change in the conjunctiva, cornea, and/or epidermis of the lid in association with an underlying sebaceous carcinoma

SGC should be considered in any patient with a history of radiotherapy to the eye or ocular adnexae or in a younger immunocompromised patient.

Differential Diagnosis

SGCs arising from the meibomian glands may mimic a chronic chalazion.[40] The clinician should suspect SGC in any chronic chalazion or one with atypical features (Figure 20.9). Chronic blepharoconjunctivitis, papillary hypertrophy, or cicatricial changes in the conjunctiva may all be signs of SGC. Intraepithelial disease may present as a chronic inflammatory condition. BCC, SCC, and amelanotic melanoma should also be considered in the differential diagnosis. BCCs, especially those with sebaceous differentiation, may be mistaken for SGCs. SCC and amelanotic melanoma should also be considered.

Investigation

If a SGC is suspected, the clinician must alert the pathologist prior to the processing of the biopsy sample so an Oil Red-O stain can be performed. This remains the gold standard in the diagnosis of this condition. Imaging is essential whenever orbital invasion is suspected.

Histopathology

SGC can be classified according to the site of origin, the degree of differentiation, the histopathologic pattern, infiltrative tendency, and the presence of pagetoid spread and/or carcinoma in situ spread in the epithelia of the conjunctiva, cornea, and/or skin of the lid.

SGC may be well differentiated, moderately differentiated, or poorly differentiated.

Well-differentiated tumors contain neoplastic cells that exhibit sebaceous differentiation.The cells have an abundant foamy or frothy, finely vacuolated cytoplasm. The nuclei are placed centrally or slightly displaced toward the periphery. The regions of sebaceous differentiation are seen toward the center of the tumor lobules.

Moderately differentiated tumors have fewer areas of highly differentiated sebaceous cells. Most of the tumor consists of neoplastic cells with hyperchromatic nuclei and prominent nucleoli and much basophilic cytoplasm.

Poorly differentiated tumors have cells with pleomorphic nuclei, prominent nucleoli, and scant cytoplasm. There is increased mitotic activity with atypical and often bizarre mitoses, in which the diagnosis is equivocal. A lipid stain such as the Oil Red-O stain is very helpful in determining the definitive diagnosis. The degree of differentiation correlates highly with prognosis, poorly differentiated tumors having the worse prognosis.

There are four types of histopathologic pattern, although there is no significant correlation with prognosis:

- Lobular, in which the neoplastic cells form well-delineated lobules of varying sizes
- Comedocarcinoma, in which the tumor lobules are of varying sizes and are characterized by a prominent central necrotic area where the cells stain for lipid
- Papillary, in which tumors have papillary projections of neoplastic cells mainly on the conjunctival surface
- Combined patterns, involving tumors with a combination of lobular and comedocarcinoma-like areas or a papillary pattern associated with either comedocarcinoma or lobular patterns

Infiltrative Features

Tumors can be classified according to the presence of minimal, moderate, or high infiltration. The degree of infiltration correlates significantly with prognosis and, indeed, mortality. Moderate and highly infiltrative tumors are associated with an increased mortality.[39] Highly infiltrating tumors have cords of tumor cells forming single rows of cells arranged in single file.

Intraepithelial Carcinoma

There are two types of intraepithelial carcinomatous change: pagetoid appearance and Bowenoid appearance. Tumors may display either or both of these changes.

Pagetoid spread resembles the intraepithelial spread of ductal carcinoma into the surrounding areolar and skin (as in Paget's disease of the breast). Pagetoid cells have abundant pale cytoplasm with hyperchromatic nuclei and are seen in squamous epithelium in small clusters of cells or singly among the surrounding nonneoplastic epithelial cells.

Bowenoid spread refers to diffuse spread and replacement of the entire surface epithelium by neoplastic cells, resembling Bowen's disease of the skin. Bowenoid changes are also characterized by focal or diffuse proliferation of large pleomorphic, hyperchromatic cells with mitotic activity replacing the normal cells of the epithelium.

These epithelial changes are typically seen in tumors that are moderately or highly infiltrative and arise from either meibomian glands or the glands of Zeis. There may be widespread intraepithelial disease not associated with marked invasion; however, tumors associated with intraepithelial carcinoma tend to have a worse prognosis.[39]

Orbital Invasion

Tumors with moderate to high infiltrative growth patterns tend to invade the orbit, lymphatic, and vascular channels—a development associated with a poor prognosis. The incidence of orbital invasion by SGCs is reported to be approximately 6%.[41]

Management

Surgery is the recommended treatment in SGC,[36,39] and wide excision of the tumor with clear margins offers a better prognosis than a simple excision.

Radiotherapy alone or prior to surgery is associated with a mortality rate of 78% and thus is not recommended.[39]

In cases of SGC associated with orbital invasion, excision of the tumor with exenteration of the orbit is recommended. The mortality rate associated with this group is 38%.[39]

Patients with evidence of metastases in the preauricular or cervical regions may be treated with a combination of radical surgery and radiation.[39]

Potential Complications

SGC is one of the most malignant eyelid tumors. It has a recurrence rate of 32%, a rate of regional lymph node metastases of 17%, and a mortality rate of 6%.[41]

Prognosis and Follow-up

SGC is a highly malignant and potentially lethal tumor. There is a significant mortality when there is associated orbital invasion. Follow-up is lifelong.

MELANOMA

Melanoma of periocular skin is a relatively rare tumor that accounts for approximately 1% of eyelid malignancies and less than 1% of all skin melanomas.[39] Melanoma may arise from the skin of the eyelid or from the conjunctiva and extend in either direction. Eyelid melanoma that involves the conjunctiva tends to behave in a more aggressive manner than melanoma confined to the eyelid skin.[42]

There are three types of cutaneous melanoma, differing in behavior and prognosis. Melanoma of the skin may arise from a Hutchinson's melanotic freckle or lentigo maligna, from an area of premalignant melanosis or superficial spreading melanoma, or as a nodular melanoma, which may arise from a preexisting nevus or de novo. Cutaneous melanoma of the eyelid occurs almost exclusively in Caucasians. It is thought that exposure to ultraviolet radiation plays a role in the etiology of melanoma.

Clinical Features

Of the three types of melanoma, nodular melanoma is the type most likely to be associated with orbital invasion. Clark suggests a classification into three types, based on clinical and histologic grounds[43,44]:

Melanoma Arising from Hutchinson's Melanotic Freckle or Lentigo Maligna

This type appears as an invasive nodule in an area of macular pigmentation that is irregular in outline with areas of irregular pigmentation. The lentigo maligna can regress and advance. It is usually found in skin exhibiting areas of solar degeneration, particularly in the elderly. It may be present for years before an area of invasive melanoma appears. Melanomas arising in

Hutchison's melanotic freckles tend to have a low grade of malignancy. The lower lid and canthal areas are commonly involved in lentigo maligna. When dermal invasion occurs, the surface becomes irregular, the lesion becomes elevated and forms a dark brown to black nodule. The incidence of malignant transformation in lentigo maligna is thought to be 25 to 30%. There is a characteristic biphasic growth pattern. The initial radial or horizontal, intraepithelial growth phase may last from months to years and is rarely associated with metastases. The vertical growth phase, involving an invasion of the dermis, is associated with metastatic disease in 35 to 75% of cases.[33] The clinician should suspect the vertical growth phase when there is a clinical change in the lesion such as a change in color or shape; surface changes such as crusting, bleeding, or ulceration; erythema of the surrounding skin; or new symptoms such as tenderness, pain, or itching.

Melanoma Arising from Areas of Premalignant Melanosis or Superficial Spreading Melanoma

This melanoma type usually presents in an area that is more circumscribed than Hutchinson's melanotic freckle, indicating there has been invasion of the dermis. This usually occurs months rather than years after the onset. This lesion may occur in both sun-exposed and unexposed skin and may occur on the conjunctiva.

Nodular Melanoma

Nodular melanoma may arise from a preexisting junctional nevus or it may arise de novo. Unexposed skin is affected as well as exposed skin, and this type of melanoma also occurs on mucosal membranes such as the conjunctiva. The lesion appears as a palpable blue-black or amelanotic nodule that rapidly increases in size. Nodular melanoma is immediately invasive and is most likely to be associated with orbital invasion. There is a higher grade—usually grade 3—of melanoma cells or anaplastic cells. Nodular melanoma has a higher proportion of invasion into deeper tissues and a less favourable prognosis than the other types of melanoma.[45]

Melanoma is usually pigmented. However, it may be nonpigmented or amelanotic, especially in recurrent tumors (Figure 20.10).

Risk Factors for Orbital Invasion

Melanoma is a potentially lethal tumor with a tendency to invade local tissues such as the orbit and to metastasize widely. Its growth occurs in a radial or vertical pattern. A vertical growth pattern is regarded as the most important negative prognostic factor in the behavior of melanomas.[46]

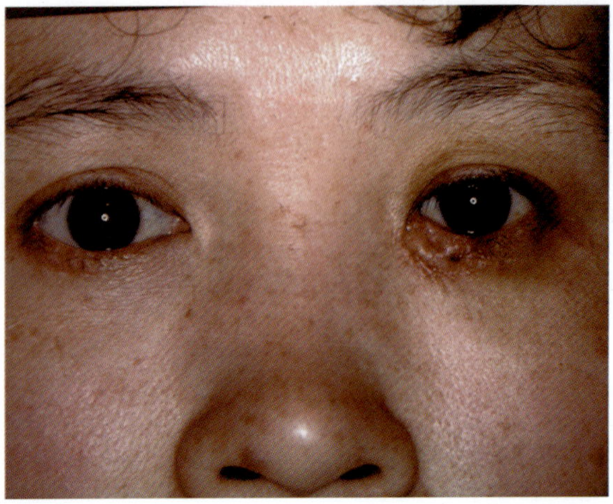

FIGURE 20.10. A 32-year-old pregnant Asian female with a 12 mm nodular amelanotic melanoma. The patient presented with a 2-month history, and the lesion was widely resected with clear margins. Two years later, the patient re-presented with a mass in the inferior fornix extending into the nasolacrimal duct.

Differential Diagnosis

Pigmented BCC may be confused with melanoma.[47] SCC and SGC may be confused with an amelanotic melanoma. Metastatic tumors to the eyelid and orbit should also be considered in differential diagnosis.

A highly aggressive, but rare, variant of melanoma is the clinicopathologic entity of desmoplastic malignant melanoma, which may invade the orbit. It is sometimes confused clinically with a recurrent chalazion.[48]

Investigation

Imaging of the orbit with CT scan or MRI is essential. Patients with orbital invasion from melanoma should also be screened systemically because of the high incidence of distant metastases. The patient should be referred to a melanoma unit for a thorough workup.

Sentinel lymph node mapping with scintillography and subsequent selective lymphadenectomy may be useful in determining lymphatic spread and subsequent treatment.[49]

Histopathology

Melanoma can be classified according to morphology, morphologic depth of invasion according to the Clark–McGovern classification, measurement of the depth of invasion according to Breslow's scheme, the presence of pigmentation, and the mitotic index.[50] All cutaneous melanomas develop initially from a neoplastic transformation of intraepidermal melanocytes. There is an initial horizontal proliferation of melanocytes followed by an invasive vertical growth.

Histopathologically, *lentigo maligna* consists of diffuse hyperplasia of atypical, pleomorphic melanocytes throughout the basal cell layer of the epidermis and extending into the outer sheaths of the pilosebaceous structures. The invading melanoma cells may have fascicles of spindle-shaped cells.

Superficial spreading melanoma consists of atypical melanocytes exhibiting pagetoid features. The cells are found at all layers of the epidermis. In the invasive vertical growth phase, the malignant melanoma cells vary in size and shape and may appear epithelioid, spindle shaped, or nevus-like; mixtures of cell types also are seen.

Nodular melanoma appears microscopically as large anaplastic epithelioid cells with evidence of dermal invasion even at the outset. This type of melanoma grows rapidly and has a more extensive depth of invasion than the other types of malignant melanoma. It is the most likely to cause orbital invasion.

Five levels of melanoma growth are identified[44,51]:

I. Tumor is entirely epidermal.
II. Tumor reaches into the papillary dermis.
III. Tumor fills the papillary dermis and impinges on the reticular dermis without invading it.
IV. Tumor invades the reticular dermis.
V. Tumor invades the subcutaneous fat.

Management

Primary treatment should be surgical with wide local excision of the tumor. The exact nature of the surgery depends on the individual case: the type of melanoma, Clark level, the thickness of the tumor, the stage of the disease, and the extent of orbital invasion. Complete excision with wide margins is recommended, depending on the depth of the lesion and its proximity to vital structures.[52,53]

Most cases of melanoma invading the orbit require exenteration.

If there is evidence of regional lymph node metastasis, parotidectomy or neck dissection and/or adjuvant chemotherapy or external beam radiotherapy is recommended.

Prognosis and Follow-up

Melanoma has a guarded prognosis. Two-thirds of deaths from skin cancers are due to the spread of melanoma. One of the most important factors affecting survival rates is the depth of invasion of the tumor. Breslow found that lesions measuring 0.76 mm or less histopathologically were associated with a 5-year survival rate of 100%.[54] In comparison, later workers reported a survival rate of only 50 to 60% for patients with tumors having a depth of more than 1.5 mm.[55]

Tumor thickness has been shown to be the most significant factor in the prognosis of melanoma. Tahery et al. found that cutaneous tumors involving the lid margin have a worse prognosis than those not involving the lid margin or conjunctiva and that melanomas of mucous membranes are more aggressive than cutaneous melanomas.[56]

A thickness occurring at Clark level IV or greater, or at a Breslow thickness greater than 1.5 mm, indicates a poor prognosis for eyelid melanoma.

THE SYDNEY EYE HOSPITAL EXPERIENCE

In a retrospective study of periocular skin tumors at the Sydney Eye Hospital (1990–2000), 399 patients with malignant skin tumors were identified. Tumors included BCC, SCC, SGC, melanoma, neurofibromas, and undifferentiated tumors. Eight percent (32 cases) had evidence of orbital invasion; 5% required exenteration. Twenty-one of the 32 invasive cases were BCCs, the remainder comprising 6 cases of SCC, 3 SGCs and 2 melanomas.

An unpublished 1987 study of skin tumors by Dr. Peter Rogers at Sydney Eye Hospital yielded 872 cases of malignant eyelid tumors. Ninety-two percent were BCCs, 5% were SCCs, 3% were melanomas, and 2% were meibomian gland carcinomas.

CONCLUSIONS

The most significant factor in the causes of orbital invasion by periocular cutaneous malignancy is delayed diagnosis, with inadequate initial treatment. Periocular skin cancers may gain access to the orbit via direct spread, vascular or lymphatic spread, or perineural spread. Treatment should therefore be aimed at prevention of spread by early diagnosis, aggressive surgery with total tumor clearance, and adjuvant therapy as required.

Acknowledgments Dr. Roger Crouch supplied the histopathologic photographs used in this chapter. Library staff at Sydney Eye Hospital provided valuable support in locating references. Hugh Mackay, social researcher, assisted with the organization and presentation of this chapter.

References

1. Axelrod M, Serafin D, Klitzman B. Ultraviolet light and free radicals: an immunologic theory of epidermal carcinogenesis. *Plast Reconstr Surg* 1990;86:582–593.
2. Green A, Williams G, Del Mar C. The severe problem of skin cancers in late twentieth century Australia. Prime Minister's Science and Engineering Council; 15th meeting, May 30, 1997.
3. Margo C, Waltz A. Basal cell carcinoma of the eyelid and periocular skin. *Surv Ophthalmol* 1993;38:169–192.
4. Moro F, de Caro R, de Caro G, et al. Eyelid basal cell carcinoma with intracranial extension. *Ophthalmic Plast Reconstr Surg* 1998;14:50–56.

5. Howard G, Nerad J, Carter K et al. Clinical characteristics associated with orbital invasion of cutaneous basal cell and squamous cell tumours of the eyelid. *Am J Ophthalmol* 1992; 113:123–133.
6. Gorlin RJ, Goltz RW. Multiple nevoid basal cell epithelioma, jaw cysts and bifid rib: a syndrome. *N Engl J Med* 1960;262: 908.
7. Anderson T, Best P. Linear basal cell nevus. *Br J Dermatol* 1962;74:20.
8. Basex A, Dope A, Christol B. Atrophodermie folliculaire, proliferationes basocellulaires et hypotrichoses. *Ann Dermatol Syph* 1966;93:241.
9. Wiggs E. Morphea-form basal cell carcinomas of the canthi. *Trans Am Acad Ophthal Otolaryngol* 1975;79:649–653.
10. Wiggs E. Basal cell carcinoma of the medial canthus—its orbital implications. *Mod Probl Ophthalmol* 1975;14:549–552.
11. Glover A, Grove A. Orbital invasion by eyelid tumours. *Ophthalmic Plast Reconstr Surg* 1989;5:1–12.
12. Hornblass A, Stephano J. Pigmented basal cell carcinoma of the eyelids. *Am J Ophthalmol* 1988;92:193–197.
13. Rahbari H, Mehregan A. Basal cell carcinoma in children and teenagers. *Cancer* 1982;49:350–353.
14. de Potter P, Shields J, Shields C. Secondary orbital tumours. In: eds. *MRI of the Eye and Orbit*. Philadelphia: JB Lippincott; 1995:255–268.
15. Veness M, Biakin S. Perineural spread leading to orbital invasion from skin cancer. *Australas Radiol* 2000;44:296–302.
16. Yanoff M, Fine B. *Ocular Pathology: A Text and Atlas*. 3rd ed. Philadelphia: JB Lippincott; 1989:192–202.
17. Putterman A. Orbital exenteration with spontaneous granulation. *Arch Ophthalmol* 1986;104:139–140.
18. Bartley G, Garrity J, Waller R, et al. Orbital exenteration at the Mayo clinic 1967–1986. *Ophthalmology* 1989;96:468–474.
19. Günalp I, Gündüz K, Duruk K. Orbital exenteration: a review of 429 cases. *Int Ophthalmol* 1996;19:177–184.
20. Rathbun J, Beard C, Quickert M. Evaluation of 48 cases of orbital exenteration. *Am J Ophthalmol* 1971;72:191–199.
21. Hanke C, Wolf R, Hochman S et al. Perineural spread of basal cell carcinoma. *J Dermatol Surg Oncol* 1983;9:742–747.
22. Reifler D, Hornblass A. Surgical management of squamous cell carcinoma of the lid. *Ophthalmic Plast Reconstr Surg* 1986;2:75–82.
23. Reifler D, Hornblass A. Squamous cell carcinoma of the eyelid. *Surv Ophthalmol* 1986;6:349–365.
24. Duke Elder S. The ocular adnexae. In: Duke-Elder S, ed. *System of Ophthalmology*. Vol 8. St Louis: CV Mosby; 1974:423.
25. Csaky K, Custer P. Perineural invasion of the orbit by squamous cell carcinoma. *Ophthalmic Surg* 1990;21:218–220.
26. Caya J, Hidayat A, Weiner J. A clinicopathologic study of 21 cases of adenoid squamous cell carcinoma of the eyelid and periorbital region. *Am J Ophthalmol* 1985;99:291–297.
27. Mohs F, Lathrop T. Modes of spread of cancer of the skin. *Arch Dermatol* 1952;66:427–439.
28. Reese A. *Tumours of the Eye*. 3rd ed. Hagerstown, MD: Harper & Row; 1976:3.
29. Aurora A, Blodi F. Lesions of the eyelids: a clinicopathologic study. *Surv Ophthalmol* 1970;15:94–104.
30. Ferry A. The biological behavior and pathological features of carcinoma metastatic to the eye and orbit. *Trans Am Ophthalmol Soc* 1973;71:373—425.
31. Trobe J, Hood C, Parsons J, et al. Intracranial spread of squamous cell carcinoma along the trigeminal nerve. *Arch Ophthalmol* 1982;100:608–611.
32. Ballantyne A, McCarten A, Ibanez M. The extension of cancer of the head and neck through peripheral nerves. *Am J Surg* 1963;106:651–667.
33. Cottel W. Perineural invasion by squamous cell carcinoma. *J Dermatol Surg Oncol* 1982;8:589–600.
34. McNab A, Francis I, Benger R, et al. Perineural spread of cutaneous squamous cell carcinoma via the orbit: clinical features and outcome in 21 cases. *Ophthalmology* 1997;104: 1457–1462.
35. Kass L, Hornblass A. Sebaceous carcinoma of the ocular adnexa. *Surv Ophthalmol* 1989;33:477–490.
36. Straatsma B. Meibomian gland tumours. *Arch Ophthalmol* 1958;56:71–93.
37. Honavor S, Shields C, Maus M, et al. Primary intraepithelial sebaceous gland carcinoma of the palpebral conjunctiva. *Arch Ophthalmol* 2001;119:764–767.
38. Boniuk M, Zimmerman L. Sebaceous carcinoma of the eyelid, eyebrow, caruncle and orbit. *Trans Am Acad Ophthalmol Otolaryngol* 1968;72:619–641.
39. Rao N, McLean I, Zimmerman L. Sebaceous carcinoma of eyelids and caruncle: correlation of clinicopathologic features with prognosis. In: Jakobiec F, ed. *Ocular and Adnexal Tumours*. Birmingham, Alabama: Aesculapius Publishing; 1978:461–476.
40. Martin P, Rogers P. Adenocarcinoma of the meibomian gland. *Aust J Ophthalmol* 1982;10:63–67.
41. Ginsberg J. Present status of meibomian gland carcinoma. *Arch Ophthalmol* 1965;73:271–277.
42. Collin J, Garner A, Allen L, et al. Malignant melanoma of the eyelid and conjunctiva. *Aust N Z J Ophthalmol* 1986;14: 29–34.
43. Naidoff M, Bernardino V, Clark W. Melanocytic lesions of eyelid skin. *Am J Ophthalmol* 1976;82:371–382.
44. Clark W, Mihm M. Lentigo maligna and lentigo-maligna melanoma. *Am J Pathol* 1969;55:39–46.
45. McGovern V. The classification of melanoma and its relationship with prognosis. *Pathology* 1970;2:85–98.
46. Wick M. Prognostic factors for cutaneous melanoma. *Am J Clin Pathol* 1998;110:713–718.
47. Resnick K, Sadun A, Albert D. Basal cell epithelioma: an unusual case. *Ophthalmology* 1981;88:1182–1185.
48. Sutula F, Dortzbach R, Bolles J. Desmoplastic malignant melanoma of the upper eyelid. *Ann Ophthalmol* 1982;14:141–143.
49. Esmaeli B. Sentinel lymph node mapping for patients with cutaneous and conjunctival malignant melanoma. *Ophthalmic Plast Reconstr Surg* 2000;16:170–172.
50. Grossniklaus H, McLean I. Cutaneous melanoma of the eyelid: clinicopathologic features. *Ophthalmology* 1991;98:1867–1873.
51. Bernardino E, et al. Histogenesis and biologic behaviour of primary human malignant melanoma of the skin. *Cancer Res* 1969;29:705–727.
52. Rodriguez-Sains R, Jakobiec F, Iwamoto T. Lentigo maligna of the lateral canthal skin. *Ophthalmology* 1981;88:1186–1192.
53. Pitman G, Kopf A, Bart R, et al. Treatment of lentigo maligna and lentigo maligna melanoma. *J Dermatol Surg Oncol* 1977; 9:727–737.
54. Breslow A. Thickness, cross-sectioned areas and depth of invasion in the prognosis of cutaneous melanoma. *Ann Surg* 1970;172:902–908.
55. Cook B, Bartley G. Epidemiologic characteristics and clinical course of patients with malignant eyelid tumours in an incidence cohort in Olmsted County, Minnesota. *Ophthalmology* 1999;106:746–750.
56. Tahery D, Goldberg R, Moy R. Malignant melanoma of the eyelid: a report of eight cases and a review of the literature. *J Am Acad Dermatol* 1992;27:17–21.

21

Conjunctival Tumors

Zeynel A. Karcıoglu

Although the conjunctiva can harbor many primary and secondary neoplasms (Table 21.1), the two most significant tumors that may extend into the orbit are squamous cell carcinoma (SCC) and melanoma.[1] Therefore, only these tumors are discussed in detail in this chapter.

SQUAMOUS CELL CARCINOMA

Clinical Features

The bulbar conjunctiva, particularly the limbus, is the frequent site for the occurrence of slow-growing, dyskeratotic epithelial proliferations. Similar to epithelial neoplasms elsewhere in the body, conjunctival tumors evolve through morphologic stages of dysplasia and carcinoma in situ to the invasive stage. Most of the conjunctival epitheliomas show histologic changes analogous to actinic solar keratosis of skin and follow a benign course early in their development. However, the degree of dysplasia in these lesions cannot be determined by clinical examination, therefore, it is absolutely necessary that biopsy samples be obtained and examined histopathologically. The incidence varies from 0.02 to 3.5 per 100,000 population depending on the geographic location.[2,3] SCC of the conjunctiva is predominantly a disease of the elderly that occurs most commonly during the sixth and seventh decades of life. However, it is reported to occur at a much younger age in patients with xeroderma pigmentosum.[4] Although the exact incidence of SCC in children is not known, it has been reported in individuals as young as 4 years old.[5] It has been recently recognized that SCC of the conjunctiva not only occurs more frequently in individuals who are immunosuppressed, but also develops at a younger age and behaves more aggressively (see Chapter 3).[6,7]

SCC of the conjunctiva usually presents as an elevated pinkish-gray lesion with a pearly or gelatinous appearance and surrounding feeding vessels (Figure 21.1).[8,9] The most common presenting symptoms of these interpalpebral/limbal lesions are redness and irritation of the eye with or without foreign body sensation. Although most lesions begin as a localized mass formation,[3] atypical presentations of SCC as a diffuse growth or a masquerade lesion mimicking scleral keratitis or scleromalacia have also been reported.[10] Atypical cases may show extensive invasion because of delayed treatment.

Conjunctival and invasive SCC is considered to be a low-grade malignancy that is locally invasive but rarely presents with distant metastases. When the neoplasm breaks through the basement membrane of the conjunctival epithelium and invades the subepithelial tissues and episclera, it behaves in a locally aggressive fashion.[11] Although these are slowly growing tumors, under certain conditions they are known to extend into the underlying structures, including the globe and the orbit.[10–15]

Although less frequently, SCC may originate from the tarsal conjunctiva as solitary or multifocal, slightly elevated, placoid tumors. These lesions clinically present as rough, irregular plaques with or without leukoplakic changes on the surface. Later, the lesions may grow into papillary masses or nodules. The SCC of the bulbar conjunctiva extends toward either eyelids, orbit, or into the globe (Figure 21.2). When the tarsal conjunctiva and the underlying lid layers are involved, the behavior of the tumors is similar to that of eyelid skin SCC involving the lymph and blood vessels and nerve sheaths (Figure 21.3) (see Chapter 20). These lesions may reach a significant size, and even in moderate sizes they develop easy access into the substance of the eyelid and into the orbit. Traditionally, SCC of the conjunctiva has been considered to be a low-grade malignancy accounted for about 5 to 7% of secondary orbital tumors.[16] But recently higher incidences have been reported. Conjunctival SCC comprised approximately 25% of secondary orbital tumors in an extensive study.[17] Although the initial site of tumor origin (bulbar vs tarsal conjunctiva) was not specified in this series, orbital invasion is considered to occur more often in tarsal tumors. The occurrence of orbital invasion has been approximately 10% in other series.[18]

SCC of the Lacrimal Drainage System

Malignant epithelial tumors of the lacrimal drainage system (LDS) outnumber the benign ones 3 to 1, and the majority of these tumors are SCCs.[19] In the LDS, SCC extends into the orbit early because of the thin

TABLE 21.1. Primary and Secondary Tumors and Pseudotumors of the Conjunctiva.

Dermoids/Choristomas	
Benign epithelial tumors	Papilloma Inverted papilloma Dacryoadenoma
Malignant epithelial tumors	Squamous cell carcinoma-in-situ Invasive squamous cell carcinoma
Benign mesenchymal tumors	Vascular hamartoma (mixed vascular elements) Hemangioma Lymphangioma Varix Hemangiopericytoma (benign or malignant) Fibrous histiocytoma (benign or malignant) Benign fibromatoses non–Langerhans cell histiocytoses (juvenile xanthogranuloma) Myxoma, fibromyxoma, lipoma Peripheral nerve tumors (neurofibromatosis) Schwannoma, granular cell tumor Leiomyoma
Malignant mesenchymal tumors	Angiosarcoma Hemangiopericytoma (benign or malignant) Fibrous histiocytoma (benign or malignant) Kaposis sarcoma Malignant fibromatoses Langerhans cell histiocytoses (histiocytoses X) Malignant schwannoma Alveolar soft part sarcoma Leiomyosarcoma
Melanocytic tumors	Nevus Melanosis Melanoma
Lymphoproliferative tumors	Lymphoid hyperplasia Lymphoma Leukemia (granulocytic sarcoma)
Secondary and metastatic tumors	From eyelid tumors (sebaceous gland carcinoma, basal cell carcinoma, squamous cell carcinoma From distant organs (breast, kidney, etc.)
Pseudotumors	Inclusion cysts Masses secondary to foreign bodies Inflammatory mass lesions Amyloidosis Ligneous conjunctivitis Subconjunctival hematoma (hematic cyst)

walls of the lacrimal passages. Fortunately, SCC of the LDS is not common. If these tumors can be recognized early and excised with clear surgical margins, the prognosis is good. Because of early extension into the orbital soft tissues, however, the recurrence rate is high.[19] A detailed discussion of these tumors is in Chapter 19.

One unique type of the LDS tumor is the *inverted papilloma*, which is in essence a benign papillary hyperplasia that may behave clinically in an aggressive,

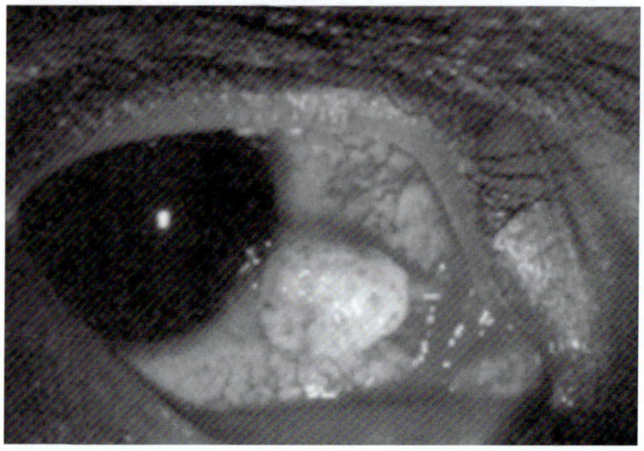

FIGURE 21.1. A nodular squamous cell carcinoma of bulbar conjunctiva.

recurrent fashion. The name *inverted* stems from its histopathologic structure, which consists of epithelial papillary proliferations inverting into the underlying stroma instead of an exophytic proliferation, which is characteristic of papillomas in general. Another distinctive feature of this tumor is the presence of numerous, small mucin-containing cysts throughout the epithelial component of the tumor. This characteristic can be best demonstrated with mucicarmine stain.[20]

Although most of these tumors originating in the conjunctiva behave as benign proliferations, approximately 40% of LDS inverted papillomas are known to develop malignant transformation ranging from dysplasia to invasive SCC.[21] Even the histopathologically benign inverted papillomas are known to recur fre-

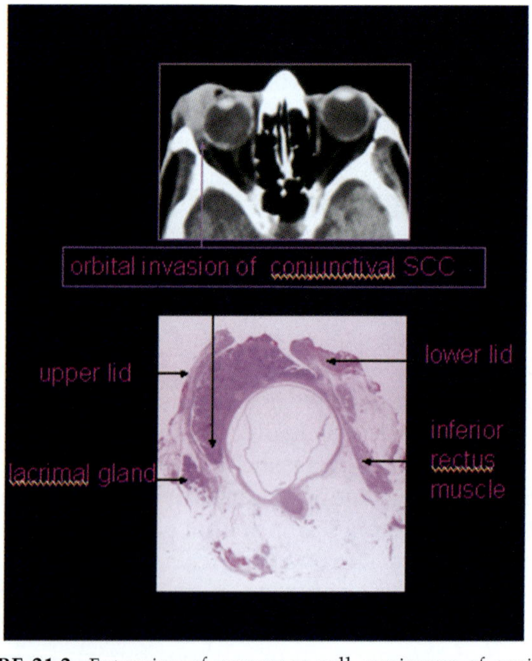

FIGURE 21.2. Extension of squamous cell carcinoma of conjunctiva into the eyelid and orbital tissues.

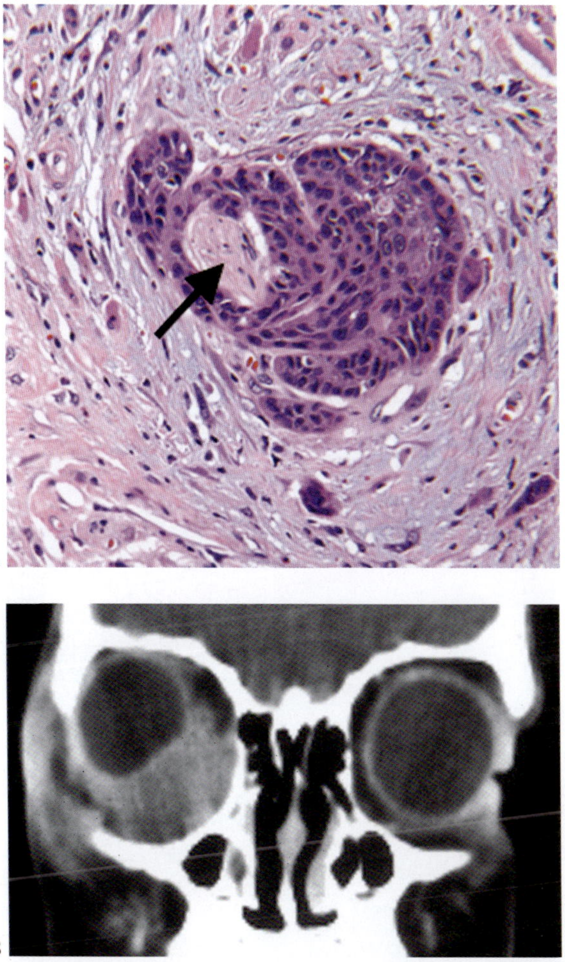

FIGURE 21.3. (A) Perineural invasion leading to the extension of squamous cell carcinoma (CC) into the orbit (B) (arrow: nerve).

quently and have been reported to invade the orbit after several recurrences (Figure 21.4).[22] These tumors are difficult to cure surgically because of their infiltrating mode of invasion and scarring.

Variations Based on Histology

Since all SCCs arise from the keratinocyte, they all display the same histopathologic appearance, whether originating in skin or other types of epithelium with squamous metaplasia potential such as the conjunctiva. In carcinoma in situ, the full thickness of the epithelium/epidermis is involved with disorderly proliferation of squamous cells (keratinocytes) with cytologic maturation. Instead, the SCC cells form sheaths of atypical, dyskeratotic groups with a scattered mitosis at all levels of the epithelium. Once the basement membrane has been violated and the tumor goes into the subepithelial/subepidermal layers, it is known as *invasive SCC*.[23] Downward growth of the neoplasm consists of irregular nests of neoplastic cells extending into the underlying tissues. Invading tumor cells are composed in varying proportions of normal-appearing and atypical squamous cells showing varying degrees of pleomorphism. The SCC may be well differentiated with keratinization horn pearls (characteristic structures composed of concentric layers of squamous cells showing gradually increasing keratinization toward the center), and intercellular bridges (desmosomes). As the tumor becomes less differentiated, these features are lost and atypical cells and mi-

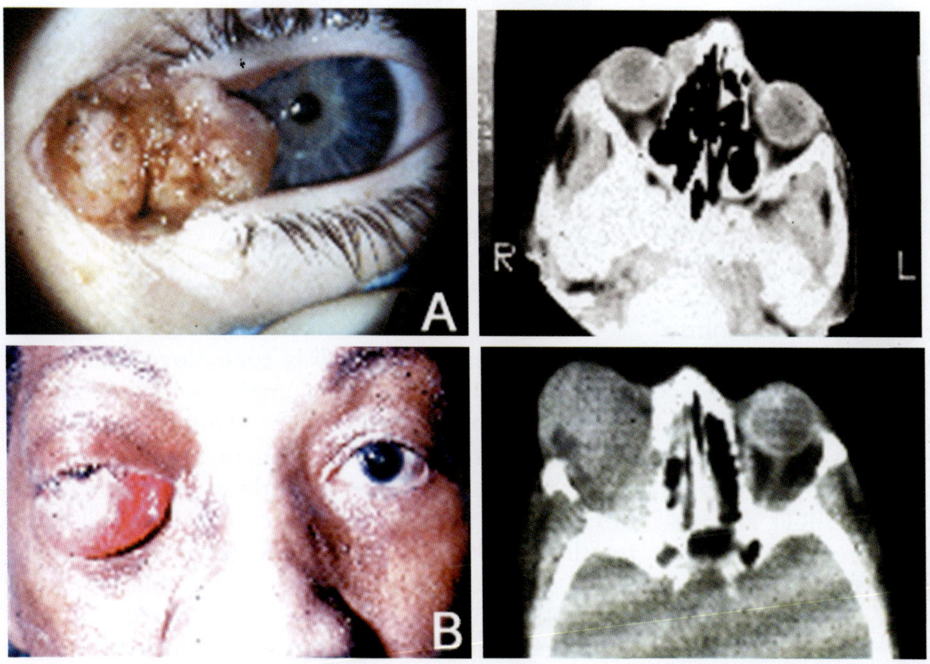

FIGURE 21.4. (A) Inverted papilloma of LDS originating from lacrimal sac as a primary lesion. (B) Secondary invasion of the orbit by inverted papilloma 20 years after its removal from the nasal cavity.

totic figures increase. Poorly differentiated tumors exhibit minimal keratinization, and their keratocyte origin may be difficult to identify histopathologically. Immunohistochemistry for cytokeratin B is an invaluable technique to identify the cell of origin of these poorly differentiated tumors.[24] Histopathologic types of conjunctival SCC, including spindle cell carcinoma,[25] mucoepidermoid carcinoma,[26,27] and adenoid squamous carcinoma (ASC),[28] are the best-known varieties. The histopathologic patterns of these tumors, which are composed of cells of different types, appear to influence the clinical course and the prognosis of the patient. Spindle cell carcinoma behaves in a rather aggressive fashion, with recurrences and invasion of the globe.[25]

Mucodepidermoid carcinoma is composed of a mixture of malignant keratinocytes and cells that secrete mucus containing acid mucopolysaccharides (Figure 21.5). These tumors behave in a more aggressive fashion than the conventional SCC, with a tendency to recur and invade ocular and orbital structures.[27] Most of the mucoepidermoid carcinomas originate in the bulbar conjunctiva, close to the limbus, and appear to look flashier and less keratinized than the conventional SCC. Recurrent lesions have a tendency to extend into the globe and orbit and metastasize.

The ASC of the conjunctiva is made of islands of malignant keratinocytes, which present in a pseudoglandular pattern and show extracellular Alcian blue positivity. Studies with transmission electron microscopy documented that ASC of the conjunctiva is different from the mucoepidermoid type.[29] ASC of the conjunctiva, like its cutaneous and oral counterparts, appears to have a worse prognosis than conventional SCC.[30]

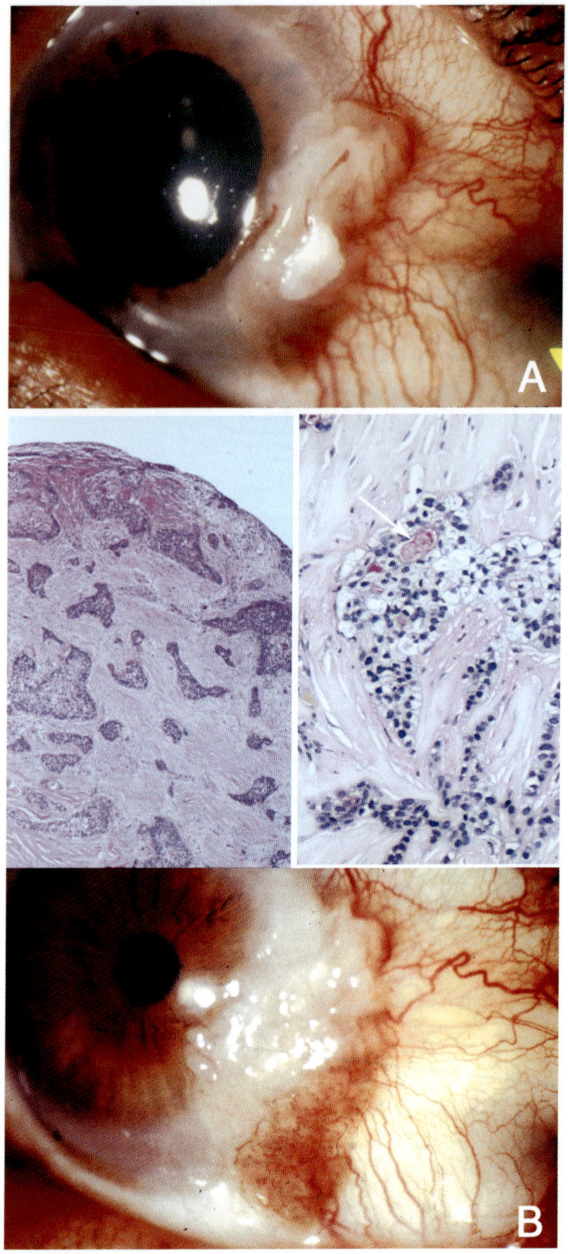

FIGURE 21.5. Mucoepidermoid carcinoma of the limbus (A) that recurred 9 months after excision (B). *Center*: Histopathology reveals nests of invading malignant squamous cells intermixed with vacuolated tumor cells containing mucin material as depicted with mucicarmine stain (arrow).

Management and Prognosis

The management of superficial disease (carcinoma in situ and/or superficial invasive SCC) includes surgical excision of the lesion with lamellar scleral keratoconjunctivectomy and cryotherapy (Figure 21.6).[31,32] Mauriello et al. also advocate the "microscopically controlled excision" technique of ASC; in this technique the lesion is resected with a no. 69 Beaver blade, and the margins of excision are treated with absolute alcohol to devitalize any residual tumor cells.[29] If the possibility of the existence of tumor cells cannot be ruled out at the deep margin, cryotherapy with a freeze–thaw–refreeze technique is advised.

Although other treatments, including brachytherapy, external beam radiation therapy (EBRT), and immunotherapy with dinitrochlorobenzene have been used, most of these methodologies do not offer a good prognosis. Currently, topical chemotherapy with mitomycin C and 5-fluorouracil has reportedly achieved good results in superficial cases.[33,34] No matter what other therapeutic modality is coemployed, an initial attempt should be made for complete surgical removal of the tumor with free margins. This is best accomplished under frozen or permanent section monitoring.[35,36] Once the ocular and orbital extension of the SCC occurs, the treatment is enucleation and exenteration, respectively, with or without postoperative EBRT. Detailed preoperative imaging studies with CT and MRI are needed to determine the extent of tumor; both procedures should be performed under frozen section control to ensure tumor-free margins.

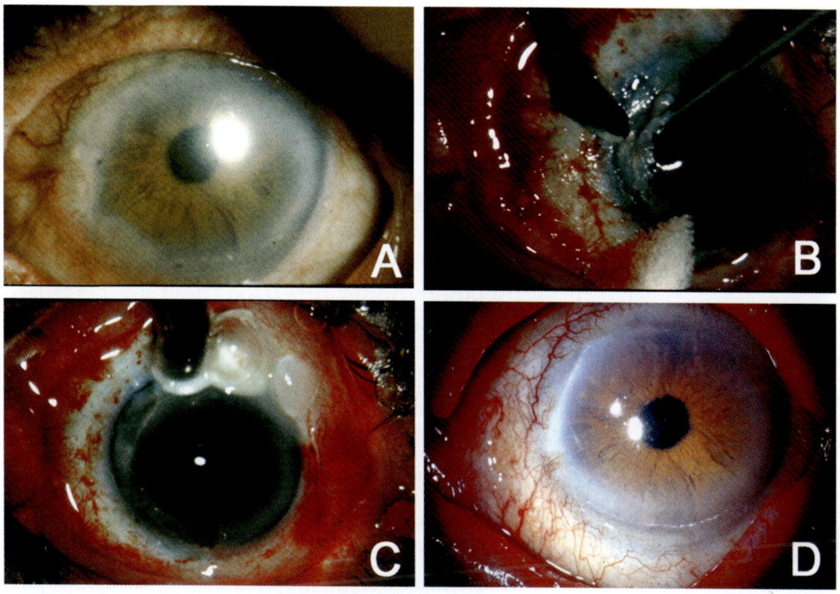

FIGURE 21.6. Treatment of the squamous cell carcinoma of conjunctiva and limbus: (A) Pretreatment appearance of a bulbar conjunctival tumor with extensive involvement into the limbus. (B) Lamellar dissection of the tumor at the limbus. (C) Cryotherapy of the tumor at the limbus. (D) Appearance of the eye approximately 9 weeks after surgery.

The biological behavior of SCC has been traditionally based on Broders's histopathologic grading system, which divides the tumors into grades based on the proportion of differentiated cells within a given SCC.[37] The premise of Broders's classification is that the more poorly differentiated the tumor, the more likely it is to invade aggressively, metastasize, and recur locally following treatment.[38] In reality, the prognosis of a given SCC is dependent on many other factors, including the site of origin and inciting cause (e.g., tumors originating from solar keratosis behave less aggressively than lesions that arise de novo).[39] SCCs originating from tissues scarred by ionizing radiation, heat, and/or chemical burns behave more aggressively.[40,41]

Other histologic features related to poor prognosis are the size of a given tumor and depth of its invasion. These two parameters should be taken into account relative to where SCC is located and the type of epithelium that it originates from. For example, a tumor measuring 1 cm in diameter may not be considered to be very deep if it is originating from the skin; on the other hand, an SCC of the same size, having ready access to the underlying vascular channels and is located in the conjunctiva, may be considered to be deeply invasive.

As our knowledge of oncogenesis expands, other risk factors are added to the histopathologic parameters just listed. Hereditary syndromes of certain types, such as xeroderma pigmentosum, albinism, epidermodysplasia verruciformis, have been associated with an increased incidence of cutaneous and conjunctival SCC. Other risk factors, including ultraviolet radiation,[42,43] oncogenes such as the gene for p53 (Figure 21.7),[44–46] human papilloma virus (HPV),[47,48] immunosuppression, and particularly acquired immunodeficiency syndrome (AIDS)[49,50] should be taken into account when one manages these patients (see Chapter 3).

CONJUNCTIVAL MELANOMA

Clinical Features

Conjunctival melanoma is a rare but aggressive ocular tumor that originates from melanocytes.[51–54] It is estimated that about 20% of conjunctival melanomas arise

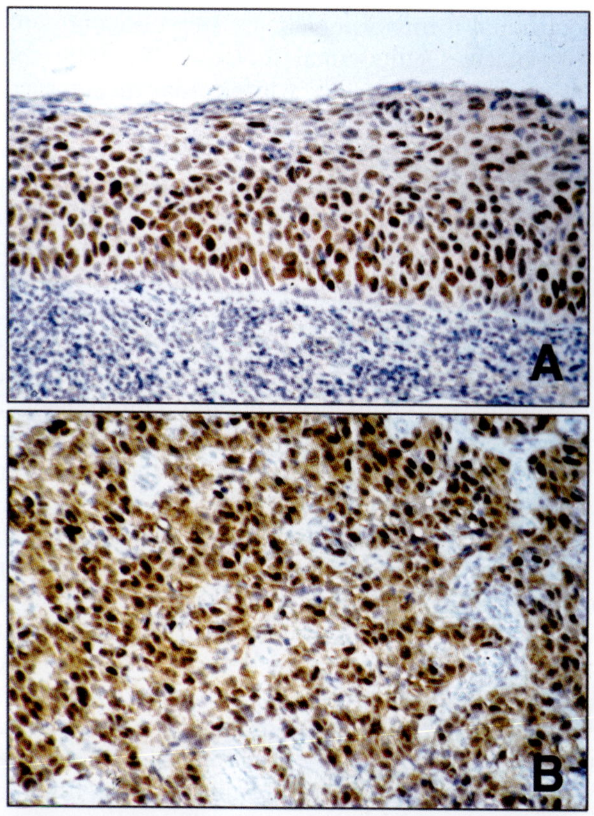

FIGURE 21.7. Squamous cell carcinoma of the conjunctiva stained with anti-p53 antibody: (A) in situ (A) and (B) in the invasive state.

from preexisting nevi, another 70% develop from primary acquired melanosis, and the rest are considered to develop de novo with no evident preexisting melanocytic lesion.[52] All three groups originate from dendritic melanocytes, the basal layer of the conjunctival epithelium.[53] Conjunctival nevi are not uncommon in children; about 50% of all nevi are encountered by the age of 20. The melanomatous transformation in the pediatric age group, however, is very rare.[55]

Variations Based on Histopathology

Melanosis

Generally speaking, melanosis refers to excessive melanocytic pigmentation occurring either as an epithelial or subepithelial lesion.[56] It is crucial to determine whether the melanosis has developed as a congenital or an acquired lesion.

Congenital melanosis typically presents at birth as grayish-blue subepithelial lesions that do not become malignant. Two main types exist: lesions in which only the globe is affected (ocular melanosis) and lesions in which ocular melanosis is accompanied by ipsilateral dermal melanosis of periorbital skin (oculodermal melanosis or nevus of Ota). Both forms appear clinically as slate-blue areas of episcleral pigmentation that may increase in size during the first few decades of life. By moving the conjunctiva over the pigmented area on slit lamp examination, one can best appreciate the depth of these lesions. In contrast, intraepithelial forms of melanosis are yellow-brown to brown-black. Oculodermal melanosis is more common in Asians and blacks, while ocular melanosis occurs more often in Caucasians.

Primary acquired melanosis (PAM) may be due to simple hyperplasia of melanocytes in the basal epithelial layer or to atypical melanocytic hyperplasia. The latter form is considered a precursor of malignant acquired melanosis. Clinically, these lesions are unilateral, tannish-brown or black, flat, localized or patchy tumors occurring in the later decades of life. Often, the pigmentation in one area of the conjunctiva disappears spontaneously and simultaneously with the development of new lesions in an adjacent zone. Clinical experience tells us that about one-third of these lesions may eventually become melanomas, but the process is slow, usually taking several decades.

Malignant acquired melanosis refers to development of melanoma within a preexisting PAM. These tumors appear as darkly pigmented, thickened areas arising within preexisting flat lesions, often with nodules and inflammation. Because the precursor lesions are multicentric, melanoma may appear in several areas at once, or it may develop stepwise. Thus, it is essential to examine the entire conjunctiva carefully, including upper and lower fornices. These lesions may remain superficially invasive for a long time, with orbital extension and metastasis to regional lymph nodes occurring only in the late stages.

Nevus

The nevus is the most frequently encountered as a melanocytic growth of the conjunctiva; approximately 30% of these lesions are detected before puberty and 90% by age 30.[56] Depending on the histopathologic location of melanocytic proliferation, nevi are classified as junctional (proliferation at the epithelial–subepithelial interface), subepithelial (proliferation with subepithelial tissues), or compound (both junctional and subepithelial proliferation). Most conjunctival nevi are compound or subepithelial.

Nevi are often located on the bulbar conjunctiva within the interpalpebral fissure. Those at the limbus tend to be flat and may extend onto the cornea, while those in the other zones of the bulbar conjunctiva, particularly on the plica and caruncle, appear more bulky and elevated. Approximately 30% of nevi are salmon colored rather than dark-brown–black; pigmentation may increase during pubery and pregnancy and with other hormonal stimuli.

On slit lamp examination, small cystic structures are seen within the subepithelial matrix of the lesion. These represent epithelial inclusion cysts lined with conjunctival epithelium and mucus-producing goblet cells (Figure 21.8). As these inclusions gather secretions and grow, they may give the impression of lesional transformation into malignancy. The nevus may also exhibit secondary inflammation with subsequent increase in size and vascularity. In many cases, these changes are accompanied by pigmentary alterations, which again may suggest malignant transformation. Although these changes are known to occur during hormonally active periods, it is advisable to perform a biopsy to sample the changing lesion. The follow-up of the nevi is best done with serial slit lamp photographs. It is advisable to see these patients every 3, 6, and 12 months initially; if the lesion proves to be stable, the patient may be seen once a year from there on.

Melanoma

Conjunctival melanomas are uncommon ocular neoplasms with an estimated incidence of 5 cases per million persons.[52] The incidence of melanoma in general is much lower in the nonwhite population.[57] Conjunctival melanoma as well is seen extremely rarely in the black population. In the series of Grossniklaus et al., the black-to-white ratio was given as 1:13.6.[58,59] Melanoma of the conjunctiva, like melanoma of the skin, has a predilection for non-sun-exposed areas (e.g., palms, soles of the feet, fornices in the conjunctiva).[60]

The rapid growth, high vascularity, spontaneous bleeding, and fixation to underlying tissues of mela-

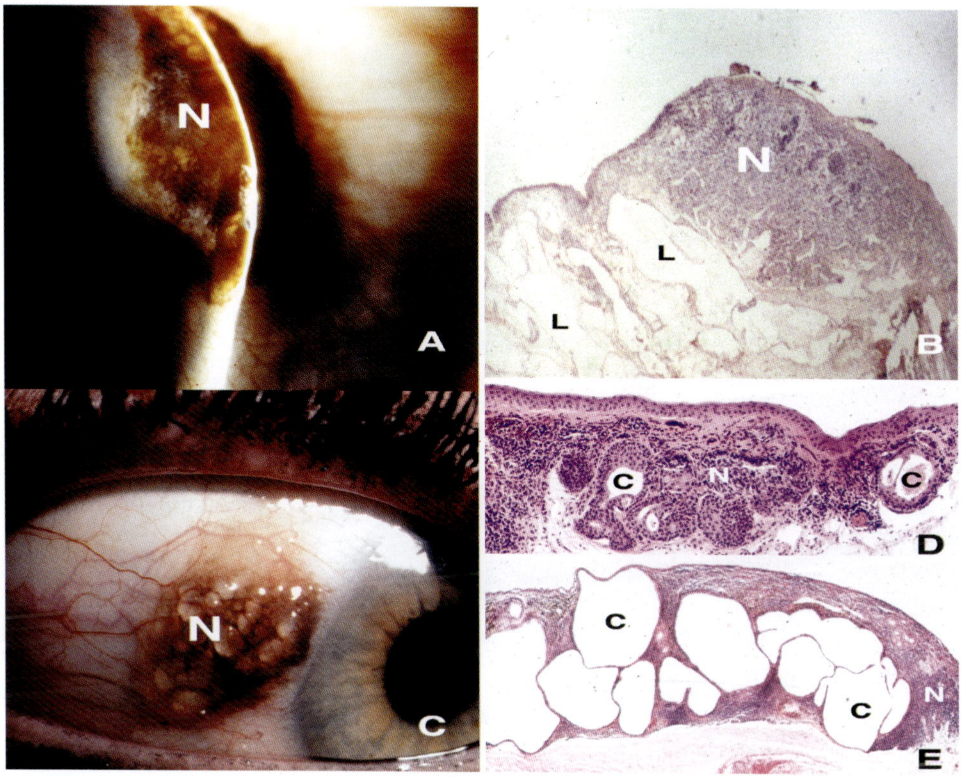

FIGURE 21.8. Nevi masquerading as melanoma because of clinical enlargement of the lesion. (A,B) Multicolored, dome-shaped bulbar nevus (N) appears to be enlarging because of the lymphangiectasis (L) with lymph/stasis developing under the lesion (B). (C,E) Enlargement of cystic nevus (N) secondary to the distension of the cystic structures (C, D).

nomas differentiates them clinically from nevi. Any long-standing conjunctival nevus that suddenly changes its size, color, or appearance should be excised for histopathologic examination, with margins of the excised specimen specifically marked for proper orientation. This can be very useful for surgical planning if involved margins necessitate the further removal of additional tissue.

Melanomas are said to arise de novo when there is no clinical or histologic evidence of a precursor lesion within the epithelium adjacent to the tumor. The terms *nodular melanoma* (borrowed from dermatologic literature) and de novo melanoma are often used synonymously.

Clinically, the de novo melanoma develops as a tumor mass with increased pigmentation, surrounded by mild inflammation and prominent blood vessels. The growth rate of melanoma is quite variable. In early stages, these lesions are not deeply invasive into the underlying tissues, and surgical excision is easy (Figure 21.9). As they grow, however, they may become fixated to underlying structures and eventually invade the LDS, globe and/or orbit (Figures 21.10, 21.11, and 21.12). An extrascleral extension of a choroidal melanoma may take the form of an epibulbar pigmented tumor mass; this should not be confused with conjunctival melanoma (Figure 21.13). If there is any suspicion that a deeply located pigmented lesion represents an extrascleral extension of a ciliary body tumor, an echographic examination with A and B scans and/or MRI should be done immediately.

Management and Prognosis

The current management of early conjunctival melanoma is surgical excision under frozen section control followed by alcohol epitheliectomy and cryotherapy to the margins of excision. Cryotherapy, which is usually applied as a double freeze–thaw technique to the excision margins of the lesion, has proven value for local tumor control, but does not seem to change the incidence of metastatic disease.[61] The cryotherapy should preferably be done to the excision margins of the conjunctiva; this application does not cause significant ad-

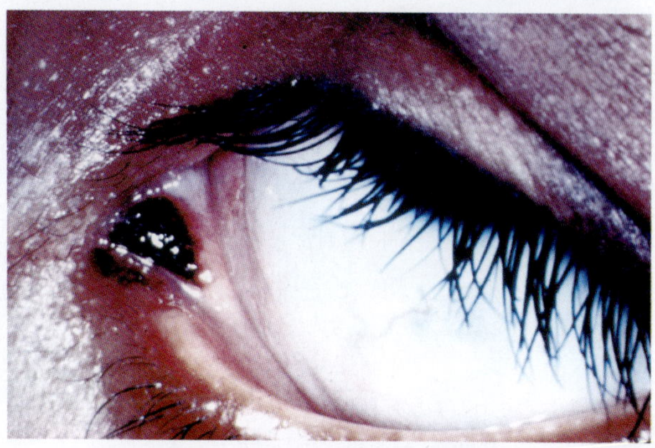

FIGURE 21.9. Melanocytic lesion at the caruncle. Although this tumor was a nongrowing nevus for many years, when the patient was about 45 years old, the lesion became thicker and darker. An excisional biopsy revealed a conjunctival melanoma, developing within a nevus. Caruncular melanoma is known to have a worse prognosis than melanoma originating from bulbar conjunctiva.

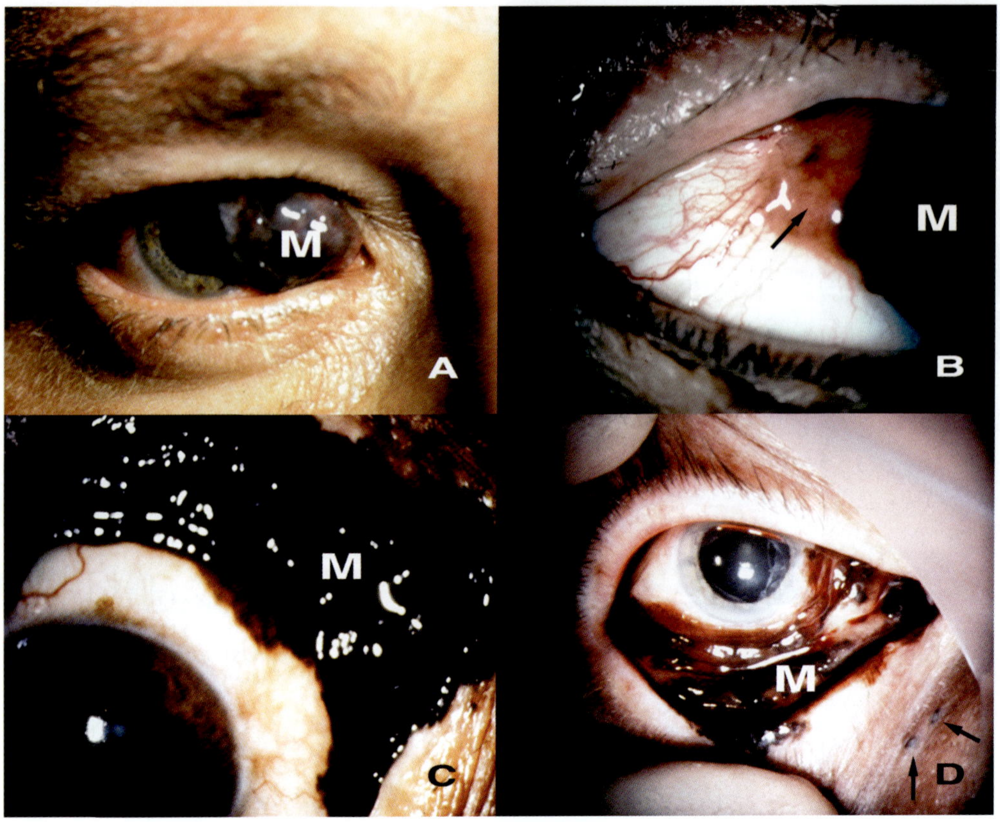

FIGURE 21.10. Large conjunctival melanomas (M). (A) Large nodular melanoma originating from bulbar conjunctiva. Despite the size of the lesion, surgical excision alone successfully treated this patient; no recurrence or any other lesions had been identified in the conjunctiva many years after excision. (Courtesy of Dr. Delmar R. Caldwell, New Orleans.) (B) Extensive conjunctival melanoma involving the bulbar conjunctiva and cornea. Note that the tumor is salmon colored (arrow) in parts and very darkly pigmented in other areas. Melanomas without pigmentation may be confused with lymphoproliferative lesions of the conjunctiva. (C) Diffuse, darkly pigmented melanoma originating from primary acquired melanosis. (D) Conjunctival melanoma originating from PAM extending into the subconjunctival, tarsal, and orbital soft tissues. The vascular spread can be seen in periorbital cutaneous lymphatics, clinically (arrows).

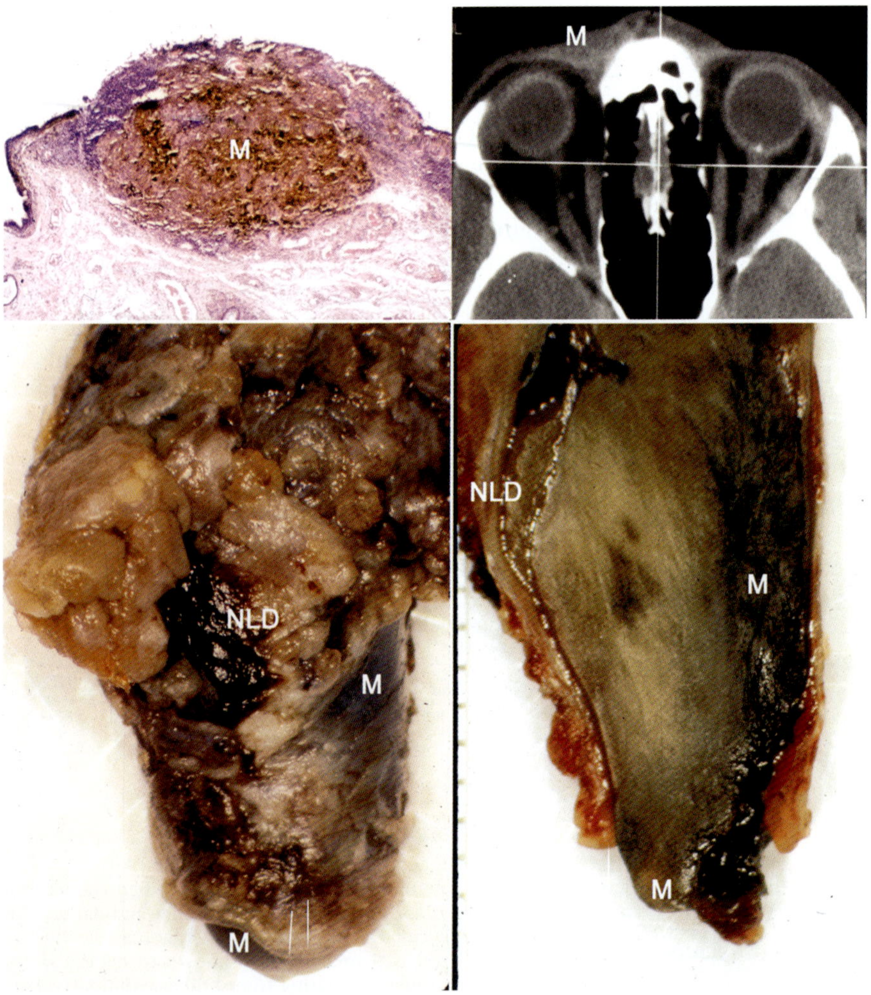

FIGURE 21.11. Recurrent multifocal conjunctival melanoma (M) documented with multiple biopsies eventually developed a large LDS tumor contained within the sac and nasolacrimal duct (NLD). It was impossible to determine whether the LDS tumor originated from an independent focus in the lacrimal sac epithelium or secondary to seeding from conjunctival lesions. The tumor was excised, and postoperative radiation was given; no recurrence of LDS was encountered (double arrows: surgical excision margin of NLD).

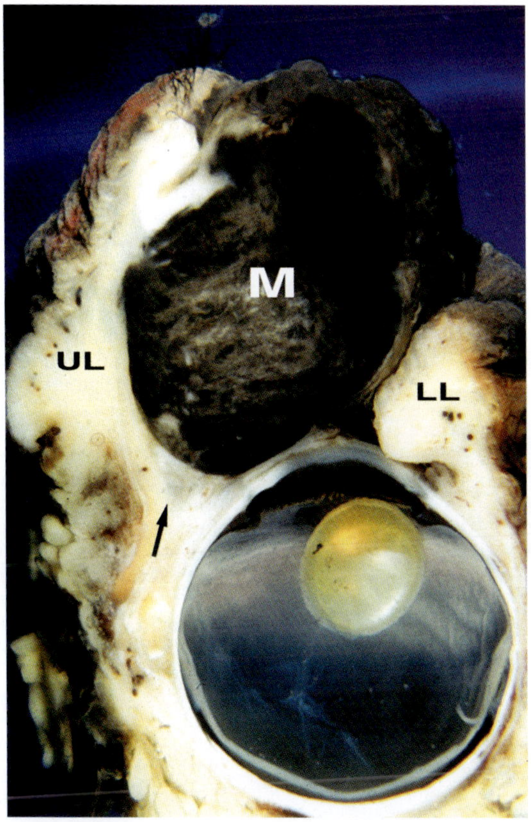

FIGURE 21.12. Exenteration specimen depicting a large, densely pigmented conjunctival melanoma extending into upper (UL) and lower (LL) eyelids and orbital soft tissues (arrow). (Courtesy of Dr. Jerry Shields, Philadelphia.)

verse effects. However, it should be sparingly applied to the scleral base of the tumor because of the risk of damage to the underlying ocular components.[52] It is believed that cryotherapy cures the clinically invisible extent of the tumor because patients who are treated with tumor excision alone have a higher recurrence rate than those who are treated with the combination of surgery and cryotherapy.[31,61,62]

Flat pigmented lesions that remain stable in size and appearance can usually be safely checked at 6-month intervals. Bulbar lesions are usually diagnosed earlier and monitored easily with sequential slit lamp examinations every 6 months. On the other hand, the tumors that originate from tarsal conjunctiva, caruncle, and fornices are usually recognized late and have a greater tendency to invade the orbit.[63] If a tumor changes its size, shape, thickness, or pigmentation pattern, it should be subjected to biopsy or excised. If the lesion is small enough, it should be entirely removed, with generous margins (1–2 mm) as an excisional biopsy. This biopsy sample is placed flat on a piece of cardboard and its margins properly identified before it is sent to the pathology laboratory. If one margin shows tumor involvement and the others do not, additional tissue may be excised from the involved margin, while healthy conjunctival tissue in other margins is preserved; hence the importance of margin orientation. In large tumors, one can safely make an initial incisional biopsy to determine the nature of the lesion. Biopsies should be performed on the thickest, most irregular, and most pigmented parts of the melanoma, with particular care not to crush or cauterize the sample, especially if it is a small one.

In larger lesions, particularly those that are recurrent, the extent of surgical excision of the tumor is individualized. In general, the surgical approach should employ wider and deeper excision for melanomas on the surface of the eye. Enucleation or exenteration should be considered for tumors with ocular or orbital invasion.[63] In patients with large tumors, the regional lymph nodes should be sampled for staging purposes (see Chapter 12).[64]

The management plan of conjunctival melanoma and the time of implementation of different treatment modalities depend on the clinical presentation and the recurrence pattern. Several histopathologic features observed in excisional and punch biopsies samples of conjunctival melanomas indicate the likelihood of recurrent and disseminated tumor (Figure 21.14). These features include invasive melanoma thickness more than 0.8 mm, lack of inflammatory cell response at

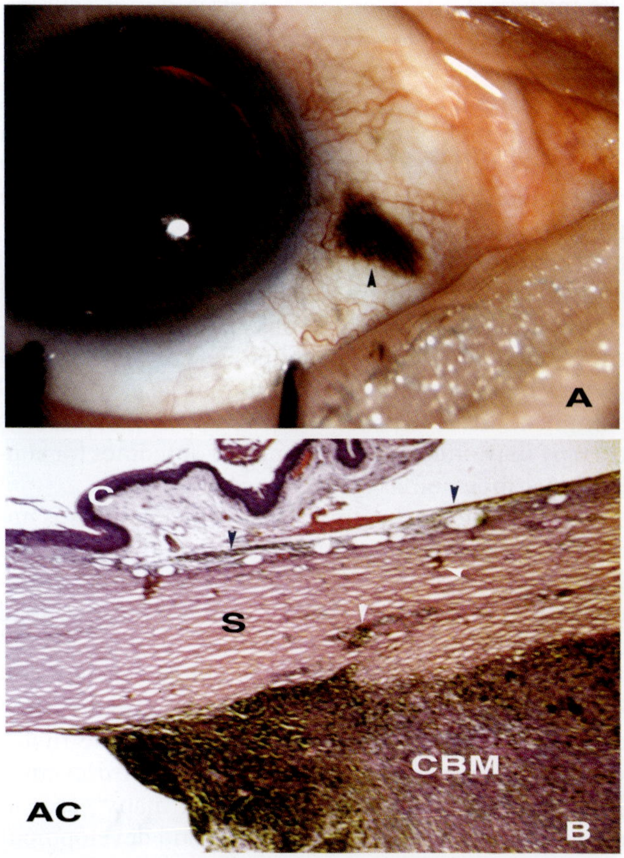

FIGURE 21.13. (A) A ciliary body melanoma (CBM) that presented as an enlarging pigmented bulbar conjunctival lesion (arrowhead). (B) Histopathology shows the lesion (arrowheads) in relation to the CBM, the anterior chamber (AC), the conjunctiva (C), and the sclera (S).

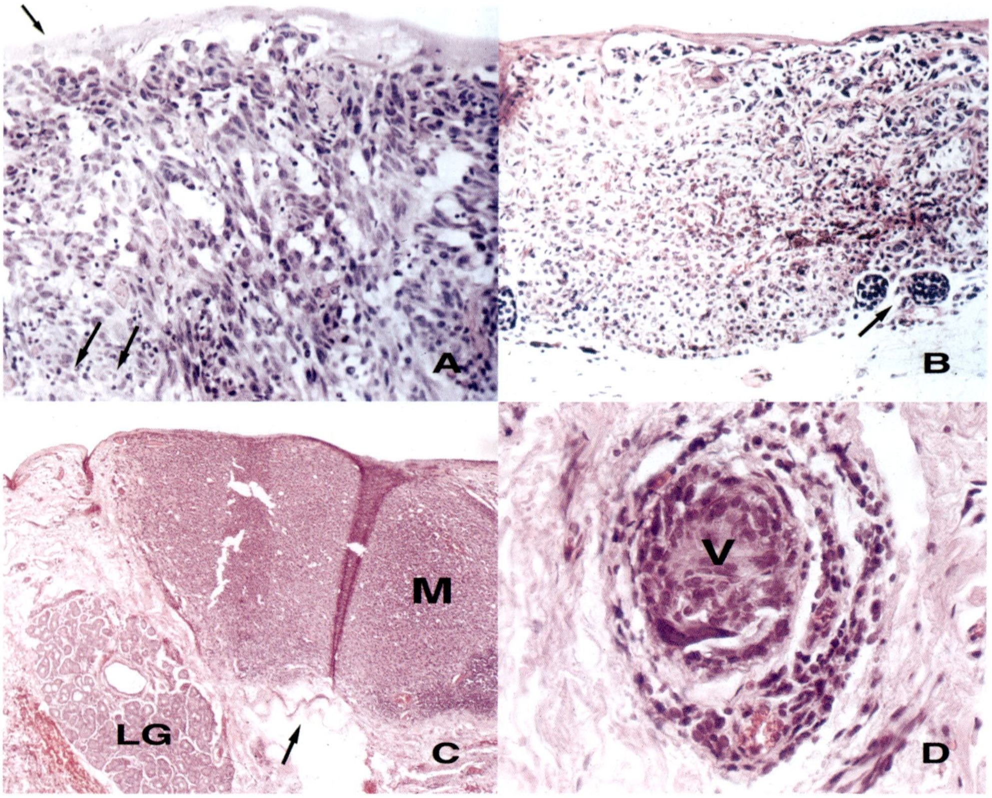

FIGURE 21.14. Histopathologic appearances of conjunctival melanoma. (A) Conjunctival melanoma invading the entire thickness of the epithelium (single arrow) with invasion of subepithelial layers (double arrows). Melanomas that invade deeper than 1 mm have a poor prognosis. (B) Conjunctival melanoma with significant invasion into subepithelial tissues forming an early nodule; rounded nests of tumor cells (arrow) can be identified at the advancing edge of the tumor. (C) Large, invasive melanoma (M) of the conjunctiva (C) extending into the soft tissues of the orbit and lacrimal gland (LG). (D) Melanoma cells within the lumen of a blood vessel (V).

the invasive front, 5 or more mitotic tumor cells per 10 high-power fields (HPF), involvement of caruncle and orbital soft tissues with melanoma, and involvement of lateral and deep margins (of the excisional biopsy) with melanoma. If the margins are positive for tumor, the patient should receive additional treatment with wider excision, cryotherapy, brachytherapy, or local antimetabolites. For one or more other findings, the patient should be followed clinically every 3 months for 1 to 2 years to detect early recurrence.[65]

Although radiotherapy has been tried on conjunctival melanomas, these tumors are not very responsive to radiation, and the EBRT may lead to several complications.[66] Recent work suggests that brachytherapy may offer better therapeutic outcomes for conjunctival melanoma.[67,68]

Topical chemotherapy with antimetabolites is another type of treatment under current investigation. Data are limited but promising; in particular, mitomycin C may be beneficial in treatment of superficial conjunctival melanomas.[69]

Conjunctival melanomas should be closely followed after treatment because approximately half these patients develop recurrences within the first 5 years after primary treatment and one third eventually develop disseminated disease. In many cases of recurrence, there is orbital invasion and development of the signs and symptoms of rapidly developing space-occupying lesions. These patients should be evaluated for regional lymph node involvement and disseminated disease to distant organs. CT and MRI can be invaluable to determine the extent of secondary orbital invasion, and the systemic workup should be done in consultation with an ocular oncologist. Although it is believed that regional lymph nodes are the initial site of metastasis, the pathways of dissemination are not well established.[70]

For a tumor that extends into the orbit, local resection of the lesion is no longer feasible and exenteration may be indicated. In a recent study of over 150 patients, 65% had no tumor recurrence after treatment and 35% experienced at least one recurrence; 5 or more recurrences were seen in 3% of the cases.[71,72] Twenty out of 150 patients (13%) developed orbital extension to different degrees and were treated with exenteration. Of the 20 exenterations, 7 were performed as initial procedures, 6 were done after the first recurrence, and 7 after multiple recurrences. The investigators concluded that exenteration became indicated in 8% of their patients by the 5-year follow-up and 32% of their patients by the 15-year follow-up.

Although the orbital exenteration has been a time-honored treatment for advanced cases of conjunctival melanoma, there is still no consensus on its indications and surgical technique. In the 1950s, early exenteration with complete removal of the globe and orbital soft tissues was advocated as the preferred treatment.[73,74] The idea of performing extensive, mutilating surgery was later challenged, and the exenteration was performed only for tumors involving the fornices or extending to the eyelid skin and tumors that did not respond to EBRT.[75,76] Others suggested that in cases of diffuse melanoma involving the caruncle, the exenteration should be combined with radical neck dissection.[77] Later it was realized that prophylactic lymph node dissection did not help to improve the incidence of disseminated disease. The technique was thus abandoned.[78] Today lymph node dissection is performed only for staging purposes when evidence exists of metastatic disease.[79] Recent investigation of regional lymph node metastasis in conjunctival melanoma performed with sentinel lymph node mapping and biopsy indicated that preauricular lymph nodes were most commonly involved (see Chapter 12). A recent clinical study by Esmaeli and coworkers found approximately 40% involvement of regional lymph nodes within about 3 years of initial diagnosis.[70] The most commonly involved lymph nodes were preauricular nodes in approximately 75% of the 11 patients with lymph node disease. It was concluded that sentinel lymph node biopsy may develop as a potential test for early detection of microscopic nodal metastasis, and therefore, these results may be used as another piece of information in decision making for exenteration. Other clinical features predictive of orbital extension of conjunctival melanoma were reported as follows: visual acuity of 20/200 or worse, extralimbal location, amelanotic tumors, caruncular lesions, and tumors that present with the histopathologic invasion deeper than 1 mm.[72] It has been noted that lesions with invasion deeper than 2 mm do not respond well even to orbital exenteration in terms of avoiding dissemination of the tumor. Paridaens and coworkers reported that mortality ranges between 33 and 50% for melanomas thicker than 1 mm invasion despite exenteration.[79] The same authors indicated that invasion of the lymphatics, blood vessels, and sclera as well as the incomplete excision at the time of initial treatment indicated very poor outcomes.

References

1. Shields JA, Shields CL. *Atlas of Eyelid and Conjunctival Tumors*. Philadelphia: Lippincott, Williams & Wilkins; 1999.
2. Newton R, Ferlay J, Reeves G, et al. Effects of ambient solar ultraviolet radiation on incidence of squamous cell carcinoma of the eye. *Lancet* 1996;347:1450–1451.
3. Lee GA, Williams G, Hirst LW, Green AC. Risk factor in the development of ocular surface epithelial dysplasia. *Ophthalmology* 1994;101:360–364.
4. Gaasterland DE, Rodriguez MM, Moshell AN. Ocular involvement in xeroderma pigmentosum. *Ophthalmology* 1982;89:980–986.
5. Elsas FJ, Green WR. Epibulbar tumors in childhood. *Am J Ophthalmol* 1975;79:1001–1007.
6. Karp CL, Scott IU, Chang TS, et al. Conjunctival intraepithelial neoplasia: a possible worker for immunodeficiency virus infection. *Arch Ophthalmol* 1996;114:257–261.
7. Lewallen S, Shroyer KR, Keyser RB, Liomba G. Aggressive conjunctival squamous cell carcinoma in three young Africans. *Arch Ophthalmol* 1996;114:215–218.
8. Lee GA, Hirst LW. Ocular surface squamous neoplasia [review]. *Surv Ophthalmol* 1995;39:429–450.
9. Cha SB, Shields JA, Shields CL, Wang MX. Squamous cell carcinoma of the conjunctiva [review]. *Intl Ophthalmol Clin* 1993;33:19–24.
10. Mahmood MA, Al-Rajhi AA, Riley F, Karcioglu ZA. Scleral keratitis. An unusual presentation of squamous cell carcinoma of the conjunctiva. *Ophthalmology* 2001;108:553–558.
11. Iliff WJ, Marback R, Green WR. Invasive squamous cell carcinoma of the conjunctiva. *Arch Ophthalmol* 1995;93:119–122.
12. Lee BA, Hirst LW. Retrospective study of ocular surface squamous cell carcinoma. *Australian N Z J Ophthalmol* 1997;25:269–276.
13. Nicholson DH, Herschler J. Intraocular extension of squamous cell carcinoma of the conjunctiva. *Arch Ophthalmol* 1977;95:843–846.
14. Johnson E, Tabarra KF, Weatherhead RG. Secondary squamous cell carcinomas of the orbit. *Arch Ophthalmol* 1997;115:75–78.
15. Tabbara KF, Kersten R, Daouk N, Blodi FC. Metastatic squamous cell carcinoma of the conjunctiva. *Ophthalmology* 1988;95:318–321.
16. Shields JA, Bakewell B, Augsburger JJ, et al. Classification and incidence of space-occupying lesions of the orbit. A survey of 645 biopsies. *Arch Ophthalmol* 1984;120:1606–1611.
17. Günalp I, Gündüz K. Secondary orbital tumors. *Ophthalmic Plast Reconstr Surg* 1997;13:31.
18. Rootman J. Secondary tumors of the orbit. In: Rootman J, ed. *Diseases of the Orbit*. Philadelphia: JB Lippincott; 1988.
19. Ryan SJ, Font RL. Primary epithelial neoplasms of the lacrimal sac. *Am J Ophthalmol* 1973;76:73–88.
20. Hyams DJ. Papillomas of the nasal cavity and paranasal sinuses. *Ann Otol Rhinol Laryngol* 1971;80:192.
21. Karcioglu ZA, Caldwell DR, Reed HT. Papillomas of the lacrimal drainage system: a clinicopathological study. *Ophthalmic Surg* 1984;15:670.
22. Karcioglu ZA, Wesley RE, Greenidge KC, McCord CD. Proptosis and pseudocyst formation from inverted papilloma. *Ann Ophthalmol* 1982;14:443–448.
23. Stern JB. In: Karcioglu ZA, Someren A, eds. *Practical Surgical Pathology*. Lexington, MA: Collamore Press; 1985:921–993.
24. Cooper D, Schermer A, Sun TT. Classification of human epithelia and neoplasms using monoclonal antibodies to keratins: strategies, applications and limitations. *Lab Invest* 1985;52:253–255.
25. Cohen DH, Green R, Iliff NT, et al. Spindle cell carcinoma of the conjunctiva. *Arch Ophthalmol* 1980;98:1809–1813.
26. Brownstein S. Mucoepidermoid carcinoma of the conjunctiva with intraocular invasion. *Ophthalmology* 1981;88:1226–1229.
27. Gamel JW, Eiferman RA, Guibor P. Mucoepidermoid carcinoma of conjunctiva. *Arch Ophthalmol* 1984;102:730–731.
28. Caya JG, Hidayat AA, Weiner JM. A clinicopathologic study of 21 cases of adenoid SCC of the eyelid and periorbital region. *Am J Ophthalmol* 1985;99:291–297.
29. Mauriello JA, Abdelsalam A, McLean IW. Adenoid squamous carcinoma of the conjunctiva. A clinicopathological study of 14 cases. *Br J Ophthalmol* 1997;81:1001–1005.
30. Batsakis JG, Husser J. Squamous carcinoma with gland-like (adenoid) features. *Ann Otol Rhinol Laryngol* 1990;99:87–88.
31. Shields JA, Shields CL, De Potter P. Surgical approach to conjunctival tumors. *Arch Ophthalmol* 1997;115:808–815.
32. Fraunfelder FT, Wingfield D. Management of intraepithelial

conjunctival tumors and squamous cell carcinoma. *Am J Ophthalmol* 1983;95:359–363.
33. Frucht-Pery J, Rozenman Y. Mitomycin C therapy for corneal intraepithelial neoplasia. *Am J Ophthalmol* 1994;117:164–168.
34. Shields CL, Naseripour M, Shields JA. Topical mitomycin C for extensive, recurrent conjunctival–corneal squamous cell carcinoma. *Am J Ophthalmol* 2002;133:601–606.
35. Buus DR, Tse DT, Folberg R. Microscopically controlled excision of conjunctival squamous cell carcinoma. *Am J Ophthalmol* 1994;117:97–102.
36. Karcioglu ZA, Caldwell DR. Frozen section diagnosis in ophthalmic surgery. *Surv Ophthalmol* 1984;28:323–332.
37. Broders AC. Practical points on microscopic grading of carcinoma. *N Y J Med* 1932;32:667–671.
38. Friedman HI, Cooper PH, Wanebo JH. Prognostic and therapeutic use of microstaging of cutaneous squamous cell carcinoma of the trunk and extremities. *Cancer* 1985;56:1099–1105.
39. Lund HC. How often does squamous cell carcinoma of the skin metastasize? *Arch Dermatol* 1965;92:635–637.
40. Martin H, Strong E, Shapiro RH. Radiation induced skin cancer of the head and neck. *Cancer* 1970;25:61–71.
41. Brennan JA, Mao L, Hruban RH, et al. Molecular assessment of histopathological staging in squamous cell carcinoma of the head and neck. *N Engl J Med* 1995;332:429–435.
42. Sun EC, Fears TR, Goerdert JJ. Epidemiology of squamous cell conjunctival cancer. *Cancer Epidemiol Biomarkers Prev* 1997;6:73–77.
43. Newton R, Ferlay J, Reeves G, et al. Effect of ambient ultraviolet radiation on incidence of squamous cell carcinoma of the eye. *Lancet* 1996;347:1450–1451.
44. Lane DP. p53 and human cancers. *Br Med Bull* 1994;50:582–599.
45. Toth J, Karcioglu ZA, Moshfeghi AA, et al. The relationship between human papillomavirus and p53 gene in conjunctival squamous cell carcinoma. *Cornea* 2000;19:59–62.
46. Karcioglu ZA, Toth J. Relation between p53 over-expression and clinical behavior of ocular/orbital invasion of conjunctival squamous cell carcinoma. *Ophthalmic Plast Reconstr Surg* 2000;16:443–449.
47. Karcioglu ZA, Issa TM. HPV in neoplastic and non-neoplastic conditions of the external eye. *Br J Ophthalmol* 1997;81:595–598.
48. McDonnell JM, McDonnell PJ, Mounts P, et al. Demonstration of papillomavirus capsid antigen in human conjunctival neoplasia. *Arch Ophthalmol* 1986;104:1801–1805.
49. Maclean H, Dhillon B, Ironside J. Squamous cell carcinoma of the eyelid and the acquired immunodeficiency syndrome. *Am J Ophthalmol* 1996;121:219–221.
50. Lewallen S, Shroyer KR, Keyser RB, Liomba G. Aggressive conjunctival squamous cell carcinoma in three young Africans. *Arch Ophthalmol* 1996;114:215–218.
51. Campbell RJ. Tissue diagnosis: eyelid and conjunctiva. In: Karcioglu ZA, ed. *Laboratory Diagnosis in Ophthalmology*. New York: Macmillan; 1987:1–23.
52. Seregard S. Conjunctival melanoma. *Surv Ophthalmol* 1998;42:21–50.
53. Folberg R, McLean IW, Zimmerman LE. Malignant melanoma of the conjunctiva. *Hum Pathol* 1985;16:136–143.
54. Liesegang TJ,Campbell RJ. Mayo Clinic experience with conjunctival melanoma. *Arch Ophthalmol* 1980;98:1385.
55. McDonnell JM, Carpenter JD, Jacobs P, et al. Conjunctival melanocytic lesions in children. *Ophthalmology* 1989;96:986–993.
56. Folberg R, McLean W, Zimmerman LE. Conjunctival melanosis and melanoma. *Ophthalmology* 1984;91:673–678.
57. Crombie IK. Racial differences in melanoma incidence. *Br J Cancer* 1979;40:185–193.
58. Grossniklaus HE, Green WR, Luckenbach M, Chan CC. Conjunctival lesions in adults. A clinical and histopathologic review. *Cornea* 1987;6:78–116.
59. Graham BJ, Duane TD. Ocular melanoma task force report. *Am J Ophthalmol* 1980;90:728–733.
60. Singh AD, Campos OE, Retigan RM, et al. *Surv Ophthalmol* 1998:43:127–133.
61. Jakobiec FA, Rine FJ, Fraunfelder FT, Brownstein S. Cryotherapy for conjunctival primary acquired melanosis and malignant melanoma. *Ophthalmology* 1988;95:1058–1070.
62. De Potter P, Shields CL, Shields JA, Menduke H. Clinical predictive factors for development and recurrence of metastasis in conjunctival melanoma: a review of 68 cases. *Br J Ophthalmol* 1993;77:624–630.
63. Shields JA. *Diagnosis and Management of Orbital Tumors*. Philadelphia: WB Saunders; 1989:63.
64. Esmaeli B. Sentinal node biopsy as a tool for accurate staging of eyelid and conjunctival malignancies. *Curr Opin Ophthalmol* 2002;13:317–323.
65. Folberg R, McLean IW, Zimmerman LE. Conjunctival melanosis and melanoma. *Ophthalmology* 1984;91:673–678.
66. Lederman M, Wybar K, Busby. Malignant epibulbar melanoma. Natural history and treatment by radiotherapy. *Br J Ophthalmol* 1984;68:605–617.
67. Lommatzsch PK, Lommatzsch RE, Kirsch I, Furmann P. Therapeutic outcome of patients suffering from malignant melanoma of the conjunctiva. *Br J Ophthalmol* 1990;74:615–619.
68. Shields JA, Shields CL, Freire JE, et al. Plaque radiotherapy for selected orbital malignancies: preliminary observations: the 2002 Montgomery Lecture, part 2. *Ophthalmic Plast Reconstr Surg* 2003;19:91–95.
69. Finger PT, Milner MS, McCormick SA. Topical chemotherapy for conjunctival melanoma. *Br J Ophthalmol* 1993;77:751–753.
70. Esmaeli B, Wang X, Youssef A, Gershenwald JE. Patterns of regional and distant metastasis in patients with conjunctival melanoma. Experience at a cancer center over 4 decades. *Ophthalmology* 2001;108:2101–2105.
71. Shields CL, Shields JA, Gündüz K, et al. Conjunctival melanoma: risk factors for recurrence, exenteration, metastasis and death in 150 consecutive patients. *Arch Ophthalmol* 2000;118:1497–1507.
72. Shields JA, Shields CL, Gündüz K, et al. Clinical features predictive of orbital exenteration for conjunctival melanoma. *Ophthalmic Plast Reconstr Surg* 2000;16:1732–1738.
73. Reese AB. Precancerous melanosis and diffuse malignant melanoma of the conjunctiva. *Arch Ophthalmol* 1938;19:354–365.
74. Reese AB. *Tumors of the Eye*. New York: Harper & Row, 1963.
75. Zimmerman LE. Discussion of pigmented tumors of the conjunctiva. In: Boniuk M, ed. *Ocular and Adnexal Tumors*. St Louis: CV Mosby; 1964:24–48.
76. Jay B. Nevi and melanomata of conjunctiva. *Br J Ophthalmol* 1965;49:169–204.
77. Tucker MA, Shields JA, Hartge P, et al. Sunlight exposure as risk factor for intraocular malignant melanoma. *N Engl J Med* 1985;313:789–792.
78. Burns JW, Jenkins HA. Melanoma of the conjunctiva. A rational approach to management. *Head Neck Surg* 1979;2:99–106.
79. Paridaens ADA, Minassian DC, McCartney ACE, et al. Prognostic factors in primary malignant melanoma of the conjunctiva: a clincopathological study of 256 cases. *Br J Ophthalmol* 1994;78:252–259.

22

Ocular Tumors

Zeynel A. Karcıoglu and Doris Hadjistilianou

Rarely, intraocular tumors extend transclerally and invade the periocular tissues and the orbit.[1–5] These tumors include retinoblastoma, uveal melanoma, malignant medulloepithelioma, retinal pigment epithelium carcinoma, and optic disk melanocytoma. The secondary involvement of orbital soft tissues with extraocular tumors is a rare condition, and the only clinically significant lesions in this group are retinoblastoma and choroidal melanoma; therefore, only these two tumors are discussed in this chapter.

RETINOBLASTOMA

Retinoblastoma (Rb) is the most common intraocular malignant tumor in childhood, with an incidence of 1 in 15,000 live births. Early diagnosis and treatment have significantly increased survival rate and organ preservation in recent years.[6] With advances in therapy, survival has risen from 30% in the 1930s to nearly 95% in the 1990s.[7]

Primary enucleation continues to be a common choice of treatment of Rb. External beam radiation therapy (EBRT) is an effective therapeutic option but unfortunately is associated with second nonocular malignancies. Historically, the use of chemotherapy has been limited to retinoblastoma with local invasion of the orbit and optic nerve in metastatic disease. Chemotherapy is now used as a conservative treatment in an effort to avoid EBRT and/or enucleation and obtain better functional results.[8,9]

Extraocular Rb is a common problem of pediatric oncology in developing countries and is almost always due to delay in diagnosis of the intraocular disease (Figure 22.1).[10,11] Extraocular extension is the most significant risk factor associated with very poor prognosis. In medically advanced countries, most cases of orbital Rb present as a recurrence following primary enucleation for intraocular tumor.[12] Orbital extension of intraocular Rb or orbital recurrence after enucleation has been reported to comprise 12% of all cases.[12,13] Orbital involvement of Rb carries a poor prognosis and is associated with a high risk of metastasis to the central nervous system (CNS), lymph nodes, bone marrow, and bones.[14] Statistically significant risk factors for orbital involvement include massive choroidal involvement, microscopic extrascleral invasion, optic nerve involvement beyond the resection margin, late enucleation, and delay in diagnosis.

Orbital invasion from advanced intraocular Rb may follow several anatomical pathways, including Schlemm canal, posterior ciliary vessels and nerves, and anterior and posterior emissary channels; it may happen, as well, by direct scleral erosion (Figure 22.2).[15]

However, surgical procedures can also allow access into the orbit for tumor cells.[16] Karcioglu et al. reported that a 25-gauge needle can seed tumor into the sclera and facilitate access into the orbit.[17] Pars plana vitrectomy in an eye with suspected retinoblastoma should be avoided. Openings in the limbus and sclera may create tissue tracts for the Rb cells to invade the orbit (Figure 22.3). Stevenson et al. reported three patients who developed recurrence in the orbit and lymph nodes after vitrectomy for unsuspected Rb.[18] Fine-needle aspiration biopsy (FNAB) is advised only in extraordinarily unusual clinical presentations.[19]

If the diagnosis of Rb is done from biopsy or vitrectomy results, efforts should be made to prevent orbital recurrence. Prophylactic chemotherapy and EBRT should be delivered in addition to enucleation to prevent systemic tumor dissemination.[20] Orbital symptoms are usually absent when extraocular extension is only microscopic. A significant orbital extension, on the other hand, produces symptoms of a retrobulbar space-occupying mass, including rapidly progressing proptosis, chemosis, and extraocular motility disturbance. Recurrent Rb following enucleation presents with displacement of the implant, difficulty in wearing an ocular prosthesis, chemosis, and cellulitis (Figures 22.4 and 22.5).[18,21]

For a correct staging of orbital involvement, all patients should undergo a careful diagnostic workup before excisional biopsy. Procedures include computed tomography (CT) and magnetic resonance imaging (MRI) of the head and orbit, bone scintigraphy, lumbar puncture with cell count and examination of the cytocentrifugate, bone marrow aspiration, and biopsy and ocular examination under anesthesia. Usually Rb extending to the orbit is less differentiated than the primary tumor, and sometimes it is difficult to dis-

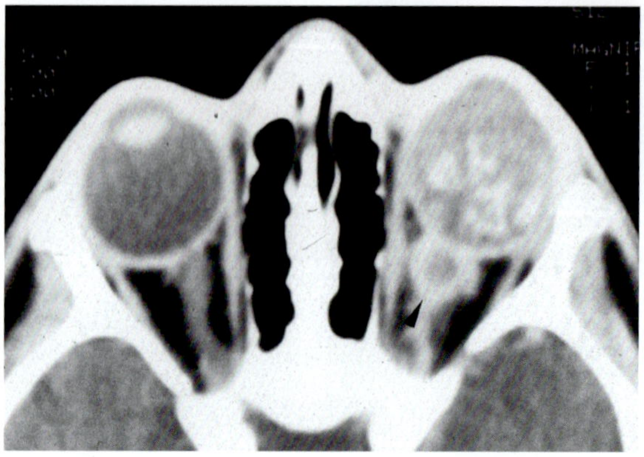

FIGURE 22.1. Axial CT scan showing a retinoblastoma of the left globe extending into the optic nerve, meninges, and orbital soft tissues (arrowhead). Note the multiple calcifications within the intraocular tumor. The secondary orbital extensions and metastatic foci of retinoblastomas very rarely show calcification.

tinguish between recurrency and second tumors (Figure 22.2).[22]

CT and MRI to document the extension of the orbital involvement are mandatory (Figures 22.1 and 22.4). At CT, large enough orbital extension appears as an intraconal mass with moderate enhancement after administration of contrast medium. On T1-weighted MRI studies, Rb produces a homogeneous to heterogeneous signal that is hyperintense to the vitreous body and to muscle and hypointense to fat, while in T2-weighted images, it appears hypointense to the vitreous and isointense to fat with variable degree of enhancement after gadolinium administration (Figure 22.6). In an attempt to improve the poor outcome of Rb cases with orbital involvement, different therapeutic protocols have been applied. Reese in the

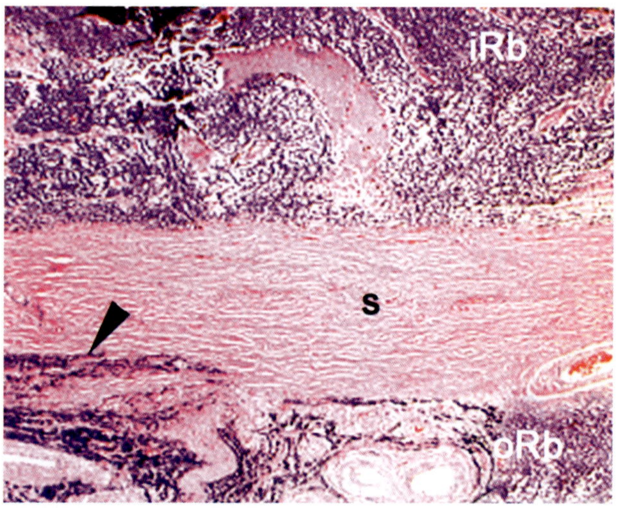

FIGURE 22.2. Histopathologic appearance of the intraocular retinoblastoma (iRb) composed of poorly differentiated small rounded cells with areas of necrosis and calcification. The tumor infiltrates (arrowhead) the sclera (S) to extend into orbital tissues. The orbital retinoblastoma (oRb) has a similar histology to its intraocular counterpart.

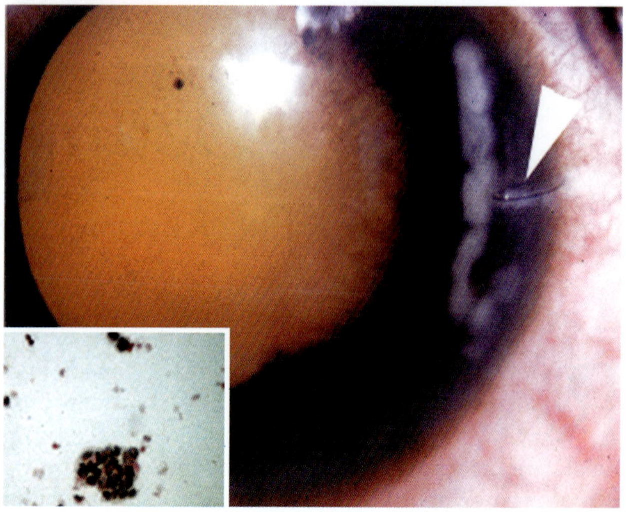

FIGURE 22.3. Retinoblastoma cells leaving the globe through the opening of vitrectomy (white arrowhead). *Inset*: Cluster of retinoblastoma cells.

1950s proposed orbital exenteration followed by EBRT, but there were no survivors among 25 children treated.[23] Orbital extension of Rb was associated with high mortality rates ranging from 94 to 100% with a mean survival of 14 months. In 1984 Mackay et al. reported that regardless of what therapy was given, affected patients died within approximately 6 months.[24] Over the past 15 years, a multidisciplinary treatment approach has improved prognosis. Different chemotherapy regimens are used for orbital Rb (Table 22.1).

Cyclophosphamide, platinum derivatives, Adriamycin, vincristine, and epipodophyllotoxins are the drugs most often used because their efficacy has been established in the treatment of other neuroectodermal tumors (neuroblastoma). Chemotherapy combined with EBRT improves survival in orbital disease.[25] Complete remission for 8 to 84 months was achieved in 5 patients with orbital recurrence after enucleation by combining excisional biopsy of the tumor with EBRT and systemic chemotherapy (cyclophosphamide, cisplatin, vincristine, methotrexate, and etoposide) and intrathecal (methotrexate) chemotherapy.[26] The use of high-dose chemotherapy regimens with autologous bone marrow transplantation has been used in patients with metastases.

Good results in terms of survival have been reported with chemotherapy and orbital EBRT. Doz et al. reported their experience in 33 patients (20 with orbital Rb and 13 with orbital Rb with metastases) who received systemic and intrathecal chemotherapy and orbital and cranial EBRT. The authors concluded that associated CNS disease still carries a bad prognosis and confirmed that intensive chemotherapy using cyclophosphamide, platinum compounds, epipodophyllotoxins, doxorubicin, and vincristine was effective in orbital Rb. In this series, the disease-free interval was longer when patients had no CNS disease.[12]

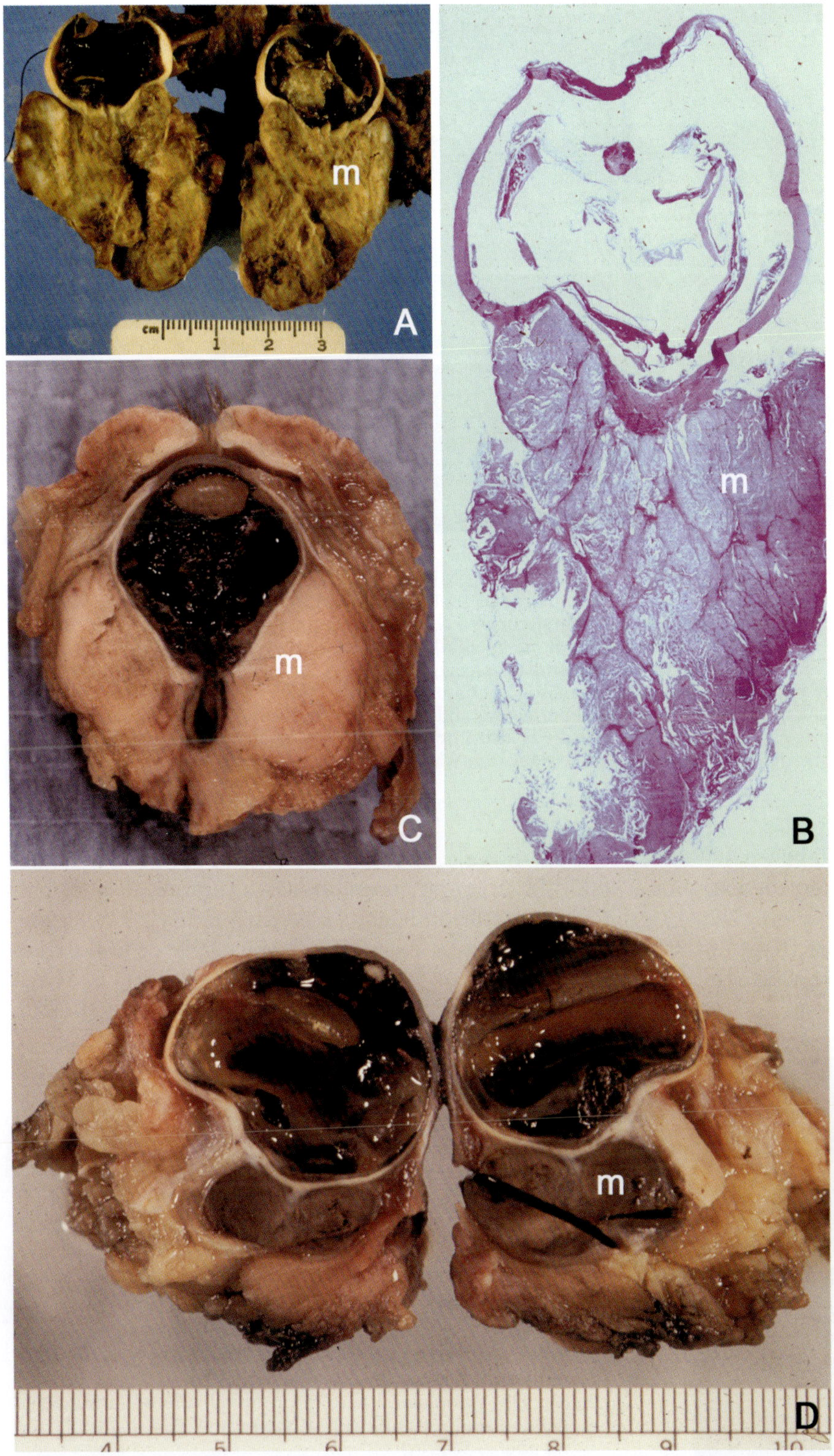

FIGURE 22.9. Gross (A, C, D) and histopathologic (B) depictions of choroidal melanomas (m) with secondary involvement of the orbital tissues. Specimens in (A) and (B) are from the same patient; a CT image of this patient's lesion appears in Figure 22.10A. Note the lobulated extension of the tumor into the orbital soft tissues in all cases. (C) The changing nature of the choroidal melanoma (m) as it extends into the optic nerve, meninges, and the orbital soft tissues. The nerve involvement is highly pigmented as opposed to the amelanotic tumor in the orbit. (D) In contrast, the tumor shows pigmented intraocular and extraocular components.

ologic characteristics when they leave the globe to invade the orbital soft tissues. For example, pigmented tumors are known to become amelanotic, and necrotic tumors develop a solid structure (Figure 22.9). This point should be kept in mind; since if a tumor happens to differentiate into an amelanotic lesion, signal characteristics of melanin will not be helpful in MRI differential diagnosis.

Extraocular extension of ciliary body melanomas, which can be seen subconjunctivally, has been described in approximately 10% of these tumors.[52,53]

It has been reported that secondary orbital mela-

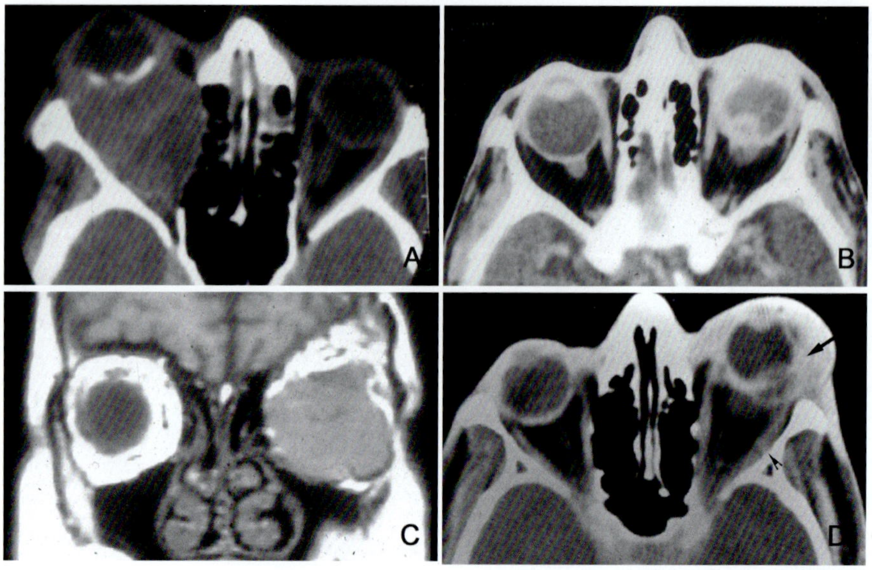

FIGURE 22.10. (A) Axial CT image showing a large, secondary orbital tumor originating from the choroidal melanoma within a phthisic eye. Note the posterior scleral calcification in the globe. The orbital tumor occupies the entire socket, extending into the ethmoidal sinus and the apex. (B) A prephthisic left globe shows a dome-shaped posterior density continuous through the sclera into the anterior orbit. The lesion could not be visualized because of a densely opaque cornea, and the clinical diagnosis was a choroidal melanoma extending into the orbit. However, histopathologic examination revealed a partially organized hematoma within the globe and the orbit. (C) T1-weighted, contrast-enhanced coronal MR image demonstrating a homogeneous, irregular choroidal melanoma revealing a signal isointense with the cerebral cortex. The extensive infiltration of the tumor into the orbital fat, medial, and inferior orbital walls and into the maxillary sinus is clearly seen. (D) A known diffuse flat choroidal melanoma on the lateral aspect of the globe extending into the lateral periocular and anterior orbital soft tissues. The lateral rectus muscle is also thickened with secondary choroidal melanoma involvement (arrowhead).

noma originating from the choroid can be treated with brachytherapy with some success when the extraocular extension is less than 3 mm thick (Figure 22.11).[43] When the melanoma nodule is greater than 3 mm in diameter, enucleation is performed to remove the melanoma nodule encased by normal-appearing orbital fat.[54] In larger and more invasive tumors, total or partial exenteration is done (see Chapter 31).[55–57] In general, extraocular extension, particularly orbital extension, is a poor prognostic indicator, with a 5-year mortality rate reported to range from 45 to 65%.[37]

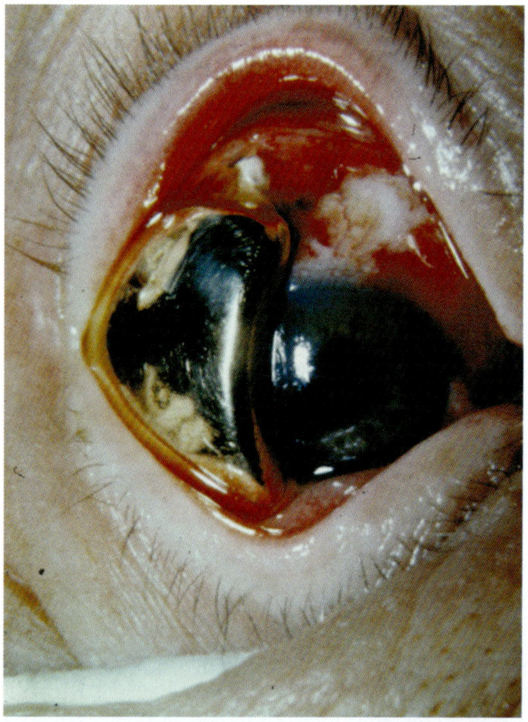

FIGURE 22.11. Treatment of extraocular melanoma with I-125 brachytherapy plaque.

References

1. Shields JA, Bakewell B, Augsberger JJ, et al. Classification and incidence of space-occupying lesions in the orbit: survey of 645 biopsies. *Arch Ophthalmol* 1984;120:1606–1611.
2. Henderson JW, Campbell RJ, Farrow GM, Garrity JA. *Orbital Tumors*. New York: Raven Press; 1994:43–52.
3. Günalp I, Gündüz K. Biopsy-proven orbital lesions in Turkey. A survey of 1092 cases over 30 years. *Orbit* 1994;13:67–79.
4. Seregard S, Sahlin S. Panorama of orbital space-occupying lesions. The 24-year experience of a referral center. *Acta Ophthalmol Scand* 1999;77:91–98.
5. Sen DK. Aetiological pattern of orbital tumors in India and their clinical presentations. A 20-year retrospective study. *Orbit* 1990;9:299–302.
6. Finger P, Harbour JW, Karcioglu ZA. Risk factors for metastasis in retinoblastoma [major review]. *Surv Ophthalmol* 2002;47:1–16.
7. Shields CL, Shields JA. Recent developments in the management of retinoblastoma. *J Pediatr Ophthalmol Strabismus* 1999;36:8–18.
8. Finger PT, Czechonska G, Demirci H, Rausen A. Chemotherapy for retinoblastoma. A current topic. *Drugs* 1999;58:983–996.
9. De Potter P. Current treatment of retinoblastoma. *Curr Opin Ophthalmol* 2002;13:331–336.
10. Belmekki M, El Bakkali M, Abdellah H, et al. Epidemiologie

des processus orbitaires chez l'enfant. *J Fr Ophtalmol;* 1999; 22:394–398.

11. Castillo BV, Kaufman L. Pediatric tumors of the eye and orbit. *Pediatr Clin N Am* 2003;50:149–172.
12. Doz F, Khelfaoui F, Mosseri V, et al. The role of chemotherapy in orbital involvement of retinoblastoma. The experience of a single institution with 33 patients. *Cancer* 1994;74:722–732.
13. Grabowski FF, Abramson DH. Intraocular and extraocular retinoblastoma. *Hematol Oncol Clin North Am* 1987;1:721–735.
14. Karcioglu ZA, Al-Mesfer SA, Jabak MH, et al. Work-up for metastatic retinoblastoma: a review of 261 patients. *Ophthalmology* 1997;104:307–312.
15. Rootman J, Hofbauer J, Ellsworth RM, et al. Orbital extension of retinoblastoma: a clinicopathological study. *Can J Ophthalmol* 1978;13:72–80.
16. Shields JA, Shields CL, Ehya H, et al. Fine needle aspiration biopsy of suspected intraocular tumors. The 1992 Urwick Lecture. *Ophthalmology* 1993;100:1677–1684.
17. Karcioglu ZA, Gordon RA, Karcioglu GL. Tumor seeding in ocular fine needle aspiration biopsy. *Ophthalmology* 1985;92: 1763–1767.
18. Stevenson KE, Hungerford J, Garner A. Local extraocular extension of retinoblastoma following intraocular surgery. *Br J Ophthalmol* 1989;73:739–742.
19. Karcioglu ZA. Fine needle biopsy for diagnosis of retinoblastoma. *Retina* 2002;22:707–710.
20. Shields CL, Honavar S, Shields JA, et al. Vitrectomy in eyes with unsuspected retinoblastoma. *Ophthalmology* 2000;107: 2250–2255.
21. Karcioglu ZA, Mullaney PB, Millar LC. Extrusion of porous polyethylene orbital implant in recurrent retinoblastoma. *Ophthalmic Plast Reconstr Surg* 1998;14:37–44.
22. Dutton JJ, Byrne SF, Proia AD. Retinoblastoma. In: *Diagnostic Atlas of Orbital Diseases.* Philadelphia: WB Saunders; 2000:136–137.
23. Reese AB. *Tumours of the Eye.* London: Cassell & Company; 1951:138.
24. Mackay CJ, Abramson DH, Ellsworth RM. Metastatic patterns of retinoblastoma. *Arch Ophthalmol* 1984;102:391–396.
25. Hungerford J, Kingston J, Plowman N. Orbital recurrence of retinoblastoma. *Ophthalmic Pediatr Genet* 1987;8:63–68.
26. Goble RR, McKenzie J, Kingston JE, et al. Orbital recurrence of retinoblastoma successfully treated by combined therapy. *Br J Ophthalmol* 1990;74:97–98.
27. Kiratli H, Bilgic S, Ozerdem U. Management of massive orbital involvement of intraocular retinoblastoma. *Ophthalmology* 1998;105:322–326.
28. Svedberg-Winholt H, Al-Mesfer SA, Riley FC. Survival trends of retinoblastoma patients with extraocular extension. Paper presented at: Congress of European Society of Ophthalmology; 1999. Abstr 502.
29. Chantada G, Fandino A, Casak S, et al. Treatment of overt extraocular retinoblastoma. *Med Pediatr Oncol* 2003;40:158–161.
30. Campbell R, Sobin LH. Histologic typing of tumors of the eye and its adnexa. *WHO International Histological Classification of Tumors.* Berlin: Springer-Verlag; 1998.
31. Shields JA, Shields CL. Massive orbital extension of posterior uveal melanoma. *Ophthalmic Plast Reconstr Surg* 1991;7: 238–251.
32. Starr HJ, Zimmerman LE. Extrascleral extension and orbital recurrence of malignant melanomas of the choroid and ciliary body. *Int Ophthalmol Clin* 1962;2:369–385.
33. Shields JA, Shields CL, Donoso LA. Management of posterior uveal melanoma. *Surv Ophthalmol* 1991;36:161–195.
34. Liarikos S, Rapidis AD, Roumeliotis A, et al. Secondary orbital melanomas: analysis of 15 cases. *J Craniomaxillofac Surg* 2000;28:148–152.
35. Shammas HF, Blodi FC. Orbital extension of choroidal and ciliary body melanomas. *Arch Ophthalmol* 1977;95:2002–2005.
36. Rini FJ, Jakobiec FA, Hornblass A, et al. The treatment of advanced choroidal melanoma with massive orbital extension. *Am J Ophthalmol* 1987;104:634–639.
37. Affeldt JC, Minckler DS, Azen SP, et al. Prognosis in uveal melanoma with extrascleral extension. *Arch Ophthalmol* 1980;98:1975–1979.
38. Shields JA, Shields CL. Orbital malignant melanoma: 2002 Sean B. Murphy Lecture. *Opthalmic Plast Reconstr Surg* 2003;19:262–269.
39. Shields CL, Shields JA, De Potter P, et al. Diffuse choroidal melanoma. Clinical features predictive of metastasis. *Arch Ophthalmol* 1996;114:956–963.
40. Collaborative Ocular Melanoma Study Group. Histopathologic characteristics of uveal melanomas in eyes enucleated from Collaborative Ocular Melanoma Study COMS Report No 6. *Am J Ophthalmol* 1998;125:745–766.
41. Shields JA. Orbital malignant melanomas. In: Hornblass A, ed. *Ophthalmic Plastic & Reconstructive Surgery.* Baltimore: Williams & Wilkins; 1988.
42. Henderson JW, Farrow GM. *Orbital Tumors.* 2nd ed, New York: BC Decker; 1980:425–450.
43. Gündüz K, Shields CL, Shields JA. Plaque radiotherapy for management of ciliary body and choroidal melanoma with extraocular extension. *Am J Ophthalmol* 2000;130:97–102.
44. Shields CL, Shields JA, Yarian DL, et al. Intracranial extension of choroidal melanoma near the optic nerve. *Br J Ophthalmol* 1987;71:172–176.
45. Shields JA, Augsburger JJ, Dougherty MJ. Orbital recurrence of choroidal melanoma 20 years after enucleation. *Am J Ophthalmol* 1984;97:767–770.
46. Shields JA, Augsburger JJ, Donoso LA, et al. Hepatic metastasis and orbital recurrence of uveal melanoma after 42 years. *Am J Ophthalmol* 1985;100:666–668.
47. Martin JA, Robertson DM. Extrascleral extension of choroidal melanoma diagnosed by ultrasound. *Ophthalmology* 1983;90: 1554.
48. Farah ME, Byrne SF, Hughes JR. Standardized echography in uveal melanoma with scleral or extraocular extension. *Arch Ophthalmol* 1984;102:1482.
49. Enochs SW, Petherick P, Bogdanova A, et al. Paramagnetic metal scavenging by melanin: MR imaging. *Radiology* 1997; 204:417–423.
50. Haik BG, Saint Louis L, Smith ME, et al. Magnetic resonance imaging in choroidal tumors. *Ann Ophthalmol* 1987;19:218–238.
51. Gormori JM, Grossman RI, Shields JA, et al. Choroidal melanomas. Correlation of NMR spectroscopy and MR imaging. *Radiology* 1986;158:443–445.
52. Shields CL, Shields JA, Karlsson U, et al. Enucleation after plaque radiotherapy for posterior uveal melanoma. *Ophthalmology* 1990;97:1665–1670.
53. Pach JM, Robertson DM, Taney BS, et al. Prognostic factors in choroidal and ciliary body melanomas with extrascleral extension. *Am J Ophthalmol* 1986;101:325–331.
54. De Potter P, Shields JA, Shields CL, Santos R. Modified enucleation via lateral orbitotomy for choroidal melanoma with orbital extension: a report of two cases. *Ophthalmic Plast Reconstr Surg* 1992;8:109–113.
55. Shields JA, Shields CL, Suvarnamani C, et al. Orbital exenteration with eyelid sparing: indications, technique, and results. *Ophthalmic Surg* 1991;22:292–297.
56. Shields JA, Shields CL, Demirci H, et al. Experience with eyelid sparing orbital exenteration: the 2000 Tullos O. Coston Lecture. *Ophthalmic Plast Reconstr Surg* 2001:17:355–361.
57. Goldberg RA, Kim JW, Shorr N. Orbital exenteration: results of an individualized approach. *Ophthalmic Plast Reconstr Surg* 2003;19:299–336.

23

Tumors of the Cranial and Nasal Cavities and Paranasal Sinuses

Zeynel A. Karcıoglu

SECONDARY ORBITAL TUMORS ORIGINATING FROM THE SINONASAL TRACT

Nasal and paranasal sinus neoplasms account for approximately 5% of tumors originating in the upper respiratory tract. Approximately half of these tumors are benign, mainly squamous papillomas, and the remainder are malignancies, of which squamous cell carcinoma (SCC) comprises approximately 75% (Table 23.1).[1,2]

Epithelial Tumors

Benign epithelial tumors of the nose and paranasal sinuses include squamous and inverted papilloma and pleomorphic adenoma originating from minor salivary glands.[2,3] Papillomas of the sinonasal tract originate from squamous or Schneiderian epithelium. Although they are benign, these tumors, which most commonly occur in white males after 50 years of age, may expand beyond their site of origin and invade the adjacent structures, including the orbit. Furthermore, these lesions recur when they are not excised completely and may show transition into squamous cell carcinoma.[3–5] An associated malignancy, usually SCC, has been reported in approximately 10 to 15% of patients with inverted papilloma.[6,7] Inverted papillomas may also develop in the lacrimal drainage system (LDS).[5] Some of the benign lesions, including the inverted papillomas of the sinonasal tract and the LDS, are known to invade the orbit secondarily (Figure 23.1).[6,8]

Although malignant tumors of the nose and paranasal sinuses constitute only about 1% of all malignancies in the body, their influence on the neighboring orbit and ocular tissues is significant. Approximately 10% of all orbital mass lesions consist of secondary tumors originating from the nose and paranasal sinuses.[9–11] Sinonasal malignancies occur more often in white males.[12]

Epidemiologic studies emphasize the influence of inhaled carcinogens, and there is also evidence that human papillomavirus (HPV) infection is an oncogenic factor in the development of paranasal upper respiratory tract neoplasms, more often in benign than in malignant lesions.[13–15]

Squamous Cell Carcinoma

SCC is the most common malignant tumor of the sinonasal tract.[2,16] Maxillary and ethmoid sinuses give origin to approximately 85% of SCC; the frontal and sphenoid sinuses are rarely involved with this tumor. In many instances, SCC has been associated with preexisting chronic sinusitis or may create secondary sinusitis owing to the obstruction of the sinusoidal ostium. Therefore, it is important to differentiate a malignancy from a coexistent inflammation.

Other malignant epithelial sinonasal tumors include adenocarcinoma and adenoid cystic carcinoma of minor salivary glands.[7]

Clinical Features

The most common clinical manifestations of the sinonasal tumors are similar if not identical to the symptoms caused by inflammatory sinus disease, including fullness, pain, nasal airway obstruction, and nasal discharge. The physical examination of the sinonasal region and orbit should include a direct fiberoptic endoscopy, which also offers an opportunity to obtain tissue for diagnosis. Tissue material from these tumors can be collected with sinus lavage/cytology, fine-needle aspiration biopsy (FNAB) and transnasal biopsy with direct or endoscopic approaches.

Once a tumor has extended into the orbit, however, the symptoms change somewhat and become more related to the eye and adnexal structures (Figures 23.2 and 23.3). Extension of the tumor usually takes place as an infiltrating fashion to create a space-occupying mass in the orbit with surrounding inflammatory reaction leading to proptosis, extraocular muscle motility disturbance, visual acuity and field loss, and edema of the eyelids and conjunctiva; epiphora may develop as a late symptom. The proptosis of the eye secondary to the infiltration of sinus tumors into the orbit is usually nonaxial and associated with a great deal of pain and paresthesia in about

TABLE 23.1. Tumors of Sinonasal Tract that May Involve the Orbit Secondarily.

	Benign	*Malignant*
Epithelial tumors	Inverted (Schneiderian) papilloma Nasal papilloma	Squamous cell carcinoma Transitional cell carcinoma Adenoid cystic carcinoma Esthesioneuroblastoma
Mesenchymal tumors	Neural tumors Fibroma, fibromyxoma Osteoma Hemangioma	Soft tissue sarcomas Osteogenic sarcoma
Lymphoproliferative tumors	Lymphoid hyperplasia	Lymphoma Burkitt's tumor Plasmacytoma Chloroma
Other tumors and tumor-like conditions	Histiocytosis Pseudotumor	Histiocytosis

75% of the cases. Metastatic disease to the orbit from distant organs, on the other hand, is painful in fewer cases and the proptosis is usually axial.[17]

An unusual inflammatory condition, which may mimic secondary orbital neoplasm, is allergic fungal disease of the nose and paransasal sinuses.[18,19] This bizarre inflammatory process of the sinonasal tract may extend into the orbit (Figure 23.4). Frequently, an *aspergillus* species is the causative organism, but other fungal species, including *Fusarium* and *Rhizomucor*, have also been incriminated.[20]

Although this allergic entity is considered to be confined to the lumen, without mucosal involvement, it nevertheless is known to spread from one paranasal cavity to the other and to the orbit.[21] Computed tomography (CT) and magnetic resonance imaging (MRI) show bony expansion and remodeling of the involved cavity and focal bony erosion. The mucoid content of

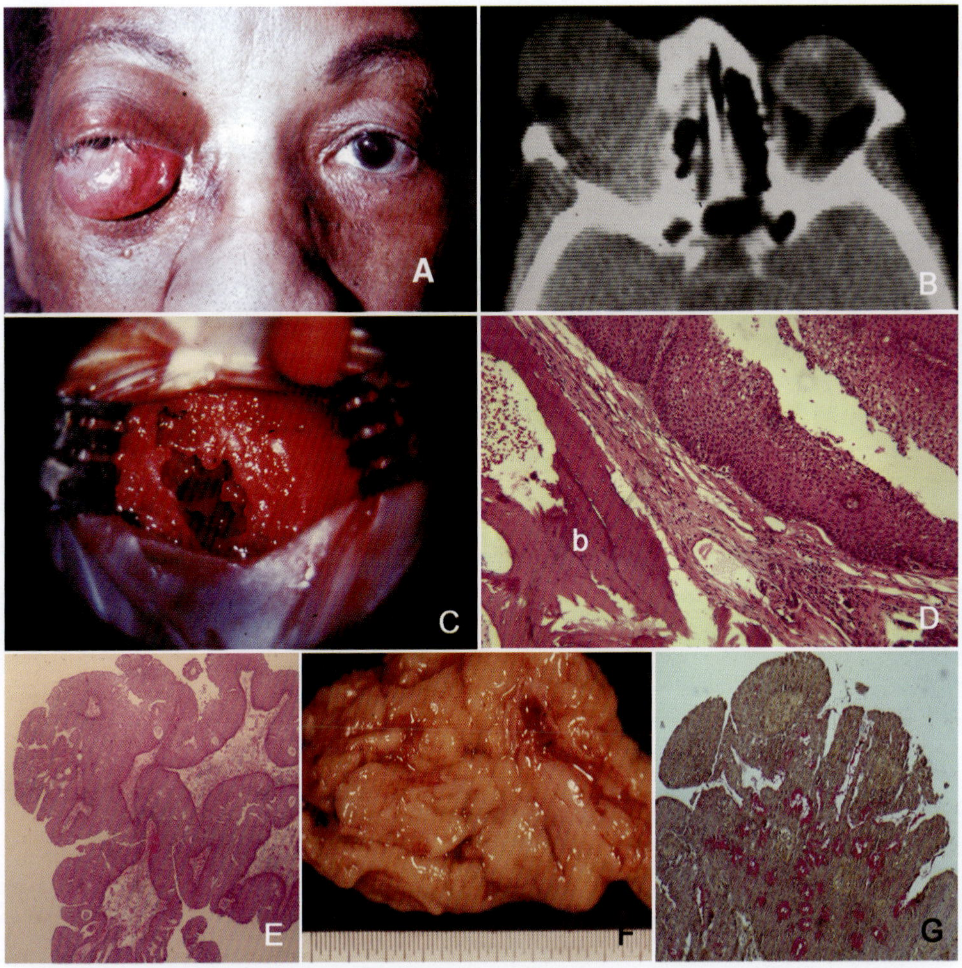

FIGURE 23.1. A 60-year-old woman with multiple recurrences over the years of a nasal inverted papilloma. Although the lesion was histopathologically benign, it presented with multiple recurrences and invasion of the adjacent paranasal sinuses and the orbit. (A) Facial photograph. (B) Axial image. (C) Intraoperative photo showing a papillary appearance with pseudocyst formations. (D) Microscopic pathology of the lesion: although the epithelial element of the tumor reveals minimal atypia, it is known to infiltrate the bone (b) during its expansion. (E–G) Gross pathology. (F) The papillary surface, with multiple invaginations (E,G). The papillary growth of the epithelium, with deep, multiple invaginations into the stroma labeled the tumor as "inverted papilloma." Within papillary proliferations of the epithelium are small cystic accumulations of mucin, as depicted with mucicarmine stain (G).

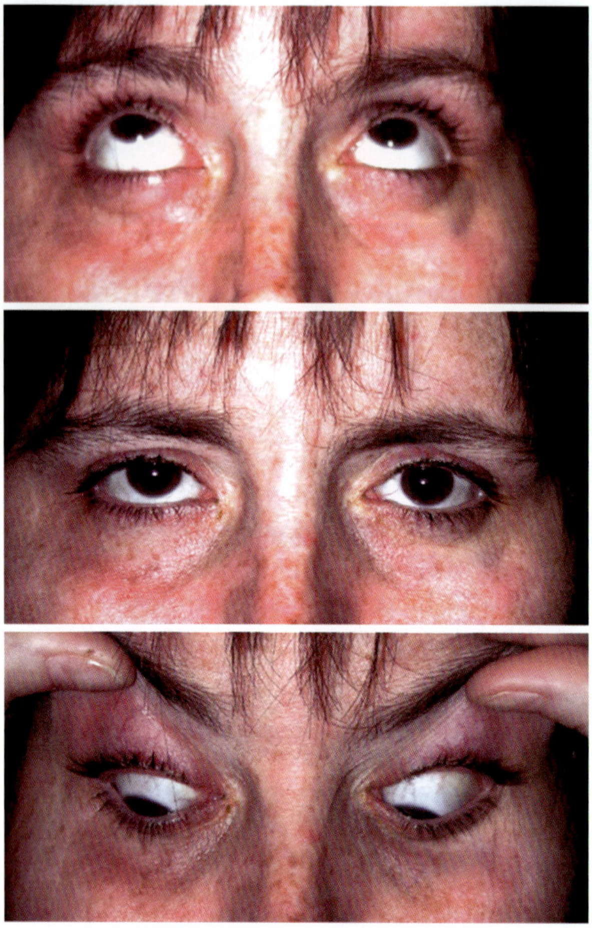

FIGURE 23.2. A 40-year-old woman with squamous cell carcinoma of the orbit originating from the maxillary sinus. Although the tumor could be palpated in the inferior orbit, proptosis and motility disorders of the right eye were minimal.

the paranasal sinuses mixed with fungus balls produces low signal intensity in the MRI. The extensive bony expansion and irregular remodeling, coupled with bony erosion, may simulate an invasive tumor of the nose or the sinus, with secondary orbital invasion, such as esthesioneuroblastoma, leukemia/lymphoma, or Burkitt's lymphoma. The histopathology shows mucoid debris intermixed with numerous eosinophils and hyphae of the causative fungus, most of the time *Aspergillus* species.[20,21]

Radiologic Features

Radiologic imaging is essential for the evaluation of the patient with plain films of the orbit and surrounding structures, as well as CT and MRI.[12,22,23] In a great majority of the cases of SCC with orbit involvement, the bony wall of the orbit demonstrates erosion. CT provides better images of bone destruction, however, it does not reliably reveal the details of soft tissue invasion (Figure 23.3). In contrast, MRI provides a more accurate evaluation of the soft tissues, although it may be difficult to distinguish a tumor limited to the periorbita from early invasion. The involvement of the periorbita, however, cannot be assessed preoperatively even with the most sensitive imaging techniques and endoscopy.

Although bone destruction is considered to be pathognomonic of malignancy, not all malignant tumors destroy the adjacent bone. Some sinonasal sarcomas, lymphomas, and plasmacytomas remodel the adjacent bone by chronic compression. Therefore, if soft tissue detail is not available, one should remem-

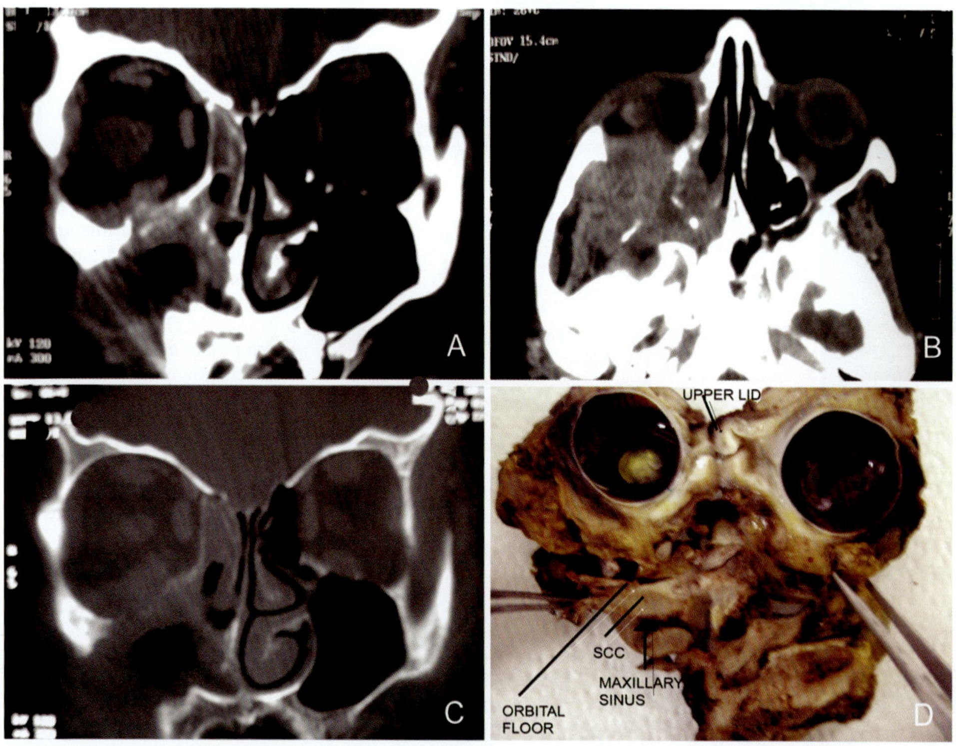

FIGURE 23.3. (A–C) coronal and axial CT images reveal a large, partially necrotic maxillary sinus tumor extending into the adjacent paranasal sinuses and the orbit. Coronal, noncontrast CT scan depicts soft tissue mass in the right maxillary sinus extending into the nasal cavity, ethmoidal sinus, and orbit. The destruction of the orbital floor is clearly seen in the regular CT (A) and bone windows (C). Axial, noncontrast CT scan (B) also shows the extensive infiltration of the maxillary sinus tumor; nonhomogeneous soft tissue density fills the maxillary sinus and extends into the orbit and nasal cavity. The tumor's mottled appearance is mostly likely due to necrosis because of presurgery radiation treatment. An exenteration specimen (D) from the same patient shows the extension of the squamous cell carcinoma from maxillary sinus into the orbital floor.

ber that tumors with benign-appearing bone changes may be aggressive, yet some other lesions that cause bone destruction, such as pyogenic or allergic fungal sinusitis, inflammatory pseudotumor, and mucocele, may be benign (Figure 23.4).[23] Inflammatory pseudotumor of the maxillary sinus, unlike its orbital counterpart, may present with aggressive bone erosion into the orbit and mimic a secondary SCC.[24]

MRI, particularly with T2-weighted images, can be extremely useful in mapping the sinonasal tumors because of the inherent differences of signal intensity between SCC and inflammatory sinus disease. The sinonasal carcinomas usually present with homogeneous intermediate signal intensity on both T1- and T2-weighted images because of their uniform cellular pattern.[25] MRI may not help to differentiate a tumor as benign or malignant; however, it provides excellent delineation of the tumor from its surrounding inflammatory tissue.[26] Sinonasal tumors obstruct the flow of mucosal secretions usually present with clinical symptoms before the secretion becomes desiccated and therefore, offer a high signal intensity on T2-weighted images. In contrast, a great majority of sinonasal tumors are hypercellular and contain less water than the inflamed mucosa and noninspissated secretions; therefore, such tumors manifest with intermediate to low signal intensity on T2-weighted images. To confuse the issue, about 5% of sinonasal tumors such as neural and vascular tumors may have high signal intensity with T2 weighting. Enhancement of SCC with gadolinium chelate is particularly helpful on T1-weighted images in most sinonasal tumors.

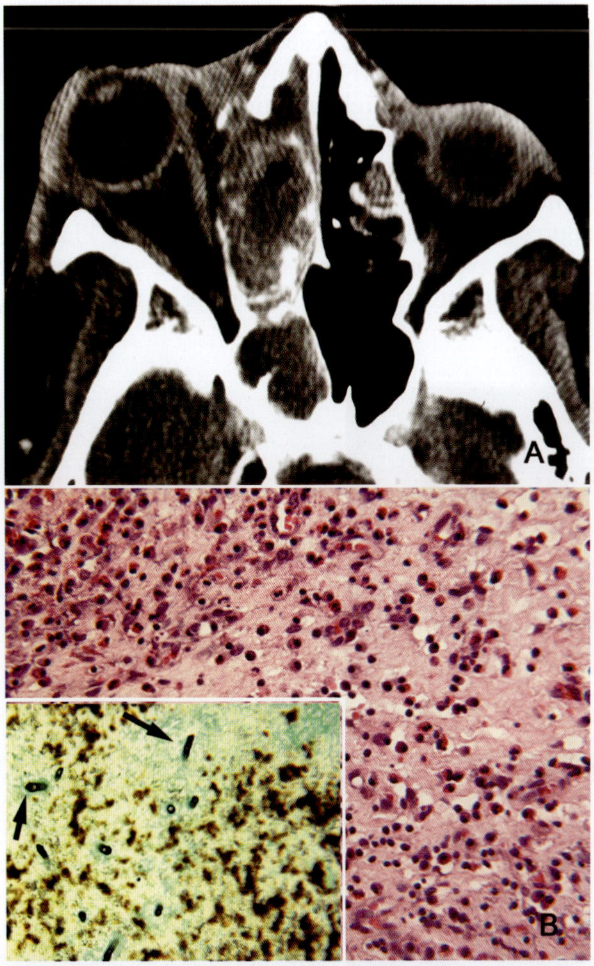

FIGURE 23.4. (A) Axial CT image showing allergic sinonasal aspergillosis with expansion and remodeling of ethmoidal bones and the medial wall of orbit. (B) Histopathologic appearance shows acute inflammatory reaction with numerous eosinophils. *Inset*: Gomori silver methanamine stain showing many *Aspergillus* hyphae (arrows).

The incidence and the presentation of orbital involvement by malignancies of the sinonasal tract vary with the site of origin and the type and aggressiveness of the tumor. SCC of the maxillary sinus involves the orbit in most cases through anatomic pathways such as the nasolacrimal duct or infraorbital fissure or by following neurovascular structures such as ethmoidal or infraorbital nerves.[27] Direct invasion of the orbit by the destruction of the bone and periorbita is also commonly seen. Over the decades, surgeons have observed that the periorbita provides a resistant barrier against the infiltration of SCC, which becomes a very significant issue in the formation of the management plan. If the periorbita is not involved, the globe and the vital orbital tissues may be preserved. The invasion of the orbital periostium can best be documented during surgery by the use of frozen section.

The majority of the cases with orbital invasion attest to a relatively slow-growing tumor that went undetected until it became obvious with orbital symptoms. Orbital involvement, particularly with soft tissue invasion, represents the late presentation of the disease, with very poor prognosis.[28]

Management and Prognosis

The conventional treatment of the nasosinal SCC with extension into orbital soft tissues has been maxillectomy with orbital exenteration followed with or without radiation therapy. Even with extensive surgery and radiation, only 10 to 50% of these patients have disease-free survival periods. Some have indicated that the preservation of the orbit through "planned exenteration" when there is localized invasion would not compromise the cure rate of these patients.[29–32] Currently it is believed that localized invasion does not downgrade the outcome as long as the full thickness of the periorbita is not involved with tumor. It is also believed that preoperative or postoperative radiation therapy does not improve thc survival ratc in patients with total or partial exenterations.

Adenocarcinoma

Adenocarcinomas and adenoid cystic carcinomas of the sinonasal tract make up approximately 5% of all its tumors.[33] Although these carcinomas are rare, once they occur, they almost always invade neighboring structures, including the orbit.[2]

Esthesioneuroblastoma

Esthesioneuroblastoma is a rare neoplasm that originates from the progenitor cells of the olfactory epithelium. Histopathologic diagnosis is difficult; antigen expression detected through a panel of antibodies by immunohistochemistry may be helpful. Expression of HASH as revealed by reverse transcriptase polymerase chain reaction (RT PCR) studies could be a specific marker of esthesioneuroblastoma.[34] It occurs during the first and second, fifth, and sixth decades in a bimodal fashion, and its prognosis depends on the extent of the lesion. Tumor extending into the orbit and into the anterior cranial fossa is staged as T3 according to the UCLA classification (Figure 23.5).[35,36] A combination of surgery and radiotherapy seems to be the optimum approach to treatment.[37] The exact role of chemotherapy is unclear. Disease-free survival at 5 years averages 45% for stage 3 disease.[38]

Mesenchymal Tumors

Fibrous, fibromyxomatous, and fibro-osseous lesions are common benign tumors of the sinonasal tract. Although their growth is usually slow, they are known to extend into the orbit if they are located in an adjacent site (Figure 23.6).[7,39]

Malignant mesenchymal tumors including rhabdomyosarcoma, smooth muscle and neurogenic sarcomas, fibrosarcomas, alveolar soft part sarcoma, osteogenic sarcoma, malignant hemangiopericytoma, and, rarely, angiosarcoma are known to occur in the sinonasal tract and may invade the orbit secondarily.[2]

Lymphoproliferative Tumors

Lymphomas of the sinonasal tract are usually of the non-Hodgkin's type that usually present in the very young and the very old.[40] In adults, in whom the lymphoma rarely affects the orbit, the 5-year survival is approximately 45%. In children, the 5-year survival rate reaches to 70 to 80% if Burkitt's lymphoma is excluded.

Burkitt's lymphoma, which represents one of the most common types of pediatric non-Hodgkin's lymphomas, is a highly aggressive, extranodal B-cell tumor (Figure 23.7). It is characterized by translocation and deregulation of the c-*myc* gene on chromosome 8. Endemic cases, which are usually seen in Africa, involve the cranial skeleton and mostly bear Epstein–Barr virus genomes. These are the tumors that usually present with orbital involvement (Figure 23.8). Sporadic cases, which are more often seen in the United States, usually involve the gastrointestinal and genitourinary systems. Non-Hodgkin's lymphomas, including Burkitt's lymphoma, develop in immunosuppressed individuals at a greater risk.[41] Plasmacytoma as a part of systemic disease or a solitary lesion is also known to involve the bones of the nasal cav-

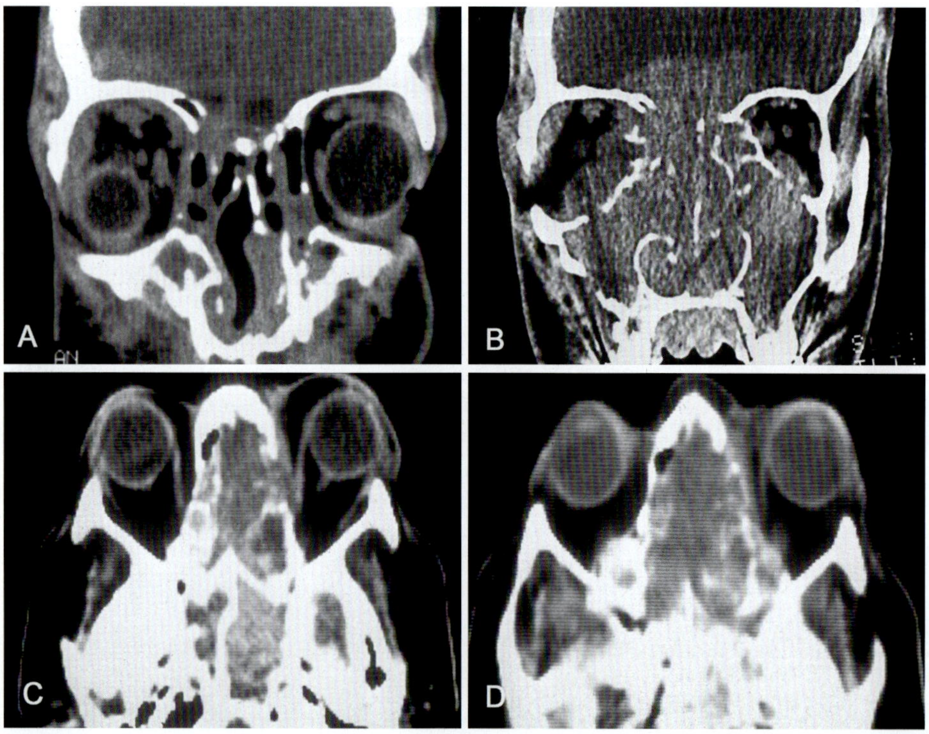

FIGURE 23.5. Two rapidly expanding esthesioneuroblastomas originating from the olfactory cells of the nose and involving the adjacent perinasal sinuses, orbits, and the brain. (A,B) Coronal and (C,D) axial CT images.

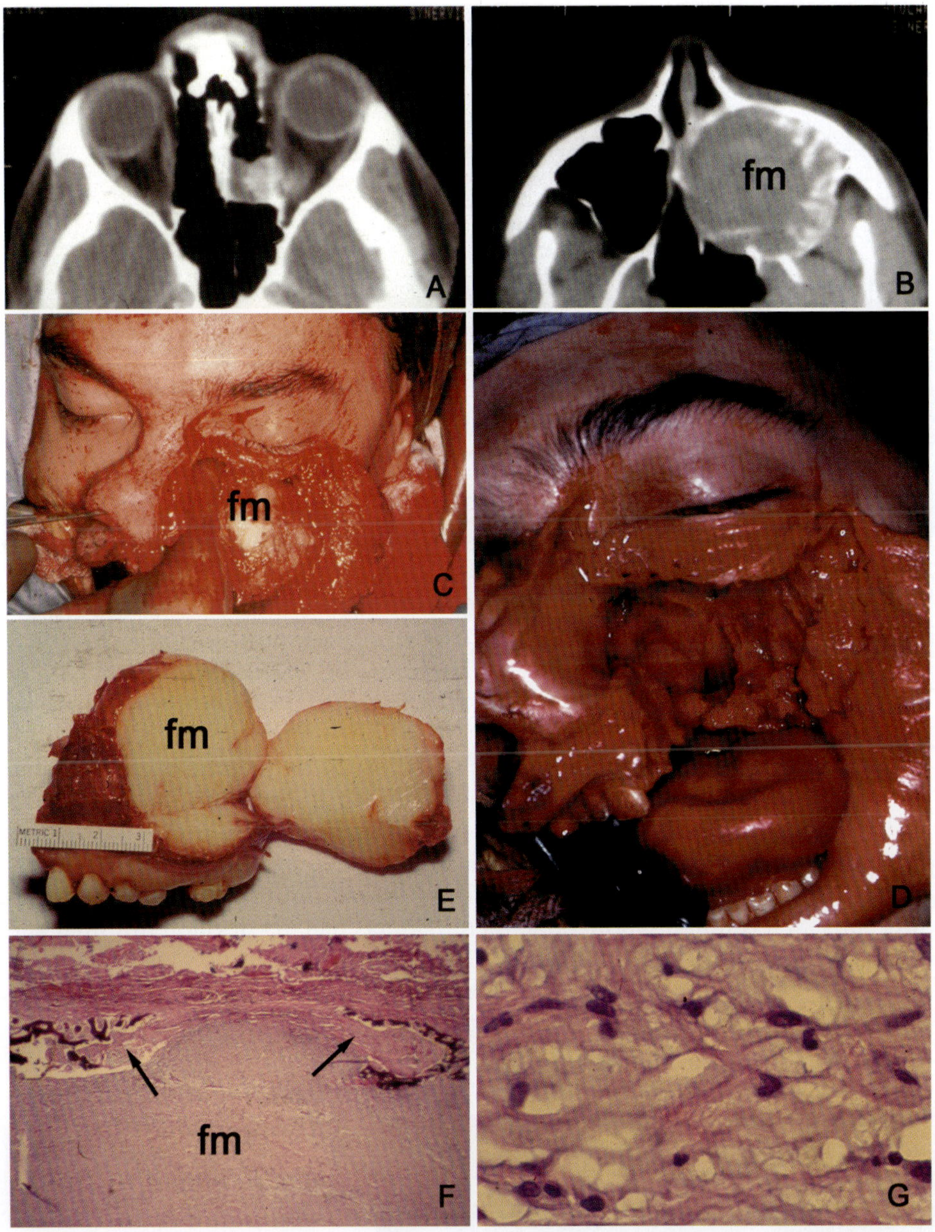

FIGURE 23.6. Benign fibromyxoma (fm) originating from maxillary bone involving the orbit (A) and maxillary sinus (B). Although the tumor was well circumscribed with a thin, fibrous capsule, the neighboring structures were involved because of its progressive growth and size (C–E). Histopathologically, the fibromyxoma was composed of myxoid spindle cell proliferation alternating with fibrous elements (F,G). Although the tumor was benign, it was eroding through the bone of the orbital floor (arrows).

ity, paranasal sinuses, and the orbit. The bones of the head and neck region have an affinity to be the site of extramedullary plasmacytoma; 80 to 90% of the cases are found in the head and neck region, 40% of which originates in the sinonasal tract.

Other Tumors and Tumorlike Conditions

Inflammatory pseudotumor (myofibroblastic inflammation) is a space-occupying lesion that occurs in the paranasal sinuses. The pathogenesis of the lesion is not known.[42] Histopathologically, it consists of fascicles of myofibroblastic cells mixed with nonspecific chronic inflammatory infiltrates consisting of lymphocytes and plasmacytes. Inflammatory pseudotumor is primarily seen in the lungs, but extrapulmonic forms may be encountered in the nose and paranasal sinuses. Although their histopathologic appearance is benign, these lesions may present a malignant biologic behavior with local aggression and even metastasis. Maxillary and ethmoidal pseudotumors may extend into the orbit through bony infiltration and thereby simulate squamous cell carcinoma. Biopsy is the only way to confirm the diagnosis.[43]

Langerhans cell and non–Langerhans cell histiocytoses commonly affect the nose, paranasal sinuses, and the orbit. Detailed discussion of this subject is given in Chapter 21.

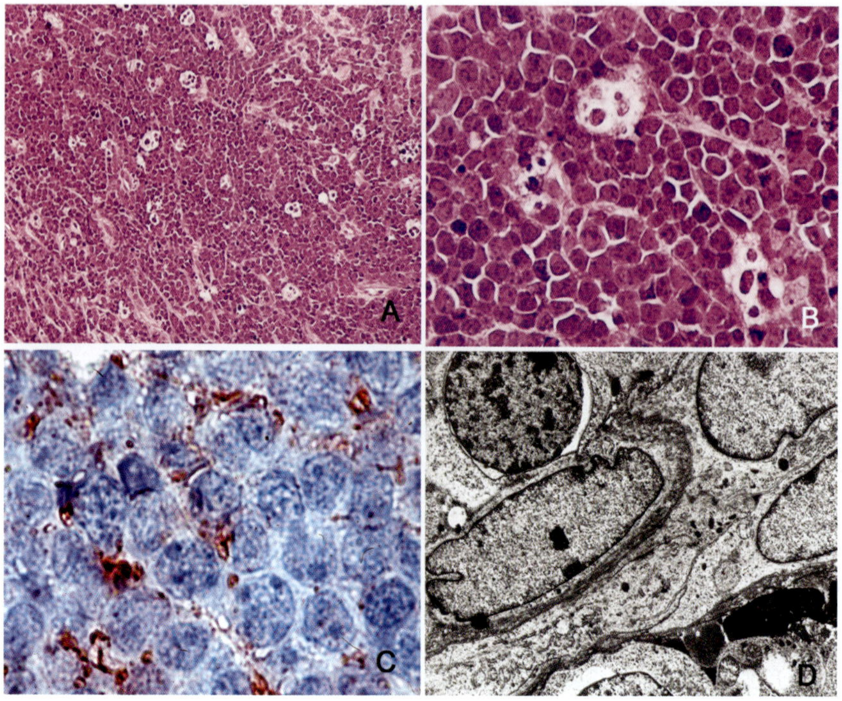

FIGURE 23.7. Burkitt's lymphoma is composed of a proliferation of medium-sized, noncleaved lymphocytes with scattered "tingible" macrophages presenting the classical "starry-sky" appearance (A,B). (C) An immunohistochemical specimen revealing κ light chain positivity of tumor cells. (D) Transmission electronmicroscopy shows detail of noncleaved neoplastic lympocytes.

SECONDARY ORBITAL TUMORS ORIGINATING FROM THE CRANIUM

Intracranial neoplasms, including sphenoid ridge meningioma and other cranial bone tumors, pituitary gland adenoma, craniopharyngioma, chiasmal tumors, and cysts, rarely extend into the orbit.[43–46]

Sphenoid Ridge Meningioma

Meningiomas of the sphenoid bone often lead to secondary invasion of the orbit.[47] These tumors usually invade the superior orbital fissure and the optic canal and may compress the optic nerve and vascular structures, leading to venous congestion and orbital edema disproportional to the size of the space-occupying lesion in the orbit. Patients with optic canal and sphenoid bone meningiomas usually develop minimal and late proptosis that often becomes noticeable after severe visual loss. Proptosis occurs only when the tumor ruptures the dura and forms a space-occupying lesion within the orbit (Figure 23.9).

Meningioma of the sphenoid ridge most often presents as an "en plaque" neoplasm that slowly grows

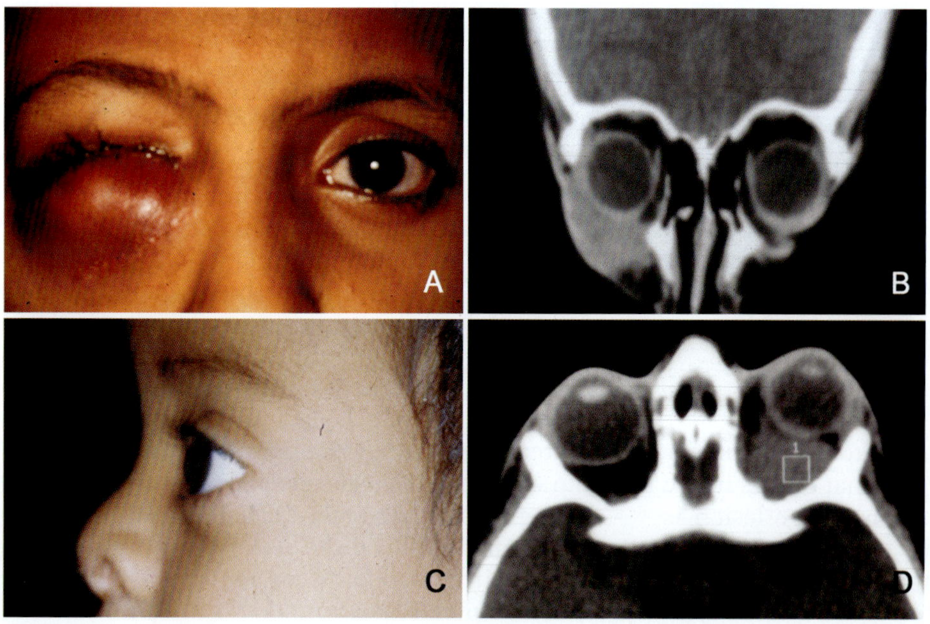

FIGURE 23.8. Endemic Burkitt's lymphoma. (A,B) a patient whose rapidly expanding maxillary tumor involved the orbit secondarily. (C,D) A patient whose nasal cavity, ethmoid sinus, and the orbit were involved at the time of presentation.

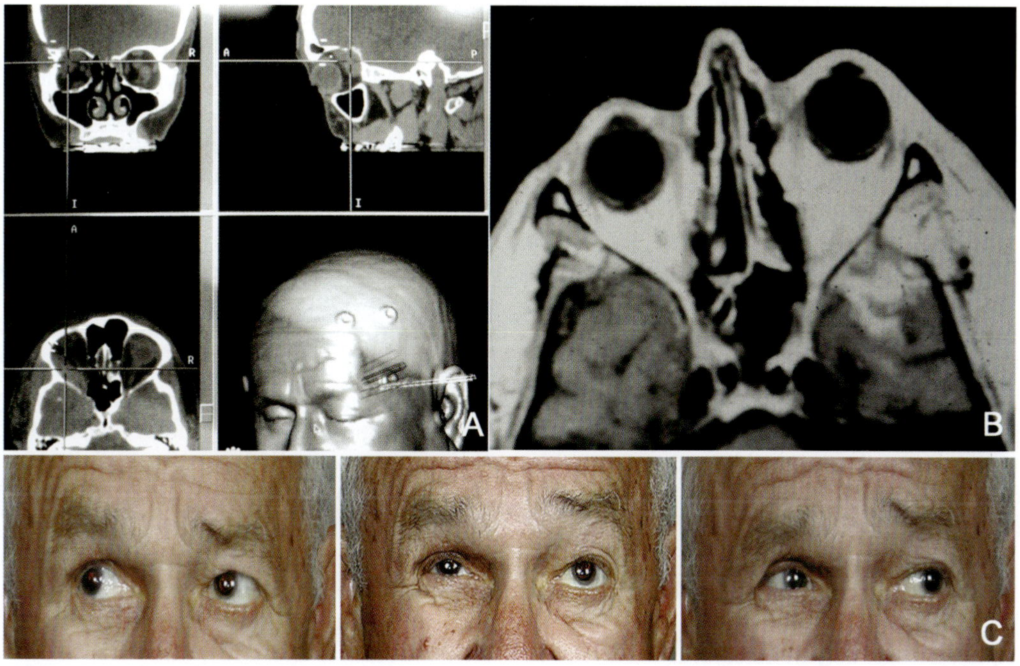

FIGURE 23.9. Sphenoid ridge meningioma. (A) Intraoperative stereotactic views of the CT scan showing the extension of a left frontal lobe meningioma into the superior and lateral orbit. (B) T1-weighted, contrast-enhanced axial MR image shows irregular homogeneous enhancement within the brain; the extension of the meningioma into the lateral orbit caused marked proptosis. (C) Gaze photographs, obtained 6 months postoperatively, show residual proptosis and extraocular motility deficit of the left eye.

as a flat lesion along the dural surface, extending into the foramina of the orbit (Figure 23.10). Depending on the location of the growth, it may extend into the optic canal and the superior and/or inferior orbital fissures, causing blindness, extraocular motility disturbance, and venous congestion in the orbit. Meningiomas of the ridge and the suprasellar area may present with bilateral papilledema, as opposed to the more commonly encountered unilateral disk edema of the optic nerve meningioma. Intracanalicular meningioma produces early unilateral blindness. Olfactory groove meningioma, on the other hand, rarely produces early blindness because these lesions must become very large before they compress the visual system. Another presentation often associated with the meningioma of the olfactory groove is Foster–Kennedy syndrome, in which the tumor causes atrophy of one optic nerve early in its growth; later, the increased in-

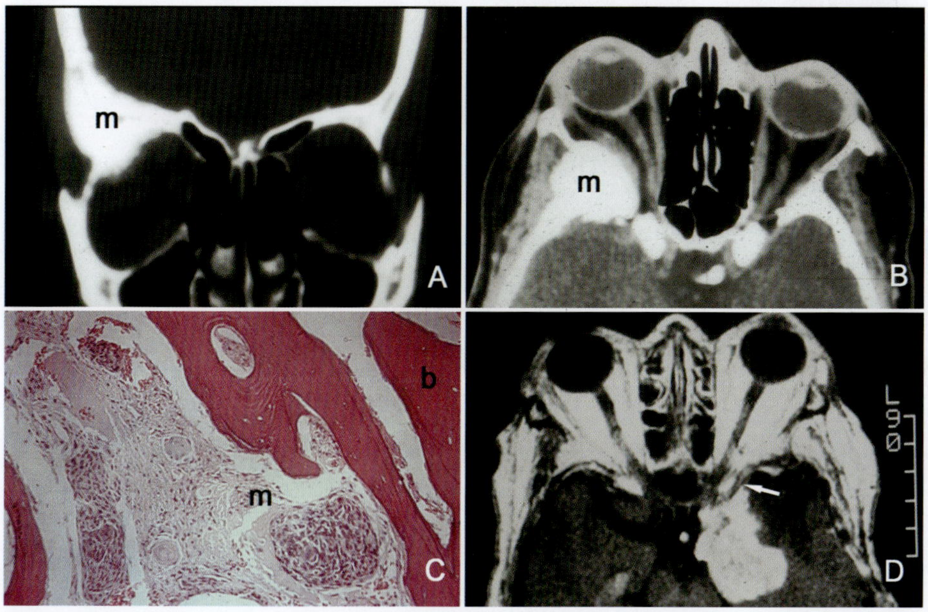

FIGURE 23.10. Hyperdense meningiomas originating from the dura of the frontal lobe (A) and the sphenoid ridge (B) are shown on coronal and axial CT scans, respectively. Note the marked compression of the meningioma (m) onto the lateral rectus muscle and optic nerve (B). (C) Histopathologic appearance of meningoendothelial cell clusters (m) from the same patient shown in (B): the clusters extend into the bone (b). (D) Axial, T1-weighted, contrast enhanced image showing the clearly visible homogeneous meningioma enhancement with a "knotty" tumor outline; the lesion extends into the orbit posteriorly (arrow).

tracranial pressure leads to edema of the fellow optic disk.[48] Although Foster–Kennedy syndrome has been most commonly associated with meningiomas, this phenomenon is also seen with optic nerve gliomas, craniopharyngiomas, and other space-occupying lesions of the orbit and the cranium, including abscesses.[49] Color vision abnormalities, afferent pupillary defect, and visual field loss are also seen with secondary meningeal tumors in the orbit. In some cases, with minimal or no proptosis, the visual field deficit and diminished vision are incorrectly attributed to glaucoma or optic neuritis.

Ultrasonography is not helpful in differential diagnosis of secondary meningiomas because most of these lesions are located deep in the posterior orbit. Approximately 50% of all cranial meningiomas appear in the sphenoid wing; another 20% are located in the sellar area. Therefore, the secondary effect of these neoplasms on the orbit, optic nerve, and other ocular structures is immense.

Because of their high cell density and tendency to develop calcification, meningiomas of the sphenoid ridge and sellar region present as hyperdense lesions on CT; diffuse hyperostosis of en plaque meningioma is particularly apparent on CT.[50,51] Since en plaque lesions grow in diffuse fashion, knowledge of the anatomy of the region as revealed by MRI, including the shape of the basal cisterns, orbital foramina, and blood vessels is required to determine accurately the extent of the disease. Most meningiomas, particularly the aggressive, angioblastic type, develop intense enhancement after the intravenous injection of contrast medium.[52] Although MRI usually does not produce a good image contrast between the tumor and the adjacent soft tissues in the orbit, it is superior to CT in the study of sellar and juxtasellar areas.[53]

Sphenoid ridge meningiomas are difficult lesions to diagnose clinically because they may mimic glaucoma, optic neuritis, and other intraorbital and intracranial neoplasms, metastatic tumors, and lymphomas.[54] One should also keep in mind that nonspecific neurologic findings such as headache, changes in mental status and personality, hypothalamic abnormalities, and seizures may very well be seen in meningiomas, particularly with intrasphenoidal ridge and perisellar tumors.[55] Intracranial meningiomas extending into the orbit through the foramina may also mimic the clinical features of myasthenia gravis. Therefore, patients with atypical presentations of myasthenia limited to ocular and/or cranial musculature should be thoroughly evaluated to rule out an intracranial mass lesion.[56]

Ectopic Meningioma

Ectopic meningioma is a rare tumor that seems to appear to originate from ectopic arachnoidal tissue outside the central nervous system in skin, scalp, nasal cavity and paransal sinuses, and in other viscera.[57–59] Among other sites, ectopic meningiomas also develop within the orbit.[60–63] Ectopic orbital meningiomas have been described in children and adults, with a sig-

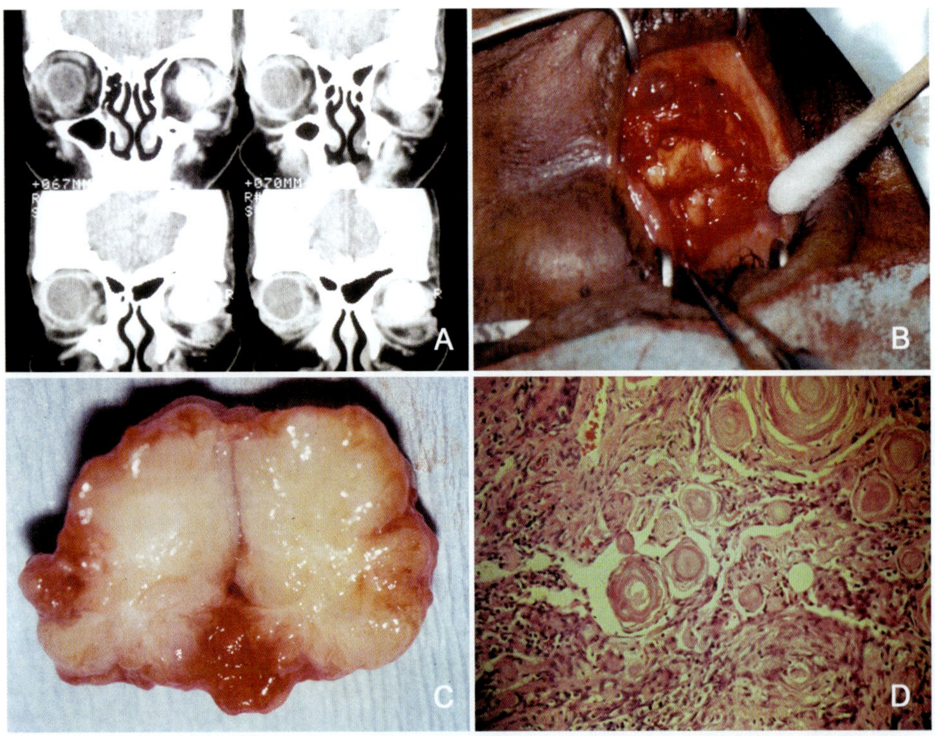

FIGURE 23.11. (A) Multiple coronal CT scans showing dense, oval inferior orbital mass, which at the time of excisional biopsy (B) were found to represent a firm and irregular tumor. (C) The grayish white, glistening surface of the meningioma. (D) Proliferation of meningioendothelial cells with numerous psammoma bodies, as revealed histopathologically.

nificant male predominance. These tumors presented space-occupying lesions, primarily in the medial orbit. The histopathogenesis of the ectopic orbital meningioma is not clear. The most conceivable of many hypotheses is that these lesions originate from regressed orbital meningoceles with leftover arachnoidal tissue, trapped within orbital soft tissues.[59,60]

The role of trauma may also explain the pathogenesis of some cases. It is possible that penetrating trauma can dislodge meningeal tissues within the orbit that later serve as a nidus for the development of meningiomas.[64] In the author's personal experience of two patients with ectopic orbital meningioma, one had a history of trauma that resulted in the enucleation of the globe and the other did not but had a superior–medial eyelid/orbit mass that had been growing slowly and ultimately caused mechanical upper lid ptosis. In the patient with the history of trauma, the tumor developed 20 years later within the inferior orbit with no other evidence of dislocated meningeal tissue (Figure 23.11). Ectopic meningiomas usually present with a meningotheliomatous histology and respond well to total surgical excision.

Craniopharyngioma

Craniopharyngiomas are benign, epithelial tumors of the sellar area that present as partially cystic, partially solid masses in children and adolescents. These tumors originate from the Rathke pouch epithelium and account for approximately 2 to 5% of all intracranial tumors. Craniopharyngiomas do not present a gender preference but do have a bimodal age distribution with one peak for children and adolescents and another one for adults.[65]

Craniopharyngiomas are divided into two basic clinical pathologic types: adamantinomatous and capillary. Capillary craniopharyngiomas present as solid tumors, are found more often in adults, and cause occlusive hydrocephalus, which produces frequent symptoms of headaches, nausea, vomiting, and papilledema. Endocrine deficiencies, including diabetes insipidus and dwarfism, are also seen in a great majority of the patients, primarily in children with the adamantinomatous type. However, the visual disturbances secondary to compression of optic structures and invasion of the orbit are more frequently seen in adults (Figure 23.12).[66,67] The adamantinomatous type of craniopharyngioma is primarily seen in children and often presents with partially calcified cystic lesions. CT and MRI are indicated to diagnose and define the extent of these tumors; MRI enables a better delineation of the tumor extent, especially on coronal and sagittal views. Differential diagnosis of these masses should include cystic pituitary adenomas, suprasellar meningiomas, dermoid cysts, gliomas of

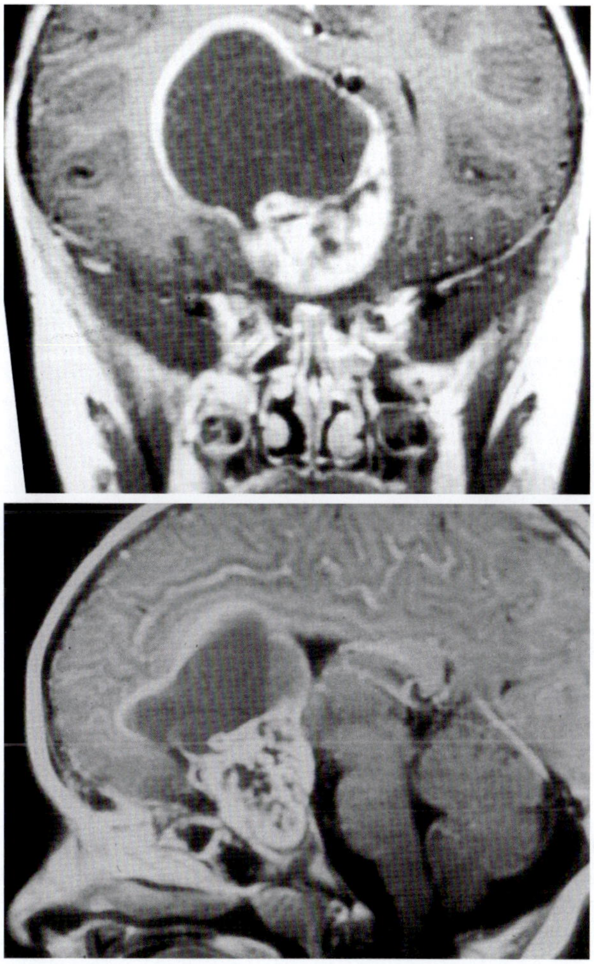

FIGURE 23.12. MR images of an 11-year-old boy who presented with headache and visual deficit bilaterally. The coronal MRI (*top*) is a T1-weighted, contrast-enhanced view in which the cyst wall and the inferior solid portion of the tumor reveal strong signal enhancement. The midsagittal, T1-weighted view (*bottom*) shows the marked enlargement of the sella by the tumor; optic chiasm cannot be identified.

the optic chiasm, and granulomatous inflammatory lesions such as sarcoidosis.

Pituitary Adenoma

Pituitary adenomas rarely involve the orbit secondarily. The prolactin-secreting type (prolactinoma) is known to extend into the posterior orbit occasionally (Figure 23.13).[46] These lesions are histopathologically benign but invasive tumors that typically present with amenorrhea and galactorrhea in women and hypogonadism and space-occupying lesions in men. "Giant" prolactinomas are invasive; these tumors are defined as lesions larger than 4 cm at the greatest diameter that produce serum prolactin in excess of 1000 ng/mL. Some become very large and invade perisellar structures and beyond; superior extension is most common, but these lesions are also known to extend laterally,

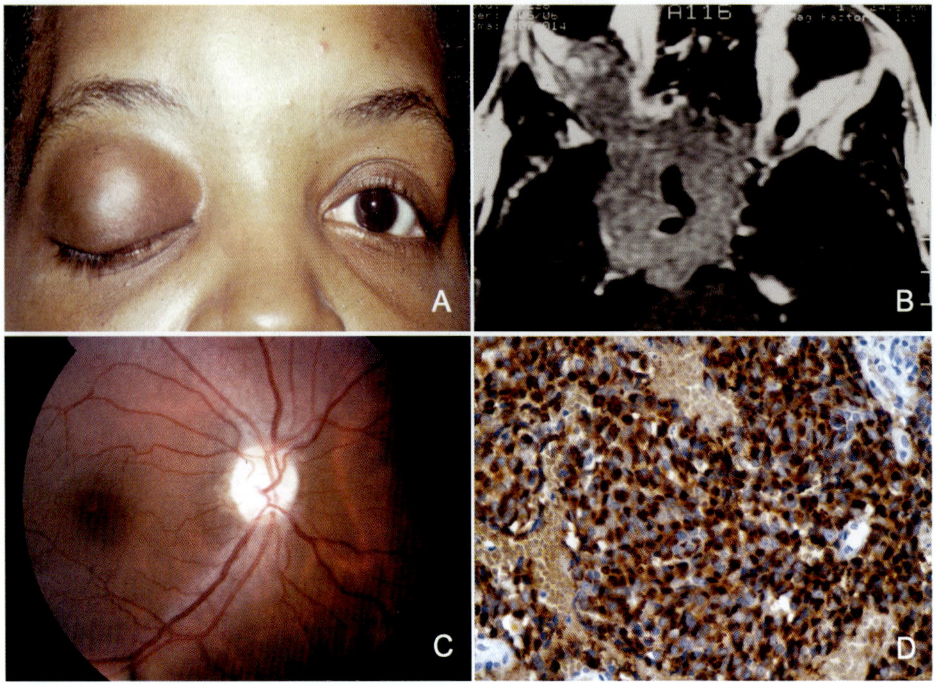

FIGURE 23.13. A large prolactinoma extending into perisellar structures, right frontal lobe, cavernous sinus, and orbit, causing massive proptosis, visual deficit, and multiple cranial nerve palsies. (A) Facial photograph. (B) Axial image. (C) The atrophy of the optic nerve. (D) Immunohistochemical stain shows the positive reaction of tumor cells with prolactin (brownish cytoplasmic staining).

posteriorly, inferiorly, and, less often, anteriorly into adjacent anatomic structures such as cavernous sinus and orbit.[68,69]

When the orbit is involved, the tumor causes proptosis, extraocular motility disturbances, orbital congestion, and increased intraocular pressure. If the orbit has been extensively invaded by the pituitary adenoma, the prognosis is poor. However, if the orbital invasion can be detected early, prior to compressive optic neuropathy, potentially disastrous visual damage can be reversed with a combination of surgery and medical treatment with bromocriptine, which is known to reduce the size of the tumor effectively and lower the levels of serum prolactin.[70]

References

1. Sisson GA, Toriumi DN, Atiyah RA. Paranasal sinus malignancy: a comprehensive update. *Laryngoscope* 1989;99:143.
2. Carrau RL, Myers EN. Neoplasms of the nose and paranasal sinuses. In: Bailey BJ, ed. *Head and Neck Surgery: Otolaryngology.* 2nd ed. Philadelphia: Lippincott-Raven; 1998:1445–1469.
3. Hyams ZJ. Papillomas of the nasal cavity and paranasal sinuses: a clinicopathological study of 315 cases. *Ann Otol Rhinol Otolaryngol* 1971;80:192.
4. Vrabec DP. The inverted Schneiderian papilloma: 25 year study. *Laryngoscope* 1994;104:582–605.
5. Karcioglu ZA, Caldwell DR, Reed TH. Papillomas of lacrimal drainage system: a clinicopathologic study. *Ophthalmic Surg* 1984;15:670.
6. Lawton AW, Karesh JW, Gray WC. Proptosis from maxillary sinus inverted papilloma with malignant transformation. *Arch Ophthalmol* 186;104:874–877.
7. Batsakis JG. *Tumors of the head and neck. Clinical and Pathological Considerations.* Baltimore: Williams & Wilkins; 1979: 130–176.
8. Karcioglu ZA, Greenidge K, Wesley R, McCord C. Proptosis and pseudocyst formation from inverted papilloma. *Ann Ophthalmol* 1982;14:443.
9. Shields JA, Bakewell B, Augsburger JJ, et al. Classification and incidence of space-occupying lesions in the orbit: survey of 645 biopsies. *Arch Ophthalmol* 1984;120:1606–1611.
10. Seregard S, Sahlin S. Panorama of orbital space-occupying lesions. The 24-year experience of a referral center. *Acta Ophthalmol Scand* 1999;77:91–98.
11. Wilson M, Grossniklaus H. Orbital disease in North America. *Ophthalmol Clin N Am* 1996;4:539–547.
12. Tabb HG, Barranco SJ. Cancer of the maxillary sinus: an analysis of 108 cases. *Laryngoscope* 1971;81:81.
13. Hernberg S, Westerholm P, Schultz-Larsen K, et al. Nasal and sinonasal cancer: connection with occupational exposures in Denmark, Finland and Sweden. *Scand J Work Environ Health* 1989:9:315.
14. Toth J, Karcioglu ZA, Moshfeghi AA, et al. The relationship between human papillomavirus and *p53* gene in conjunctival squamous cell carcinoma. *Cornea* 2000;19:59–62.
15. Karcioglu ZA, Toth J. Relation between *p53* over-expression and clinical behavior of ocular/orbital invasion of conjunctival squamous cell carcinoma. *Ophthalmic Plast Reconstr Surg* 2000;16:443–449.
16. Weiland H. Upper respiratory tract and ear. In: Karcioglu ZA, Someren A, eds. *Practical Surgical Pathology.* Lexington, MA: Collomore Press; 1985:10–41.
17. Rootman J. Robertson WD. Tumors. In: Rootman J, ed. *Diseases of the Orbit.* Philadelphia: JB Lippincott; 1988:427–432.
18. Chang WJ, Shields CL, Shields JA, et al. Bilateral orbital involvement with massive allergic fungal sinusitis. *Arch Ophthalmol* 1996;114:767–768.
19. Dunlop IS, Billson FA. Visual failure in allergic aspergillus sinusitis: case report. *Br J Ophthalmol* 1988;72:127–130.

20. Torres C, El Naggar AK, Sim SJ, et al. Allergic fungal sinusitis: a clinicopathological study of 16 cases. *Hum Pathol* 1996; 27:793–799.
21. Michaels L, Lloyd G, Phelps T. Origin and spread of allergic fungal disease of the nose and paranasal sinuses. *Clin Otolaryngol Allied Sci* 2000;25:518–525.
22. Graamans L, Slootweg PJ. Orbital exenteration in surgery of malignant neoplasms of the paranasal sinuses; the value of preoperative computed tomorgraphy. *Arch Otolaryngol Head Neck Surg* 1989;115:977–980.
23. Mosesson RE, Som PM. The radiographic evaluation of sinonasal tumors. *Otolaryngol Clin North Amer* 1995;28: 1097–1115.
24. Som PN, Brandwein MS, Maldjian C, et al. Inflammatory pseudotumor of the maxillary sinus: CT and MR findings in six cases. *AJR Am J Roentgenol* 1994;163:689–692.
25. Shapiro MD, Som PM. MRI of the paranasal sinuses and nasal cavity. *Radiol Clin North Am* 1989;27:447–475.
26. Som PM, Dillon WP, Sze G, et al. Benign and malignant sinonasal lesions with intracranial extension: differentiation by MR imaging. *Radiology* 1989;172:763–766.
27. Hesselink JR, Weber AL. Pathways of orbital extension of extraorbital neoplasms. *J Comput Assist Tomogr* 1982;6:593–597.
28. Akyol MU, Karcioglu ZA. Secondary orbital tumors originating from nasal cavity and paranasal sinuses: review of 71 cases. *Orbit* 1992;3:131–135.
29. McCarny WS, Levine PA, Cantrell RW. Preservation of the eye in the treatment of sinonasal malignant neoplasms with orbital involvement: a confirmation of the original treatise. *Arch Otolaryngol Head Neck Surg* 1996;122:657–659.
30. McNab TI, Flores AD, Anderson DS. Treatment of paranasal sinus malignancy: the BCCA experience. J Otolaryngol 1992; 21:244–248.
31. Xuexi W, Pingzhang T, Yongfa Q. Management of the orbital contents in radical surgery for squamous cell carcinoma of the maxillary sinus. *Chin Med J* 1995;108:123–125.
32. Waitz G, Wigand ME. Results of endoscopic sinus surgery for the treatment of inverted papillomas. *Laryngoscope* 1992; 102:917–922.
33. Goepfert H, Luna MA, Lindberg RD, White AK. Malignant salivary gland tumors of the paranasal sinuses and nasal cavity. *Arch Otolaryngol* 1983;109:662.
34. Miyagami M, Katayma Y, Kinukawa N, Sawada T. An ultrastructural and immunohistochemical study of olfactory neuroepithelioma with rhabdomyoblasts. *Med Electron Microsc* 2002;35:160–166.
35. Levine PA, McLean WC, Cantrell RW. Esthesioneuroblastoma: the University of Virigina experience. 1960–1985. *Laryngoscope* 1986;96:742.
36. Snyderman CH, Aydogan B, D'Amico F. A comparison of staging systems for esthesioneuroblastoma. *Otolaryngol Head Neck Surg*. 2004.
37. Girod D, Hanna E, Marentette L. Esthesioneuroblastoma. *Head Neck* 2001;23:500–505.
38. Bradley PJ, Jones NS, Robertson I. Diagnosis and management of esthesioneuroblastoma. *Curr Opin Otolaryngol Head Neck Surg* 2003;11:112–118.
39. Barnes L. *Surgical Pathology of the Head and Neck*. New York: Dekker; 1985.
40. Abbondanzo SL, Wenig BM. Non-Hodgkin's lymphoma of the sinonasal tract: a clinicopathologic and immunophenotypic study of 120 cases. *Cancer* 1995;45:1281–1291.
41. Doll DL, List AF. Burkitt's lymphoma in a homosexual patient. *Lancet* 1982;1:1026–1027.
42. Karakok M, Ozer E, Sari I, et al. Inflammatory myofibroblastic tumor (inflammatory pseudotumor) of the maxillary sinus mimicking malignancy: a case report of an unusual location (is that a true neoplasm?). *Auris Nasus Larynx* 2002;29:383–386.
43. Batsakis JG, el-Naggar AK, Luna MA, et al. Inflammatory pseudotumor: What is it? How does it behave? *Ann Otol Rhinol Laryngol* 1995;104:329–331.
44. Limburgh R, Walsh FB, Sacks JG. *Neuropathology of Vision. An Atlas*. Philadelphia: Lea & Febiger; 1973:190–195.
45. Wilson WB. Meningiomas of the anterior visual system. *Surv Ophthalmol* 1981;26:109.
46. Karcioglu ZA, Aden LB, Cruz AA, et al. Orbital invasion with prolactinoma: a clinical review of 4 patients. *Ophthalmic Plast Reconstr Surg* 2002;18:64–71.
47. Wilson WB, Gordon M, Lehman RAW. Meningiomas confined to the optic canal and foramina. *Surg Neurol* 1979;12:21–28.
48. Cushing HC, Eisenhart MD. *Meningiomas*. New York: Hafner; 1962:250–282.
49. Jarus GD, Feldon SE. Clinical and computed tomography findings in the Foster–Kennedy syndrome. *Am J Ophthalmol* 1982;93:317–322.
50. Sartor K. *MR Imaging of the Skull and Brain. A Correlative Text-Atlas*. Berlin: Springer-Verlag; 1992.
51. Louis DN, Scheithauer BW, Budka H, et al. Meningiomas. In: Kleihues P, Cavenee WK, eds. *Pathology and Genetics. Tumors of the Nervous System*. Lyons, France: International Agency for Research on Cancer; 2000:176–184.
52. Osborn A. Meningiomas and other nonglial neoplasms. In: Osborn A, ed. *Diagnostic Neuroradiology*. St. Louis: CV Mosby; 1994:579–625.
53. Lee BCT, Deck MDF. Sellar and juxtasellar lesion detection with MRI. *Radiology* 1985;157:143–147.
54. Karcioglu ZA, Yulug A, Haik BG. Tumors of the optic nerve. In: Margo CE, Hamed LM, Mames RN, eds. *Diagnostic Problems in Clinical Ophthalmology*. Philadelphia: WB Saunders; 1994:105–114.
55. Anderson D, Khalil M. Meningioma and the ophthalmologist: a review of 80 cases. *Ophthalmology* 1981;88:1004–1009.
56. Moorthy G, Behrens MM, Rachmann DD, et al. Ocular pseudomyasthenia or ocular myasthenia plus: a warning to clinicians. *Neurology* 1989;39:1150–1154.
57. Hanada M, Kitajima K. Primary ectopic meningioma in the right ethmoid sinus: a case report. *Auris Nauss Larynx* 1997; 24:321–324.
58. Falleni M, Roz E, Dessy E, et al. Primary intrathoracic meningioma: histopathological, immunohistochemical and ultrastructural study of two cases. *Virchows Arch* 2001;439:196–200.
59. Lopez C, Silvers VN, Helwig ED. Cutaneous meningiomas, a clinicopathological study. *Cancer* 1974;34:728–744.
60. Farah SE, Konrad H, Huang DT, et al. Ectopic orbital meningioma: a case report and review. *Ophthalmic Plast Reconstr Surg* 1999;15:463–466.
61. Johnson TE, Weatherhead RG, Nasr AM, et al. Ectopic (extradural) meningioma of the orbit: a report of two cases in children. *J Pediatr Ophthalmol Strabismus* 1993;30:43–47.
62. Karp LA, Zimmerman LE, Borit A, et al. Primary intraorbital meningiomas. *Arch Ophthalmol* 1974;91:24–28.
63. Arai H, Sato K, Matsumoto T. Free-lying ectopic meningioma within the orbit. *Br J Neurosurg* 1997;11:560–563.
64. Black PM. Meningiomas. *Neurosurgery* 1990;32:643–657.
65. Crotty TB, Scheithauer BW, Young WF Jr, et al. Papillary craniopharyngioma: a clinical study of 48 cases. *J Neurosurg* 1995; 83:206–214.
66. Sartoretti-Schefer S, Wichmann W, Aguzzi A, et al. MR differentiation of adamantinous and squamous–capillary craniopharyngioma. *AJNR Am J Neuroradiol* 1997;18: 77–87.
67. Kucharczyk W, Montanera W, Ebcker LE. The sella turcica and parasellar region. In: Atlas SW, ed. *Magnetic Resonance Imag-*

ing of the Brain and Spine. Philadelphia: Lippincott-Raven; 1996:871–930.
68. Sammartino A, Bonavolonto G, Pettinato G, et al. Exophthalmos caused by an invasive pituitary adenoma in a child. *Ophthalmologica* 1979;179:83–89.
69. Spiegel PH, Karcioglu ZA. Orbital invasion by pituitary adenoma. *Am J Ophthalmol* 1994;117:270–271.
70. Bernardini FP, Kersten RV, Moin M, et al. Unsuspected recurrent pituitary adenoma presenting as an orbital mass. *Ophthalmic Plast Reconstr Surg* 2001;17:140–143.

24

Metastatic Tumors

J. Oscar Croxatto and Zeynel A. Karcıoglu

Compared with orbital diseases and other conditions in patients who seek consultation in ophthalmic practice, metastases to the orbit are rare. Nevertheless, the ophthalmologists confronted with presumed orbital metastases play an important role in the diagnosis and management of these patients. Up to 35% of patients with orbital metastasis present with no known history of primary tumor at the time of ophthalmologic examination.[1,2] The ophthalmologist should be able to identify symptoms and signs more commonly associated with metastatic orbital disease, recognize the results of imaging studies, know the most frequent primary sites that disseminate to the eye and orbit, and implement appropriate management according with the original tumor and stage of the disease.

INCIDENCE AND EPIDEMIOLOGY

In biopsy-proven series, the frequency of metastatic tumors among orbital mass lesions ranges from 2.5 to 10%.[3–5] The ratio between orbital metastases and ocular metastases varied from 1:8 in histopathologic series to 1:1.4 in more recent clinical series.[6–9]

Almost any primary tumor originating elsewhere in the body has been reported to metastasize to the orbit.[10,11] The most frequent primary sites are those most common in the adult and older populations, including breast, lung, prostate, and malignant melanoma.[12–15] Metastases from the liver and gastrointestinal tract are seen more frequently in Japan than in the United States and Europe, reflecting geographical, environmental, or genetic susceptibilities.[16] From clinical ophthalmologic practice, tumors with more aggressive behavior, like metastatic carcinoma from the lungs, tend to be underrepresented. At the time of presentation of orbital metastasis, patients with lung carcinoma are usually in poor clinical condition. Metastatic cancer from an unknown primary site is a clinical challenge for all physicians. In a recent series, the primary tumors remained undetected in 10% of patients without history of primary tumor at the time of ophthalmologic examination.[15]

In developed countries, because of the trend toward early diagnosis of cancer and the use of more sophisticated imaging studies, most patients with metastatic orbital lesions present with a known history of primary tumors. In approximately one out of four patients with presumed orbital metastases, the orbital specialist may be the first physician to demonstrate the dissemination of the tumor.[15] The time lag between the diagnosis of the primary tumor and orbital manifestation varies according to the biologic behavior of the tumors. Carcinomas from the breast, thyroid, and kidney have relatively long delays between diagnosis of the primary and the manifestation of metastasis, but this time lapse is very difficult to determine accurately.

Contrary to what one might expect from metastatic disease, most orbital metastases present as unilateral, solitary masses. Only 10% of orbital metastases are bilateral.[13,17] Bilateral disease is more frequent in breast carcinoma (19%) than other tumors (2–5%). In a combined case series,[10] 47% have demonstrated concurrent involvement of other sites, including the eye. Combined ocular and orbital metastases have been observed in 21% of cases from an ophthalmologic practice.[15] Concurrent involvement of the central nervous system is less than 5%.[18]

CLINICAL FINDINGS

Two recent series reported average ages of 44.8 and 62 years, but age may vary depending on the primary tumor.[15,16] In other published cases, the average age was 59 years for breast, 58 years for lung, 70 years for prostate, and 45 years for malignant melanoma.[5,10,11,19] The sex predominance is also dependent on the origin of the metastatic tumors. Amemiya et al. reported 74 males and 52 females, but the most frequent primary site was the lung.[16] In contrast, Shields and coworkers found 60 females and 40 males in a series with predominant breast carcinomas.[15]

The most frequent complaints of patients with presumed metastatic disease to the orbit are proptosis, ocular motility disturbances and diplopia, pain, palpable mass, ptosis, and lid swelling. Visual acuity may not be affected during the early phases of the disease. The duration of symptoms varies from one to a few months in lung primaries to more than a year in slow-growing carcinoid tumors, depending on the growth rate of the tumor. A distinguishing feature of orbital metastasis is the progressive course associated with motor and sensory deficits. These deficits may be significant, even with small metastatic orbital masses because of their rapid development. Slow-growing lesions (e.g., pleomorphic adenomas), would not cause as much orbital dysfunction, even when they reach much larger sizes.

Individual symptoms reflect particular tissue involvement within the orbit. Tumors that infiltrate fat and extraocular muscles produce proptosis.[20–25] When muscle involvement is early, the presenting complaint is diplopia. Pain is usually associated with periosteal and bone involvement. Pulsation may be the result of either bone destruction or highly vascular tumors like unusual cases of renal carcinoma. A rare sign is enophthalmos, observed in approximately 10% of cases in some series.[10] It is generally related to the fibroblastic response associated with breast carcinoma and other tumors with a schirrous stromal component (Figure 24.1). Enophthalmos may also result from fat atrophy.[20]

Information obtained from clinical, imaging, and surgical studies indicates that the lateral orbit is the most common location of orbital metastasis (39%), followed by the superior (32%), medial (20%), and inferior (12%) quadrants.[10] Goldberg and coworkers summarize the clinical presentation of metastatic orbital disease in five generalized types.[10]

1. *Mass formation.* More than 65% of the patients present with mass formation (Figure 24.2). Primary mass effect presents with axial or nonaxial proptosis because of displacement of the globe. The mass may be palpable in anteriorly located tumors. Posterior lesions may present with papilledema and pressure on the posterior globe.
2. *Infiltration.* Approximately 25% of the patients present diffuse or localized infiltration of orbital tissues characterized by diplopia, increased resistance to retrodisplacement of the globe, and, rarely, enophthalmos.
3. *Functional.* Predominant decrease in cranial nerve function not related to the size of the mass or degree of infiltration.
4. *Inflammation.* Acute or subacute orbital and periocular inflammatory signs.
5. *Silent.* No orbital signs or symptoms.

Metastatic disease may present as focal nodular muscle enlargement without compromise of other orbital tissues.[21–25] One or more muscles may be affected, and even bilateral involvement has been reported. The horizontal rectus muscles are more commonly affected than the vertical recti and oblique muscles. In some cases diffuse muscle enlargement may resemble an inflammatory pseudotumor or thyroid orbitopathy.[23] The differential diagnoses of muscle enlargement include Graves ophthalmopathy, orbital myositis, lymphoma, vascular malformations, amyloidosis, and specific inflammatory diseases.[25] A transient response to steroid treatment may be misleading because it can occur in metastatic lesions of the orbit. The two most frequent metastatic tumors associated with extraocular muscle involvement are breast carcinoma (55%) and melanoma (21%).[25]

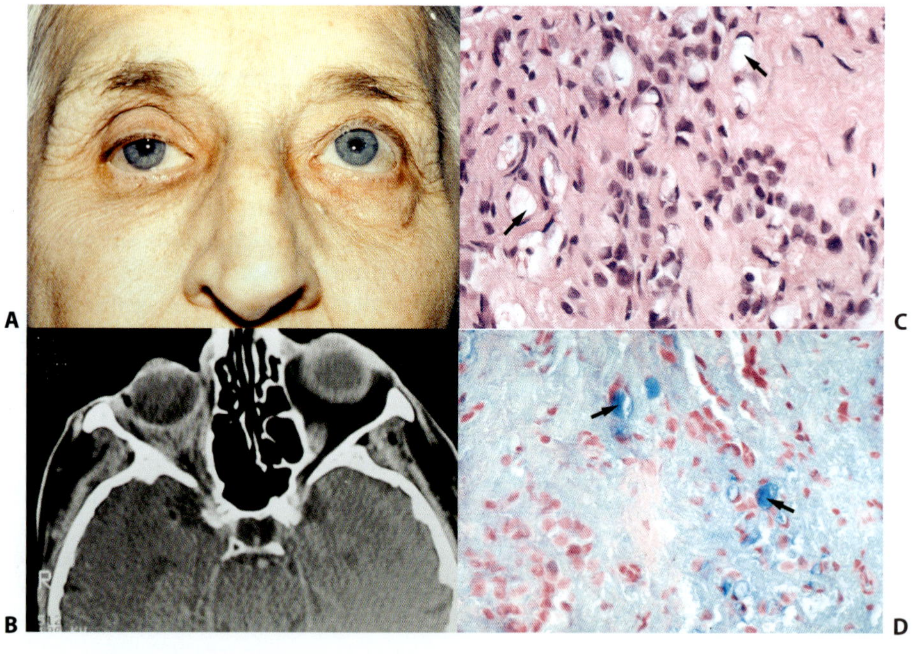

FIGURE 24.1. (A) Schirrous-type breast carcinoma metastatic to the right orbit causing enophthalmos. Note that the right eye, which is enophthalmic, remains at straight gaze when the patient looks up. (B) CT scan depicts a diffuse fibrous component of the tumor, diffusely infiltrating the intraconal space of the right orbit. (C,D) Histopathology reveals multiple, adenocarcinoma cells ("signet-ring" cells) containing intracytoplasmic mucin (arrows) scattered within the fibrous stroma of the tumor. (D) Histopathologic specimen shows tumor cells (arrows) stained with Alcian blue.

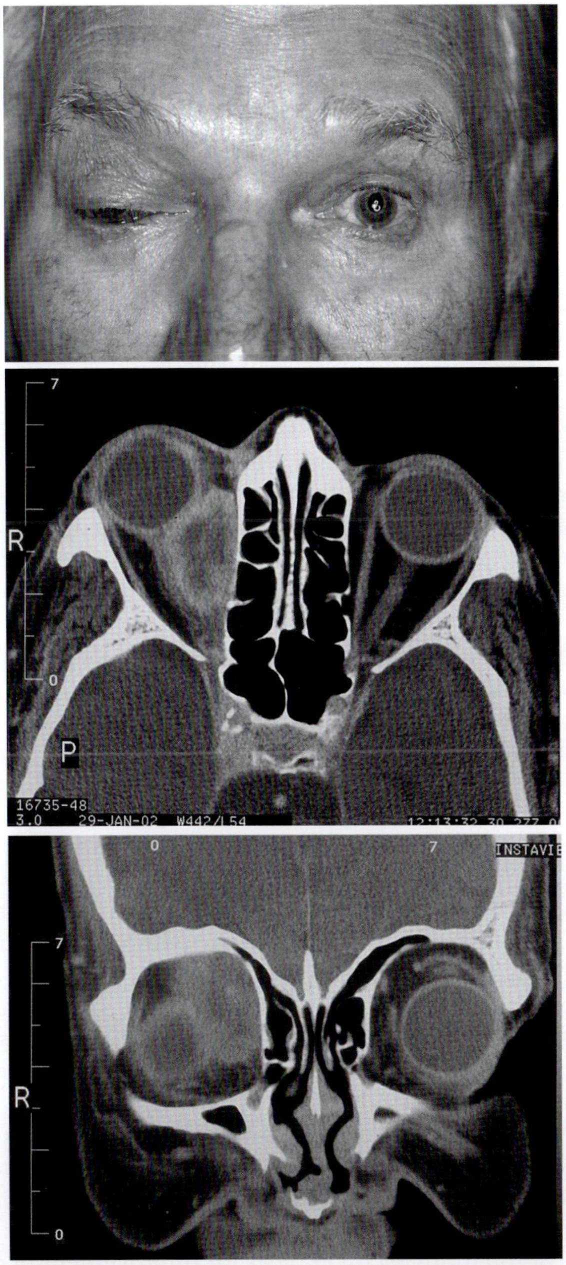

FIGURE 24.2. Mass formation of a metastatic tumor (squamous cell carcinoma), presenting as a large space-occupying lesion, superior medial to the globe in the right orbit. The axial CT image reveals the necrotic nature of the tumor core, indicating a rapid growth. The mass was causing inferior lateral proptosis and extraocular motility problems. The primary of this lesion was unknown despite extensive workup, including thorough consultations with ear, nose, and throat specialists.

DIAGNOSTIC PROCEDURES

Orbital Imaging

Computed tomography (CT) and magnetic resonance imaging (MRI) provide information regarding tissues involved with tumor. Growth pattern is either a well-delineated mass or a diffuse lesion with irregular margins. Multifocal nodularity of the muscles, which may be demonstrated by CT scan or MRI, is more consistent with the diagnosis of a metastatic process (Table 24.1).[24,25] The relative frequency of each presentation is as follows: orbital mass 58%, bone 25%, muscle 9%, and/or diffuse involvement 8%. Although classic presentations have been described, carcinomas from the same primary site may disclose a discrete mass in some patients and a diffuse pattern in others.

On CT scan, metastatic lesions are very similar in density to extraocular muscles.[26] Muscle involvement usually discloses a solitary mass with irregular borders; other findings include bone destruction with or without intracranial or sinus extension. Evidence of direct intracranial extension has been demonstrated in 46% of patients with orbital metastasis.[26]

CT scans are particularly useful in suspected cases of prostate carcinoma and other metastatic tumors with bone involvement. The bone lesions may be either hyperostotic (osteoblastic) or hypostotic (oseolytic). In general, prostate carcinoma causes a hyperostotic (osteoblastic) response (Figure 24.3).

T1-weighted MR images provide excellent resolution to differentiate muscle involvement from the hyperreflective orbital fat.[27,28] T1-weighted images with fat suppression allow better visualization and resolution of soft tissue growth pattern and location. T2-weighted images are less specific; metastatic tumors are hyperreflective with these studies, particularly after gadolinium injection (see Chapters 9 and 10).

Echography of the orbit is useful to measure enlarged muscles and may occasionally show cystic degeneration of necrotic tumors but is not very helpful in most instances.

The most important point in the evaluation of patients with presumed metastatic disease is guided history taking. Elderly patients who had primary tumors in other body sites treated several years prior to orbital manifestations may forget or intentionally deny any history of cancer.

A systemic workup should be done by a medical oncologist in confirmed cases for the evaluation of other metastatic sites and staging. The ophthalmolo-

TABLE 24.1. Diagnosis of Metastatic Disease of the Orbit.

History	Previous history of cancer Family history of cancer Use of "cancer medication"
Ophthalmic examination	Unilateral, diffuse infiltrative lesion Nodular, extraocular muscle involvement Osteolytic or osteoblastic orbital bone lesion in an elderly patient
Systemic evaluation	Medical oncology consultation CT/MRI of chest and abdomen Bone marrow biopsy Laboratory workup
Tissue diagnosis	Fine-needle aspiration biopsy with or without CT guidance or ultrasonography Excisional biopsy

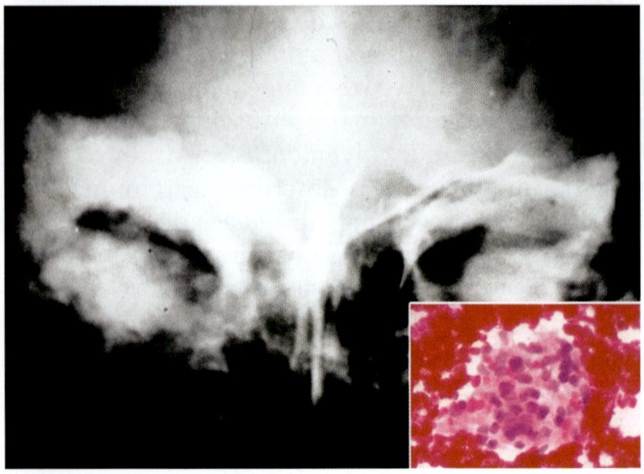

FIGURE 24.3. Hyperostosis of the superior orbital rim in a patient with metastatic prostate carcinoma. *Inset*: Groups of malignant epithelial cells consistent with prostate carcinoma obtained with FNAB.

gist should clearly state the presumed diagnosis as metastatic orbital tumor.

Rarely, the orbital specialist may request other laboratory tests and radiographic studies as part of the initial workup in a patient suspected to have an orbital metastasis. Specific tests are particularly useful in tumors that elaborate or are associated with an elevation of measurable substances in serum or urine, such as prostate carcinoma and carcinoid tumors. Carcinoid tumors have an affinity for uptake of the radiopharmaceutical [^{131}I]metaiodobenzylguanidine (MIBG). Hanson et al. reported a patient with a known carcinoid tumor who developed a left orbital mass that demonstrated abnormal uptake of [^{131}I]MIBG indicative of metastatic carcinoid tumor of the orbit.[29]

Tissue Diagnosis

Fine-needle aspiration biopsy (FNAB) (see Chapter 12) of the orbit is a simple but effective method for confirmation of the orbital metastasis (Figure 24.3).[30–32] FNAB may be performed as an ambulatory procedure or in the operating room after superficial exposure of the tumor. In both situations the procedure is rapid and cost-effective. An adequate specimen usually provides material for routine studies and in some cases for special stains. The optimal setting of FNAB is guidance of the procedure by means of CT and preparation and evaluation of the specimens by an experienced cytopathologist with knowledge of orbital disease. Negative results or the presence of inflammatory cells may be misleading. Metastatic tumors with a prominent stromal component may result in nonrepresentative samples.[33] The observation of a few lymphocytes as the only cells present should not rule out a metastatic disease because infiltrative orbital lesion may show a chronic inflammatory response. Bloody samples in a patient suspected of harboring orbital metastasis should be carefully examined to detect individual, atypical cells or isolated clusters of tumor cells. Melanoma and renal carcinoma are commonly associated with hemorrhage.[34] False negative results vary according to the location of the lesion within the orbit and the type of lesion, but no false positive results have been reported in FNABs for the diagnosis of orbital metastasis.[1,33,34]

An incisional biopsy is indicated either when FNAB results in nonrepresentative samples or when FNAB cannot be performed because of location or because ample tissue is required for special studies. Currently, most differential diagnoses are resolved by immunohistochemical staining techniques using tissue-specific antibodies. Electron microscopy is rarely used for the diagnosis of specific tumor cell types. Special studies include hormonal receptors, proliferative factors, major chemotherapy resistance gene expression, and fusion gene expression. In these instances, the orbital surgeon should communicate with the pathologist in advance regarding the required size and handling of tissue samples.

MANAGEMENT AND PROGNOSIS

The behavior and management of orbital metastases is largely dependent on the primary tumor. Although the prognosis of the patient with orbital metastasis is poor, long survival after treatment of certain neoplasms may occur. Nevertheless, even in hopeless situations, treatment to restore or maintain visual function may provide a better quality of life.

Management of orbital metastatic disease includes palliative irradiation, hormone therapy, chemotherapy, surgical excision, and observation, depending on clinical circumstances (Table 24.2). Radiotherapy is one of the more useful choices for improvement of orbital signs and symptoms and recovery of vision.[35,36] Irradiation doses are divided over periods of two to four weeks for a total dose of 30 to 50 Gy (see Chap-

TABLE 24.2. Management of Patients with Metastasis to the Orbit.

Treatment	*Application*
Observation	Advanced disease, asymptomatic orbital metastasis
Radiotherapy	Diffuse tumors, extraocular muscle involvement, bone involvement
Hormonal therapy	Hormonally sensitive tumors
Chemotherapy	Widespread disease or systemic metastasis
	Simultaneous treatment of primary and metastatic tumors
Surgical excision	Localized, solitary, orbital metastasis
Surgical debulking	Compromise of the globe or optic nerve

ter 33). The success rate in published series is 70 to 90%. The use of adequate doses, delivery through the lateral orbital wall, and eye protection may reduce complications. In one large series, 12 patients experienced acute, transient keratoconjunctivitis; as late side effects, two cases of cataract were observed during a period of observation of 37 and 117 months.[37] In advanced cases of orbital metastases, which may also involve adjacent structures, high-dose radiation (HDR) brachytherapy may be used for palliative purposes.[38]

Hormonal therapy is an alternative to more aggressive methods of treatment in tumors that show estrogen and progesterone surface receptors. Breast carcinoma and prostate carcinoma have been treated solely with hormonal therapy with good results. Prostate carcinoma may be responsive to orchiectomy or diethylstilbestrol.

Chemotherapy with antimetabolites is indicated in tumors that are unresponsive to hormonal therapy and in premenopausal women. Dramatic reduction of signs and symptoms has been observed with systemic chemotherapy alone.

If the only site of metastasis is the orbit, or if a solitary, circumscribed orbital mass is present, surgical excision of the tumor may relieve the clinical manifestations in some patients and even provide a reasonable tumor-free period. Experience with patients who have undergone biopsy has shown that a slow-growing carcinoid may be amenable to surgical excision. Surgical debulking may be required in patients with tumors resistant to other treatment modalities.

Observation without specific treatment of the orbital tumor is a reasonable choice for patients with asymptomatic orbital metastasis but otherwise advanced systemic disease. The prognosis of patients with orbital metastases is poor. Among patients with sufficient follow-up, 95% died of metastasis, with overall mean survival of 15 months, ranging from 3 to 96 months after diagnosis.[1,15]

ORIGINS OF METASTASES TO ORBIT

Breast Carcinoma

Breast carcinoma is the most common primary source of orbital metastases. The ophthalmologist should be aware that incidences of breast cancer have increased approximately 30% in the past two decades.[39] The frequency of breast carcinoma among orbital metastases varies from 29 to 51%. Breast primaries are almost always identified either before or simultaneously with the metastatic disease. Rarely, an orbital metastatic focus will precede the diagnosis of a nonpalpable primary breast carcinoma.[40] A long delay between the diagnosis of the primary tumor and orbital manifestation is not uncommon. The average time is 4.5 to 6.5 years.[40] Longer delays up to 25 years have been reported, however.[40,41]

Patients with breast carcinoma that has metastasized to the orbit are predominantly females, although a few cases in males have been described.[42] The median age at the time of presentation is in the sixth decade.[43] Bilateral orbital involvement is seen in 20% of the cases, exceeding the average incidence of bilateral metastases from other primary neoplasms.

Although symptoms and signs of breast carcinoma do not basically differ from metastases from other primary tumors, certain presentations are quite characteristic. Most breast carcinomas are invasive and infiltrate the fat and muscle. Isolated extraocular muscle involvement is more common in breast carcinoma, and the eyelid may also be affected. Slowly progressive enophthalmos with reduced motility is nearly pathognomonic of metastatic scirrhous breast carcinoma (Figure 24.1).[44] Nearly 54% of patients present with an infiltrative or inflammatory syndrome that should be differentiated from such other conditions as idiopathic inflammatory pseudotumor, myositis, and cellulitis.[45–47]

Clinical examination should include physical examination of the breasts and axillary and supraclavicular lymph nodes. Mammography may be of help in female patients without history of prior cancer. Rarely, patients may present with metastatic disease from an unknown breast primary.[48]

Invasive ductal carcinoma is the most frequent breast cancer histologic type; it includes mucinous, papillary, and scirrhous variants. Other cell types are lobular invasive and undifferentiated carcinomas. Lobular carcinoma has a tendency toward multicentric and bilateral mammary gland involvement. In a literature review of orbital breast metastases, the histopathologic subtypes of 54 carcinomas were as follows: 9 invasive ductal, 5 invasive lobular, 5 scirrhous, and 35 undifferentiated.[46] Scirrhous and lobular carcinoma of the breast may pose a challenge for histopathologic diagnosis because the yield of FNAB is low. The dominance of fibrous tissue in these tumors may lead to nondiagnostic results. Some authors favor the use of an incisional biopsy in suspected cases with enophthalmos or inflammatory presentations. At the time the tumor tissue is surgically removed, estrogen-receptor (ER) and progesteron-receptor (PR) status should be determined, and it is good practice to save fresh tissue for further analysis, including expression of *HER2-neu*.

Patients with breast cancer and orbital metastases are classified in stage IV of the system of the American Joint Committee on Cancer, which includes patients with any status of the primary tumor and lymph nodes, and distant metastases (see Chapter 30).[49] Goals of treatment include improving quality of life and prolonging life. The median survival is 18 to 24 months, but some patients may experience longer survivals.[37] Treatment of metastatic breast cancer will usually involve hormone therapy and/or chemotherapy with or without trastuzumab (Herceptin). Radiation therapy and/or surgery may be indicated for patients with limited symptomatic metastases. The rate of regression after palliative radiotherapy of orbital lesions has been 60 and 79% in different series.[37,50,51]

Hormone therapy should generally be considered as initial treatment for a postmenopausal patient with newly diagnosed metastatic disease if the patient's tumor is ER positive, PR positive, or ER/PR unknown. Hormone therapy is especially indicated if the disease involves only bone and soft tissue and the patient either has not received adjuvant antiestrogen therapy or has been off such therapy for more than a year. Therapy with tamoxifen has been reported to reduce eyelid and orbital metastases of carcinoma of the breast.[52] In patients whose tumors overexpress *HER2-neu*, administration of Herceptin as a single agent resulted in a significant response rate. Patients whose tumors have progressed despite hormone therapy are candidates for chemotherapy with antimetabolites. Patients with EP/PR-negative tumors and those with visceral metastases are also candidates for chemotherapy.

Miscellaneous Primary Sites

According to different series, the other common cancers metastatic to the orbit include lung (Figure 24.4),[53–56] prostate (Figure 24.5),[57,58] and hepatic carcinoma (Figure 24.6).[59–62] Because of the occult lesion and a symptomatic growth of the primary tumor, orbital metastasis may be the first manifestation of disseminated diseases in 20% of cases.[4,6] Many patients have a fulminant course with short survival.

In patients with prostate carcinoma, the diagnosis of metastastic orbital disease is facilitated by the demonstration of osteoblastic and/or osteolytic bone lesions that are associated with pain. In cases of primary manifestation of the disease, confirmation is provided by the measurement of prostate-specific antigen (PSA) in serum or the expression of the same antigen in tissue sections from the metastatic tumor.[17,63]

Hepatocellular carcinoma is the most frequent metastatic orbital tumor in Japan, but it is rarely seen in Western countries.[16] The patients are predominantly males with an average age of 56 years.[16] Metastasis to the orbit is usually associated with advanced disease and early mortality; the mean survival after diagnosis is about one year. In a majority of the cases, the proptosis is associated with pain because of early periosteal involvement. The differential diagnosis of painful proptosis should include malignant schwannoma, adenoid cystic carcinoma of the lacrimal gland, and perineural invasion of the orbit by cutaneous squamous cell carcinoma.[64–66] FNAB material is usually sufficient for diagnosis, particularly if enough tissue is recovered for immunohistologic chemical stains. Positive stainings of bile canaliculi with polyclonal carcinoembryonic antigen (CEA) marker confirms the diagnosis of hepatocellular carcinoma. α-Fetoprotein (AFP) has been reported to be positive in about 80% of hepatocellular carcinomas.[67]

Metastatic melanoma of the orbit may be seen in several clinical settings.[68–71] Most frequently, the patient has had a cutaneous melanoma excised, or an active, nonocular melanoma (Figure 24.7). Rarely, a history or clinical signs of a spontaneously regressed

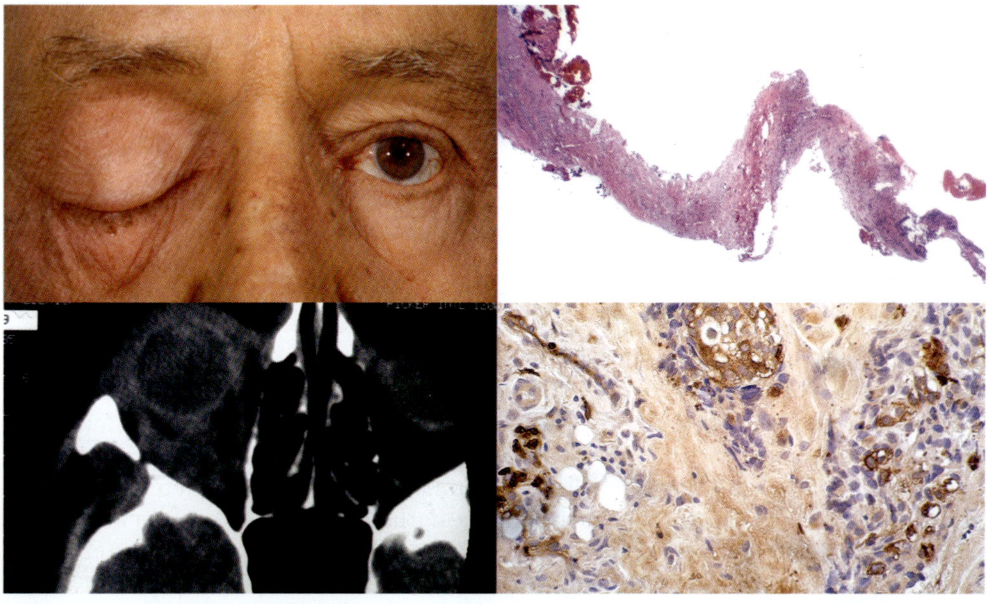

FIGURE 24.4. Metastatic squamous cell carcinoma of the lung in the right orbit causing mild proptosis; ptosis of the upper lid and extraocular motility disturbance was secondary to diffuse infiltration of the tumor into the soft tissues of the right orbit. FNAB revealed poorly differentiated carcinoma. Immunohistochemistry demonstrated the presence of cytokeratin, revealing the tumor to be poorly differentiated squamous cell carcinoma (lower right).

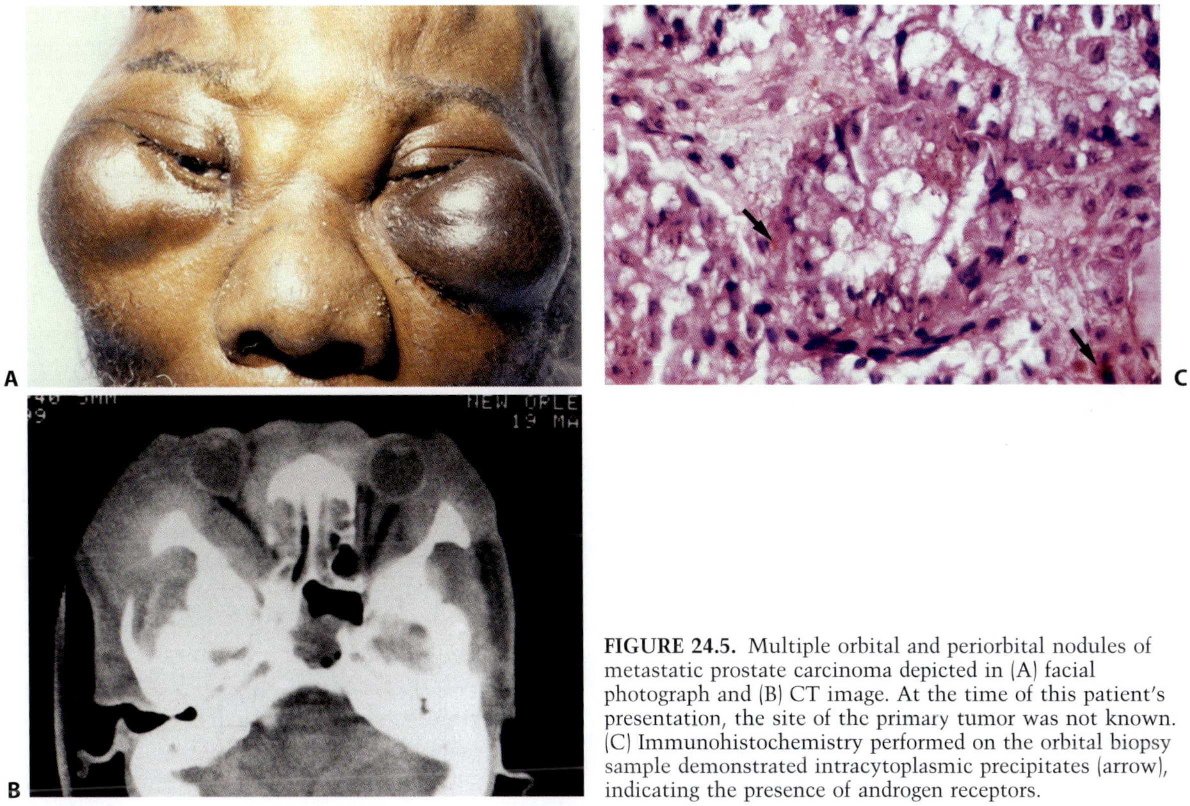

FIGURE 24.5. Multiple orbital and periorbital nodules of metastatic prostate carcinoma depicted in (A) facial photograph and (B) CT image. At the time of this patient's presentation, the site of the primary tumor was not known. (C) Immunohistochemistry performed on the orbital biopsy sample demonstrated intracytoplasmic precipitates (arrow), indicating the presence of androgen receptors.

malignant melanoma of the skin lesion may be documented. In the few remaining cases, no primary site can be demonstrated after comprehensive dermatologic and oncologic workup. The most frequent primary sites for orbital metastases are the upper arms and trunk. Metastases of melanoma are commonly discrete and well circumscribed. The melanoma cells may grow predominantly within an extraocular muscle. Contralateral orbital metastasis from choroidal melanoma have been reported.[69–71] Although advanced metastatic melanoma is relatively resistant to therapy, several biologic response modifiers and cytotoxic agents can result in longer survival times. In some cases, excision of isolated orbital metastasis may be associated with prolonged survival.

Other less frequent primary sites of metastatic tumors to the orbit are gastrointestinal tract and salivary glands,[72–75] kidney,[76,77] thyroid,[78,79] urinary

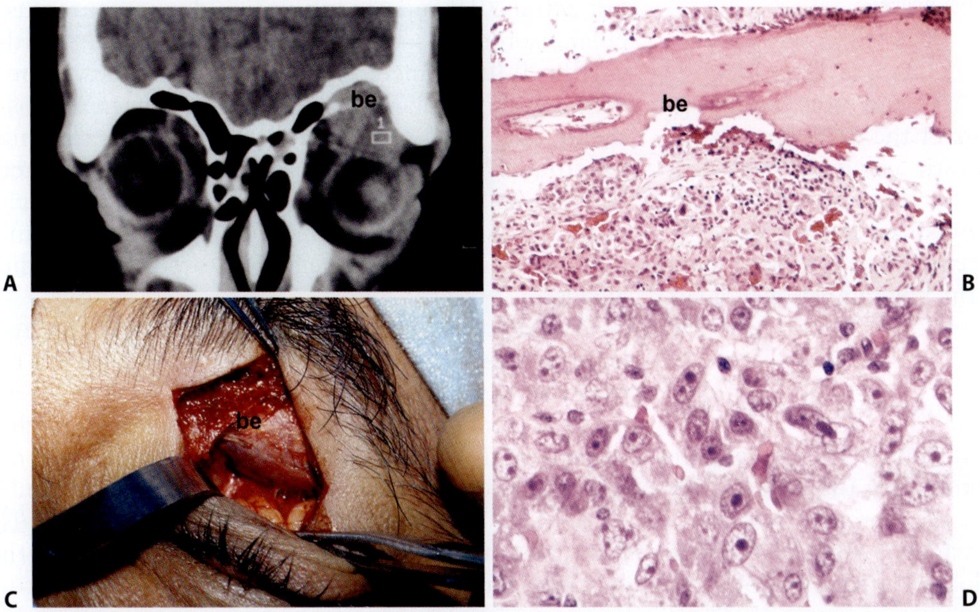

FIGURE 24.6. (A) Coronal CT, (C) intraoperative photograph, and (B,D) histopathology specimen showing extensive bony erosion (be) secondary to hepatocellular carcinoma metastatic to the orbit. (D) Large polygonal hepatocellular carcinoma cells with granular cytoplasm; large nuclei with prominent nucleoli are visible.

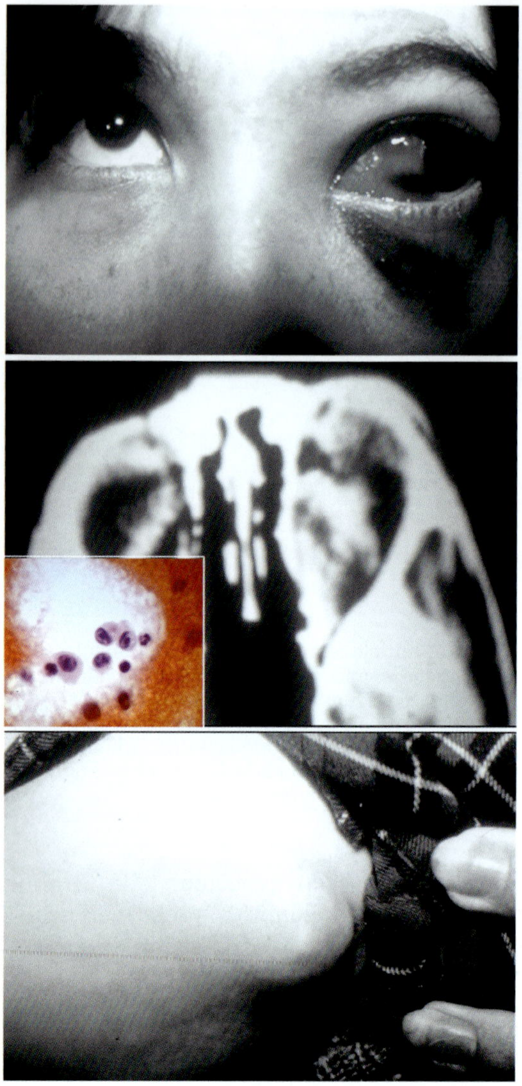
A
B
C

FIGURE 24.7. (A,B) Cutaneous melanoma metastatic to the orbits bilaterally. The predominant tumor load was in the left orbit, and, therefore, the left eye appears to be more proptotic. (B) The extraocular motility of the right orbit was full at the time of the CT scan. *Inset*: Melanoma cells obtained with FNAB. (C) Enlarged, melanoma-laden, left axillary lymph nodes.

bladder,[80] genital organs,[81,82] and soft tissue tumors.[83–87] Carcinoid tumors of the orbit may be primary or metastatic. Metastatic carcinoid tumors to the orbit are characterized by slow growth, circumscribed appearance, and long survival after local[88–94] surgical excision. Surgical removal of carcinoid metastatic in the orbit is one of the few indications for surgery because of longer survival.

Metastatic Cancer from Unknown Primary Site

In 10% of metastastic orbital tumors, the origin of the primary tumor remains unknown at the time of diagnosis.[13–15] This rate represents approximately 2.5 to 3.5% of orbital metastases, which is similar to the percentage of histologically documented carcinomas in any body location in which the origin is not identified clinically (Figure 24.2). This situation is known as "carcinoma of unknown primary site" (CUPS) or occult primary malignancy.

The minimal criteria to define CUPS include biopsy of the tumor, complete physical examination, chest x-ray, chest and abdominal CT/MRI, complete blood cell count, urinalysis, and examination of the stool for occult blood.[95] Most instances of CUPS are adenocarcinomas or undifferentiated tumors. The majority of the patients with CUPS are over age 60.

The pathologist plays a pivotal role in the identification of the primary tumor. Immunohistochemical studies, histochemistry, polymerase chain reaction sequencing, chromosomal analysis, and electron microscopy may provide useful information to confirm or rule out certain tumors.[96,97] A favorable group for therapy has been identified in patients younger than 50 years, with elevated serum levels of β human chorionic gonadotropin (hCG) and AFP, presence of neurogranules, and rapid growth rate.

The overall prognosis of CUPS is poor with a median survival of about 6 months. Tumors of the lung, breast, prostate, and thyroid represent approximately 15% of CUPS.[98,99] CUPS in which the cell type is identified are treated with standard chemotherapy and hormonal therapy regimens already indicated for such tumors. In the remaining cases, several combined protocols have been used but without much success.[99]

Paraneoplastic Orbital Syndrome

Paraneoplastic syndromes with ocular and adnexal involvement are rare. In general, paraneoplastic syndromes are seen in less than 1% of patients with cancer.

Ocular muscle palsy and ptosis may occur without extraocular muscle infiltration due to neuromuscular disorders associated with cancer.[95] Patients with small-cell lung cancer may develop antibodies to prevent neuromuscular transmission resulting in a myasthenic-like syndrome (Lambert–Eaton myasthenic syndrome).[100] Other malignancies that may produce similar signs and symptoms include renal cell carcinoma, bronchial carcinoma, lymphoma, malignant thymoma, and transitional cell carcinoma of the bladder.

A rare clinical presentation, apparently not related to direct tumor invasion, has been observed in patients with seminoma and in one patient with paran-glioma.[101–104] This unusual syndrome might present with bilateral nonspecific inflammation or Graves-like orbitopathy and thickening of the four extraocular rectus muscles. The mechanism of this disorder is unknown and has been associated with elevated serum levels of hCG. In one case, histopathologic examination of the orbit did not reveal any evidence of tumor infiltation.[103] Regression of signs and symptoms has been observed after excision of the primary tumor and in response to corticosteroids. Retinal abnormalities ranging from atrophy to hypopigmentation have been reported in lung cancers and other types of malignant disease.[105,106] Since orbital metastases often take place during advanced stages of a malignant process, it is advisable to keep the possibility of retinal dysfunction in mind and examine the patient accordingly.

References

1. Char DH, Miller T, Kroll S. Orbital metastases: diagnosis and course. *Br J Ophthalmol* 1997;81:386.
2. Ferry AP, Font RL. Carcinoma metastatic to the eye and orbit. I. A clinicopathologic study of 227 cases. *Arch Ophthalmol* 1974;92:276–286.
3. Kennedy RE. An evaluation of 820 orbital cases. *Trans Am Ophthalmol Soc* 1984;82:134.
4. Shields JA, Bakewell B, Augsburger JJ, Flanagan JC. Classification and incidence of space-occupying lesions of the orbit: a survey of 645 biopsies. *Arch Ophthalmol* 1984;102:1606.
5. Rootman J. *Diseases of the Orbit. A Multidisciplinary Approach.* Philadelphia: JB Lippincott; 1988:405–427.
6. Jensen OA. Metastatic tumors of the eye and orbit: a histopathologic analysis of a Danish series. *Acta Pathol Microbiol Scand* 1970;212(suppl):201.
7. Font RL, Ferry AP. Carcinoma metastatic to the eye and orbit. III. A clinicopathologic study of 28 cases metastatic to the orbit. *Cancer* 1976;38:1326.
8. Freedman MI, Folk JC. Metastatic tumors to the eye and orbit: patient survival and clinical characteristics. *Arch Ophthalmol* 1987;105:1215.
9. Bullock JD, Yanes B. Metastatic tumors of the orbit. *Ann Ophthalmol* 1980;12:1392.
10. Goldberg RA, Rootman J, Cline RA. Tumors metastatic to the orbit: a changing picture. *Surv Ophthalmol* 1990;35:1.
11. Katz SE, Rootman J, Goldberg RA. Secondary and metastatic tumors of the orbit. In: Tasman W, Jaeger EA, eds. *Duane Ophthalmology CD-ROM Edition.* Hagerstown, MD: Lippincott, Williams & Wilkins; 2001;2:46.
12. Shields CL, Shields JA, Peggs M. Tumors metastatic to the orbit. *Ophthalmic Plast Reconstr Surg* 1988;4:73.
13. Henderson JW, Campbell RJ, Farrow GM, Garrity JA. *Orbital Tumors.* 3rd ed. New York: Raven Press; 1993:361–375.
14. Günalp I, Gündüz K. Metastatic orbital tumors. *Jpn J Ophthalmol* 1995;39:65.
15. Shields JA, Shields CL, Brotman HK, et al. Cancer metastatic to the orbit: the 2000 Robert M. Curts Lecture. *Ophthalmic Plast Reconstr Surg* 2001;17:346–354.
16. Amemiya T, Hayashida H, Dake Y. Metastatic orbital tumors in Japan: a review of the literature. *Ophthalmic Epidemiol* 2002;9:35–47.
17. Carriere VM, Karcioglu ZA, Apple DJ, Inser MS. A case of prostate carcinoma with bilateral orbital metastases and the review of the literature. *Ophthalmology* 1882;89:402–406.
18. Tijl J, Koornneef L, Eijpe A, et al. Metastatic tumors to the orbit—management and prognosis. *Graefes Arch Clin Exp Ophthalmol* 1992;230:527.
19. Goldberg RA, Rootman J. Clinical characteristics of metastatic orbital tumors. *Ophthalmology* 1990;97:620.
20. Cline RA, Rootman J. Enophthalmos: a clinical review. *Ophthalmology* 1984;91:229.
21. Ashton N, Morgan G. Discrete carcinomatous metastases in the extraocular muscles. *Br J Ophthalmol* 1974;58:112.
22. Capone A, Slamovits TL. Discrete metastasis of solid tumors to extraocular muscles. *Arch Ophthalmol* 1990;108:237.
23. Divine RD, Anderson RL. Metastatic small cell carcinoma masquerading as orbital myositis. *Ophthalmic Surg* 1982;14:483.
24. Trokel SL, Hilal SK. Recognition and differential diagnosis of enlarged extraocular muscles in computed tomography. *Am J Ophthalmol* 1979;87:503.
25. Slamovits TL, Burde RM. Bumpy muscles. *Surv Ophthalmol* 1988;33:189.
26. Healy JF. Computed tomographic evaluation of metastases to the orbit. *Ann Ophthalmol* 1983;15:1026.
27. Han JS, Benson JE, Bonstelle CT, et al. Magnetic resonance imaging of the orbit: a preliminary experience. *Radiology* 1984;150:755.
28. Peyster RG, Shapiro MD, Haik BG. Orbital metastasis: role of magnetic resonance imaging and computed tomography. *Radiol Clin North Am* 1987;25:647.
29. Hanson MW, Schneider AM, Enterline DS, et al. Iodine-131-metaiodobenzylguanidine uptake in metastatic carcinoid tumor to the orbit. *J Nucl Med* 1998;39:647–650.
30. Kennerdell JS, Dekker A, Johnson BL, et al. Fine needle aspiration biopsy: a report of its use in orbital tumors. *Arch Ophthalmol* 1979;97:1315.
31. Dresner SD, Kennerdell JS, Dekker A. Fine needle aspiration biopsy of metastatic orbital tumors. *Surv Ophthalmol* 1983;27:397.
32. Kennerdell JS, Slamovits TL, Dekker A, et al. Orbital fine needle aspiration biopsy. *Am J Ophthalmol* 1985;99:547.
33. Krohel GB, Tobin DR, Chavis RM. Inaccuracy of fine needle aspiration biopsy. *Ophthalmology* 1985;92:666.
34. Liu D. Complications of fine needle aspiration biopsy of the orbit. *Ophthalmology* 1985;92:1768.
35. Huh SH, Nisce LZ, Simpson LD, et al. Value of radiation therapy in the treatment of orbital metastasis. *AJR Am J Roentgenol* 1974;120:589.
36. Glasburn JR, Klionsky M, Brady LW. Radiation therapy for metastatic diseases involving the orbit. *Am J Clin Oncol* 1984;7:145.
37. Amichetti M, Caffo O, Minatel E, et al. Ocular metastases from breast carcinoma: a multicentric retrospective study. *Oncol Rep* 2000;7:761–765.
38. Levenday PC. Cancer in the head and neck: the role of brachytherapy in local control [abstract]. *Intl Brachyther* 1995:24–29.
39. Surveillance Epidemiology and End Results. *SEER Cancer Statistics Review, 1973–1994: Tables and Graphs.* Bethesda, MD: National Cancer Institute; 1997. NIH Publication No 97-2789.
40. Reeves D, Levine MR, Lash R. Nonpalpable breast carcinoma presenting as orbital infiltration: case presentation and literature review. *Ophthalmic Plast Reconstr Surg* 2002;18:84–88.
41. Hart WM. Metastatic carcinoma to the eye and orbit. *Int Ophthalmol Clin* 1962;2:465–482.
42. Schlaen ND, Naves AE. Orbital and choroidal metastases from carcinoma of the male breast. *Arch Ophthalmol* 1986;104:1344.
43. Bullock JD, Yanes B. Ophthalmic manifestations of metastatic breast cancer. *Ophthalmology* 1980;87:961.
44. Lagreze WD, Wesendahl TA, Kommerell G. Enophthalmos caused by orbital metastasis of breast carcinoma. *Klin Monatsbl Augenheilkd* 1997;211:68–69.
45. Mottow-Lippa L, Jakobiec FA, Iwamoto T. Pseudoinflammatory metastatic breast carcinoma of the orbit and lids. *Ophthalmology* 1981;88:575.
46. Toller KK, Gigantelli JW, Spalding MJ. Bilateral orbital metas-

tases from breast carcinoma. A case of false pseudotumor. *Ophthalmology* 1998;105:1897–1901.

47. Reifler DM, Davidson P. Histochemical analysis of breast carcinoma metastatic to the orbit. *Ophthalmology* 1986;93:254.
48. Wolstencroft SJ, Hodder SC, Askill CF, et al. Orbital metastasis due to interval lobular carcinoma of the breast. *Arch Ophthalmol* 1999;117:1419–1421.
49. National Cancer Institute. Breast cancer: treatment. http://www.cancer.gov/cancerinfo/pdq/treatment/breast/HealthProfessional#7.40 Last modified November 2002.
50. Burmeister BH, Benjamin CS, Childs WJ. The management of metastases to the eye and orbit from carcinoma of the breast. *Aust N Z J Ophthalmol* 1990;18:187.
51. Ratanatharathorn V, Powers WE, Grimm J, et al. Eye metastasis from carcinoma of the breast: diagnosis, radiation treatment and results. *Cancer Treat Rev* 1991;18:261.
52. Saitoh A, Amemiya T, Tsuda N. Metastasis of breast carcinoma to eyelid and orbit of a postmenopausal woman: good response to tamoxifen therapy. *Ophthalmologica* 1997;211:362–366.
53. Rosenbluth J, Laval J, Weil JV. Metastasis of bronchial adenoma to the eye. *Arch Ophthalmol* 1960;63:47.
54. Whyte AM. Bronchogenic carcinoma metastasizing to the orbit: a case report. *J Maxillofac Surg* 1978;6:277–279.
55. Spaide RF, Granger E, Hammer BD, et al. Rapidly expanding exophthalmos: an unusual presentation of small cell lung cancer. *Br J Ophthalmol* 1989;73:461.
56. Kubota K, Furuse K, Kawahara M, et al. A case of malignant pleural mesothelioma with metastasis to the orbit. *Jpn J Clin Oncol* 1996;26:469.
57. Boldt HC, Nerad JA. Orbital metastasis from prostate carcinoma. *Arch Ophthalmol* 1988;106:1403.
58. Sher JH, Weinstock SJ. Orbital metastasis of prostatic carcinoma. *Can J Ophthalmol* 1983;18:248.
59. Lubin JR, Grove AS Jr, Zakov ZN, et al. Hepatoma metastatic to the orbit. *Am J Ophthalmol* 1980;89:268.
60. Zubler MA, Rivera R, Lane M. Hepatoma presenting as a retro-orbital metastasis. *Cancer* 1981;48:1883.
61. Schwab L, Doshi H, Shields JA, et al. Hepatocellular carcinoma metastatic to the orbit in an African patient. *Ophthalmic Surg* 1994;25:106.
62. Font RL, Maturi RK, Small RG, et al. Hepatocellular carcinoma metastatic to the orbit. *Arch Ophthalmol* 1998;116:942–945.
63. Kopelman JE, Shorr N. A case of prostatic carcinoma metastatic to the orbit diagnosed by fine needle aspiration and immunoperoxidase staining for prostate-specific antigen. *Ophthalmic Surg* 1987;18:599–603.
64. Jakobiec FA, Font RL, Zimmerman LE. Malignant peripheral nerve sheath tumor of the orbit: a clinicopathologic study of 8 cases. *Trans Am Ophthalmol Soc* 1985;83:17–35.
65. Font RL, Gamel JW. Adenoid cystic carcinoma of the lacrimal gland: a clinicopathologic study of 79 cases. In: Nicholson DH, ed. *Ocular Pathology Update*. New York: Masson; 1980:277–283.
66. Alonso PE, Bescansa E, Solar J, et al. Peripheral spread of cutaneous squamous cell carcinoma manifesting as ptosis and ophthalmoplegia (orbital apex syndrome). *Br J Plast Surg* 1995;48:564–568.
67. Kojiro H, Kawano Y, Isomura T. Distribution of albumin and/or alpha-fetoprotein positive cells in hepatocellular carcinoma. *Lab Invest* 1981;44:221.
68. Orcutt JC, Char DH. Melanoma metastatic to the orbit. *Ophthalmology* 1988;95:1033.
69. Shields JA, Shields CL, Shakin EP, Kobetz LE. Metastasis of choroidal melanoma to the contralateral choroid, orbit and eyelid. *Br J Ophthalmol* 1988;72:456.
70. Coupland SE, Sidiki S, Clark BJ, et al. Metastatic choroidal melanoma to the contralateral orbit 40 years after enucleation. *Arch Ophthalmol* 1996;114:751.
71. Abramson DA, Servodidio CA. Metastatic choroidal melanoma to the contralateral orbit 40 years after enucleation. [letter]. *Arch Ophthalmol* 1997;115:134.
72. Seretan EL. Metastatic adenocarcinoma from the stomach to the orbit. *Arch Ophthalmol* 1981;99:1469.
73. Leske JM, Zhan J, Mown LA. Metastatic gastroesophogeal junction adenocarcinoma to the extraocular muscle. *Ophthalmology* 2003;110:318–321.
74. Snidermann HR. Orbital metastases from tumor of the pancreas: report of two cases with necropsy findings. *Am J Ophthalmol* 1942;25:1215.
75. Saxena RB, Mathur RN, Sonani SZ. Orbital metastasis of mixed parotid tumor. *Indian J Ophthalmol* 1975;23:23.
76. Denby P, Harvey L, English MG. Solitary metastasis from an occult renal cell carcinoma presenting as a primary lacrimal gland tumor. *Orbit* 1986;5:21.
77. Bersani TA, Costello JJ, Mango CA, Streeten BW. Benign approach to a malignant orbital tumor: metastatic renal cell carcinoma. *Ophthalmic Plast Reconstr Surg* 1994;10:42.
78. Betharia SM. Metastatic orbital carcinoma of the thyroid. *Indian J Ophthalmol* 1985;33:191.
79. Hornblass A, Kass LG, Reich R. Thyroid carcinoma metastatic to the orbit. *Ophthalmology* 1987;94:1004.
80. Smiley SS. An orbital metastasis from the urinary bladder. *Arch Ophthalmol* 1965;74:809.
81. Rush JA, Older JJ, Richman AV. Testicular seminoma metastatic to the orbit. *Am J Ophthalmol* 1981;91:258.
82. Ballinger WH Jr, Wesley RE. Seminoma metastatic to the orbit. *Ophthalmic Surg* 1984;15:120.
83. Drake ET, Dobben GD. Leiomyosarcoma of the uterus with unusual metastases. *JAMA* 1959;170:1294.
84. Abdalla MI, Ghaly AF, Hosni F. Liposarcoma with orbital metastases: case report. *Br J Ophthalmol* 1966;50:426.
85. Stewart WB, Newman NM, Cavender JC, et al. Fibrous histiocytoma metastatic to the orbit. *Arch Ophthalmol* 1978;96:871.
86. Burnstine MA, Frueh BR, Elner VM. Angiosarcoma metastatic to the orbit. *Arch Ophthalmol* 1996;114:93.
87. Walton RC, Ellis GS Jr, Haik BG. Rhabdomyosarcoma presumed metastatic to the orbit. *Ophthalmology* 1996;103:1512.
88. Rush JA, Walker RR, Campbell RJ. Orbital carcinoid tumor metastatic from the colon. *Am J Ophthalmol* 1980;89:636.
89. Harris AL, Montgomery A. Orbital carcinoid tumor. *Am J Ophthalmol* 1980;90:875.
90. Riddle PJ, Font RL, Zimmerman LE. Carcinoid tumors of the eye and orbit: a clinicopathologic study of 15 cases, with histochemical and electron microscopic observations. *Hum Pathol* 1982;13:459.
91. Divina RD, Anderson RL, Ossoinig KC. Metastatic carcinoid unresponsive to radiation therapy presenting as a lacrimal fossa mass. *Ophthalmology* 1982;89:516.
92. Shields CL, Shields JA, Eagle RC, et al. Orbital metastases from a carcinoid tumor: computed tomography, magnetic resonance imaging and electron microscopic findings. *Arch Ophthalmol* 1987;105:968.
93. Shetlar DJ, Font RL, Ordonez N, et al. A clinicopathologic study of three carcinoid tumors metastatic to the orbit. *Ophthalmology* 1990;97:257.
94. Fan JT, Buettner H, Bartley GB, Bolling JP. Clinical features and treatment of seven patients with carcinoid tumor metastatic to the eye and orbit. *Am J Ophthalmol* 1995;119:211.
95. Muir C. Cancer of unknown primary site. *Cancer* 1995;75:353–356.
96. Ruddon RW, Norton SE. Use of biological markers in the di-

agnosis of cancer of unknown primary tumor. *Semin Oncol* 1993;20:251–260.

97. Motzer RJ, Rodriguez E, Reuter VE, et al. Molecular and cytogenetic studies in the diagnosis of patients with poorly differentiated carcinomas of unknown primary site. *J Clin Oncol* 1995;13:274–282.
98. Neumann KH, Nystron JS. Metastatic cancer of unknown origin: nonsquamous cell type. *Semin Oncol* 1982;9:427–434.
99. Altman E, Cadman E. An analysis of 1539 patients with cancer of unknown primary site. *Cancer* 1986;57:120–124.
100. Rojas-Marcos I, Rene R, Graus F. Paraneoplastic syndromes in otoneuro-ophthalmology. *Rev Neurol* 2000;31:1206–1212.
101. Mann AS. Bilateral exophthalmos and seminoma. *J Clin Endocrinol Metabol* 1967;27:1500–1502.
102. Leyson JF. Mediastinal seminoma associated with exophthalmos and gynecomastia. *Urology* 1974;3:366–369.
103. Taylor JB, Solomon BH, Levine RE, et al. Exophthalmos in seminoma: regression with steroids and orchiectomy. *JAMA* 1978;240:860–861.
104. Spraul CW, Lang GE, Lang GK. Orbital myopathy in metastatic malignant paraganglioma: a paraneoplastic syndrome? *Klin Monatsbl Augenheilkd* 1996;209:153–157.
105. Thirkill CE, Keltner JL, Tyler NK, Roth AM. Antibody reactions with retina and cancer-associated antigens in 10 patients with cancer-associated retinopathy. *Arch Ophthalmol* 1993;111:931–937.
106. Kim RY, Retsas S, Fitzke FW, et al. Cutaneous melanoma-associated retinopathy. *Ophthalmology* 1994;101:1837–1843.

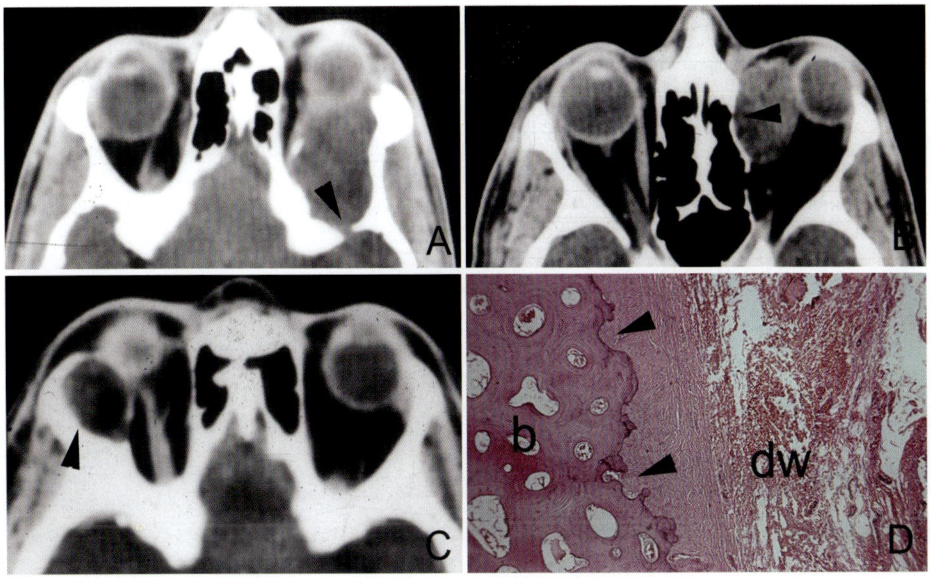

FIGURE 25.2. Dermoids located in different parts of the orbit causing bony erosion. (A) A large posterior dermoid occupying almost the entire orbit, extending into the middle cranial fossa. (B) An oval dermoid eroding into the medial wall of the orbit. (C) A superior lateral dermoid causing erosion into the wall of the lacrimal gland fossa. (D) Histopathologic example of the relationship between the dermoid wall (dw) and bone (b). Arrowheads point to bony erosion.

pointense to extraocular muscles in T1-weighted images (Figure 25.5). Because of the fat content, however, the signal varies on T1-weighted images, which may show two or more signal intensities within one lesion. The specific nature of the fatty, luminal contents is best demonstrated when diffusion-weighted imaging (DWI) is used, which enables specific definition by signal enhancement.[26–29]

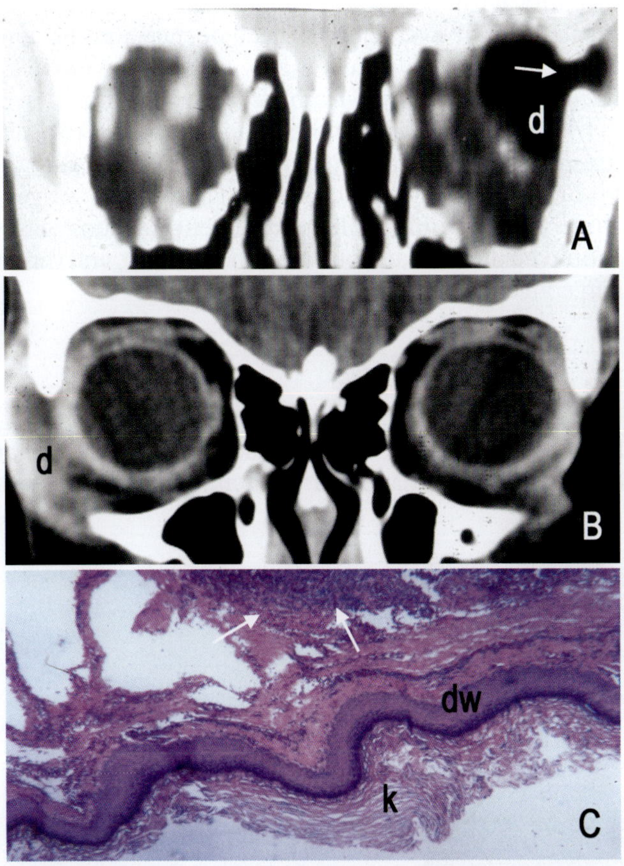

FIGURE 25.3. (A,B) Two dumbbell-shaped dermoids (d) located partially in the orbit and partially in the temporal fossa. The widening of the frontozygomatic fissure (arrow) by the expanding dermoid is shown in (A). (C) A chronic inflammatory reaction (arrows) adjacent to a leaking dermoid wall (dw); k = keratin.

Small dermoids and epidermoids do not need immediate treatment and can be observed until the second or third year of life and sometimes even longer. However, when the lesion reaches a certain size, it should be surgically removed; whenever possible, removal of these lesions should be conducted with special care to avoid rupture of the cyst wall.[11] The surgical removal should be performed before the lesion becomes large enough to displace the eyelid and orbital structures. The growth of the dermoid is primarily due to the increase of its secretions within the lumen, which in turn leads to distension of the cyst wall with focal thinning. The luminal contents may leak out through the weakened areas of the wall and cause chronic inflammatory foreign body reaction. Another issue to consider is that as a child grows and becomes more active, the chance of the dermoids becoming traumatized increases, particularly in the case of the superficial ones. If the lesion is sufficiently large, even a minor trauma may cause the rupture of the tumor with leakage of keratin material into adjacent soft tissues, causing a severe, localized, anaphylactoid reaction. Again, removal should be performed prior to rupture of the cyst, which makes complete excision of the tumor difficult.

Superficial orbital dermoids that are located superiorally can easily be reached through a lid crease incision, which allows good exposure of the tumor, even if it is not located immediately below the lid crease.[30,31] Since it is important to remove the dermoid with an intact wall, the surgeon should take time in dissecting around the lesion in a blunt fashion, using cotton tip applicators and blunt curved hemostats to push and spread the adherent soft tissues

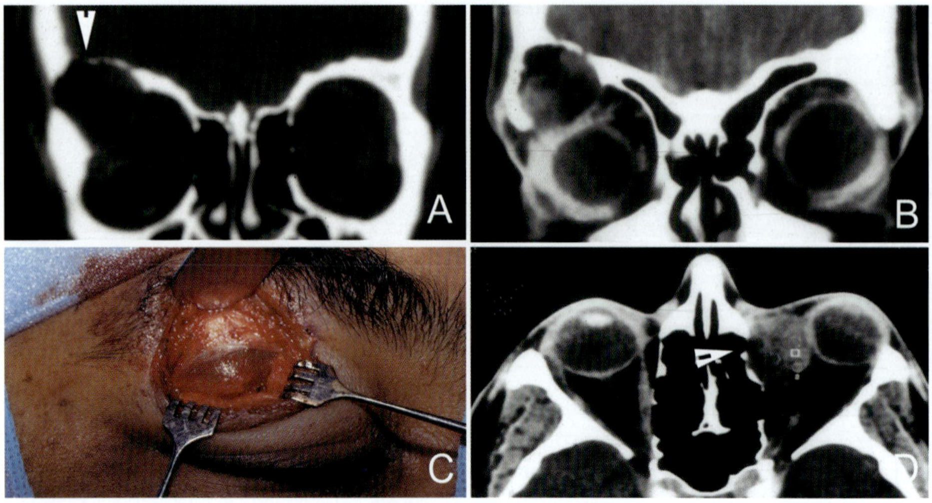

FIGURE 25.4. Extension of the dermoid into the cranium (A–C) and into the ethmoidal sinus (D). Intraoperative photograph (C) shows the purplish-red dermoid lesion underneath the frontal bone.

away from the wall. During this procedure, it is important to look for areas of firm connection between the dermoid wall and the bone, which may represent vestigial portions of the originally entrapped epidermis. If these adherences are left behind, the likelihood of recurrence increases. Application of the cryoprobe during the dissection is suggested by some authors; however, the cryoprobe is usually not necessary for the excision of superficial lesions that readily present themselves. The effectiveness of the cryoprobe to adhere itself to a deeper dermoid is limited; because of the fatty content of the cyst, only a superficial iceball is created between the tip of the probe and the wall of the lesion. At times the cryoprobe may very well be a disadvantage because if applied to a weak portion of the wall, it may create a break in the capsule and make the intact removal more difficult.

The surgical removal of deep orbital dermoids is more difficult.[32] The decision to remove these lesions depends on the size and location of the tumor and its potential to lead to functional deficit. If the tumor compresses the globe and the optic nerve or causes extraocular motility disturbance, which in turn leads to amblyopia, removal is indicated and should be done without delay. The rule just given for the removal of superficial dermoids applies to deep orbital lesions, as well: that is, the surgeon should first attempt to remove the lesion with an intact capsule. However, in deep lesions, this is not as easy as with superficial ones because of limited visibility, presence of vital structures adjacent to the lesion, and the possible adherence of the base of the long-standing lesion to the bone. In these situations, if the lesion cannot be removed in toto, the luminal contents may be removed carefully without too much spillage into the soft tissues. Once the cyst wall has been opened and the contents completely cleaned, it may be easier to mobilize the lesion for removal from its bony attachments. If the lesion is too large and extends into adjacent cavities including the nose, paranasal sinuses, and the cranium, removal of the lesion through orbital surgery alone may be impossible; treatment in such cases should be undertaken jointly with ear, nose, and throat surgeons and neurosurgeons.

DERMOLIPOMA

Dermolipoma is another choristomatous lesion that contains skin and adnexal elements surrounded by a

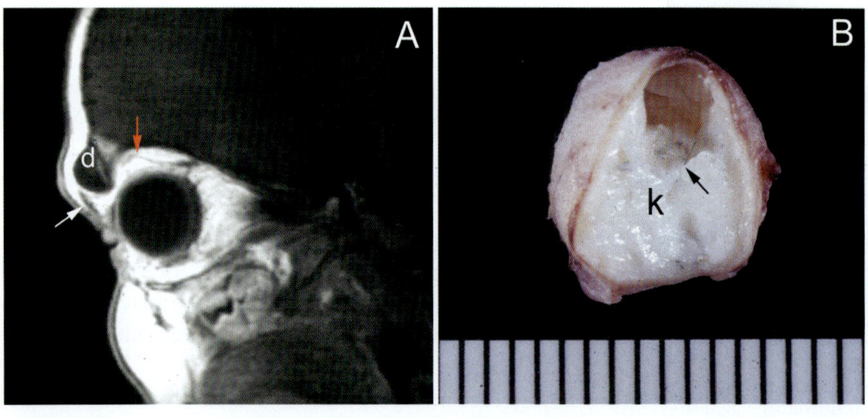

FIGURE 25.5. (A) A T1-weighted, sagittal MRI image showing a superior anterior dermoid (d). Note that the levator muscle is distorted with a kink posterior to the lesion (red arrow) and the septum is pushed inferiorly and anteriorly (white arrow). (B) The appearance of dermoid after surgical removal; contains a considerable amount of keratin (k) and a few hairs (black arrow).

disproportionate amount of fat within conjunctival, episcleral, and anterior orbital tissues. These lesions are not cystic. Because of the superiolateral location of these lesions, the lacrimal gland, its ductules, and the lateral rectus muscle may be affected by sufficiently large dermolipomas (Figure 25.6). Most of these lesions in children are discovered accidentally by parents; a common presentation is as a yellowish-white superiotemporal mass partially covered with a thin web of blood vessels.

Dermolipomas are frequently associated with a number of congenital developmental disorders including Goldenhar syndrome, Treacher–Collins syndrome, hemifacial microsomia, and linear nevus sebaceous syndrome.[33–36] Unless dermolipomas reach a very large size, enough to distort the eyelid anatomy, or unless they contain hairs on their surface that cause persistent foreign body sensation, they should be observed and managed conservatively.[37,38] Even when surgical management is elected, partial excision of the symptomatic portion should be employed rather than complete resection of the tumor. Serious complications have been reported as a result of overzealous dermolipoma excisions, including damage to the palpebral lobe of the lacrimal gland and its ductules, as well as strabismus and pseudostrabismus.[39,40] With a conservative approach, serious complications such as extraocular disturbance with diplopia, upper eyelid ptosis, and dry eyes are likely to be avoided.

Other lesions that can be encountered in the superior lateral fossa include complex choriostomas, which are made of a variety of ectopic tissues including lacrimal gland, conjunctival, and respiratory tract epithelium as well as central nervous system tissue.[41–47] Cystic dilatation of the lacrimal gland ductules known as *dacryops* may also present as space-occupying lesions in the lacrimal fossa (Figure 25.7).[48,49] Dacryops may occasionally present as a congenital lesion (Figure 25.8).

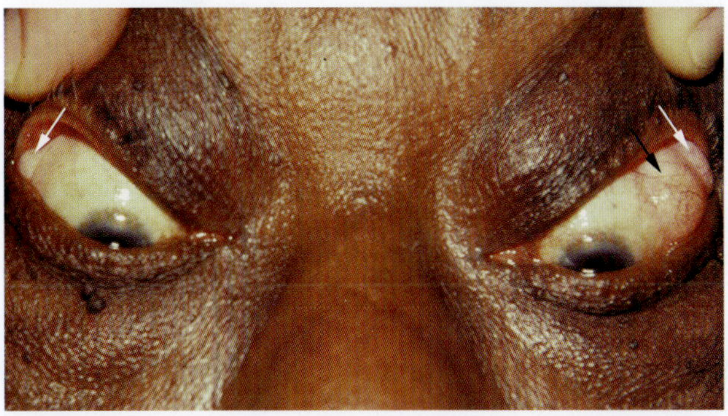

FIGURE 25.6. A dermolipoma of the left superior orbit and periocular tissues (black arrow) in an adult. The lacrimal glands are marked with white arrows bilaterally. The patient had had this lesion since childhood.

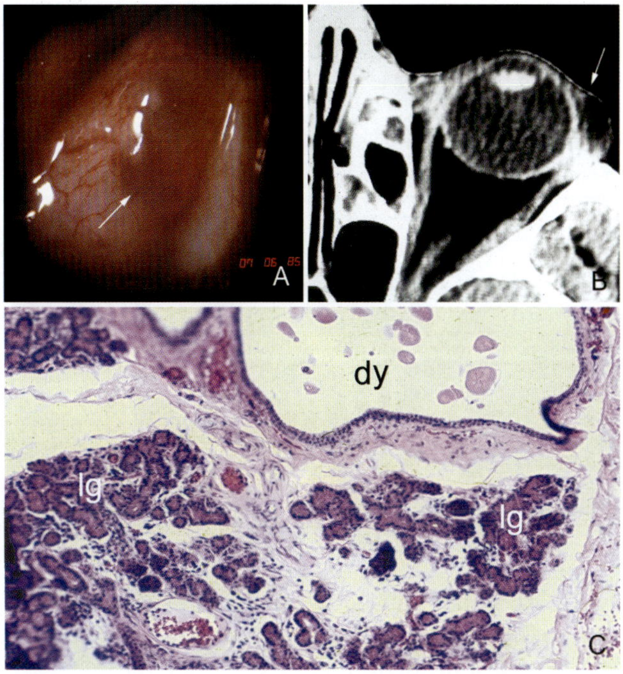

FIGURE 25.7. (A) Slit lamp view and (B) axial CT image of dacryops reveal its thin, transparent wall (arrows). (C) Histopathologic appearance shows the distended dacryops (dy) lumen lined by two layers of columnar epithelium and containing a small amount of pinkish proteinaceous material. Partially atrophic lacrimal gland acini (lg) are scattered around the distended ductule.

TERATOMA

Teratoma is a germ cell tumor that contains tissues derived from the endoderm, ectoderm, and mesoderm (Figure 25.9).[50,51] Therefore, these lesions may contain skin, bowel, lung, brain, thyroid, cartilage, and bone tissues. Most teratomas develop unilaterally and in girls. A great majority of these congenital tumors are benign. Occasional reports have documented malignant transformation within orbitocranial teratomas. These tumors continue to grow 6 to 12 months after birth because of the collection of secretions from different tissues into the partially cystic spaces of the tumor. Some teratomas create massive proptosis, and most can be treated only by exenteration. Recently, however, some of these lesions have been removed surgically, with preservation of the globe and other vital orbital structures reported.[52]

If the teratoma extends beyond the orbit into the cranium, radical surgical efforts including craniotomy are indicated.[53] Although most orbital teratomas are small, some reach alarming sizes with marked distortion of the craniofacial anatomy. Large teratomas may displace the globe severely, to the degree that the tumor may be completely invisible, with total loss of vision secondary to compression of the globe and/or the optic nerve. These lesions may be solid or cystic, and the cystic ones tend to grow because of the accumulation of secretory elements within the cysts of the teratoma. In a great majority of the cases, the growth of

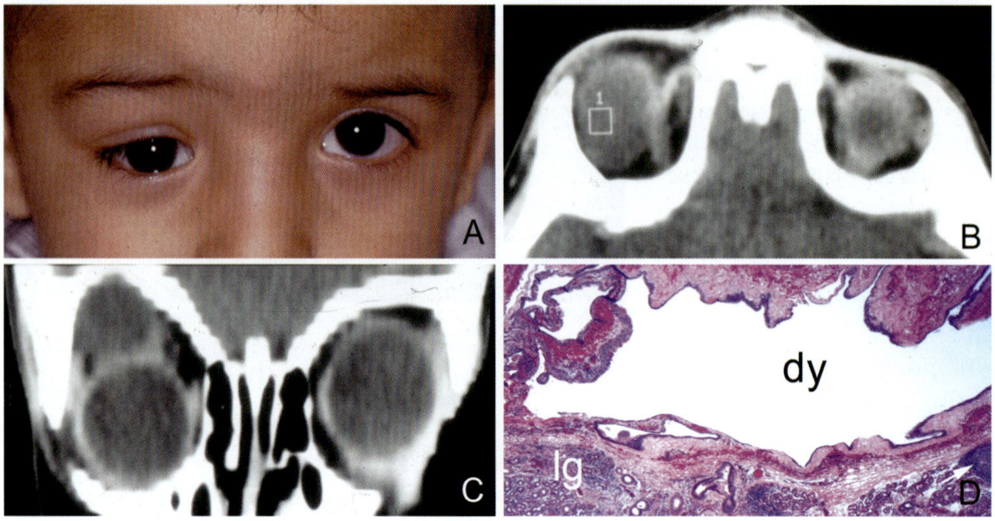

FIGURE 25.8. (A) Eighteen-month-old boy who was born with a congenital dacryops in the superior orbit displacing the right globe inferiorly. The cystic lesion is depicted in (B) axial and (C) coronal views of the CT scan. (D) Histopathologic appearance reveals the lumen of the dacryops (dy) partially lined by choroidal cells and surrounded by atrophic lacrimal gland (lg) tissue and chronic inflammation forming germinal centers (arrow).

the lesion is not caused by malignant behavior; however, recurrence and malignant transformation have been reported in incompletely excised teratomas.[54,55]

MASS LESIONS SECONDARY TO ORBITOCRANIAL MALDEVELOPMENTS

Cephalocele results from the herniation of maldeveloped tissues of the central nervous system (CNS), including meninges (meningocele), brain parenchyma (encephalocele), and the combination of the two (meningoencephalocele) into the orbital cavity.[44,56] Intraorbital cephaloceles may develop anteriorly at the suture lines of orbital bones or posteriorly extending into the orbit from orbital fissures and the optic canal. Depending on the combination of these herniations, they contain brain and/or meningeal tissues (Figures 25.10 and 25.11). Herniation of the CNS tissue and meninges into the orbit occurs with a high incidence

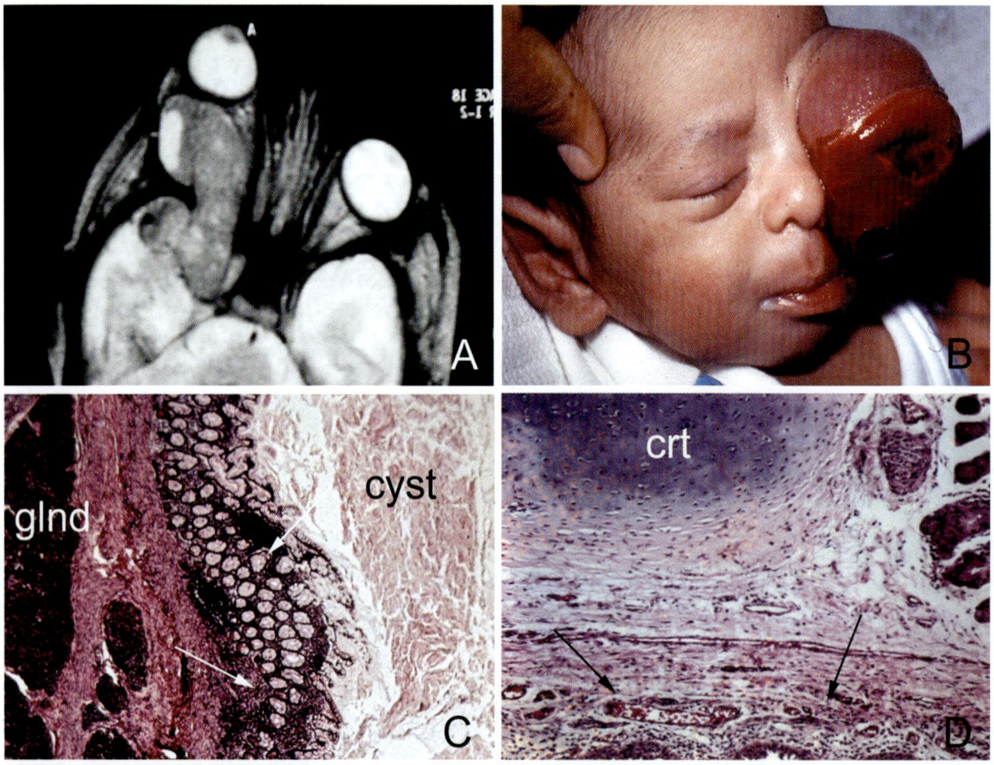

FIGURE 25.9. Orbitocranial teratomas may reach incredibly large size to the point of distorting the craniofacial anatomy. (A,B) Teratomas that had successful surgical procedures without any recurrence. (C,D) Teratomas may contain different types of tissues including intestinal mucosa (white arrows), glandular tissue (glnd), cartilage (crt) and (cyst) intermixed with fibrous tissue and blood vessels (black arrows).

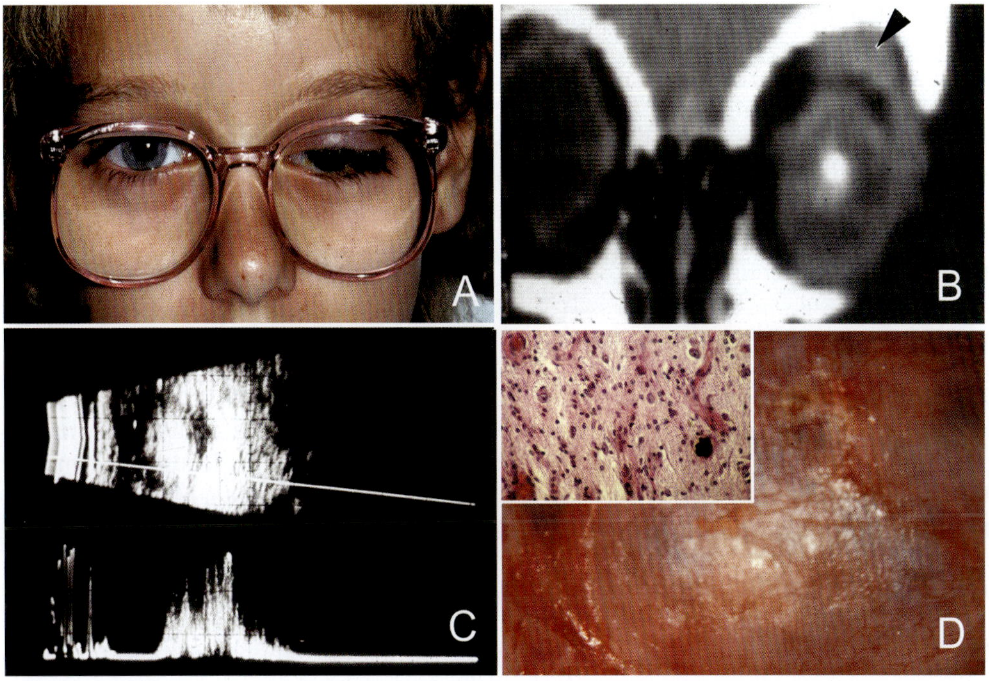

FIGURE 25.10. (A,B) Superiorly located, partially calcified encephalocele causing inferior dislocation of the left eye and blepharatosis of the left upper eyelid. The left globe was prephthisical at the time of presentation, with total disorganization of its internal structure and partial calcification. (C) The combined A and B scans show the disorganized globe with multiple calcified foci causing the spikes on A scan. (D) The bluish-purple, glossy surface of the encephalocele after removal. *Inset*: Histopathologic appearance of the encephalocele showing brain tissue with focal calcifications.

among children with congenital craniofacial clefting abnormalities.[36] Orbital meningoencephaloceles are considered to be developmental abnormalities that occur secondary to the lack of fusion or delayed fusion between orbital bones.

Anterior meningoencephalocele most commonly herniates through an opening between the frontal and lacrimal bones, which characteristically presents shortly after birth. The mass clinically presents as a fluctuant bluish lesion between the nose and the medial canthal. On palpation, these lesions are felt to be softer than other developmental cysts.[57] The globe and the lacrimal drainage system are usually displaced laterally, and some patients may have epiphora.[58]

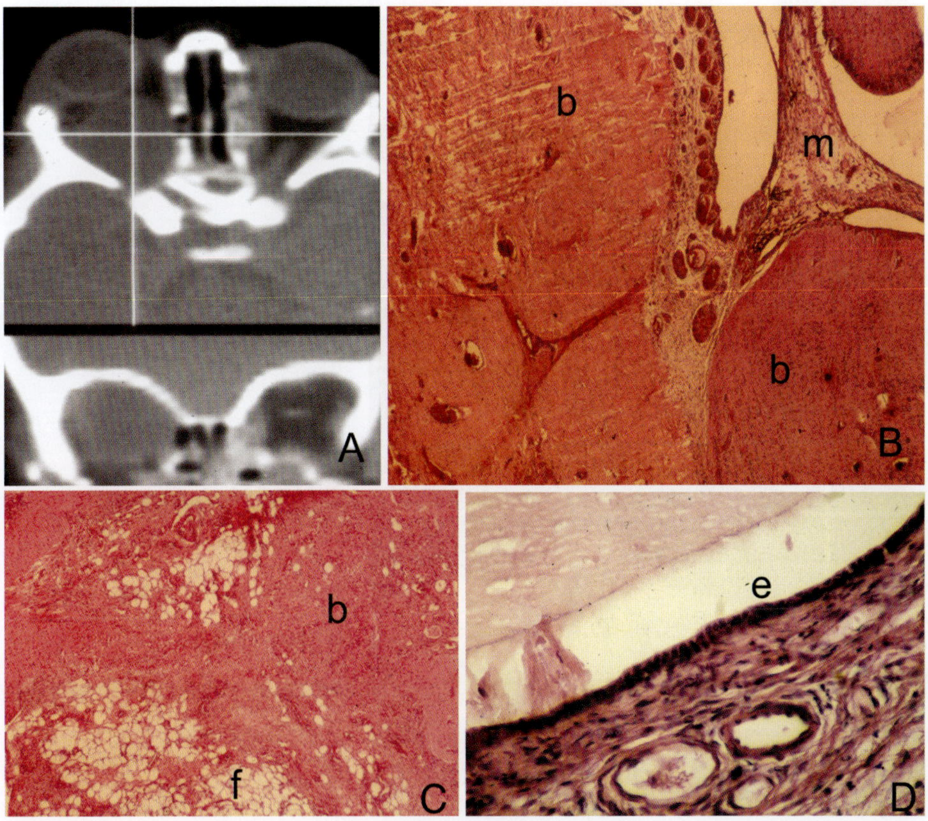

FIGURE 25.11. (A) A large, partially cystic meningoencephalocele occupying the posterior orbit and causing axial proptosis. (B–D) Histopathologic photographs from different parts of the same lesion show haphazard coexistence of different types of tissue, including brain (b), meninges (m), and fat (f). Some of the cystic lesions are lined by ciliated ependymal cells (e).

When the meningoencephalocele is posteriorly located, it usually herniates through the superior orbital fissure and/or optic canal. The symptoms of the posterior meningoencephalocele are less dramatic than those of its anterior counterpart. It usually presents with slowly progressive proptosis, and displacement of the globe and extraocular motility disturbances. Both anterior and posterior meningoencephaloceles may present with pulsating proptosis, depending on the size of the bony defect. In some instances, the pulsation ceases because fibrosis or fusion of the bony defect has cut off the CNS tissue herniation from its connection to the brain, and the lesion becomes an isolated orbital mass. Aberrant fibroglial tissue has also been described in the orbit.[59]

Grossly, meningoceles and meningoencephaloceles are well-circumscribed masses that appear to be grayish-white and glistening on the cut surface. Histopathologic examination may or may not reveal meningeal tissue around the herniated mass. The mass itself is usually composed of brain tissue that sometimes contains tiny calcified psammoma bodies.

The osseous defect can usually be demonstrated by CT, which is the most useful imaging study. The connection of the encephalocele contents to the brain tissue may also be demonstrated with CT and MRI. The treatment of orbital cephaloceles demands a multidisciplinary surgical approach, primarily relying on the input of neurosurgeons and craniofacial surgeons.[60,61]

CONGENITAL CYSTS

Anophthalmos/Microphthalmos

When the globe is abnormally developed, *microphthalmos, congenital cystic eye* and, extremely rarely, *anophthalmos* occur. *Microphthalmos* is usually seen as a unilateral condition; in about 10% of cases it is associated with other craniofacial malformations, including agenesis of the corpus callosum, polymicrogyria, and midline arachnoidal cysts. Microphthalmos may be seen as a part of several genetically determined neuronal migration disorders such as Walker–Warburg syndrome, Aicardi syndrome, and Fukuyama congenital muscular dystrophy.

In microphthalmos and anophthalmos, the orbit may be well formed at birth but does not develop to a full adult volume because of the abnormal eye and/or cyst formation (Figure 25.12). The mechanism by which the presence of the globe affects the growth of the orbit is not well understood.[62,63] This cystic struc-

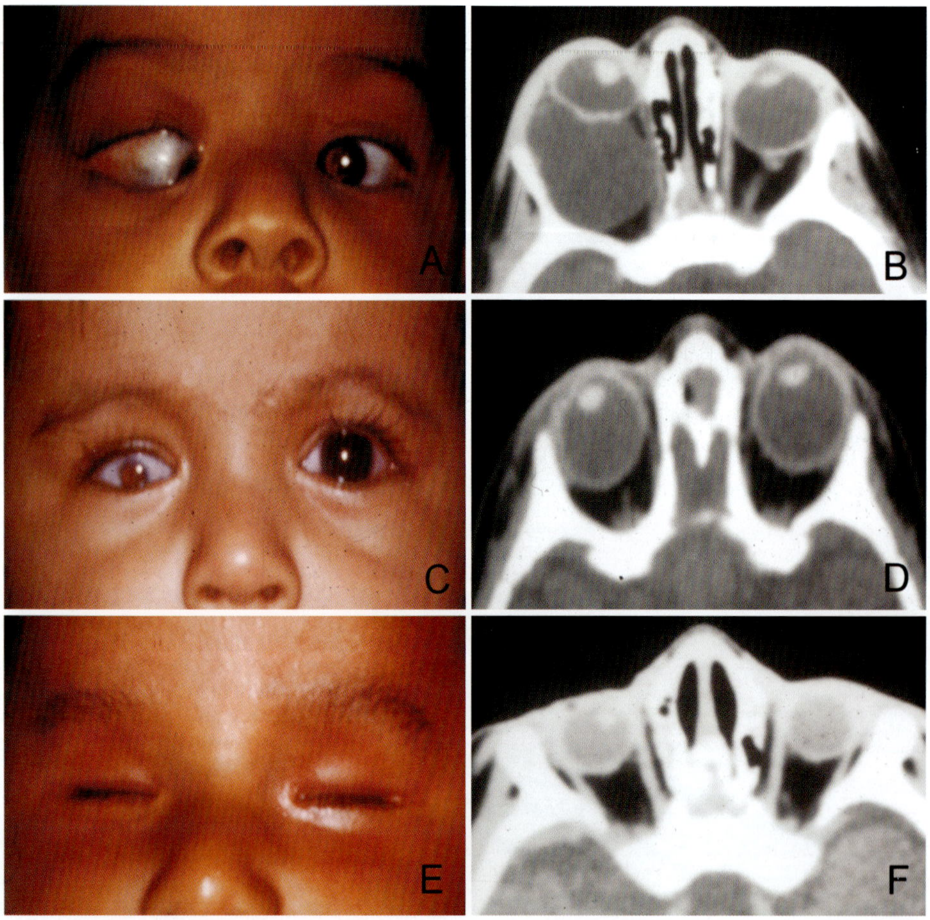

FIGURE 25.12. Three patients with malformed eyes showing (right eye) microphthalmia with a colobomatos cyst (A, B), (right eye) microphthalmia without a cyst (C, D), and bilateral microphthalmia without cyst (E, F). (B) Note the enlargement of the right orbit secondary to large cyst formation. (D) In the patient with microphthalmia without cyst, the right orbit is smaller than the left. (F) In the third patient, both orbits are small but symmetrical.

ture may increase rapidly in size to overshadow the abnormal globe, leading to potential confusion with a neoplasm. When cystic lesions in the orbit are suspected, imaging studies should be performed—not only to look for other intracranial abnormalities but also to establish the possible connection of the cyst to the colobomatous globe and/or to abnormally formed meninges.[64]

The size of the cyst varies depending on the degree of embryonic maldevelopment. The early failure of the closure of the embryonic optic fissure leads to large colobomatous defects with a large congenital cystic component, easily identified at birth (Figure 25.13).[65] The larger the cyst at birth, the smaller and more abnormally developed is the globe. These congenital cysts are commonly unilateral; but bilateral cysts have been reported in association with 131 deletion syndrome and trisomy 18.[66,67] The degree of proptosis is usually moderate, with an anterior superior displacement of the globe. Examination with transillumination and B-scan ultrasonography can help to differentiate these lesions from solid congenital mass lesions, including teratomas and cephaloceles. Imaging with CT and MR will confirm the presence of the cyst and establish the position of the cyst within the orbit in relation to the abnormal globe.[68,69] CT is also useful to identify any associated bony abnormalities of the orbit.

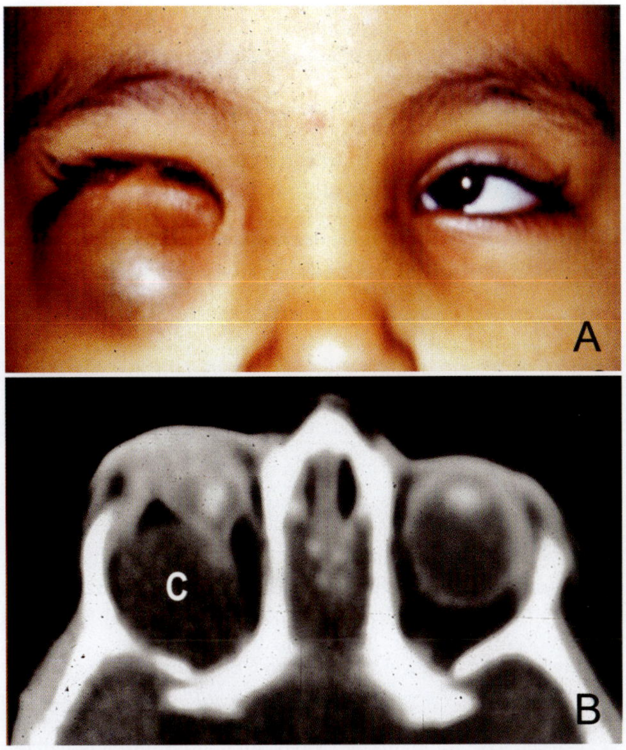

FIGURE 25.13. (A,B) A microphthalmic, maldeveloped right eye with a colobomatous cyst (c). Note the inferiorly located cyst formation with thin, purplish-blue overlying skin. These cysts usually transilluminate well with a muscle light.

Most of the microphthalmic eyes have a poor visual prognosis. If they are accompanied with large cysts, the best treatment is enucleation with complete excision of the cyst. Smaller cysts associated with a reasonably well-developed globe, which may continue to grow and maintain the growth of the orbit, may not require enucleation. Instead, the orbital cyst is excised by itself.[70]

The differential diagnosis of the congenital medial cystic mass should also include dacryocystocele; rarely, encepholocele and the lacrimal drainage system malformations may occur together.[71]

OTHER CYSTS

Mucocele

Orbital mucocele is a rare lesion in the pediatric age group. Most mucoceles in children originate from the ethmoid sinuses, as opposed to the common occurrence of the adult mucocele from the frontal sinus. This is most likely due to delayed formation of the frontal sinus, which begins to aerate around the age of 10. Mucocele is covered in detail elsewhere in the book (see Chapter 29). It should be kept in mind that pediatric orbital mucoceles may develop into common pediatric disorders of children: allergic rhinitis and cystic fibrosis.[72,73] The treatment is surgical drainage and removal, which can occasionally be done endoscopically.[74,75]

Arachnoidal Cyst

The arachnoidal cyst is a rare, benign distension of the meningeal tissues, which surround the optic nerve.[76,77] Histopathologically, the wall consists of dura and epidural tissue with proliferation of the underlying meningothelial cells.[77] This lesion may be encountered in all age groups and presents with compressive optic neuropathy with decreased visual acuity and visual field loss due to atrophy of the optic nerve. Cystic masses of the optic nerve sheath have also been reported to develop as a result of trauma.[78]

References

1. Grove AS Jr. Orbital disorders: diagnosis and management. In: McCord CD Jr, ed. *Oculoplastic Surgery*. New York: Raven Press; 1995:274.
2. Illif WJ, Green WR. Orbital tumors in children. In: Jakobiec FA, ed. *Ocular and Adnexal Tumors*. Birmingham, AL: Aesculapius Publishing; 1978:669–684.
3. Crawford JS. Diseases of the orbit. In: Crawford JS, Morin JD, eds. *The Eye in Childhood*. New York: Grune & Stratton; 1983:361–394.
4. Shields JA, Bakewell B, Augsburger JJ, et al. Space occupying orbital masses in children. A review of 250 consecutive biopsies. *Ophthalmology* 1986;93:379–384.

5. Rootman J. Frequency and differential diagnosis or orbital disease. In: Rootman J, ed. *Diseases of the Orbit*. Philadelphia: JB Lippincott; 1988:124.
6. Kodsi SR, Shetlar DJ, Campbell RJ, et al. A review of 340 orbital tumors in children during a 60-year period. *Am J Ophthalmol* 1994;117:177–182.
7. Nicholson DH, Green WR. *Pediatric Ocular Tumors*. New York: Masson; 1981.
8. Brown HH, Kersten RC, Kulwin DR. Lipomatous hamartoma of the orbit. *Arch Ophthalmol* 1991;109:240.
9. Shields JA, Augsburger JJ, Donoso LA. Orbital dermoid cyst of conjunctival origin. *Am J Ophthalmol* 1986;101:726.
10. Smirniotopoulo JG, Chiechi MV. Teratomas, dermoids and epidermoids of the head and neck. *Radiographs* 1995;15:1437–1455.
11. Shields JA, Kaden IH, Eagle RV Jr, Shields CL. Orbital dermoid cysts: clinicopathologic correlations, classification and management. The 1997 Josephine E. Schueler Lecture. *Ophthalmic Plast Reconstr Surg* 1997;13:256–276.
12. Lacey M, Gear AJ, Lee A. Temporal dermoids: three cases and a modified treatment algorithm. *Ann Plast Surg* 2003;51: 103–109.
13. Kivela T, Tarkkanen A. Orbital germ cell tumors revisited: a clinicopathological approach to classification. *Surv Ophthalmol* 1994;38:541–554.
14. Shield JA, Bakewell B, Augsburger JJ, et al. Classification and incidence of space-occupying lesions of the orbit. A survey of 645 biopsies. *Arch Ophthalmol* 1984;102:1606–1611.
15. Sathananthan N, Moseley IF, Rose GE, et al. The frequency and clinical significance of involvement in outer canthus dermoid cysts. *Br J Ophthalmol* 1993;77:789–794.
16. Colombo F, Holbach LM, Naumann GO. Chronic inflammation in dermoid cysts: a clinicopathologic study of 115 patients. *Orbit* 20;19:97–107.
17. Pollard ZF, Calhoun J. Deep orbital dermoid with draining sinus. *Am J Ophthalmol* 1975;79:310–313.
18. Wilkins RB, Byrd WA. Intraconal dermoid cyst. A case report. *Ophthalmic Plast Reconstr Surg* 1986;2:83–87.
19. Grove AS. Giant dermoid cysts of the orbit. *Ophthalmology* 1979;86:1513–1518.
20. Rochels R, Nover A, Hackelbusch R. Echographische Befunde und differential Diagnostik bei (peri-orbitalen Dermoidzyste) [Echographic findings and differential diagnosis in (peri-orbital dermoid cysts)]. *Klin Monatsbl Augenheilkd* 1986;188:101–104.
21. Junwu G, Jun W. B-ultrasound and computed tomography scan diagnosis of 32 cases of intraorbital dermoid cysts. *Trop Doct* 2001;31:49–50.
22. Tadmor RR, New PF. Computed tomography of the orbit with special emphasis on coronal sections. II. Pathological anatomy. *J Comput Assist Tomogr* 1978;2:35–44.
23. Wende S, Aulich A, Nover A, et al. Computed tomography of orbital lesions. A comparative study of 210 cases. *Neuroradiology* 1977;13:123–134.
24. Samuelson TW, Margo CE, Levy MH, Pusateri TJ. Zygomaticofrontal suture defect associated with orbital dermoid cyst. *Surv Ophthalmol* 1988;33:127–130.
25. Chawda SJ, Moseley IF. Computed tomography of orbital dermoids: a 20-year review. *Clin Radiol* 1999;54:821–825.
26. Günalp I, Gündüz K. Cystic lesions of the orbit. *Int Ophthalmol* 1996;20:273–277.
27. Dechambre S, Duprez T, Lecouvet F, et al. Diffusion-weighted MRI postoperative assessment of an epidermoid tumor in the cerebellopontine angle. *Neuroradiology* 1999;1:829–831.
28. Kaufman LM, Villablanca JP, Mafee MF. Diagnostic imaging of cystic lesions in the child's orbit. *Radiol Clin North Am* 1998;36:1149–1163.
29. Müller-Forell WS. *Imaging of Orbital and Visual Pathway Pathology*. Berlin: Springer-Verlag; 2002:128–129.
30. Wolfley DE. The lid crease approach to the superomedial orbit. *Ophthalmic Surg* 1985;16:652–656.
31. Kronish JW, Dortzbach RK. Upper eyelid crease surgical approach to dermoid and epidermoid cysts in children. *Arch Ophthalmol* 1988;106:1625–1627.
32. Carta F, Siccardi D, Cossu M, et al. Removal of tumours of the orbital apex via a postero-lateral orbitotomy. *J Neurosurg Sci* 1998;42:185–188.
33. Beard C. Congenital heredity abnormalities of the eyelids, lacrimal system and orbit. *Transactions of the New Orleans Academy of Ophthalmology*. St. Louis: CV Mosby; 1968.
34. Hertle RW, Quinn GE, Katowitz JA. Ocular and adnexal findings in patients with facial microsomias. *Ophthalmology* 1992;99:114–119.
35. Waugh MS, Chong WK, Sonksen P. Neuroimaging in children with congenital disorders of the peripheral visual system. *Dev Med Child Neurol* 1998;40:812–819.
36. Fries PD, Katowitz JA. Congenital craniofacial anomalies of ophthalmic importance. *Surv Ophthalmol* 1990;35:87–119.
37. Beard C. Dermolipoma surgery, or, "an ounce of prevention is worth a pound of cure." *Ophthalmic Plast Reconstr Surg* 1990;6:153–157.
38. Fry CL, Leone CR Jr. Safe management of dermolipomas. *Arch Ophthalmol* 1994;112:1114–1116.
39. François P, Lekieffre M, Wiillez M, Ryckewaert M. Complications of dermolipoma ablation. *Bull Soc Ophtalmol Fr* 1989;89:289–290.
40. Kiratli H, Tatlipinar S, Sanac AS, Bilgic S. Pseudo-Brown's syndrome secondary to a growing conjunctival dermolipoma. *J Pediatr Ophthalmol Strabismus* 2001;38:112–113.
41. Porkony KS, Hyman BM, Jakobiec FA, et al. Epibulbar choristomas containing lacrimal tissue: clinical distinction from dermoids and histologic evidence of an origin from the palpebral lobe. *Ophthalmology* 1987;94:1249–1261.
42. Green WR, Zimmerman LE. Ectopic lacrimal gland tissue: report of eight cases with orbital involvement. *Arch Ophthalmol* 1967;78:318–325.
43. Margo CE, Naugle TC, Karcioglu ZA. Ectopic lacrimal gland tissue of the orbit and sclerosing dacryoadenitis. *Ophthalmic Surg* 1985;16:178.
44. Newman NJ, Miller NR, Green WR. Ectopic brain in the orbit. *Ophthalmology* 1986;93:268–272.
45. Newton C, Dutton JJ, Klintworth GK. A respiratory epithelial choristomatous cyst of the orbit. *Ophthalmology* 1985; 92:1754–1757.
46. Call NB, Baylis HI. Cerebellar heterotropia in the orbit. *Arch Ophthalmol* 1980;98:717–719.
47. James CRH, Lyness R, Wright JE. Respiratory epithelium lined cysts presenting in the orbit without associated mucocele formation. *Br J Ophthalmol* 1986;70:387–390.
48. Bullock JD, Fleishman JA, Rosset JS. Lacrimal duct cysts. *Ophthalmology* 1986;93:1355–1360.
49. Monica, M. Long DA, Karcioglu ZA. Bilateral dacryops. *Ann Ophthalmol* 1988;20:259–263.
50. Kivela T, Tarkkanen A. Orbital germ cell tumors revisited: a clinicopathological approach to classification. *Surv Ophthalmol* 1994;38:541–554.
51. Lacey NA, McWilliams S, Jan W, et al. Case of the month: congenital unilateral proptosis. *Br J Radiol* 2002;75:191–192.
52. Itani K, Tranoulsi EL, Karim FWA, et al. Conservative surgery in orbital teratoma. *Orbit* 1986;5:61–65.
53. Weiss AH, Greenwald MJ, Margo CE. Primary and secondary orbital teratomas. *J Pediatr Ophthalmol Strabismus* 1989; 26:4–49.
54. Garden JW, McManis JC. Congenital orbitointracranial teratoma with subsequent malignancy: case reports. *Br J Ophthalmol* 1986;70:111–113.
55. Soares BJC, Lopes K, Andrade J, et al. Orbital malignant teratoma: a case report. *Orbit* 1983;2:235–242.

56. Suwanwela C, Suwanwela N. A morphological classification of sinciputal encephalomengingoceles. *J Neurosurg* 1972; 36:201.
57. Ackers TE. Encephalocele. *Arch Ophthalmol* 1965;73:84–85.
58. Rashid ER, Bergstrom TJ, Evans RM, et al. Anterior encephalocele presenting as nasolacrimal obstruction. *Ann Ophthalmol* 1986;18:132–136.
59. Grossniklaus HE, Wojno T. Orbital aberrant fibroglial tissue associated with microphthalmos. *J Pediatr Ophthalmol Strabismus* 1994;31:338–340.
60. Lello GE, Sparrow OC, Gopal R. The surgical correction of fronto-ethmoidal meningoencephalocele. *J Craniomaxillofac Surg* 1989;17:293–298.
61. Koopman CF, Reynolds AF. Combined neurosurgical-otolaryngologic operative approach to a massive nasoepithelial encephalomeningocele. *Otolaryngol Head Neck Surg* 1981: 89:545–549.
62. Barishak YR. *Embryology of the Eye and Its Adnexa*. 2nd ed. Basel: S Karger; 2001:15.
63. Ozanics V, Jakobiec F. Prenatal development of the eye and its adnexae. In: Jakobiec F, ed. *Ocular Anatomy, Embryology and Teratology*. New York: Harper & Row; 1982:11–96.
64. De Potter P, Shields JA, Shields CL. *MRI of the Eye and Orbit*. Philadelphia: JB Lippincott; 1995.
65. Waring GO, Roth AM, Rodrigues MM. Clinicopathologic correlations of microphthalmos with cyst. *Am J Ophthalmol* 1976;8:714–721.
66. Guterman C, Abbout E, Mets MB. Microphthalmos with cyst and Edwards' syndrome. *Am J Ophthalmol* 1990;109:228–230.
67. Warburg M. An update on microphthalmos and coloboma: a brief survey of genetic disorders with microphthalmos and coloboma. *Ophthalmic Paediatr Genet* 1991;12:57–63.
68. Mafee MF. Eye and orbit. In: Som PM, Curtin HD, eds. *Head and Neck Imaging*. Vol II. 3rd ed. St Louis: CV Mosby; 1996:1009–1128.
69. Weiss A, Greenwald M, Martinez C. Microphthalmos with cyst: clinical presentations and computed tomographic findings. *J Pediatr Ophthalmol Strabismus* 1985;22:6–12.
70. Polito E, Leccisotti A. Colobomatous ocular cyst excision with globe preservation. *Ophthalmic Plast Reconstr Surg* 1995;11: 288–292.
71. Hakin KN, Rose GE, Sullivan TJ. Combined congenital dacryocele and anterior orbital hydroencephalocoele. *Orbit* 2000; 19:1–5.
72. de Juan E Jr, Green WR, Iliff NT. Allergic periorbital mucopyocele in children. *Am J Ophthalmol* 1983;96:299–303.
73. Robertson DM, Henderson JW. Unilateral proptosis secondary to orbital mucocele in infancy. *Am J Ophthalmol* 1969; 68:845–847.
74. Thome DC, Voegels RL, Cataldo de la Cortina RA, Butugan O. Bilateral ethmoidal mucocele in cystic fibrosis: report of a case. *Int J Pediatr Otorhinolaryngol* 2000;55:143–148.
75. Hartley BE, Lund VJ. Endoscopic drainage of pediatric paranasal sinus mucoceles. *Int J Pediatr Otorhinolaryngol* 1999;50: 109–111.
76. Akor C, Wojno TH, Newman NJ, Grossniklaus HE. Arachnoidal cyst of the optic nerve. *Ophthalmic Plast Reconstr Surg* 2003;19:466–469.
77. Spencer WH. Primary neoplasms of the optic nerve and its sheaths: clinical features and current concepts in pathogenic mechanisms. *Trans Am Ophthalmol Soc* 1972;70:490–528.
78. Hupp SL, Buckley EG, Byrne SF, et al. Posttraumatic venous obstructive retinopathy associated with enlarged optic nerve sheath. *Arch Ophthalmol* 1984;102:254–256.

26

Malignant Pediatric Tumors

Doris Hadjistilianou and Zeynel A. Karcıoglu

Based on several large series published during the past three decades, the incidence of orbital malignancies in children and adolescents ranges from approximately 8 to 18% of all orbital lesions in this age group.[1–6] The most common orbital malignancy in the United States and western European series is rhabdomyosarcoma, which accounts for approximately 40% of all pediatric orbital malignant tumors. In the developing countries and the underdeveloped regions of the world, however, the most common orbital malignancies in the pediatric group are not primary malignant tumors, but secondary and metastatic lesions, such as retinoblastoma, Burkitt's lymphoma, and leukemias.[7–10] Other tumors, including mesenchymal malignancies (Ewing's sarcoma, osteogenic sarcoma, fibrosarcoma, alveolar soft part sarcoma, malignant hemangiopericytoma), fibrohistiocytoses (Langerhans cell histiocytosis), lacrimal gland tumors (adenoid cystic carcinoma), and secondary metastatic tumors (neuroblastoma and esthesioneuroblastoma) also develop within the pediatric orbit, leading to proptosis, extraocular motility disorders, and compressive optic neuropathy. Although it is a low-grade malignancy, optic nerve glioma (grade I and II astrocytoma) should also technically be considered to be a malignant lesion of the pediatric orbit.

This chapter details the more commonly encountered primary and secondary malignant tumors of the pediatric orbit, including rhabdomyosarcoma, orbital myeloid sarcoma (granulocytic sarcoma), neuroblastoma, and the optic nerve glioma. Other tumors, listed by way of introduction, are covered elsewhere in this book (Chapters 5, 15, 17, 18, and 22).

PRIMARY TUMORS

Orbital Rhabdomyosarcoma

Once considered to be a very rare malignancy, orbital rhabdomyosarcoma (RMS) has emerged as the most common malignant mesenchymal orbital tumor of childhood. It accounts for about 5% of all cancers in the pediatric population. Rhabdomyosarcoma of the neck and the head usually appears in the first decade of life.

Orbital RMS accounts for about 10 to 20% of all the rhabdomyosarcomas. Males are more affected than females, and the mean age at diagnosis is 8 years. A history of trauma is frequently associated with the clinical presentation of the tumor.[11,12] The histopathologic types include embryonal, alveolar, spindle cell, and botryoid tumors (Box 26.1). The embryonal type is the most common; the alveolar is less common and carries the worst prognosis (Figures 26.1 and 26.2).[13] Another type of RMS, called the pleomorphic type, is extremely rare in the orbit. Tumor location correlates with histology: embryonal and differentiated types are more commonly located in the superonasal quadrants, whereas the alveolar type originates within the inferior orbit.[14]

Orbital RMS can present insidiously, mimicking other lesions clinically and radiologically. The most characteristic presenting features of orbital RMS are a fairly rapid onset and progression of proptosis and displacement of the globe (Box 26.2). The upper inner quadrant is the most common site of origin. Intracranial extension and invasion of the paranasal sinuses are rather uncommon at presentation, whereas changes in the adjacent bone have frequently been reported.[15]

The best way of arriving at a diagnosis is to suspect rhabdomyosarcoma whenever one observes the clinical presentation of a rapidly progressive unilateral exophthalmos in a child. However, RMS may also present as a palpable nodular subconjunctival or lid mass with edema of the lids and conjuctiva (Figure 26.3). Symptoms depend on the origin and site of the tumor mass. Posterior tumors rapidly develop edema of the optic disk, choroidal folds, and some degree of ophthalmoplegia (Figure 26.4). When RMS is situated in the inferior and anterior portions of the orbit, it often causes obvious chemosis and swelling of the eyelids. The superior nasal quadrant of the orbit is the most common site of origin of this tumor.[13]

Once ophthalmologists believed that orbital RMS arose from the extraocular muscles; now, however, it is accepted that the condition develops from undifferentiated mesenchymal cells that have the capacity to differentiate into striated muscle.[16] The clinical differential diagnosis includes most causes of proptosis in childhood. The important lesions to be considered

BOX 26.1. Proposed Classification for Childhood Rhabdomyosarcoma

I. Superior prognosis
   a. Botryoid RMS
   b. Spindle cell RMS
II. Intermediate prognosis
   a. Embryonal RMS
III. Poor prognosis
   a. Alveolar RMS
   b. Undifferentiated sarcoma
IV. Subtypes whose prognosis cannot be evaluated at present

include benign and malignant conditions such as capillary hemangioma, dermoid cyst, orbital cellulitis, eosinophilic granuloma, and metastatic neuroblastoma (Box 26.3).[17,18]

Computed tomography (CT) and magnetic resonance imaging (MRI) play important roles in the preoperative evaluation to determine location and size and also in evaluating residual or recurrent disease. Particular attention should be given to the presence of bone erosion and intracranial extension.[19] CT demonstrates a moderately well-defined homogeneous orbital mass isodense to the extraocular muscles, which often shows enhancement after contrast administration; bone destruction is relatively frequent and can

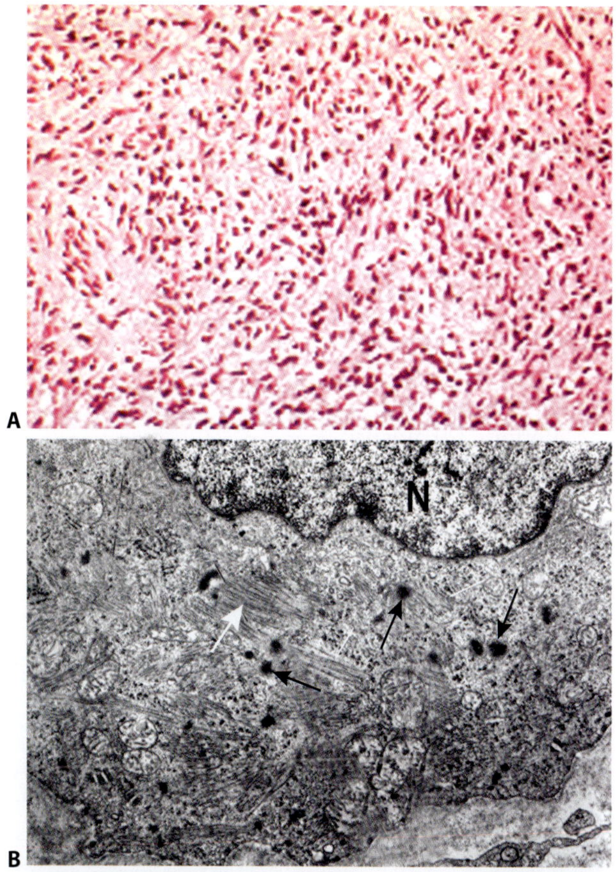

FIGURE 26.2. Photomicrographs of embryonal rhabdomyosarcoma. (A) Light microscopy shows a mixture of pleomorphic malignant cells, some of which are elongated and tadpole shaped. (B) Electron microscopy is invaluable to identify the myofilaments (white arrows) and Z bands (black arrows) (B). N: nucleus.

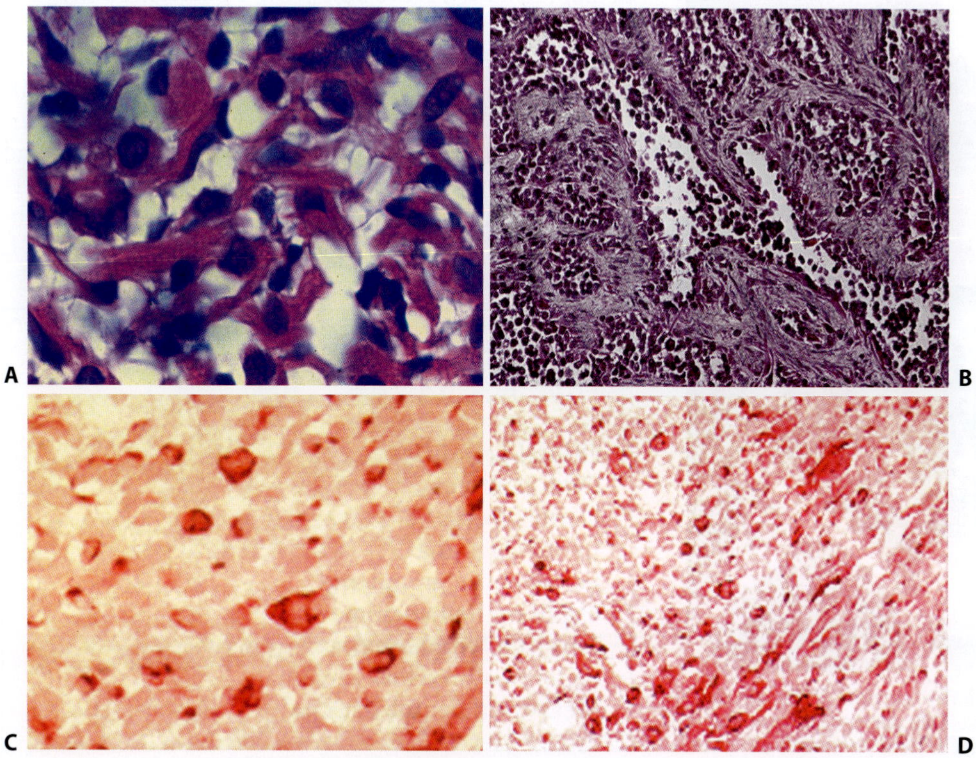

FIGURE 26.1. Light microscopic appearance of embryonal (A) and alveolar (B) histopathology patterns. In the embryonal type, relatively well-differentiated "strap" cells contain intracytoplasmic cross-striations that correspond to myosin and actin filaments. The alveolar pattern, on the other hand, presents a distinctive architecture in which the cells are interspersed within a branching network of connective tissue trabeculae. In many areas, a single layer of tumor cells adheres to the fibrous septae, and in other areas, loosely cohesive cells occupy the spaces within the fibrous skeleton. Immunohistochemical stains reveal positivity for desmin (C) and actin (D) within the cytoplasm of rhabdomyosarcoma cells.

BOX 26.2. Orbital Rhabdomyosarcoma: Clinical Presentation

Proptosis
Globe displacement
Blepharoptosis
Palpable mass
Conjunctival and eyelid swelling
Pain
Ophthalmoscopic findings
  Optic disk edema
  Choroidal folds
  Venous tortuosity

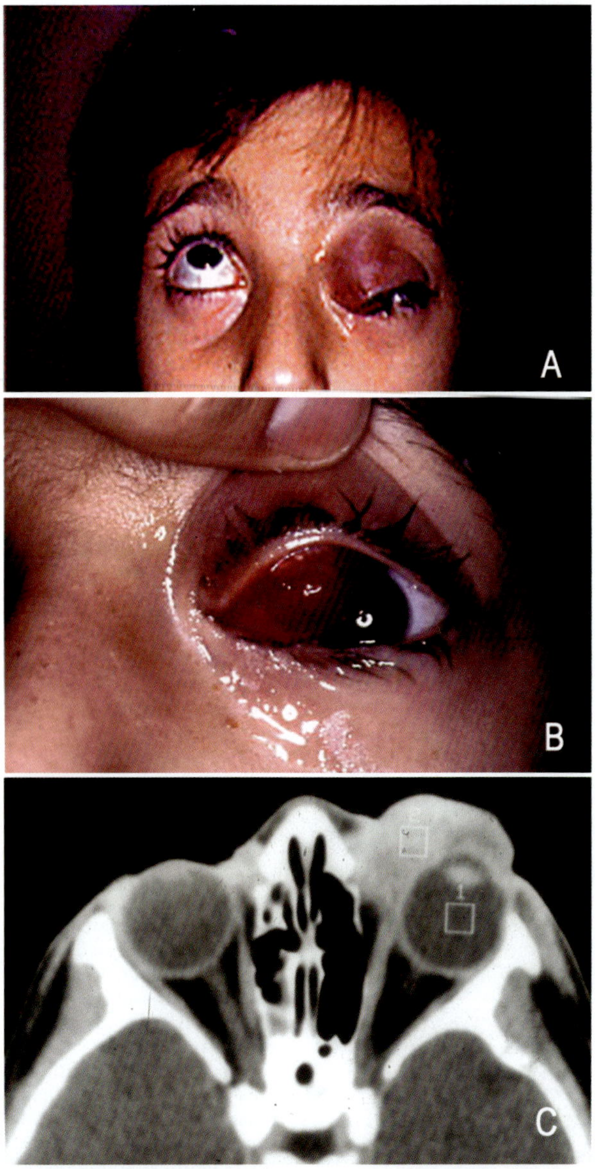

FIGURE 26.3. Symptoms of rhabdomyosarcoma depend on the site and the growth rate of the tumor. This patient's tumor involved the superior medial orbit, upper eyelid, and conjunctiva.

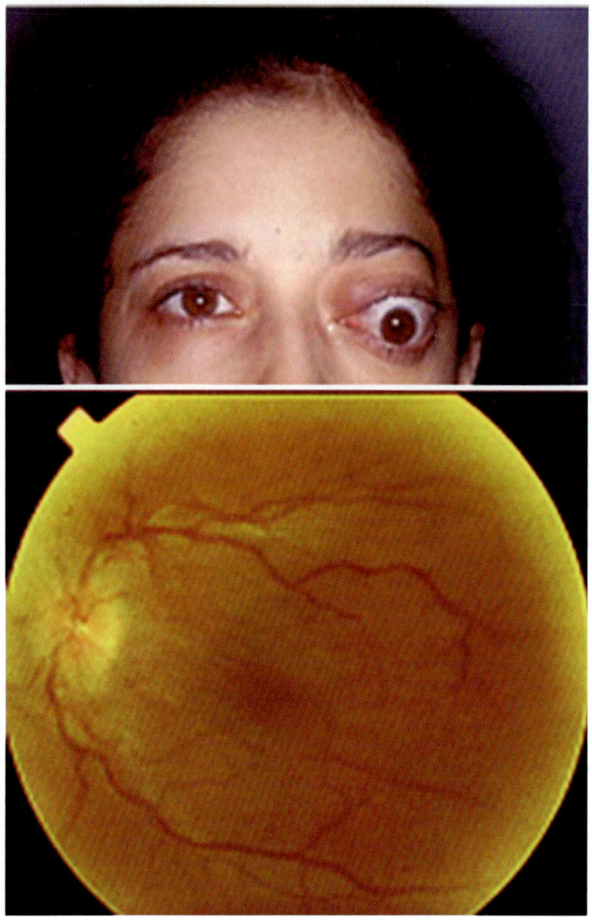

FIGURE 26.4. Large posterior tumor causing marked proptosis of the left eye with choroidal folds of the fundus.

be appreciable (Figure 26.5). On T1-weighted MR images the tumor may appear iso- to hyperintense to the extraocular muscles and hypointense with respect to the orbital fat. On proton density and T2-weighted MR images, hypointensity, isointensity, and even hyperintensity with respect to both extraocular muscles and orbital fat may be appreciable (Figure 26.6). On T1-weighted, contrast-enhanced MR images, rhab-

BOX 26.3. Differential Diagnosis of Orbital RMS

Orbital cellulitis
Orbital abscess
Dermoid cyst
Lymphangioma
Eosinophilic granuloma
Capillary hemangioma
Burkitt's lymphoma
Chloroma (myeloid sarcoma)
Metastatic neuroblastoma

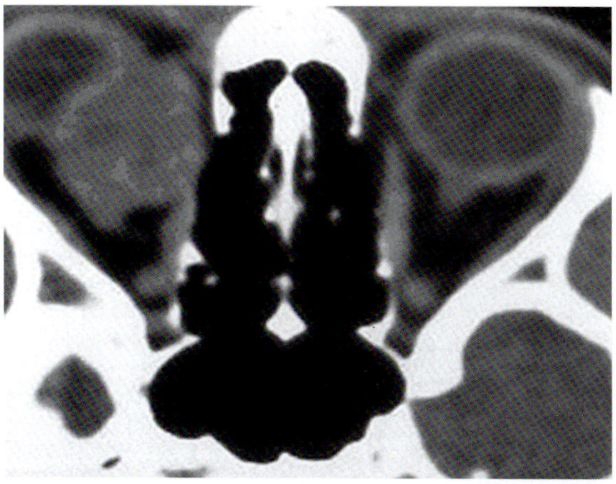

FIGURE 26.5. Axial CT image shows a rather well-circumscribed homogeneous mass, isodense to the extraocular muscles in the superior portion of the right orbit.

TABLE 26.1. Staging by the Intergroup Rhabdomyosarcoma Study Group.

Group	Description
I	Completely resected localized disease implying gross impression resection and microscopic confirmation of complete resection with absence of regional lymph node involvement
Ia	Confirmed to muscle or organ of origin
Ib	Contiguous involvement outside the muscle or organ of origin
II	Residual disease and/or regional lymph node involvement
IIa	Grossly resected localized tumor with microscopic residual disease and no evidence of gross residual tumor or regional lymph node involvement
IIb	Completely resected regional disease with no microscopic residual tumor
IIc	Grossly resected regional disease with microscopic residual tumor
III	Incomplete resection with biopsy or gross residual disease
IV	Distant metastatic disease present at onset

domyosarcomas show moderate to marked enhancement, even though in some cases a highly vascular internal architecture mimicking a capillary hemangioma may be demonstrated.[20]

The staging of RMS proposed in the third Intergroup Rhabdomyosarcoma Study is summarized in Table 26.1.[20] The simplification of this classification by Shields et al. can also be applied to cases of orbital RMS.[21] Exenteration was the standard surgical treatment for orbital rhabdomyosarcoma up to the 1970s. Orbital exenteration is now confined to the treatment of patients with recurrent disease.[21] The poor prognosis for children with orbital rhabdomyosarcoma following orbital exenteration suggested the use of radiotherapy. In fractionated doses, 4000 cGy offered satisfactory tumor control.[22] Chemotherapy, introduced subsequently, also succeeded in reducing these lesions (Figure 26.7). Vincristine, actinomycin D, and, recently, ifosfamide and etoposide following conservative surgery and combined with radiotherapy (5000 cGy) allow a survival rate of 90%.

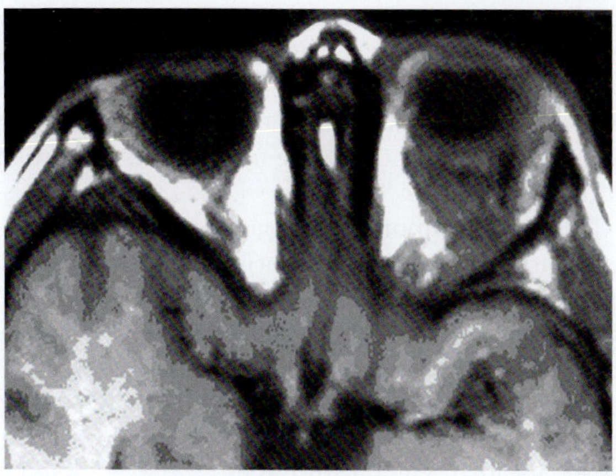

FIGURE 26.6. Axial T1-weighted MR image of a rhabdomyosarcoma in a patient with neurofibromatosis type 1. The tumor shows isodensity with respect to the muscles and hypodensity with respect to the orbital fat. The belly of the lateral rectus muscle is involved with the tumor, which extends posteriorly into the superior orbital fissure. In this case, the greater wing of the sphenoid bone was absent because of neurofibromatosis.

The role of surgery in the management of orbital RMS is still controversial. Some centers perform extensive surgery while others prefer to do incisional biopsy only. The surgical approach should be planned according to the clinical and radiographic findings. When possible, a complete or near complete tumor excision is suggested without damaging vital structures (optic nerve and/or extraocular muscles) (Figures 26.8 and 26.9). If the suspected orbital RMS is located deep in the orbit, an incisional biopsy is appropriate. Fine-needle aspiration biopsy is usually unrepresentative and may be misleading.

Advances in chemotherapy and radiotherapy have significantly improved survival rates. The excellent survival rate has allowed following survivors for many years and observing the late effects of radiotherapy on both facial growth (bony hypoplasia of the orbit and facial asymmetry) and visual function (cataracts, keratopathy, retinopathy).[23,24]

The challenge for the future should be to identify the characteristics of patients who can safely be treated with primary chemotherapy alone to reserve radiotherapy for the remaining patients in an attempt to reduce late effects.[25–27] Further reduction in radiation sequelae may derive from the use of three-dimensional conformal radiation therapy techniques, by minimizing the inclusion of normal structures in the treated volume.[28]

Optic Nerve Glioma

Optic pathway gliomas account for 0.6 to 1.2% of all intracranial tumors (see Chapter 7).[29] The incidence

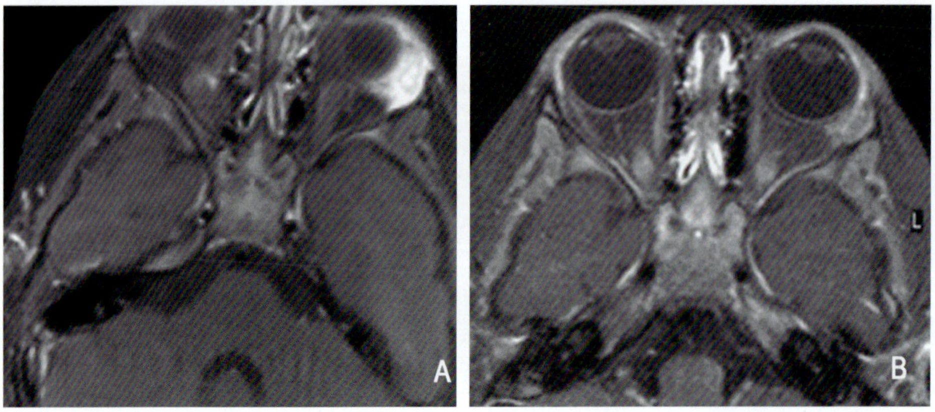

FIGURE 26.7. Axial T1-weighted, fat-suppressed MR images with contrast reveal an orbital tumor before chemotherapy (A) and afterward (B). The tumor, which was proven to be an alveolar rhabdomyosarcoma, shows marked reduction of enhancement after therapy.

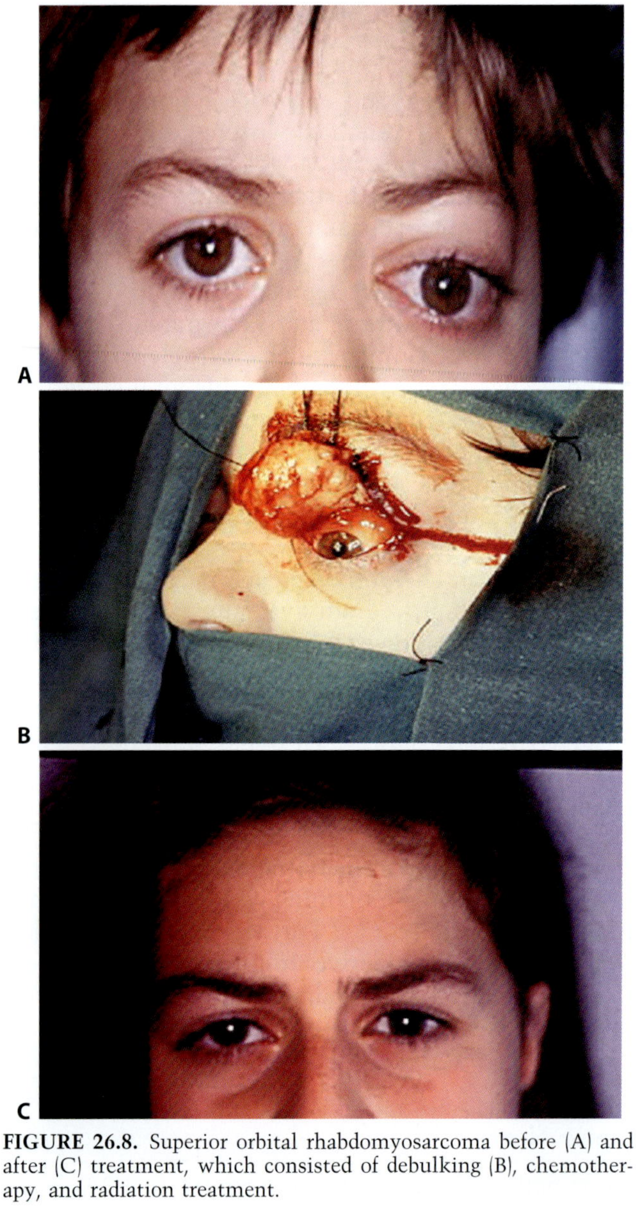

FIGURE 26.8. Superior orbital rhabdomyosarcoma before (A) and after (C) treatment, which consisted of debulking (B), chemotherapy, and radiation treatment.

is 1 in 100,000 patients, with 90% presenting in the first two decades and 65% in the first 5 years of life. First reported by von Graefe in 1864, gliomas of the anterior visual pathways constitute about 1 to 5% of all childhood intracranial tumors.[30] The majority of these tumors, including optic nerve gliomas, are low-grade astrocytomas. Some astrocytes present spherical or cylindrical swollen cell processes called Rosenthal fibers, which stain eosinophilic (Figure 26.10). The astrocytic nature of the tumor can be confirmed using immunohistochemical techniques with antibodies against glial fibrillary acidic protein (GFAP, MW 15 kDa).[31] Although this protein may also be present in some schwannomas, increased GFAP expression is typical for astrocytic tumors.[32]

Optic gliomas commonly occur in neurofibromatosis type 1 (NF1) and belong to the diagnostic criteria of NF1.[33–35]

The incidence of optic gliomas in children with NF1 is as high as to 15 to 20%, with symptomatic visual loss in approximately 20% of affected patients (Figure 26.11). Bilateral gliomas are most often seen in patients with NF1 (Figure 26.12). The optic nerve alone is involved in 24% of cases and the chiasm in 76% of cases; invasion of the midbrain is documented in 46% of patients.[35,36]

The most important prognostic factor is age at presentation. Early-onset optic gliomas (<6 years) grow rapidly and must be followed closely.[37,38] Primary symptoms include deterioration of visual acuity and progressive visual field defects. However, patients with NF1 seem to have a less aggressive variant of glioma. Neuro-ophthalmic aspects of optic nerve glioma are also covered in Chapter 7.[39,40]

The clinical course of optic pathway gliomas is related to the extent at diagnosis and histopathologic pattern (Figure 26.13). In pediatric patients with NF1 and optic pathway gliomas, the likelihood of visual

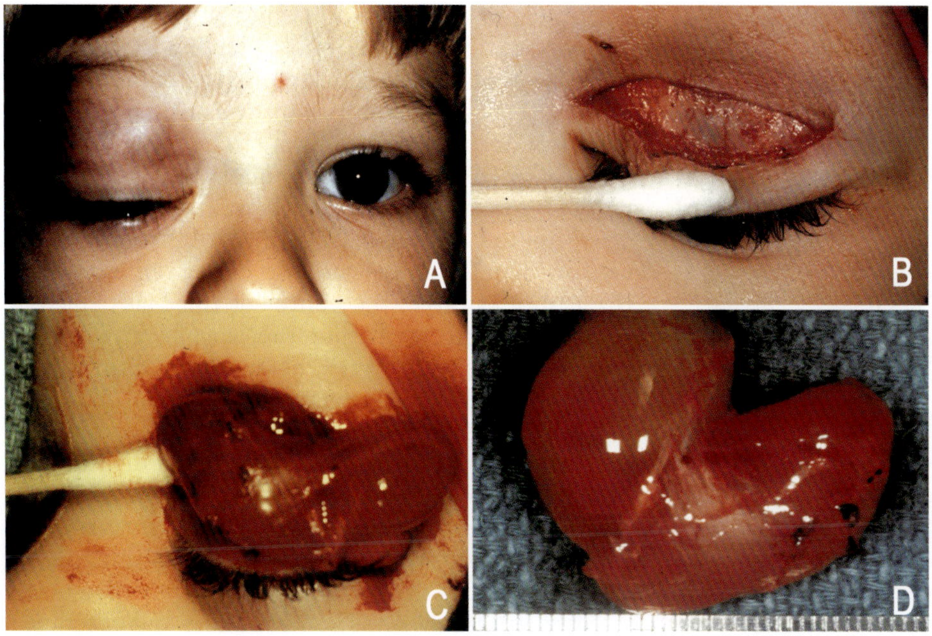

FIGURE 26.9. (A) Rhabdomyosarcoma of the superior orbit and the upper lid is removed (B) through a lid crease incision. Note the well-delineated myxoid tumor with a grayish-white glistening surface that appears to be "fleshy" like a lymphoma (C,D).

loss depends on the extent and location of the tumor as determined by MRI and is particularly associated with postchiasmal structure involvement.[40]

There is still controversy regarding the growth of optic gliomas and potential extension posteriorly to the chiasma. Hoyt and Baghdassarian suggested that optic gliomas represent congenital hamartomas with growth potential in the first years of life.[41] Progression usually occurs in the first year of presentation.[42] However, the variable and unpredictable course of these tumors makes standardization of treatment strategies difficult. Optic gliomas may undergo spontaneous regression. In a recent study, Parsa et al. documented spontaneous regression and tumor shrinkage in 12 patients with optic glioma. Regression was observed in patients with and without NF1.[43] Accurate follow-up of optic pathway gliomas to evaluate stability or progression should include a high-resolution MRI study. This is particularly helpful to evaluate the intracranial extent of optic nerve glioma.[44,45]

CT and MRI are important to establish the tumor extension, to plan treatment, and to allow radiologic

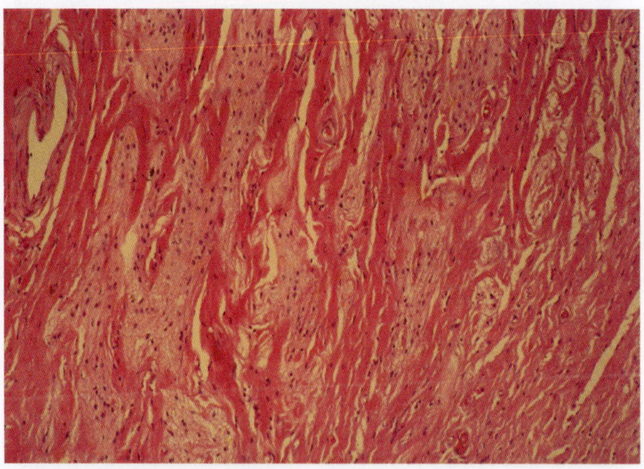

FIGURE 26.10. Histopathologic appearance of an optic nerve glioma that is composed of proliferating fibrillary astrocytes showing different degrees of pleomorphism.

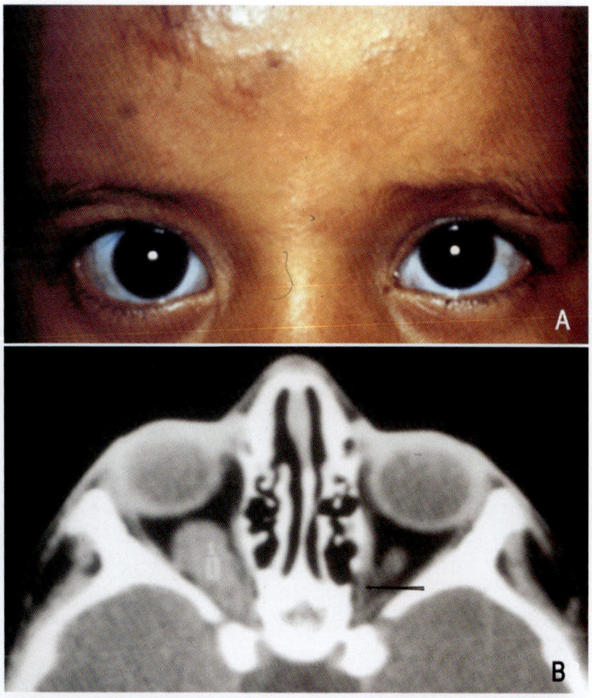

FIGURE 26.11. (A) Patient with neurofibromatosis type 1 has cutaneous neurofibromas of the forehead and slight proptosis of the right eye secondary to a unilateral optic nerve glioma. (B) Note the missing greater wing of the sphenoid bone (arrow) on axial CT image.

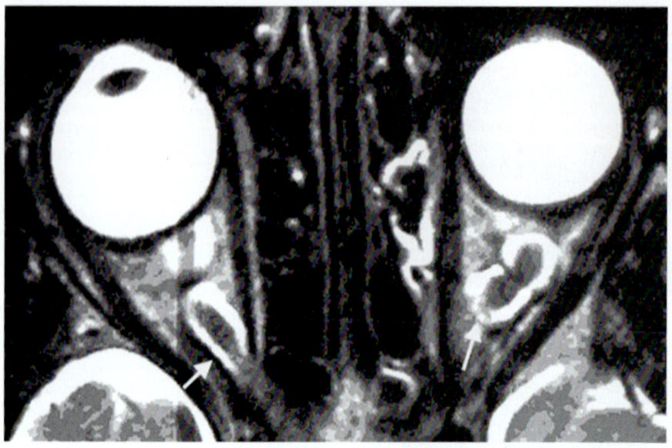

FIGURE 26.12. Bilateral optic nerve gliomas in neurofibromatosis type I. Axial T2-weighted MR image shows enlargement of both optic nerves (arrows), which presents as isointense to the gray matter and as surrounded by hyperintense cerebrospinal fluid.

and clinical follow-up. The tumor causes fusiform enlargement of the optic nerve. On CT the tumor presents an enlarged, fusiform, not calcified optic nerve mass with frequent kinking and cystic areas.[46] Uniform and marked enhancement after contrast administration is commonly observed. On T1-weighted MR images, the tumor is usually isointense to the cerebral gray matter. On T2-weighted MR-images fusiform lesions show high signal, while large lobulated tumors tend to have a more heterogeneous signal. A double-intensity "tubular thickening," with kinked and elongated optic nerves, suggests but does not prove glioma in patients with NF1 (Figure 26.14). Enlargements of the chiasm and the optic tracts are signs of intracranial involvement. T1-weighted MR images after gadolinium administration usually show variable enhancement; when the tumor is large, the center of the mass shows a marked enhancement, but the periphery is not enhanced (consistent with ectactic or hyperplastic arachnoid around the nerve). Differential diagnosis of optic nerve glioma should include idiopathic optic neuritis, sarcoidosis, demyelinating disease, and optic nerve sheath meningioma.[47,48]

Treatment strategies include observation only, surgery, irradiation, chemotherapy, or a combination of these modalities. An "observation" policy may be applied in children with anterior tumors and absence of signs of progression.

Surgical resection is successful in tumors confined to an optic nerve. Radiotherapy is usually reserved for patients with progression after surgery and for opticohypothalamic gliomas. Chemotherapy is at an experimental stage. Chemotherapy of optic nerve glioma is further covered in Chapter 34.[49,50]

A

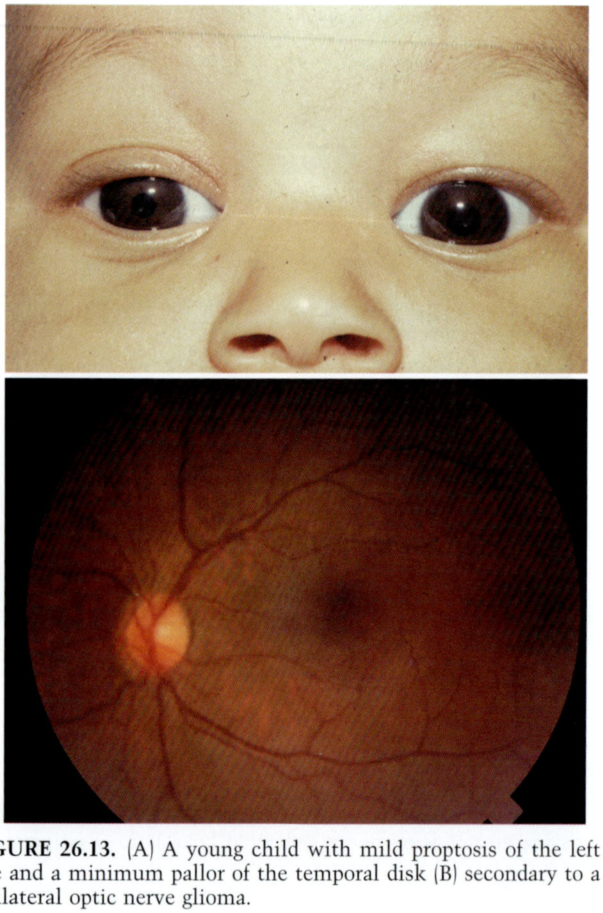

B

FIGURE 26.13. (A) A young child with mild proptosis of the left eye and a minimum pallor of the temporal disk (B) secondary to a unilateral optic nerve glioma.

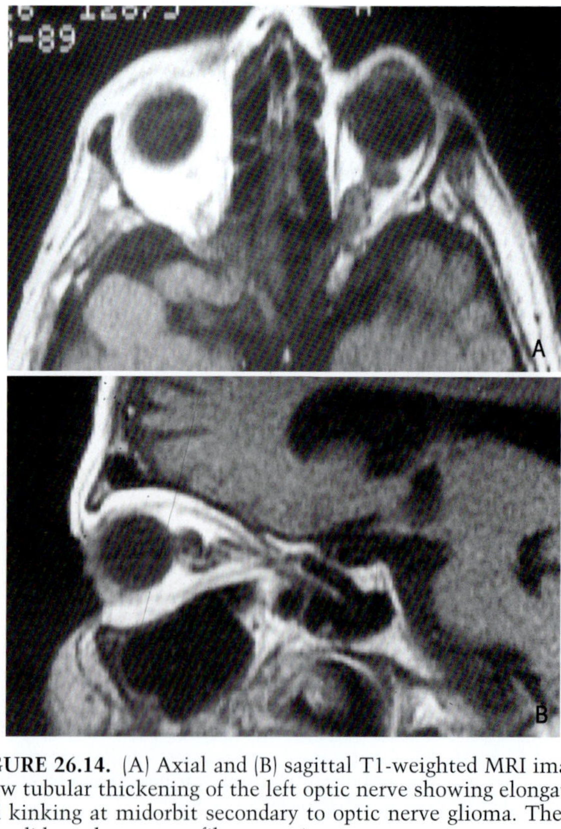

FIGURE 26.14. (A) Axial and (B) sagittal T1-weighted MRI images show tubular thickening of the left optic nerve showing elongation and kinking at midorbit secondary to optic nerve glioma. The patient did not have neurofibromatosis.

SECONDARY AND METASTATIC TUMORS

Neuroblastoma

Neuroblastoma is the most common extracranial solid tumor of childhood, accounting for 8 to 10% of all childhood cancers. It represents a malignant neoplasm of primitive neuroblast and is the most common metastatic orbital tumor, affecting children at a mean age of 2 years.[51]

Neuroblastoma arises in the abdomen, thoracic, cervical, and pelvic regions, and metastases occur by hematogenous spread. Ophthalmic manifestations are common, frequently resulting from periorbital soft tissue infiltration of the tumor.[52,53] The most common sign of orbital metastic neuroblastoma is proptosis and periorbital ecchymosis ("panda bear eyes"), followed by unilateral Horner syndrome and opsoclonus (Figure 26.15). Proptosis and periorbital ecchymosis are typical; ptosis and globe displacement are rather common. Symptoms are bilateral in 20 to 50% of cases (Box 26.4). Orbital involvement is almost exclusively associated with disseminated disease, while Horner syndrome and opsoclonus are frequently associated with localized neuroblastoma, particularly in the mediastinum.[54] Horner syndrome, secondary to tumor in the cervical sympathetic chain, may be the presenting sign.

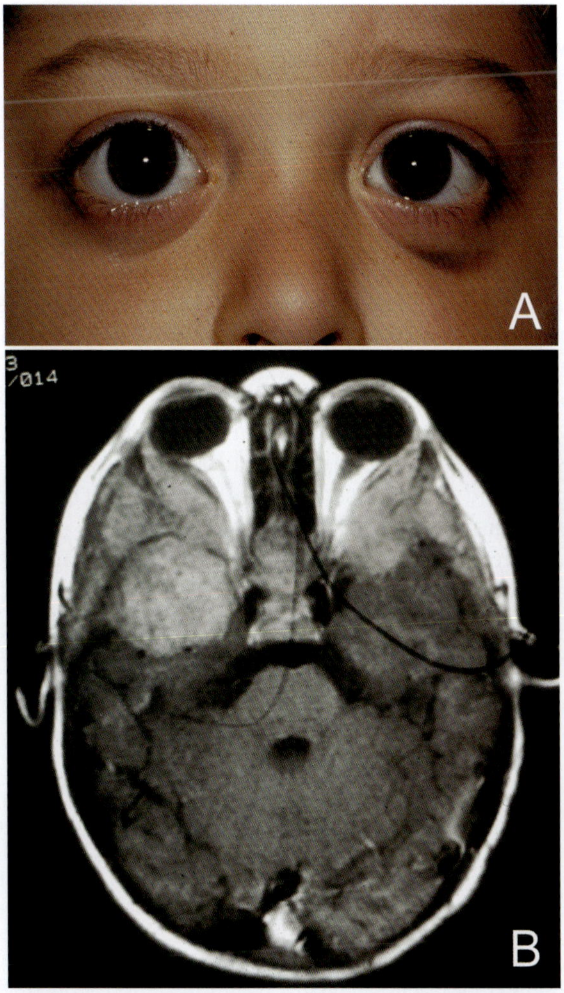

FIGURE 26.15. (A) Bilateral ecchymosis of the eyelids and periorbital skin of a patient with metastatic abdominal neuroblastoma of both orbits and brain. (B) Multiple metastatic nodules in orbits and brain are shown in T-1 weighted axial MRI image. (Courtesy of Dr. Robert A. Gordon of New Orleans, Louisiana.)

BOX 26.4. Orbital Neuroblastoma: Clinical Presentation

Proptosis
Periorbital ecchymosis ("panda bear" eyes)
Ptosis
Globe displacement
Blindness (rare)

On a retrospective review of children, ophthalmic involvement in neuroblastoma was present in 80 of 405 cases (20%). The most common site of origin was the abdomen.[51]

At CT, a soft tissue mass inhomogeneously enhancing with associated lytic bony erosions is appreciable (typically involving the zygomatic bone adjacent temporal orbit). At MRI, the tumor often is isointense to the extraocular muscles, but intratumoral hemorrhages may lead to variable appearance both on T1- and T2-weighted images, depending on the degree of hemoglobin catabolism. After gadolinium administration, variable degrees of enhancement are encountered. Histopathologically, neuroblastoma can be distinguished from most of the neurogenic tumors of the orbit by the presence of neurosecretory dense-core granules, detected by electron microscopy, and by positive neuron-specific enolase (NSE) activity, demonstrated by immunohistochemistry. Immunohistochemistry helps to differentiate a neuroblastoma from other small-cell tumors such as rhabdomyosarcoma, retinoblastoma, Ewing's sarcoma, and lymphoma.[55,56]

The prognosis in neuroblastoma is influenced mainly by age, stage, and site of origin. In children diagnosed during the first year of life, the 2-year relapse-free survival rate is 75%; it drops to 12% after the age of 2 years.[57] The survival rate in neuroblastoma has improved little in the past two decades; about 70% of the patients present with disseminated disease at the time of diagnosis. Early diagnosis is an important factor influencing the prognosis. The ophthalmologist may play a major role in the diagnosis of the disease, since 20% of the patients present with ophthalmologic involvement.[51] The treatment consists of multiagent chemotherapy; combinations of cisplatin, teniposide, vincristine, and cyclophosphamide have been employed. Radiotherapy doses vary according to the age (1500–4000 cGy) Orbital metastasis has a poor prognosis; the 3-year survival rate is 11%.

Orbital Myeloid Sarcoma (Granulocytic Sarcoma)

The orbit may be affected in all types of leukemia, but it has a greater propensity to be involved in acute myeloid leukemia (AML). Mass formation, however, is quite rare; diffuse infiltration is more common. The tumor may appear before, after, or concomitant with hematologic evidence of leukemia.[58]

The most frequent clinical manifestations include exophthalmos, ptosis, edema, and chemosis of the eyelids, with pain. Diagnosis is established by clinical and laboratory findings, imaging studies and biopsy. Granulocytic sarcoma (myeloblastoma or chloroma) is a very uncommon manifestation of acute myelocytic leukemia and presents as a focal soft tissue mass (Figure 26.16).

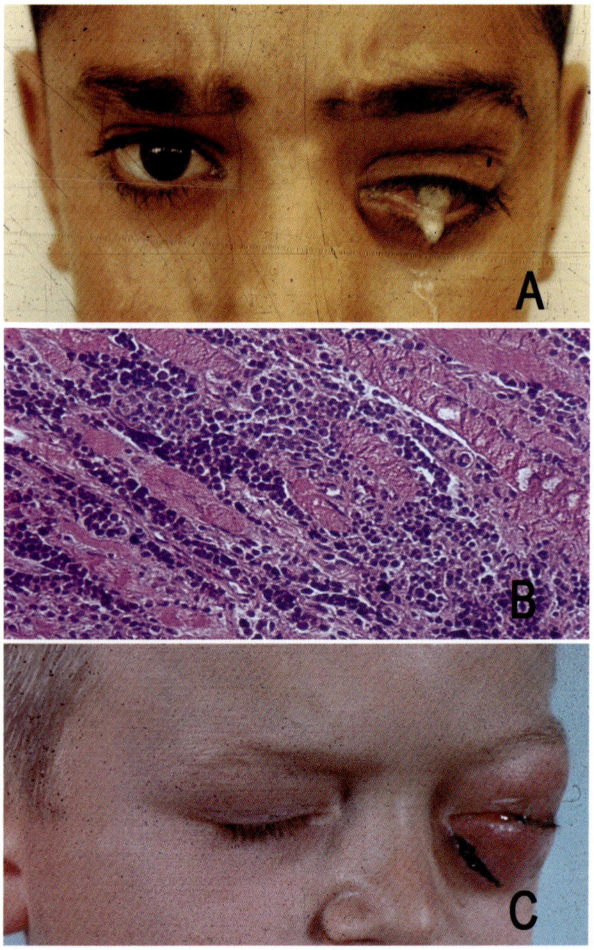

FIGURE 26.16. Granulocytic sarcoma: two patients (A,C) with orbital mass lesions of granulocytic sarcoma. Cornea of the first patient (A) was exposed because of longstanding proptosis and developed corneal ulcer. (B) Biopsy sample from the second patient (C) shows clusters of myeloid cells infiltrating the orbicularis muscle. (Courtesy of Dr. A.O. Çavdar of Ankara, Turkey.)

The term *chloroma* (green tumor) is derived from the greenish coloration of this lesion, which is due to the myeloperoxidase in cells of granulocytic lineage. On occasion, granulocytic sarcoma presents as an isolated soft tissue mass prior to the development of systemic disease. Correct diagnosis of the solitary lesion is important because it leads to early implementation of chemotherapy.[59]

While most childhood orbital tumors, such as lymphangioma, rhabdomyosarcoma, capillary hemangioma, dermoid cyst, and optic nerve glioma are unilateral, bilateral orbital involvement is observed in metastatic neuroblastoma and myeloid sarcoma.[60]

Orbital myeloid sarcoma occurs in young children and is quite rare among the orbital tumors of childhood, accounting for only 1 of 250 cases.[3]

On the basis of a review, Shields et al. calculated that about 88% of the patients with proptosis seen by an ophthalmologist have no history of leukemia at the time of presentation.[60]

Myeloid sarcomas are most common in certain subtypes of AML, in particular, M5a (monoblastic), M5b (monocytic), M4 (myelomonocytic), and M2 (myeloblastic with maturation).[61] There appears to be a very strong association of orbital myeloid sarcoma with AML cases demonstrating a t(8;21) translocation, which is associated with a good prognosis.[62,63] At T1-weighted MRI, granulocytic sarcoma is slighthy hyperintense to gray matter, muscle, and bone marrow. At T2-weighted imaging, it is isointense to white matter, muscle, and bone marrow.[64] CT shows the mass to be isodense to muscle. This tumor trends to mold to contiguous structures and demonstrates relatively little bony destruction.[65] Orbital myeloid sarcoma preferentially involves the lateral orbital wall. Imaging appearance, clinical history, and location can suggest the correct diagnosis, allowing prompt treatment before the development of systemic disease.[66]

References

1. Crawford, JS. Diseases of the orbit. In: Crawford JS, Morin JD, eds. *The Eye in Childhood.* New York: Grune & Stratton; 1983:361–394.
2. Iliff WJ, Green WR. Orbital tumors in children. In: Jakobiec FA, ed. *Ocular and Anexal Tumors.* Birmingham, AL: Aesculapius Publishing; 1978:669–684.
3. Shields JA, Bakewell B, Augsburger JJ, et al. Space occupying orbital masses in children: a review of 250 consecutive biopsies. *Ophthalmology* 1986;93:379–384.
4. Kodsi SR, Shetlar DJ, Campbell RJ, et al. A review of 340 orbital tumors in children during a 60-year period. *Am J Ophthalmol* 1994;117:177–182.

5. Rootman J. Frequency and differential diagnosis of orbital disease. In: Rootman J, ed. *Diseases of the Orbit.* Philadelphia: JB Lippincott; 1988:124.
6. Katowitz JA. *Pediatric Oculoplastic Surgery.* New York: Springer-Verlag; 2002:491–492.
7. Mesfer SA, Mullaney PB, Dowaidi ME, Karcioglu ZA. Retinoblastoma referral patterns in Saudi Arabia. *Invest Ophthamol Vis Sci* 1995;36:S428.
8. Finger P, Harbour JW, Karcioglu ZA. Risk factors for metastasis in retinoblastoma [major review]. *Surv Ophthalmol* 2002;47:1–16.
9. Templeton AC. Orbital tumors in African children. *Br J Ophthalmol* 1971;55:254–261.
10. Magrath I. The pathogenesis of Burkitt's lymphoma. *Adv Cancer Res* 1990;555:133–270.
11. Frezzotti R, Hadjistilianou T, Tosi P. Rhabdomyosarcoma of the orbit: clinical and histopathological analysis of a personal series of 19 cases. *Orbit* 1990;9:307–312.
12. Shields JA, Shields CL. Rhabdomyosarcoma: review for the ophthalmologist. *Surv Ophthalmol* 2003;48:39–57.
13. Newton WA, Gehan EA, Webber BL, et al. Classification of rhabdomyosarcomas and related sarcomas. *Cancer* 1995;76:1073–1085.
14. Warner MA, Weber AL, Jakobiec FA. Benign and malignant tumors of the orbital cavity including the lacrimal gland. In: *Imaging of the Globe, Orbit and Visual Pathway.* Philadelphia: WB Saunders, 1996:123–142.
15. Shaib SA, Moseley I, Wright JE. Orbital rhabdomyosarcoma—the radiological characteristics. *Clin Radiol* 1998;53:357–362.
16. Frayer WC, Enterline HT. Embryonal rhabdomyosarcoma of the orbit in children and young adults. *Arch Ophthalmol* 1959;62:203–210.
17. Cota N, Chandna A, Abernethy LJ. Orbital abscess masquerading as a rhabdomyosarcoma. *JAAPOS* 2000;4:318–320.
18. Mafee MF, Pai E, Binu P. Rhabdomyosarcoma of the orbit. Evaluation with MR imaging and CT. *Radiol Clin North Am* 1998;36:1215–1227.
19. De Potter P, Shields CL, Shields JA. Myogenic tumors. In: De Potter P, Shields CL, Shields JA, eds. *MRI of the Eye and Orbit.* Philadelphia: JB Lippincott; 1995:223–224.
20. Crist W, Gehan EA, Ragad AH, et al. The Third Intergroup Rhabdomyosarcoma Study. *J Clin Oncol* 1995;13:610–630.
21. Shields JA, Shields CL, Honavar SG, Demirci H. Clinical spectrum of primary ophthalmic rhabdomyosarcoma. *Ophthalmology* 2001;108:2284–2292.
22. Cassady JR. How much is enough? The continuing evolution therapy of childhood rhabdomyosarcoma and its refinement. *Int J Radiat Oncol Biol Phys* 1995;31:675–676.
23. Raney RB, Anderson JR, Kollath J, et al. Late effects of therapy in 94 patients with localized rhabdomyosarcoma of the orbit: report from the Intergroup Rhabdomyosarcoma Study (IRS)-III, 1984–1991. *Med Pediatric Oncol* 2000;34:413–420.
24. Breneman JC, Wiener ES. Issues in the local control of rhabdomyosarcoma. *Med Pediatric Oncol* 2000;35:104–109.
25. Oberlin O, Rey A, Anderson J, et al. Treatment of orbital rhabdomyosarcoma: survival and late effects of treatment. Results of an international workshop. *J Clin Oncol* 2001;19:197–204.
26. Ducrey N, Nemadov-Beck M, Spahn B. La thérapie actuelle du rhabdomyosarcome orbitaire de l'enfant. *J Fr Ophthalmol* 2002;25:298–302.
27. Fiorillo A, Migliorati R, Vassallo P, et al. Radiation late effects in children treated for orbital rhabdomyosarcoma. *Radiother Oncol* 1999;53:143–148.
28. Michalski JM, Sur RK, Harms WB, et al. Three-dimensional conformal radiation therapy in pediatric parameningeal rhabdomyosarcomas. *Int J Radiat Oncol Biol Phys* 1995;33:985–991.
29. Janss AJ, Grundy R, Caan A, et al. Optic pathway and hypothalamic/chiasmatic gliomas in children younger than age 5 years with 6 years follow-up. *Cancer* 1995;75:1051–1059.
30. von Graefe A. Geschwulste des Schenerven. *Arch Ophthalmol* 1864;10:193.
31. Dutton JJ. Gliomas of the anterior visual pathway. *Surv Ophthalmol* 1994;38:427–452.
32. Memoli VA, Brown EF, Gould VE. Glial fibrillary acidic protein (GFA) immunoreactivity in peripheral nerve sheath tumors. *Ultrastruct Pathol* 1984;7:269–275.
33. Lewis RA, Gerson LP, Axelson KA, et al. Von Recklinghausen neurofibromatosis II. Incidence of optic glioma. *Ophthalmology* 1984;91:929–935.
34. Schroder S, Baumann-Schroder U, Hazim W, et al. Langzeitverlauf von Gliomen der Sehbahn bei Neurofibromatose Typ 1. *Klin Monatsbl Augenheilkd* 1999;215:349–354.
35. Dutton J. Optic nerve glioma. In: Dutton JJ, ed. *Diagnostic Atlas of Orbital Diseases.* Philadelphia: WB Saunders; 2000:120–121.
36. Lund AM, Skouby F. Optic gliomas in children with neurofibromatosis type 1. *Eur J Pediatr* 1991;150:835–838.
37. Listernick R, Charrow J, Greenwald MJ, et al. Optical pathway tumors in children: the effect of neurofibromatosis type 1 on clinical manifestation and natural history. *J Pediatr* 1995;127:718–722.
38. Kuenzle CH, Weissert M, Roulet Bode H, et al. Follow-up of optic pathway gliomas in children with neurofibromatosis type 1. *Neuropediatrics* 1994;25:295–300.
39. Packer RJ, Bilarimk LT, Cohen BH, et al. Intracranial visual pathway gliomas in children with neurofibromatosis. *Neurofibromatosis* 1988;1:212–222.
40. Balcer L, Liu G, Heller G, et al. Visual loss in children with neurofibromatosis type 1 and optic pathway gliomas: relation to tumor location by magnetic resonance imaging. *Am J Ophthalmol* 2001;131:442–445.
41. Hoyt WF, Baghdassarian SA. Optic gliomas of childhood: natural history and rationale for conservative management. *Br J Ophthalmol* 1969;53:793–798.
42. Gaye G, Scott IU, Feuer W, et al. Long-term visual outcome in patients with anterior visual pathway gliomas. *J Neuro-Ophthalmol* 2001;21:1–7.
43. Parsa CF, Hoyt CS, Lesser RL, et al. Spontaneous regression of optic gliomas. *Arch Ophthalmol* 2001;119:516–529.
44. Sartor K. *MR imaging of the Skull and Brain. A Correlative Text-Atlas.* Berlin: Springer-Verlag; 1992.
45. Brown EW, Riccardi VM, Mawad M. MR Imaging of optic pathways in patients with neurofibromatosis. *AJNR Am J Neuroradiol* 1987;8:1031–1036.
46. De Potter P, Shields CL, Shields JA. Optic nerve and meningeal tumors. In: De Potter P, Shields CL, Shields JA, eds. *MRI of the Eye and Orbit.* Philadelphia: JB Lippincott; 1995:193–201.
47. Hollander MD, FitzPatrick M, O'Connor SG, et al. Optic gliomas. *Radiol Clin North Am* 1999;37:59–71.
48. Karcioglu ZA, Yulug A, Haik BG. Tumors of the optic nerve. In: Margo CE, Hamed LM, Mames RN, ed. *Diagnostic Problems in Clinical Pathology.* Philadelphia: WB Saunders; 1994:105–114.
49. Grabenbauer G, Schuchardt U, Buchfelder M, et al. Radiation therapy of opticohypothalamic gliomas (OHG): radiographic response, vision and late toxicity. *Radiother Oncol* 2000;54:239–245.
50. Khafaga Y, Hassounah M, Kandil A, et al. Optic gliomas: a retrospective analysis of 50 cases. *Int J Radiat Oncol Biol Phys* 2003;56:807–812.
51. Musarella M, Chan, De Boer G, Gallie B. Ocular involvement in neuroblastoma: prognostic implications. *Ophthalmology* 1984;91:936–940.

52. Belgaumi AF, Kauffman WM, Cordoba J, et al. Blindness in children with neuroblastoma. *Cancer* 1997;80:1997–2004.
53. Bullock J, Goldberg SH, Rakes SM, et al. Primary orbital neuroblastoma. *Arch Ophthalmol* 1989;107:1031–1033.
54. Mortada A. Clinical characteristics of early orbital metastatic neuroblastoma. *Am J Ophthalmol* 1967;Jun:1787–1789.
55. Jakobiec FA, Klepach GL, Crissman JD, Spoor TC. Primary differentiated neuroblastoma of the orbit. *Ophthalmology* 1987;94:255–266.
56. Dutton JJ. Neuroblastoma. In: Dutton JJ, ed. *Diagnostic Atlas of Orbital Diseases*. Philadelphia: WB Saunders; 2000:118–119.
57. Maurer HM. Current concepts in cancer. Solid tumors in children. *N Engl J Med* 1978;299:1345–1348.
58. Zimmermann LE, Font RL. Ophthalmologic manifestation of granulocytic sarcoma. The Third Pan American Association of Ophthalmology and American Journal of Ophthalmology Lecture. *Am J Ophthalmol* 1975;80:975–990.
59. Stein Wexter R, Wooton-Gorges SL, West DC. Orbital granulocytic sarcoma: an unusual presentation of acute myelocitic leukaemia. *Pediatr Radiol* 2003;33:136–139.
60. Shields JA, Stopyra GA, Marr PB, et al. Bilateral orbital myeloid sarcoma as initial sign of acute myeloid leukaemia: case report and review of the literature. *Arch Ophthalmol* 2003;121:138–142.
61. Byrd JC, Edenfield J, Shields DJ, et al. Extramedullary myeloid cell tumors in acute myeloid leukaemia. *Br J Ophthalmol* 1971;55:844–847.
62. Schwyzer R, Sherman GG, Cohn RJ, et al. Granulocytic sarcoma in children with acute myeloblastic leukaemia and t(8;21). *Med Pediatr Oncol* 1998;31:144–149.
63. Tanigawa M, Tsuda Y, Amemiya T, Yamada K. Orbital tumor in acute myeloid leukemia associated with karyotype 46 XX t(8;21) (q22;q22): a case report. *Ophthalmologica* 1998;212:202–205.
64. Pui MH, Fletcher BD, Langston JW. Granulocytic sarcoma in childhood leukaemia: imaging features. *Radiology* 1994;190:698–702.
65. Jakobiec FA. Granulocytic sarcoma. *AJNR Am J Neuroradiol* 1991;12:263–264.
66. Stein Wexter R, Wotton-Gorges SL, West DC. *Pediatr Radiol* 2003;33:136–139.

PART SIX

Tumorlike Conditions in the Orbit

27

Orbital Inflammation and Infection Versus Neoplasia

Antonio Augusto V. Cruz

The term *neoplasia* literally means "new growth," and the tissue that results from this process is called a *neoplasm*. The word *tumor* originally designated the edema caused by inflammation but is now widely used as a synonym for neoplasm.

Although patients understand that a tumor is an abnormal and harmful lesion, a precise medical definition of what characterizes a neoplasm is difficult. According to Cotran et al., a neoplasm is an abnormal mass of tissue whose growth is uncoordinated with that of the normal tissues; the mass is purposeless and preys on the host.[1] From the functional standpoint, neoplasms can be divided into two basic categories: benign and malignant. Rapid growth, local invasion, and metastasis are typical characteristics of malignancy. Since most cancers grow rapidly with infiltration and destruction of the surrounding tissues, most clinicians intuitively consider local invasiveness to be the hallmark of neoplasms.

Inflammation is a complex tissue reaction that occurs in response to specific endogenous or exogenous stimuli. The inflammatory process is characterized by increased vascular permeability that allows plasma proteins and circulating cells to leave the circulation and infiltrate the injured area. Depending on the nature of the stimulus that initiates the inflammation, the cells involved in the inflammatory process will change. Infection, for instance, is characterized by a predominance of neutrophils and polymorphonuclear leukocytes. Other infiltrates are formed by collection of epithelioid histiocytes and granuloma formation or polyclonal lymphocytes. Sometimes the cell contingent is sparse and the tissue changes are dominated by fibrous proliferation. The ultimate goal of the inflammatory reaction is to protect the organism from the initial cause of injury. However, the process of tissue repair that is closely related to inflammation can be harmful, and severe sequelae may be the final result of the inflammatory response.

Although neoplasia and inflammation are different biological processes, the clinical differentiation between the two can be difficult in the orbit. Neoplasia can induce inflammation, and some inflammatory responses may mimic malignant neoplasms.

INFLAMMATION MIMICKING NEOPLASIA

Idiopathic orbital inflammation (IOI) is a condition of unknown etiology characterized by the involvement of the orbital tissues by a nonspecific inflammatory process. Histologically, this infiltration is composed of lymphocytes, plasma cells, eosinophils, macrophages, and varying amounts of collagen deposition.[2] By definition, IOI is restricted to the orbital contents, and several patterns of tissue involvement have been described.[3] However, the same types of inflammatory change found in the orbit have been reported in other locations of the head and neck region, including larynx, mouth, tonsils, paranasal sinuses, pterygomaxillary fossa, thyroid, and parotid.[4]

Whenever there is inflammation within the boundaries of the orbit, it is not uncommon to find inflammatory changes outside the orbit as well. Table 27.1, which summarizes the clinical characteristics of 11 cases of idiopathic inflammation diagnosed around the orbits, indicates that 53.8% of the inflammatory changes are found simultaneously inside and outside the orbital limits, and bone erosion was a common finding (69.2%).[5–11] From the clinical point of view, bone erosion is a disturbing feature because it indicates an aggressive lesion with high capacity of local invasion and destruction, typical of neoplasias. Figure 27.1 shows how similar to neoplasia an idiopathic inflammation can be: the patient, a 35-year-old man, presented with a 1-month history of proptosis, diplopia, and pain in the right eye (OD). Visual acuity was normal. Hertel exophthalmometry measurements were OD 19 mm, and for the left eye (OS), 14 mm with elevation and marked inferior restriction of the right eye (Figure 27.1A). A computed tomography (CT) scan of the orbits showed an extensive infiltration along the floor involving the inferior, lateral, and medial recti. The intraconal fat between the optic nerve and the inferior rectus was also affected. The infiltration extended outside the orbit into the pterygopalatine and infratemporal fossae. The lateral wall was partially destroyed (Figure 27.1C,D). The results of the biopsy revealed mature lymphocytes associated with dense col-

TABLE 27.1. Summary of the Clinical Characteristics of 11 Cases of Idiopathic Inflammation Diagnosed Around the Orbit.

Author	Year	No. of cases	Sex	Age	Location	Image	Bone erosion	Orbital involvement
Keen et al.[5]	1986	1	M	55	PPF	CT	No	No
Weisman and Osguthorpe[6]	1988	1[a]	F	63	MS, ITF	CT	Yes	Yes
Takimoto et al.[7]	1990	1	M	83	MS, NC, PPF	CT	Yes	No
Som et al.[8]	1994	6	M	41	MS, ES, NC	CT	Yes	No
			M	63	MS, NC	CT	Yes	Yes
			M	67	MS, SS, NC	CT	Yes	No
			M	58	MS, NC	CT	Yes	Yes
			M[b]	15	MS, IFT	CT	Yes	Yes
			M	48	MS, IFT	CT	Yes	Yes
de Ruiter et al[9]	2000	1	F	48	PPF	MRI	No	No
De Miguel Garcia, F et al.[10]	1990	1	M	40	MS, NC, NPR	CT	Yes	No

MS, maxillary sinus; ES, ethmoid sinus; SS, sphenoid sinus; PPF, pterygopalatine fossa, ITF, infratemporal fossa, NC, nasal cavity.

[a]Three published cases: two were typical orbital pseudotumors and only one was a true head and neck pseudotumor.

[b]Case also published by Maldjian et al.[11]

lagen deposition (Figure 27.1E,F). The patient was treated with radiation (2000 cGy) and 1 mg/kg/day of prednisone for one month. The steroid therapy was maintained for an additional month and tapered over 8 weeks. There was a gradual improvement in ocular motility and relief of the symptoms (Figure 27.1G,H). The patient's clinical picture was indistinguishable from a malignant neoplasm of the paranasal sinuses and the pterygopalatine and infratemporal fossae; a correct diagnosis was possible only after a biopsy.

Large areas of infiltration beyond orbital limits are also suspect and can easily lead the physician to the conclusion that the orbit is being invaded by a malignant process. The patient shown in Figure 27.2A presented with a 5-month history of diplopia, pain, and proptosis in the right eye. On examination, a painful mass was palpable in the right temporal fossa. Visual acuity for both eyes was 20/40; ocular fundi and visual fields were normal. Hertel measurements were 20 mm (OD) and 13 mm (OS) with a significant limitation of right abduction. Computed tomography and magnetic resonance imaging (MRI) of the orbits showed a large mass infiltrating soft tissue structures well beyond the orbital limits. As shown in Figure 27.2B,C, the infratemporal and temporal fossae as well the lateral aspect of the right orbit were extensively involved. The infiltration was into the lateral and inferior recti muscles but did not cause bone erosion. Biopsy samples from intraorbital and temporal fossa contents showed the same histology: a chronic inflammatory process composed mainly of mature lymphocytes associated with collagen deposition, and occasional lymphoid follicles. The patient was treated with prednisone (1 mg/kg/day) tapered over 4 weeks. The clinical response to treatment was good, with pain reduction and improvement of ocular motility. A repeat CT scan showed that infiltration was less dense (Figure 27.2D).

Orbital myositis is a subgroup of IOI characterized by inflammation of the extraocular muscles (EOMs).[12] Lacey et al., in their comprehensive review of EOM disease, classified orbital myositis into acute, chronic or recurrent, and atypical forms.[13] The isolated form is characterized by a short history (days to weeks) of pain, swelling, and/or diplopia. Pain exacerbated by eye movement is the most common clinical presentation (62.5%). The recurrent form (32%) is typified by repeated acute episodes; less frequently, it has a progressive course. Rarely (5%), patients may present with features such as optic nerve dysfunction and minimal pain in atypical cases.

The differential diagnosis of myositis includes other causes of specific EOM inflammation such as sarcoidosis,[14–16] systemic lupus erythematosus,[17,18] rheumatoid arthritis,[19] Wegener's granulomatosis,[20] scleroderma,[21] infections (trichinosis, cysticercosis, Lyme disease),[22,33] Crohn's disease, celiac disease, Wipple's disease,[13,24] and neoplasias such as lymphoma[25] and metastatic tumors.[26]

The diagnosis of myositis can be straightforward. On imaging, increased EOM with muscle tendon thickening is a common finding. Orbital fat is generally not infiltrated. Because orbital myositis is usually localized to the extraocular muscles, the coexistence of myositis and infiltration of other structures not related to the EDMs creates a diagnostic dilemma that is resolved only with a biopsy. The patient described next exemplifies a nonspecific myositis with atypical findings, similar to neoplasia.

A 66-year-old woman presented with redness, foreign body sensation, and proptosis in the right eye. She had a hard nodule in the lateral aspect of the right upper lid of 3-month duration that was painful to palpation. She also complained of diplopia in right and superior gazes. Extraocular motility was decreased in abduction and infraduction of the right eye. Pupillary examination was within normal limits. Intraocular pressures were 15 mm OD and 13 mm OS. Biomicroscopy revealed a mass in the superior conjunctival fornix of the right upper lid. Arteriolar attenuation and

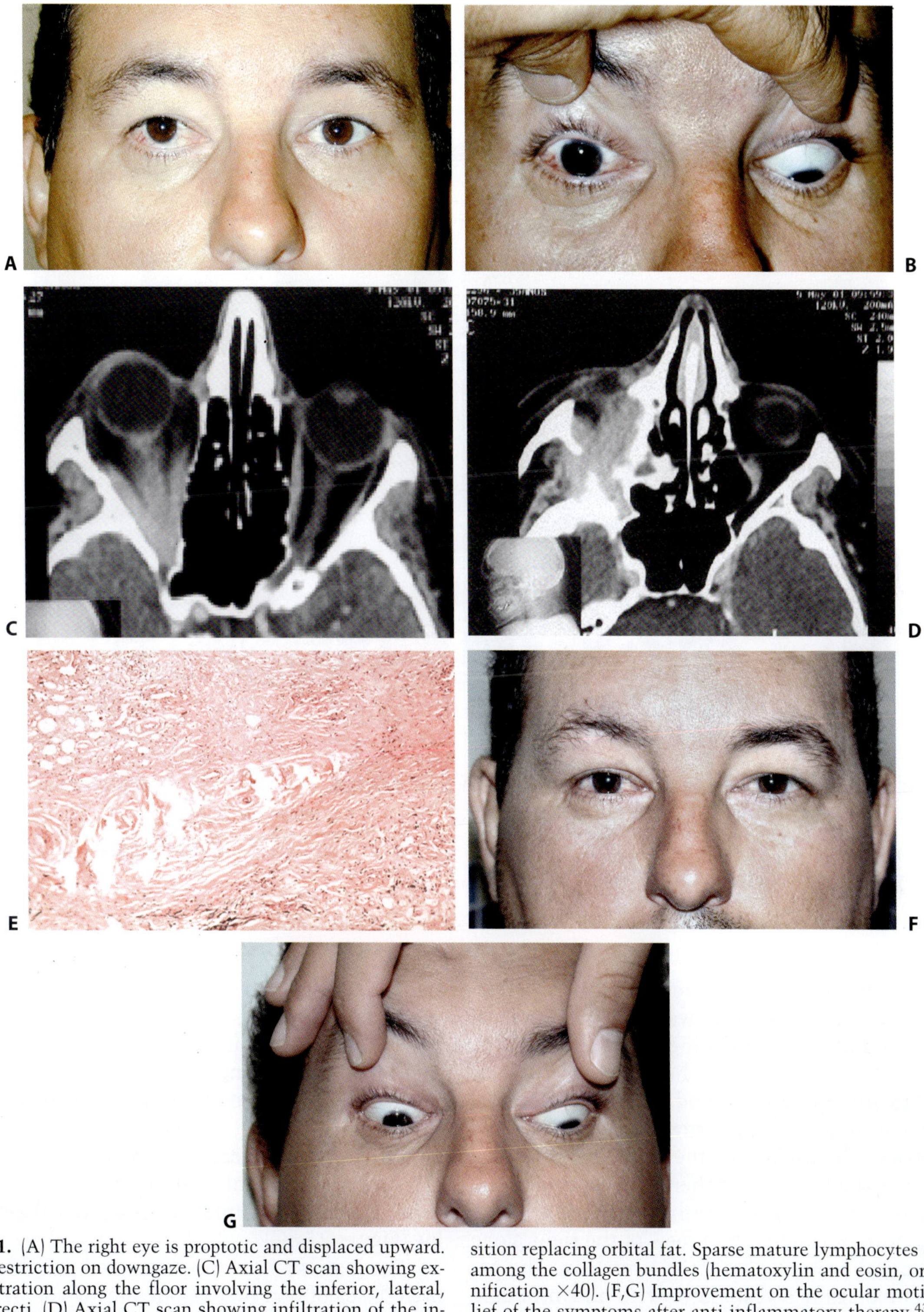

FIGURE 27.1. (A) The right eye is proptotic and displaced upward. (B) Marked restriction on downgaze. (C) Axial CT scan showing extensive infiltration along the floor involving the inferior, lateral, and medial recti. (D) Axial CT scan showing infiltration of the infratemporal fossa with bone destruction. (E) Dense collagen deposition replacing orbital fat. Sparse mature lymphocytes can be seen among the collagen bundles (hematoxylin and eosin, original magnification ×40). (F,G) Improvement on the ocular motility and relief of the symptoms after anti-inflammatory therapy.[43]

mild tortuosity of the vessels were the only significant findings on funduscopy. Hertel exophthalmometry revealed 21 mm OD and 14 mm OS.

A CT scan showed diffuse enlargement of the right lateral rectus muscle with a hyperdense lesion. The optic nerve was dislocated to the right but normal in appearance, and the right infraorbital nerve was somewhat enlarged at the level of the pterygopalatine fossa (Figure 27.3B). Thyroid function tests were normal. C-reactive protein, anti-streptolysin titers, and results of a com-

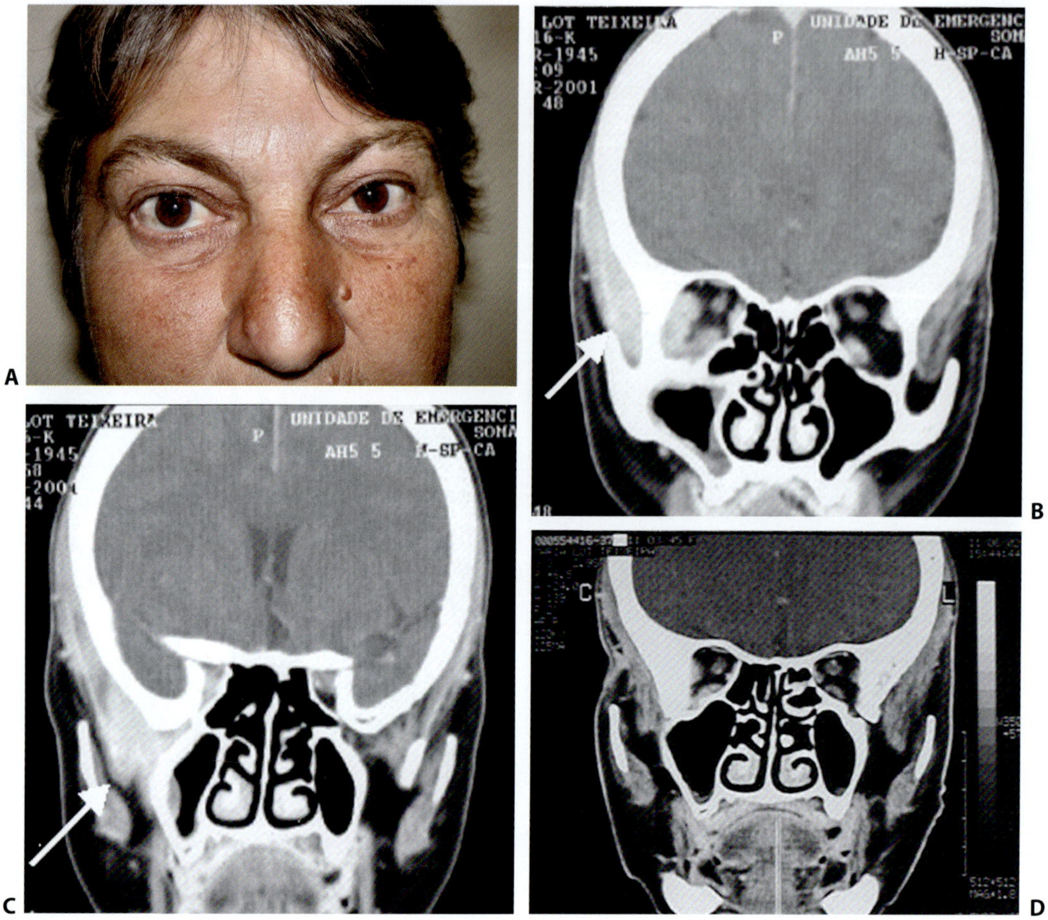

FIGURE 27.2. (A) A 56-year-old woman who had diplopia, pain, and proptosis in the right eye. (B) Coronal CT scan showing infiltration involving the lateral and inferior recti and temporal fossa (arrow) without bone erosion. (C) Coronal CT scan showing infiltration in the infratemporal fossa (arrow). (D) Coronal CT scan after anti-inflammatory therapy. The infiltration in temporal and infratemporal fossa disappeared. The inferior and lateral recti are still enlarged.[43]

plete blood cell count were normal; erythrocyte sedimentation rate was 22. Results were negative for antinuclear factor and antineutrophil cytoplasm antibody.

A diagnosis of myositis of the lateral rectus was made, and treatment was initiated with three daily oral doses of prednisone totaling 1 mg/kg/day and tapered over 3 weeks. The nodule in the right upper lid improved after just a few days of therapy. However, there was no change in diplopia or motility restriction. There was only 1 mm of residual proptosis of the right globe from her initial presentation after 4 months. The patient presented again 2 years later with a firm nodule in the right lower eyelid. Visual acuity was 20/25 with correction. Goldmann visual fields were normal in both eyes. A CT scan at this time showed enlargement of medial, lateral, and inferior recti, with the latter two being most involved (Figure 27.3C,D). The enlargement of the infraorbital nerve had significantly increased. Prednisone was again given with a good response and reduction in proptosis.

The patient was lost to subsequent follow-up for 4 years. When she presented again there was about 6 to 7 mm proptosis of the right globe with a pattern of motility restriction similar to the one she had at presentation, as well as a firm nodule in the right lower eyelid. She had been self-medicating herself with 20 mg/day of prednisone for 2 months. A CT scan performed at this time showed involvement of all extraocular muscles including the levator–superior rectus complex. There was enlargement of the infraorbital canal circumferentially from the pterygopalatine fossa to about midway along the floor of the orbit (Figure 27.3C).

The patient was again treated empirically with high doses of oral prednisone during the next 2 years, with good results. An MRI scan was also performed 3 years after treatment, which showed diffuse enlargement of all rectus muscles. The right infraorbital nerve was markedly enlarged posteriorly, near its origin and along the pterygopalatine fossa (Figure 27.3E,F).

Biopsy of the inferior oblique muscle and the infraorbital canal was performed. The infraorbital canal was so enlarged that there was no difficulty in obtaining a piece of the nerve, which showed a nonspecific chronic inflammatory infiltrate with follicle formation interspersed among the nerve

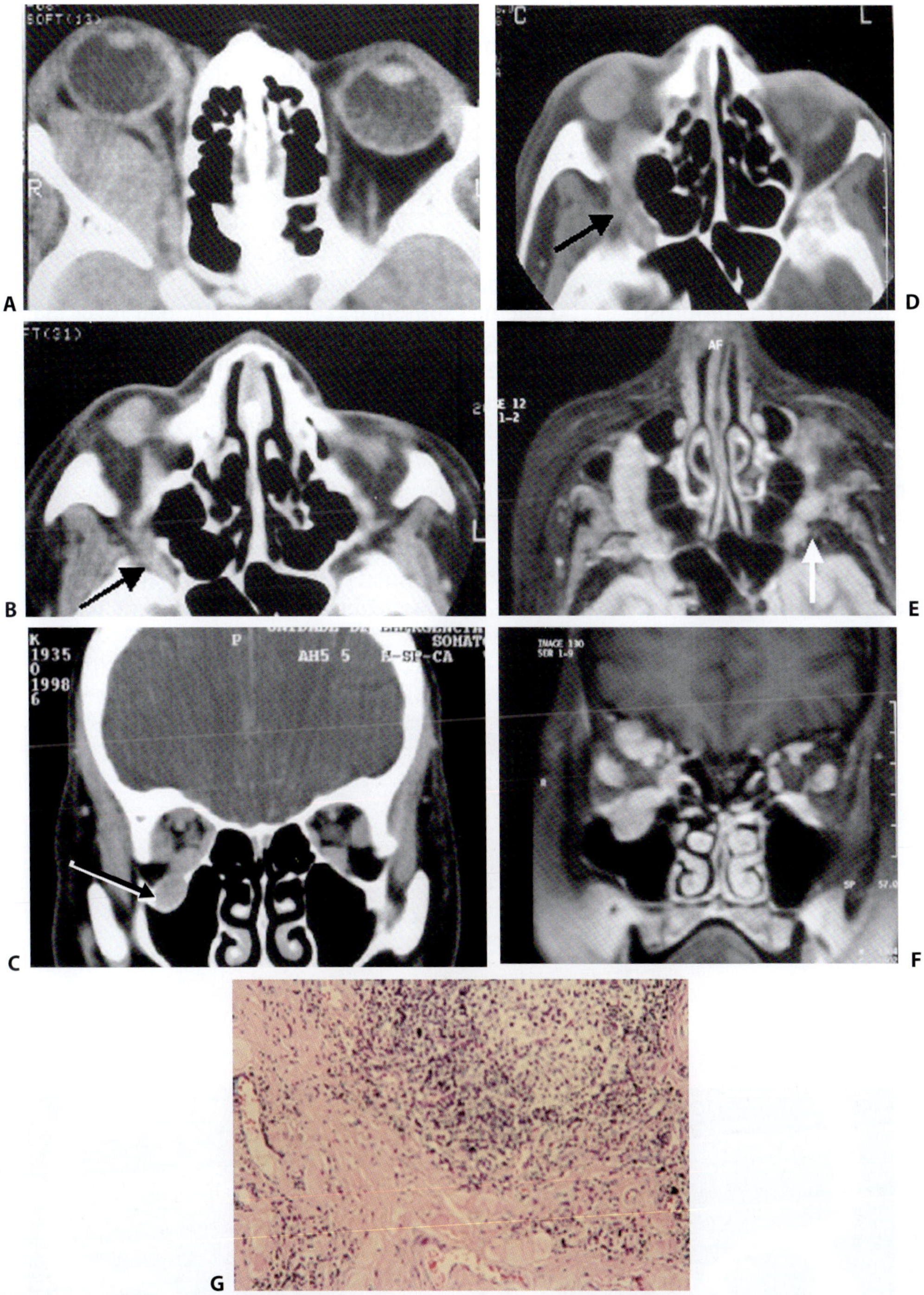

FIGURE 27.3. (A) Axial CT scan showing diffuse infiltration of the right lateral rectus muscle. The optic nerve is moved medially. (B) Axial CT scan showing enlargement of the right infraorbital nerve at the level of the pterygopalatine fossa (arrow). (C) Coronal CT scan showing enlargement of the right medial, lateral, and inferior recti muscles as well as of the right infraorbital nerve. (D) Axial CT scan: significant increment of the infraorbital nerve enlargement (arrow). (E) T1-weighted, contrast-enhanced MR image showing enlargement of all extraocular muscles and of the infraorbital nerve. (F) Unenhanced T2-weighted MR image showing the diffuse enlargement of the right infraorbital nerve and also reveals that the size of the left infraorbital nerve is increased in the pterygopalatine fossa. (G) Histopathology from biopsy of right inferior oblique muscle: lymphoid follicle in a dense collagen matrix (hematoxylin and eosin, original magnification ×1000).[44]

bundles. The muscle biopsy showed similar histology with a greater degree of fibrosis (Figure 27.3G). Immunohistochemistry revealed this infiltrate to be polyclonal and showed B κ and λ in lymphocytes as well as T lymphocytes.

NEOPLASIA MIMICKING INFLAMMATION

Patients with typical inflammatory signs may prove to be suffering from orbital neoplasia. A classic example is rhabdomysarcoma, which grows rapidly and frequently presents with infection and swelling of the eyelids. Usually, imaging and histopathologic studies disclose the true nature of these pseudoinflammatory features, and a correct diagnosis can be suggested, but the ultimate diagnosis should always be based on histopathologic examination.

In rare instances, the malignancy of an acutely inflamed orbit can be elusive and extremely difficult to prove. For instance, in childhood the classic signs of orbital inflammation such as proptosis, eyelid edema and erythema, pain, limitation of extraocular movements, and loss of vision are most often related to cellulitis due to sinusitis.[27] Less frequently, this clinical picture can be the expression of IOI or represent extremely rare cases of Tor T/natural killer cell (T/NK) sinonasal lymphomas.[28] The case presented in Figure 27.4 highlights the difficulty of diagnosing this type of lymphoma.

The patient, an 11-year-old boy, was admitted with a 2-month history of right ethmoid–maxillary sinusitis and cellulitis of the right eye. The patient had initially been managed at another hospital with intravenous antibiotics and sinus drainage without success. During the 2 weeks before admission to our hospital, the proptosis of the right eye worsened and the child lost his vision in both eyes. He presented with proptosis, eyelid edema and erythema, limitation of eye movement, and excruciating pain on the right side of the face (Figure 27.4A). There was bilateral mydriasis and no light perception in either eye. Fundoscopy was unremarkable. The boy had fever (38°C) and was extremely anxious. Orbital CT scans from his initial treatment were available and showed opacification of the right maxillary and ethmoid sinuses and progressive right EOM (Figure 27.4B). The initial CT scan after admission showed massive right extraocular muscle infiltration; EOMs were almost indistinct. There was also an infiltrate in the frontal lobe (Figure 27.4C). Biopsies were done on the right orbit and the inferior turbinate immediately. Histopathologic examination was reported to be consistent with IOI. Cultures for

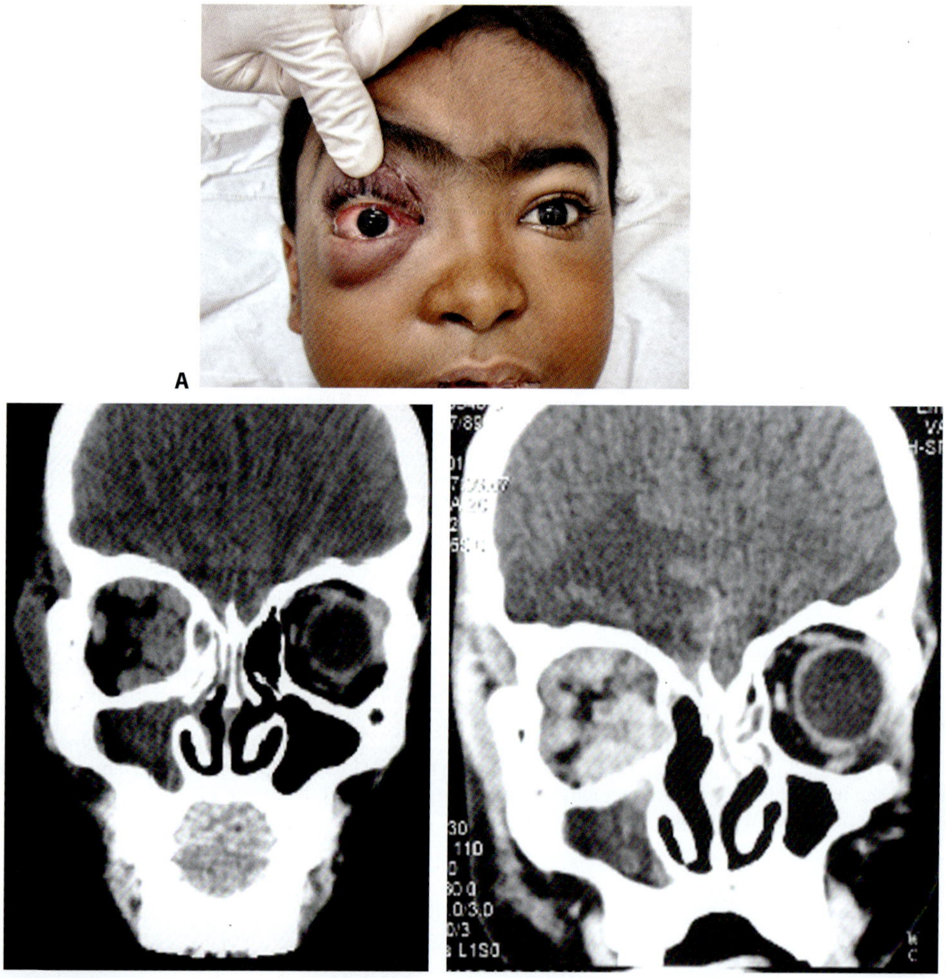

A B C

FIGURE 27.4. (A) Proptotic right orbit in an 11-year-old child. (B) Opacification of the right maxillary and ethmoidal sinuses and enlargement of the right extraocular muscle. (C) Signs of right ethmoidectomy, massive right extraocular muscle infiltration, and frontal lobe edema.

bacteria and fungi were negative. Since the clinical picture was not consistent with IOI, another biopsy was performed, but the same results were obtained. Only on the third biopsy, tissue samples from the medial rectus muscle, did orbital soft tissue and maxillary sinus show extensive tissue necrosis and an infiltrate of atypical cells, with pleomorphic nuclei and no architectural pattern permeating the nonnecrotic areas and the walls of blood vessels. The immunohistochemical study showed that these cells were positive for leukocyte common antigen (CD45), terminal deoxynucleotidyltransferase (TdT), CD3, and CD45RO, and negative for CD56, CD20, CD57, CD99, and Epstein–Barr virus. Both the morphologic and the immunohistochemical findings supported the diagnosis of T-cell lymphoma.

During the investigation period the disease progressed rapidly with development of scalp and palatal ulcers, fever, and deterioration of patient's consciousness. Blood cultures and lumbar puncture results were negative. MRI disclosed a frontal lobe area of edema and diffuse meningeal infiltration. Chemotherapy was instituted, but the child's status continued to deteriorate and he died of respiratory insufficiency.

It is interesting to note three biopsies were necessary to demonstrate the malignant cells. The scarcity of neoplastic cells in the biopsies is a typical finding in T or T/NK sinonasal lymphomas.[29] It is well to remember that the biopsy should be repeated if results are not consistent with the clinical picture. In sinonasal T/NK-cell lymphomas, the cytologic atypia is quite variable, with cells of different sizes. The immunophenotype is positive for T-cell markers (CD2, CD3, CD5, CD45RO) and/or NK-cell markers, especially CD56. In almost all cases, Epstein–Barr virus infection can be demonstrated by in situ hybridization. The difficulty in recognizing such cases as malignancies is exemplified by the fact that only recently has this entity been delineated as a lymphoma. In the past, the clinical presentation characterized by palatal ulcers, orbital swelling, and erythema was described as "lethal midline granuloma," "idiopathic midline destructive disease," "malignant granuloma," "midline malignant reticulosis," "rhinitis gangrenosa progressiva," and "polymorphous reticulosis."[30–34] Because this neoplasm typically shows an angiocentric and angiodestructive pattern of growth, usually there is extensive necrosis admixture with inflammatory cells. In this context, identification of atypical malignant cells can be difficult, especially because these cells tend to be scarce and the diagnosis of lymphoma is seldom suspected clinically. In addition, surface crusting and secondary changes due to local infection explain the need for abundant biopsy material to establish a correct diagnosis. With respect to the patient discussed in connection with Figure 27.4, positivity for T-cell markers (CD3, CD45RO) and negativity of CD56 confirmed that the case was a pure T-cell lymphoma.

"MALIGNANT" INFECTIONS

Most patients interpret cancer as an extremely harmful disease that carries a somber prognosis; a rapidly fatal course is widely seen as a hallmark of such an illness. However, some infections, even in our era of antibiotic eras, can behave like aggressive tumors and destroy the host at an astonishing pace. Sino-orbital mucormycosis is an example of an infection that can mimic an aggressive cancer. This type of infection is caused by fungi that belong to the class Zygomycetes, order Mucorales. The genera that account for most cases of mucormycosis (*Rhizopus*, *Absidia*, *Rhizomucor*, *Mucor*, and *Apophysomyces*) belong to the Mucoraceae family. Agents from other families of the Mucorales order (Cunninghamellaceae, Saksenaceae, Syncephalastraceae, and Thamnidiaceae) have also been implicated in this disease.[25]

These fungi are widely distributed in nature and are harmless in immunocompetent individuals. The disease represents an opportunistic infection that occurs in debilitated patients, especially those with diabetes and ketoacidosis.[36] Spores inhaled from the air may invade and grow in the paranasal sinuses. From this site, hyphae invade the blood vessels, provoking thrombosis and necrosis. Spread of the organisms to the orbit, face, and brain gives rise to rhino-facial-orbital-cerebral mucormycosis. The clinical course of the disease may range from rare chronic and indolent presentations[37] to fulminant fatal forms.[38] These polar extremes of the presentation spectrum of mucormycosis are illustrated in two cases presented next.

The first patient was a 65-year-old male who was seen at another hospital with a history of pain in the infraorbital region of the left eye. He had presented with edema on the left side of his face that appeared to be paretic. A CT scan demonstrated left ethmoid and maxillary sinus opacification. Serum glucose was 307 mg. The following day the local physician noted that the left side of the patient's face was clearly paretic and erythematous. A new CT scan revealed that the sinus opacification extended into the right ethmoid sinus and nasal cavity. Ceftriaxone was prescribed, but on the third day of admission the patient's status deteriorated. The left soft palate was paretic, and there was left ptosis with mydriasis in both eyes. An otolaryngologic examination disclosed an area of necrosis in the nasal mucosa, and a biopsy sample was taken. Histopathologic examination of this material revealed the presence of nonseptate hyphae typical of mucormycosis. Intravenous amphotericin B was ini-

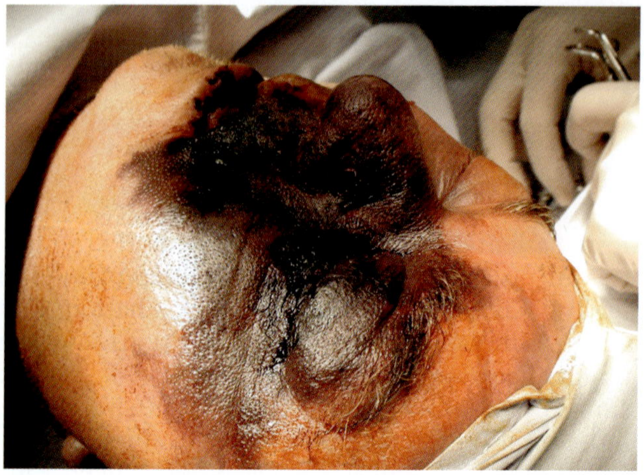

FIGURE 27.5. Extensive necrosis involving almost the entire left side of patient's face.

tiated. The following day the patient developed respiratory distress, and the entire left side of his face became necrotic (Figure 27.5). An aggressive surgical debridement was performed without success, and the patient died one day after surgery.

The clinical presentation of the next patient with rhino-orbital mucormycosis was completely different. The course of the infection was chronic and difficult to eradicate. The patient was a 70-year-old diabetic male who had a history of 10-day treatment for cellulitis at another hospital. Twenty-five days after discharge he developed ophthalmoplegia and lost vision in his left eye. On admission to our hospital, visual acuity was 20/30 in the right eye, but there was no light perception in the left eye, which showed proptotic edema and erythema in the upper eyelid. There was a large amount of secretion in the nasal cavity. The middle turbinate was necrotic. An orbital CT scan disclosed opacification of the ethmoid and sphenoid sinuses and an area of atypical infiltration along the medial wall (Figure 27.6A). The orbit and the sinuses were simultaneously operated. A combined endoscopic and transconjunctival approach was employed. A large amount of necrotic tissue was removed from both the sinuses and the orbit. Histopathologic examination of these samples revealed the nonseptate hyphae characteristic of mucormycosis. Four days after surgery the sinuses were clean and the patient was transferred to the infectious disease unit. After 2 months of treatment with amphotericin B, a new CT scan revealed an infiltration in the pterygopalatine fossa with bone destruction of the lateral wall of the maxillary sinus and erosion of the deep portions of the lateral wall of the orbit (greater wing of the sphenoid bone) (Figure 27.6B). Exenteration, plus a combined transcranial approach to the sphenoid bone, was performed. Six months after the initial presentation, the patient was being carefully followed, with no certainty that the infection was under control.

These two cases illustrate different presentations of orbital mucormycosis. In the first case, the fulminating course of the disease is an example of aggressiveness rarely encountered in cancers. The second case, in contrast, shows a disease that tends to be locally invasive with an indolent but progressive destructive pattern.

In a previously healthy child, particularly between the ages of 1 and 7 years, rapidly developing proptosis and eyelid edema, often mimicking orbital cellulitis, should always arouse suspicion of rhabdomyosarcoma, which needs to be ruled out by biopsy results. However, the masquerade syndrome may present in reversed order: namely, a child who presents with signs and symptoms of rhabdomyosarcoma may be proven by biopsy results to have infectious etiology. The boy shown in Figure 27.7 provides a good example of the reverse masquerade syndrome. This patient presented with a rapidly enlarging, well-delineated mass in the left orbit, which was worked up with the clinical diagnosis of rhabdomyosarcoma; on biopsy, however, the condition proved to be mucormycosis.

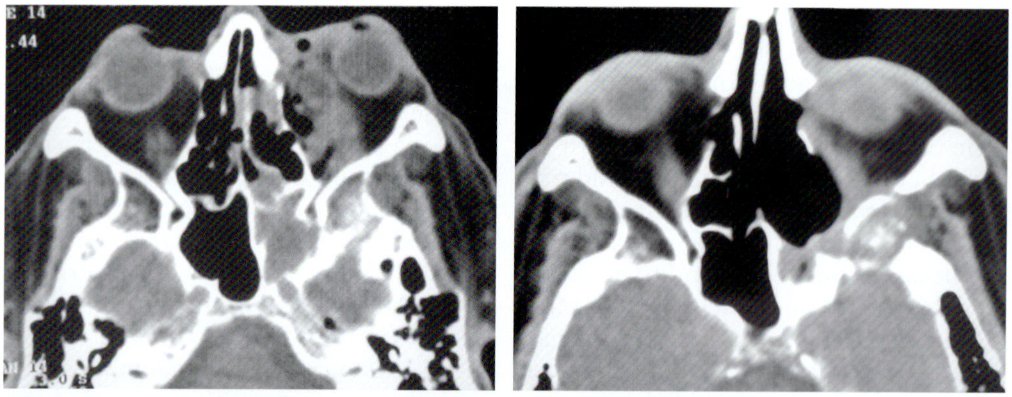

A B

FIGURE 27.6. (A) Opacification in the ethmoidal and sphenoid sinuses with an atypical area of infiltration along the left medial wall. (B) Erosion of the greater wing of the sphenoid bone.

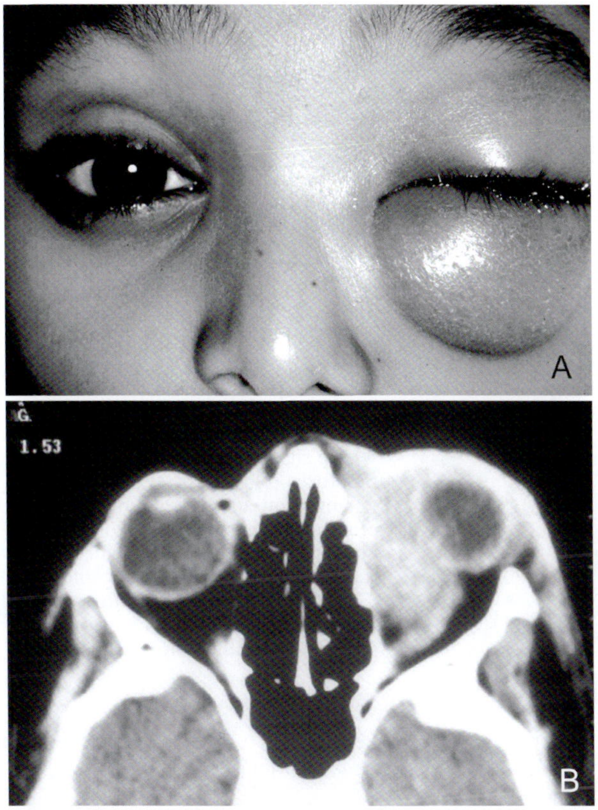

FIGURE 27.7. (A) Eyelid edema and proptosis secondary to rapidly developing medial orbital mass causing bone erosion. (B) Axial scan showing bone erosion due to orbital mass.

The upper respiratory tract involvement of mucormycosis was not obvious at the time of admission, but sinus lesions and pulmonary involvement developed after the biopsy, causing death, despite exenteration and amphotericin B treatment.

Another inflammatory condition that may mimic invasive neoplasm is the allergic fungal disease of the nose and paranasal sinuses (Table 27.2).[39,40] In this disease, the infection starts in the nasal cavity or in the lumen of a paranasal sinus and may extend into the orbit. In most instances, an *Aspergillus* species is the causative organism; other fungal species, including *Fusarium* and *Rhizomucor*, have also been incriminated.[41] Although this entity is considered to be confined to the lumina, without mucosal and submucosal invasion, it nevertheless is known to spread from one paranasal sinus cavity to the other and to the orbit.[42] Imaging studies show bony expansion and remodeling of the involved cavity and focal bony erosion. The mucoid content of the paranasal sinuses mixed with fungus balls produce low signal intensity in MR images. The extensive bony expansion and irregular remodeling, coupled with bony erosion, may simulate an invasive tumor of the nose or the sinus, with secondary orbital invasion, such as esthesioneuroblastoma or leukemia/lymphoma.

The 9-year-old girl shown in Figure 27.8A presented with right-sided proptosis and diplopia; her visual acuity was 20/40 OD, 20/20 OS. She had an initial working diagnosis of a malignant tumor, based on clinical findings. Orbital CT revealed high attenuation within the maxillary ethmoid and the sphenoid sinus. Bone destruction suggested an invasive tumor, but the diffuse nature of the process in paranasal sinuses, coupled with eosinophilia and elevated IgE levels, brought up the possibility of allergic fungal sinusitis. During ethmoidectomy/medial orbitotomy, extensively necrotic, whitish-gray, toothpastelike material was removed from the sinuses. The histopathologic examination of this material revealed a mixture of necrotic mucosal cells, eosinophils, and clusters of septate-fungal hyphae. Fungal cultures revealed the causative organism as *Aspergillus flavus*. The patient's orbital symptoms were resolved, and the visual acuity went back to normal after treatment with surgical debridement and systemic corticosteroids.

CONCLUSIONS

Inflammation and neoplasia may be extremely difficult to differentiate in the orbit. In some cases, a correct diagnosis is made only after consideration of the whole context of the pathology, including clinical presentation, pattern of disease evolution, imaging studies, and histopathologic examination.

TABLE 27.2. Imaging and Histpathologic Features of Allergic Fungal Disease of the Nose, Paranasal Sinuses and Orbit.

CT	*MR*	*Histopathology*
High attenuation	Low signal on T2	Inspissated mucus mass with fungal hyphae in the center and necrotic eosinophils at the periphery
Bony expansion and remodeling; low attenuation surrounding areas of high attenuation	Minimal enhancement of inspissated mucus centrally with subtraction Gd-DPTA study, surrounded by a thin zone of strong enhancement	Severe epithelial edema, loss of seromucineous glands, severe goblet cell hyperplasia, vascularization, and focal fibrosis of submucosa
Bony erosion with irregular bone margins with or without enhancement	Irregular bone signal on T1 and T2	Occasional presence of bony trabeculae with new bone formation; no invasion of bone or submucosal tissues with fungi

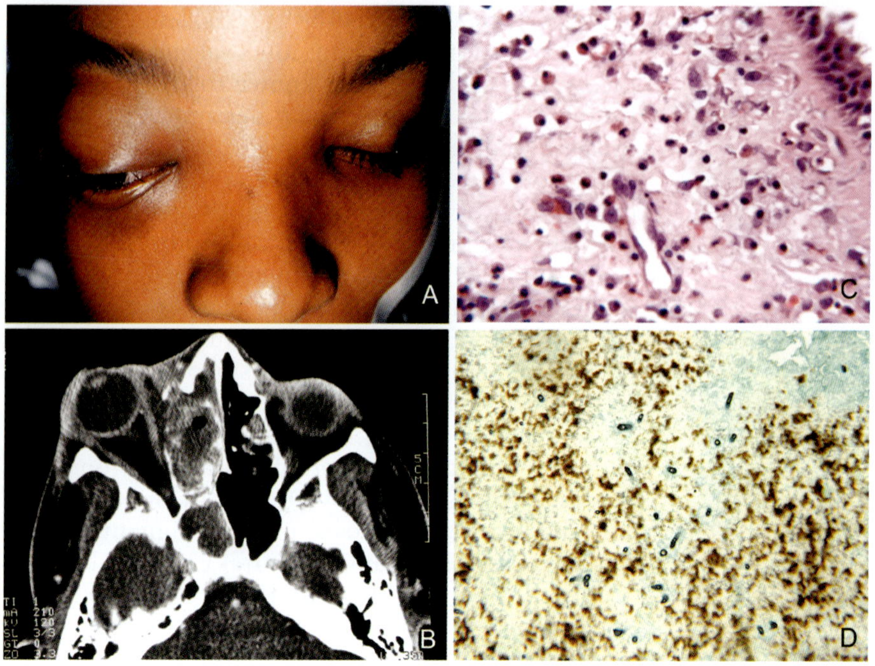

FIGURE 27.8. (A) A 9-year-old girl whose right eye showed inferior lateral proptosis. (B) Axial scan shows enlargement and remodeling of right ethmoidal sinus; bone erosion and orbital invasion are seen medially. Biopsy results revealed numerous eosinophils (C) and hyphae of *Aspergillus* species, (D) depicted clearly (Gomori silver stain (original magnification ×100).

References

1. Cotran R, Kumar V, Collins T. Neoplasia. In: Cotran RS, Kumar V, Collins T, eds. *Robbins Pathologic Basis of Disease*. Vol 1. 6th ed. Philadelphia: WB Saunders; 1999:260–327.
2. Rootman J, Nugent R. The classification and management of acute orbital pseudotumor. *Ophthalmology* 1982;89:1040–1048.
3. Nugent RA, Rootman J, Robertson WD, et al. Acute orbital pseudotumors: classification and CT features. *AJNR Am J Neuroradiol* 1981;137:957–962.
4. Hytiroglou P, Brandwein MS, Strauchen JA, et al. Inflammatory pseudotumor of the paralaryngeal space: case report and review of the literature. *Head-Neck* 1992;14:230–234.
5. Keen M, Conley J, Mutter G, et al. Pseudotumor of the pterygomaxillary space presenting as anesthesia of the mandibular nerve. *Laryngoscope* 1986;96:560–563.
6. Weisman RA, Osguthorpe JD. Pseudotumor of the head and neck masquerading as neoplasia. *Laryngoscope* 1988;96:610–614.
7. Takimoto T, Kathoh T, Ohmura T, et al. Inflammatory pseudotumor of the maxillary sinus mimicking malignancy. *Rhinology* 1990;28:123–127.
8. Som PM, Brandwein MS, Maldjian C, et al. Inflammatory pseudotumor of the maxillary sinus: CT and MR findings in six cases. *AJR Am J Roentgenol* 1994;163:689–692.
9. de Ruiter ED, Kwekkeboom DJ, Mooi WJ, et al. Inflammatory pseudotumor of the fossa pterygopalatina: diagnosis and treatment. *Neth J Med* 2000;56:17–20.
10. De Miguel Garcia F, Aiguabella MAB, Liesa RF. Pseudotumor inflamatorio de senos paranasales. *Acta Otorrinolaring Esp* 1990;41:351–353.
11. Maldjian JA, Norton KI, Groisman GM, Som PM. Inflammatory pseudotumor of the maxillary sinus in a 15-year-old boy. *AJNR Am J Neuroradiol* 1994;15:784–786.
12. Scott IU, Siatkowski RM. Idiopathic orbital myositis. *Curr Opin Rheumatol* 1997;9:504–512.
13. Lacey B, Chang W, Rootman J. Nonthyroid causes of extraocular muscle disease. *Surv Ophthalmol* 1999;44:187–213.
14. Cornblat WT, Elner V, Rolfe M. Extraocular muscle involvement in sarcoidosis. *Ophthalmology* 1993;100:501–505.
15. Patel AS, Kelman SE, Duncan GW, Rismond V. Painless diplopia caused by extraocular muscle sarcoid. *Arch Ophthalmol* 1994;112:879–880.
16. Stannard K, Spalton DJ. Sarcoidosis with infiltration of the external ocular muscles. *Br J Ophthalmol* 1985;69:562–566.
17. Grimson BS, Simons KB. Orbital inflammation, myositis, and systemic lupus erythematosus. *Arch Ophthalmol* 1983;101:736–738.
18. Weinstein GS, Dresner SC, Slamovits TL, Kennerdell JS. Acute and subacute orbital myositis. *Am J Ophthalmol* 1983;96:209–216.
19. Panfilio CB, Hernández-Cossio O, Hernández-Fustes OJ. Orbital myositis and rheumatoid arthritis. *Arq Neuropsiquiatr* 2000;58:174–177.
20. Pinchoff BS, Spahlinger BA, Bergstrom TJ, Sandall GS. Extraocular muscle involvement in Wegener's granulomatosis. *J Clin Neuro-Ophthalmol* 1983;3:163–168.
21. Suttorp-Schulten MSA, Koornneef L. Linear scleroderma associated ptosis and motility disorders. *Br J Ophthalmol* 1990;74:694–695.
22. Seidenberg KB, Leib ML. Orbital myositis with Lyme disease [see Comments]. *Am J Ophthalmol* 1990;109:13–16.
23. Jakobiec FA, Bilyk JR, Font RL. Orbit. In: Spencer WH, ed. *Ophthalmic Pathology: An Atlas and Textbook*. Vol 4. 4th ed. Philadelphia: WB Saunders; 1996:2877–2878.
24. Lin H, Burton EM, Felz MW. Orbital myositis due to Kawasaki's disease. *Pediatr Radiol* 1999;29:634–636.
25. Hornblass A, Jakobiec FA, Reifler DM, Mines J. Orbital lymphoid turmors located predominantly within extraocular muscles. *Ophthalmology* 1987;94:688–697.
26. Divine RD, Anderson RL. Metastatic small cell carcinoma masquerading as orbital myositis. *Ophthalmic Surg* 1982;13:483–487.
27. Rumelt S, Rubin PA. Potential sources for orbital cellulitis. *Int Ophthalmol Clin* 1996;36:207–221.
28. Cleary KR, Batsakis JG. Sinonasal lymphomas. *Ann Otol Rhinol Laryngol* 1994;103:911–914.
29. Jaffe ES, Chan JKC, Su IJ, et al. Report of the workshop on nasal and related extranodal angiocentric T/natural killer cell lymphomas. *Am J Surg Pathol* 1996;20:103–111.

30. Tsokos M, Fauci AS, Costa J. Idiopathic midline destructive disease—a subgroup of patients with the "midline granuloma" syndrome. *Am J Clin Pathol* 1982;77:162–168.
31. Mann WJ, Riede UN, Bocking A. Midline malignant reticulosis. *Acta Otolaryngol* 1984;97:365–372.
32. Eichel BS, Harrison EG, Devine KD, et al. Primary lymphoma of the nose including a relationship to lethal midline granuloma. *Am J Surg* 1966;112:597–605.
33. McDonald TJ, DeRemee RA, Weiland LH. Wegener's granulomatosis and polymorphic reticulosis—two diseases or one? *Arch Otol* 1981;107:141–144.
34. DeRemee RA, Weiland LH, McDonald TJ. Polymorphic reticulosis, lymphomatoid granulomatosis—two diseases or one? *Mayo Clin Proc* 1978;53:634–640.
35. Kwon-Chung KJ, Bennet JE. Mucormycosis. In: Kwon-Chung KJ, Bennet JE, eds. *Medical Mycology*. Vol 1. Philadelphia: Lea & Febiger; 1992:524–529.
36. Rootman J. Inflammatory diseases. In: Rootman J, ed. *Diseases of the Orbit*. Vol 1. 2nd ed. Philadelphia: JB Lippincott; 2003: 455–506.
37. Dooley DP, Hollsten DA, Grimes SR, Moss JJ. Indolent orbital apex syndrome caused by occult mucormycosis. *J Clin Neuro-Ophthalmol* 1992;12:245–249.
38. Kameh DS, Gonzalez OR, Pearl GS, et al. Fatal rhino-orbital-cerebral zygomycosis. *South Med J* 1997;90:1133–1135.
39. Chang WJ, Shields CL, Shields JA, et al. Bilateral orbital involvement with massive allergic fungal sinusitis. *Arch Ophthalmol* 1996;114:767–768.
40. Dunlop IS, Billson FA. Visual failure in allergic aspergillus sinusitis: case report. *Br J Ophthalmol* 1988;72:127–130.
41. Torres C, El Naggar AK, Sim SJ, et al. Allergic fungal sinusitis: a clinical pathological study of 16 cases. *Hum Pathol* 1996; 27:793–799.
42. Michaels L, Lloyd G, Phelps T. Origin and spread of allergic fungal disease of the nose and paranasal sinuses. *Clin Otolaryngol Allied Sci* 2000;25:518–525.
43. Cruz AAV, Akeishi PMS, Chahud F, Eliac Jr. J. Sclerosing inflammation in the orbit and in the pterygopalatine and infratemporal tissue. *Ophthal Plastic Reconstr Surg* 2003;19:201–206.
44. Siqueira GB, Jain A, Chahud F, Cruz AAV. Bilateral infraorbital nerve involvement in idiopathic orbital myositis. *Ophthal Plastic Reconstr Surg* 2002;18:474–478.

28

Graves Disease

Daniel Weil and Guillermo A. Fridrich

Although Graves disease (GD) is a type of orbital inflammation, certain clinical features may be confused with orbital tumors. Therefore, a brief review of GD is included in this book. Graves disease presents with a great variability of clinical signs; for this there are numerous nomenclatures and classifications in the literature. Among others, thyroid-associated orbitopathy and thyroid-related ophthalmopathy are descriptive names, even though in about 10% of the cases orbital signs are observed without chemically detectable thyroid manifestations. The name *Graves disease* is the time-honored terminology, used by many ophthalmologists. An orbital inflammation associated with GD can present diverse changes in the orbit, ranging from a cosmetic lid retraction to a loss of vision produced by the compressive optic neuropathy. Management must be directed to the systemic thyroid disease as well as to local ocular and orbital changes.[1–4]

PATHOGENESIS

The pathogenesis of GD is not completely understood; it is labeled an autoimmune process.[5,6] It occurs in a genetically preselected population, usually affecting middle-aged females four to five times more frequently than males. The propensity for development and severity of the orbital disease may be related to immunogenetic predisposition as well. The hypothesis is that circulating T cells directed against an antigen in thyroid follicular cells recognize a similar antigen in orbital tissues. The activated T cells infiltrate the orbital soft tissues and the fibers of extraocular muscles.[6] Thyroid-stimulating hormone receptor mRNA has been detected in orbital fat specimens.[7] Clinical and experimental studies suggest that the thyrotropin receptor (TSH-R) is one of the possible antigens stimulating the autoantibodies implicated in the inflammatory changes of orbital soft tissues. The antigen may be recognized by a receptor on CD4+ T lymphocytes. After antigen recognition, lymphocytes secrete cytokines that amplify the immune reaction by activating CD8+ T lymphocytes or autoantibody-producing B cells. In GD there is a predominance of T cells with a T_H1 profile [interleukin (IL)2, interferon γ, tumor necrosis factor α], although a T_H2 profile of cytokine production (IL-4, -5, -10) has also been reported.[6] The cytokines stimulate fibroblasts to synthesize and secrete glycosaminoglycans. The higher glycosaminoglycan content in GD is largely due to an excess of chondroitin sulfate and hyaluronic acid. Orbital fibroblasts may contribute to perpetuating the immune reaction by protecting T cells from apoptosis. The immune-mediated process leads to inflammation and deposition of hydrophilic mucopolysaccharides and collagen, resulting in muscle injury and scarring. The extraocular muscles are also infiltrated by lymphocytes, plasma cells, and mast cells that cause degenerative changes. Another interesting finding is the observation of degenerative muscle changes in temporal muscle biopsy samples obtained from active GD patients during decompression surgery (personal communication with Dr. Karcioglu, 2003), indicating that other musculature in the vicinity is also affected with the pathologic process. Cell-mediated immune reactions predominate in early GD, whereas humoral immunity plays a greater role in later stages.[5–7]

SYSTEMIC CLINICAL FEATURES

GD presents with different manifestations of thyroid dysfunction, including hyperthyroidism, hypothyroidism, and Hashimoto's thyroiditis; it may also be seen in euthyroid patients. Hyperthyroidism is the most frequent thyroid dysfunction related to orbital disease (90%), and its systemic signs and symptoms may include weight loss, smooth skin, tachycardia, pretibial myxedema and clubbing of the fingers and toes, and subperiosteal new bone formation (thyroid dermopathy and thyroid acropathy). When the systemic features of hyperthyroidism are present, the diagnosis is rather straightforward, especially with lid retraction or exophthalmos. GD, however, may occur in apparently euthyroid (6%) or hypothyroid (1%) patients as well as in those with thyroiditis (3%).[8] In these settings the diagnosis may be more challenging. All patients with possible thyroid-related orbital disease should be followed jointly with an endocrinologist. However, the ophthalmologist should also be fa-

BOX 28.1. Laboratory Tests to Evaluate Thyroid Function in Patients with Orbital Graves Disease

Serum triiodothyronine (T_3) and thyroxine (T_4)
Triiodothyronine (T_3) uptake and free thyroxine (T_4) index
Serum thyrotropin (thyroid-stimulating hormone, TSH)
Thyrotropin receptor antibodies (TRA)
Thyroid hormone antibodies

miliar with the thyroid function tests (Box 28.1) and the possible effects of commonly used medications on thyroid functions (Table 28.1).[3] GD is most frequent in younger women (Figure 28.1) but presents with more severe symptoms in men and patients older than 50 years of age.[9] GD may be seen in children, but they are unlikely to develop severe forms of the disease. In some cases goiter is present, especially in endemic areas. Between 30 and 35% of the patients have family history of thyroid disease. The average age at the time of diagnosis of GD is 46 with an age range of 8 to 88 years.[10,11]

ORBITAL HISTOPATHOLOGY

The histopathologic changes can be divided into two stages. The first is the active inflammatory stage, in which one can find perivascular groups of inflammatory cells in loose edematous tissue; these include plasma cells and lymphocytes. Lymphoid follicles are less frequent in GD than in pseudotumors. In the second stage, the volume of the orbital content is increased by infiltration of fibroblasts, collagen, mucopolysaccharides, and glycoproteins. The mucopolysaccharides are hygroscopic. This property leads to the edema of all orbital soft tissues, particularly muscles. Increased numbers of interstitial fibroblasts and chronic inflammatory cells infiltrate the muscle fibers. In this chronic stage, the muscles become fibrotic and the anti-inflammatory treatment is no longer effective. Fibrotic phase of the disease can be demonstrated with the absence of high signal intensity in T2-weighted magnetic resonance (MR) images.[12,13]

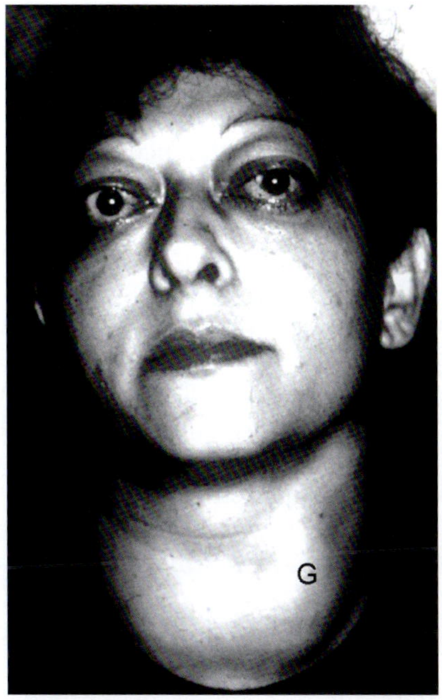

FIGURE 28.1. Bilateral proptosis due to Graves disease with a massively enlarged multinodular goiter (G).

TABLE 28.1. Effects of Some Commonly Used Drugs on Thyroid Function Tests.

	Tests			
Drugs	T_3	T_4	Free T_4	TSH
Amiodarone	↓	↑	↑	↑
Androgens	↓	↓	N	N
Cholestyramine	—	↓	↓	↑
Diphenylhydantoin	↓	↓	↑	↓
Estrogens	↑	↑	↑	N
5-Fluorouracil	↑	↑	↑	N
Furosemide	↓	↓	↑	↓
Glucocorticoids	↓	↓	N	N
Heparin	↓	↓	↑	↓
Iodine	↓	↓	↓	↑
Iron	—	↓	↓	↑
Lithium	↓	↓	↓	↑
Phenylbutazone	↓	↓	↑	↓
Propylthiouracil	↓	—	—	↑
Propranolol	↓	—	—	↑
Salicylates	↓	↓	↑	↓
Sucralfate	—	↓	↓	↑
Sulfonylureas	↓	↓	↑	↓

N, normal.

ORBITAL CLINICAL FEATURES

The orbital clinical manifestations may present in an acute, subacute, or chronic pattern and may also start with any of the different clinical signs. All the orbital clinical signs can be unilateral or bilateral, but they may present unilaterally at the outset and later become bilateral as the disease progresses. Upper lid retraction is the most frequent orbital clinical sign in early GD (75% at initial diagnosis and 90% at some point in the clinical course) and may lead to the false impression of proptosis.[14] Generally, upper lid retraction is produced by sympathetic tonicity of the Müller muscle at the beginning of the clinical course and then by the inflammation and fibrosis of the levator muscle. Less frequently, the inferior lid may also be retracted.

Bilateral proptosis is the second most frequent sign (62%); it is mainly caused by muscle enlargement, with or without active inflammation (Figure 28.2). Displacement of the globe by Hertel exophthalmometry over 20 mm or a difference between the orbits over 3 mm suggests true proptosis. An exophthalmometry measurement over 30 mm is classified as severe proptosis. The enlargement of the lacrimal gland may also increase the exophthalmos.

Restrictive extraocular palsy is present in about 40% of GD patients (Figure 28.3). It is produced by infiltration and enlargement of the ocular muscles and can be unilateral or bilateral. Medial and inferior recti are most commonly involved, but all the muscles may be affected. The impaired upward gaze is the most common extraocular muscle (EOM) limitation. Diplopia is noted at the initial examination in approximately 20% of cases.[8]

Optic nerve dysfunction (6%) may produce color deficiency and afferent papillary defect or loss of vision and field due to compressive optic neuropathy.[8] Such dysfunction is caused by the compression of the optic nerve by the EOM in the apex or by stretching of the optic nerve in severe exophthalmos. In initial stages of the optic nerve dysfunction, this neuropathy typically shows different degrees of visual field contraction (peripheral scotoma). Testing the visual field is the best way to monitor the progression of the optic neuropathy. The earliest symptoms may be the impairment of color vision or mild afferent pupillary defect. If the lids cannot close well (lagophthalmos), there may be keratitis or ulceration of the cornea, which in turn may develop into endophthalmitis and loss of vision.[14] The ocular hypertension in patients with GD is caused by the elevated intraorbital pressure associated with orbital congestion or contraction of EOM muscles. The prevalence has been reported to be approximately 20%.[14] In the select subgroup of patients with GD who required orbital decompression and strabismus surgery, a significant reduction in intraocular pressure in the early postoperative period was documented.[15]

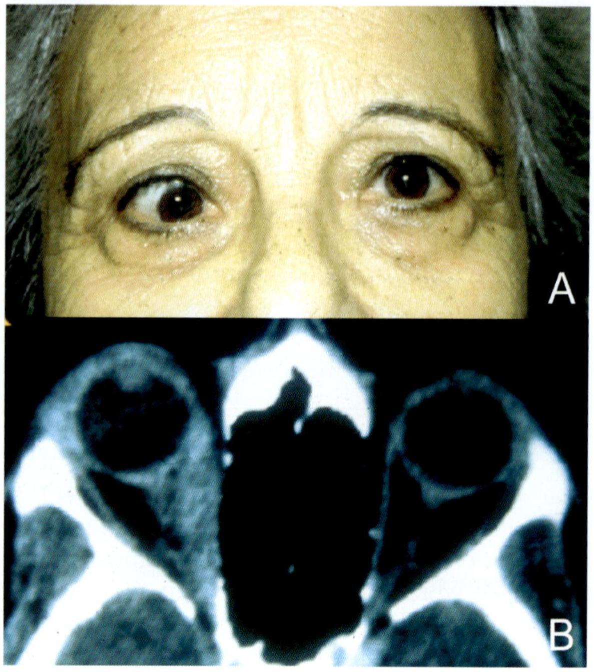

FIGURE 28.3. (A) Single-muscle involvement of Graves disease, causing esotropia of the right eye. (B) The CT scan shows enlarged right medial rectus muscle with scarring but not a significant amount of proptosis, indicating the chronic stage of the disease.

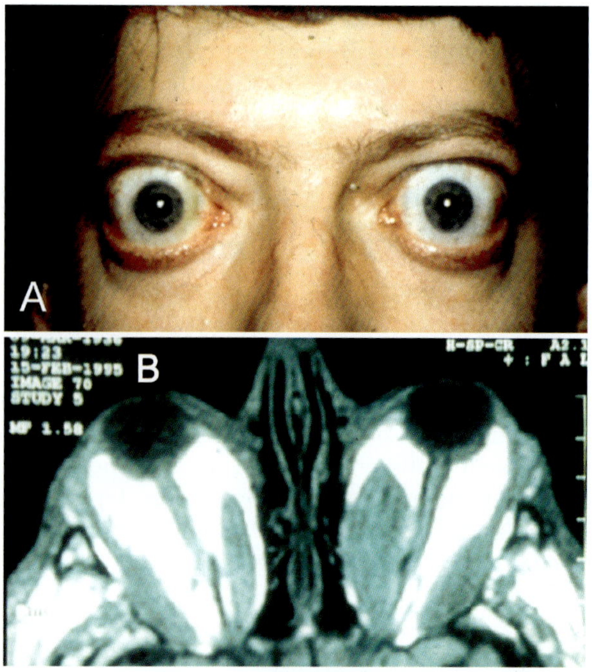

FIGURE 28.2. (A) Typical multimuscle Graves disease with severe proptosis of both eyes and retraction of upper and lower eyelids. (B) Although the left medial rectus muscle reveals the most prominent enlargement, the bilateral involvement of all horizontal recti is clearly depicted in the T1-weighted MRI image.

Pain is seldom a manifestation in GD, but patients usually complain of a retrobulbar pressure sensation. A complete constellation of typical features (hyperthyroidism, eyelid retraction, exophthalmos, restrictive extraocular myopathy, and optic nerve dysfunction) is not frequent. Smoking has been shown to be an important factor in the development of GD.[16] Several classifications of the ocular signs of GD have been reported, but none is of much use. It is very difficult to standardize the orbital variations.[17,18] The best known is the "NO SPECS" outline, which was introduced by the American Thyroid Association in 1969.[18] Other classifications include the Ophthalmology Index proposed by Donaldson in 1973 and Van Dyck's modification of NOSPECS in 1981.[19] Finally in 1992 the International Thyroid Association decided to abandon NOSPECS for clinical studies.[20]

GD can also be divided into noninfiltrative or infiltrative disease.[2] The noninfiltrative subgroup shows as part of the thyroid disease lid retraction, which may regress with the control of the thyroid endocrinopathy. In other cases lid retraction and proptosis are not related to the underlying endocrine disorder. The infiltrative disease manifests itself with soft tissue alterations and muscle disease.

RADIOLOGIC FEATURES

The best tests to evaluate the orbital changes of GD are the computed tomography (CT) scan and MR imaging (Figure 28.2B) (Boxes 28.2 and 28.3).[21–23] The CT scan is a valuable means of depicting the enlargement of the EOMs; it also helps to document infiltrative versus noninfiltrative disease. The axial films show the medial and the lateral recti and their relationship to the optic nerve. The coronal sections are more useful to evaluate the enlargement of the muscles and the orbital apex. "Crowded" apex is an apt name to describe the hypertrophy of the muscles in the posterior orbit that may lead to compressive optic neuropathy (Figure 28.4). MR imaging is more useful than CT to evaluate the nature of the pathology within the muscle, especially in cases of EOM enlargement due to pseudotumor or metastasis.

Orbital ultrasonography can also be helpful in establishing the diagnosis of GD by showing intramuscular changes (Figure 28.5). Although muscle enlargement typically presents as a bilateral condition, affecting multiple extraocular muscles, it may begin as an asymmetrical presentation with significant changes in one orbit and none in the other. Echography is particularly useful here because this technique can reveal very early changes in the orbit. The most commonly enlarged muscles as detected by echography are the superior rectus–levator complex and the medial rectus, followed by inferior and lateral recti. On the other hand, the most common clinical motility problem in GD is the limitation of the superior gaze, indicating the involvement of the inferior rectus muscle.[24] The internal reflectivity of the involved muscle in GD is typically medium during the active inflammatory phase; it becomes high when the muscle develops fibrosis in later stages of the disease (Figure 28.5B).[25] Echography can be done in the clinic quickly and inexpensively. However, ultrasonography is not effective for evaluating the posterior orbit, particularly the apex area.

Echography may also be helpful to differentiate myositis from GD. Although myositis may involve multiple muscles, unlike GD, it typically presents acutely and with severe pain.[26] The involved muscle in myositis shows diffuse thickening, in the muscle itself and in its tendon. In contrast, in thyroid disease the tendon is classically spared. The internal reflec-

BOX 28.2. The CT Features of Graves Disease

- Enlargement of muscle body (70–75% have muscle hypertrophy, mainly medial and inferior recti)
- Compression of optic nerve in the orbital apex by the enlarged extraocular muscles
- Increased orbital fat volume
- Convex shape of ethmoidal wall in chronic disease
- Image of the enlargement of the inferior rectus in back third of orbit in axial views may mimic orbital tumor
- Elongation of the globe and stretch of the optic nerve secondary to proptosis

BOX 28.3. MRI Features of Graves Disease

- Increased volume of intra- and extraconal space
- Heterogeneous fat in T1-weighted image due to vascularization and congestion (hypointense signal)
- Hypointense signal in the middle of the muscle (fat and inflammatory cell infiltration) with T1-weighted image
- Hyperintense signal of the muscle with T2-weighted image
- Increased muscle vascularization with GDPA

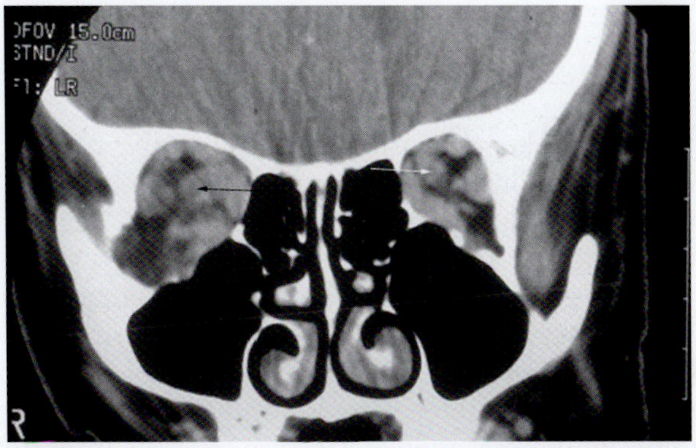

FIGURE 28.4. Coronal CT scan show bilateral "crowding" of the orbital apex with compression of the muscles onto the optic nerves (arrows).

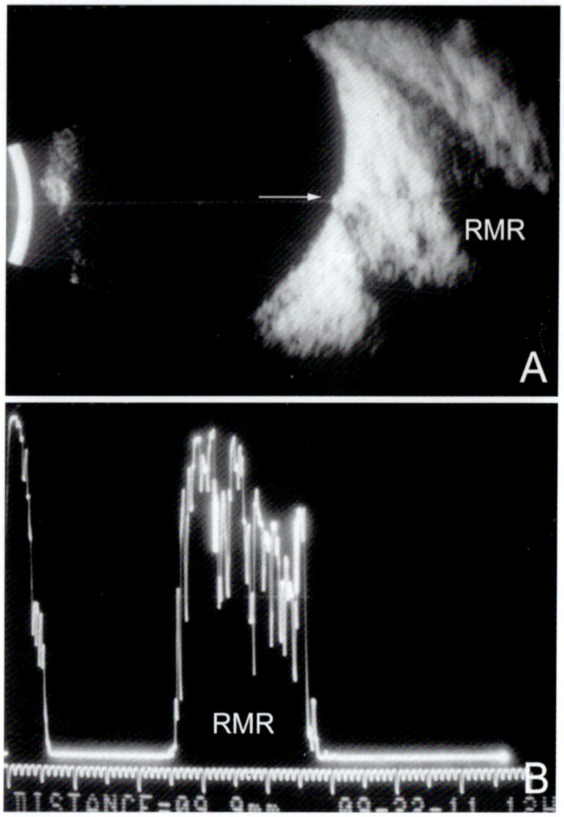

FIGURE 28.5. Echograms of an enlarged right medial rectus muscle (RMR) in a patient with Graves disease.

tivity in myositis is usually low during the acute stages of the disease; however, it may change to medium or high when fibrosis has developed within the muscle after several episodes of myositis.

Echography can also be useful to differentiate neoplastic diseases of extraocular muscles from inflammatory pathology. Metastatic tumors to the intraocular muscles usually present with rapidly developing unilateral proptosis involving a single muscle.[27] Color Doppler imaging can be used to monitor patients with GD for alterations in orbital blood flow parameters and their correlations with EOM enlargement, proptosis, and intraocular pressure.[28,29]

DIFFERENTIAL DIAGNOSIS

It should be kept in mind that GD is the most frequent cause not only of bilateral proptosis but also of unilateral proptosis as well (Figure 28.6). The early presentation of the disease may be with asymmetrical proptosis, secondary to more active disease in one orbit. Slowly progressive unilateral presentation of GD may be confused with orbital pseudotumors (orbital myositis, fibrosclerosis) and neoplasia (lymphoma, leukemia, metastatic tumors).[30,31] In certain instances, solitary vascular lesions, such as an orbital varix, may also be confused with GD.[32] When the clinical presentation of GD consists of bilateral proptosis with lid retraction, chemosis, and vascular tortuosity at the insertion sites of extraocular muscles, along with the typical complaint of burning sensation and tearing and pressure behind the globe, diagnosis is not difficult. In other instances, patients may develop asymmetrical proptosis, and there will be absence of congested conjunctiva and upper eyelid ptosis instead of lid retraction. These cases may be confused with the tumors of the orbit. The retraction of the upper eyelid must be distinguished from the pseudoretraction, which may occur in an effort to overcome ptosis. The most confusing picture may be an isolated enlargement of an extraocular muscle. Myositis usually presents with pain, and the imaging workup reveals the enlargement of the muscle insertion (tendon). Another feature of the pseudotumor is its rapid response to steroid treatment.[33] Lymphoma is another tumor that needs to be considered in unilateral GD.[34] Careful examination of imaging studies usually reveals that the lymphoproliferative process is not limited to the muscle but homogeneously extends into other soft tissues of the orbit.

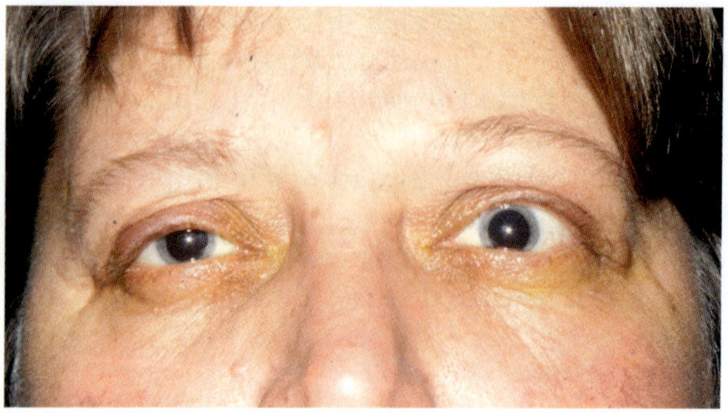

FIGURE 28.6. Unilateral proptosis of a patient who presented with asymmetrical Graves disease. However, 11 months after initial diagnosis, she developed bilateral involvement of all horizontal recti.

Orbital metastatic disease may be confusing if it limits itself to the EOM, in which case, the imaging workup depicts nodular enlargement on CT and MRI (Figure 28.7). Irregular intramuscular neoplastic for-

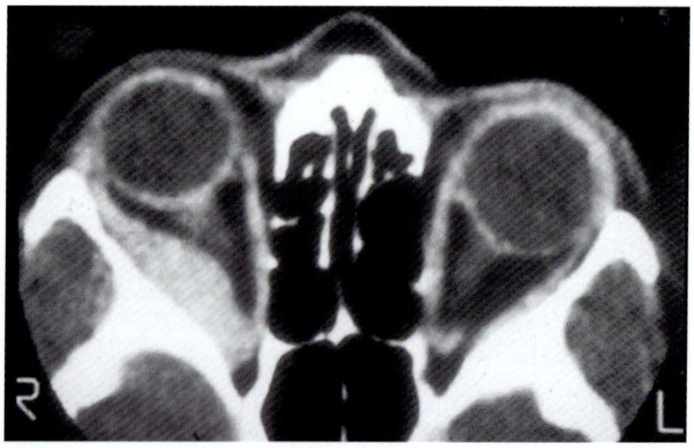

FIGURE 28.7. An enlarged right lateral rectus muscle, secondary to metastatic colon cancer, showing slight proptosis of the right eye. Note the heterogeneity of the belly of the muscle, due to infiltrating carcinoma. All other muscles are within normal limits.

mations are best depicted with T2-weighted hypersignal of MRI. Systemic workup to identify a possible primary tumor should be started immediately in these cases.

MANAGEMENT AND PROGNOSIS

A detailed discussion of GD management is not within the scope of this book. It is briefly mentioned, however, that there are different therapies for GD. The orbital disease may have a self-limited course from 6 months to 3 years, but the evolution of the disease cannot be predicted. Medical therapies include artificial tears and ointments, elevation of the head during sleep, and ice compress. Oral and intravenous corticosteroid treatments are recommended by some for acute or subacute advancing disease that affects the cornea and the optic nerve.[35–38] In case of severe neuropathy, it may be necessary to use intravenous corticosteroid pulse (Tg/day) 1 g methyprednisolone for 3 days. Peribulbar triamcinolone (20 mg of triamcinolone into each orbit every week for 4 weeks) may be effective to improve proptosis and diplopia, especially in acute cases.[39] The peribulbar administration does not cause local or systemic adverse effects. A poor response to local or systemic steroids does not exclude a good response to radiation. Radiotherapy has been used for many years with mixed benefits, especially for optic neuropathy, but recent reports question its effectiveness.[40,41]

Decompression is the time-honored surgical treatment for reducing exophthalmos and for optic neuropathy.[42–44] EOM imbalance, which may develop as a manifestation of the disease or as a complication of orbital decompression, requires surgery after 6 months of stability.[45] Eyelid surgery may be used as the last surgical intervention for retraction and cosmesis.[46]

In 1996 Bartley reported that about 75% of 120 patients required either no therapy or only supportive measures, 6% were treated with systemic corticosteroids, and 20% underwent one or more surgical procedures.[11]

References

1. Char DH. *Thyroid Eye Disease.* Baltimore: Williams & Wilkins; 1995.
2. Rootman J, ed. *Diseases of the Orbit.* Philadelphia: JB Lippincott; 1988.
3. Felig P, Baxter JD, Frohman LA. *Endocrinology and Metabolism.* 3rd ed. New York: McGraw-Hill; 1995.
4. Pérez Moreiras José V, Prada Sánchez MC. *Oftalmopatia Distiroidea.* Barcelona: Edika Med; 1997.
5. Warwar R. New insights into pathogenesis and potential therapeutic options for Graves orbitopathy. *Curr Opin Ophthalmol* 1999;10:358–361.
6. Diez J. Therapy of Graves' ophthalmopathy: a novel application of somatostatin analogues. *Expert Opin Pharmacother* 2001-2;9:1361–1365.
7. Bradley E. Graves' ophthalmopathy. *Curr Opin Ophthalmol* 2001;12:347–351.
8. Bartley G, et al. Clinical features of Graves' ophthalmopathy in an incidence cohort. *Am J Ophthalmol* 1996;121:284–290.
9. Kendler DL, Lippa J, Rootman J. The initial clinical characteristics of Graves' orbitopathy vary with age and sex. *Arch Ophthalmol* 1993;111:197–201.
10. Bartley G, et al. The chronology of Graves' ophthalmopathy in an incidence cohort. *Am J Ophthalmol* 1996;121:426–434.
11. Bartley G, et al. Long-term follow-up of Graves' ophthalmopathy in an incidence cohort. *Ophthalmology* 1996;103:958–962.
12. Ohnishi T, Noguchi S, Murakami N, et al. Extraocular muscles in Graves' ophthalmopathy: usefulness of T2 relaxation time measurements. *Radiology* 1994;190:857–862.
13. Utech CI, Khatibnia U, Winter PF, Wulle KG. MR T2 relaxation time for the assessment of retrobulbar inflammation in Graves' ophthalmopathy. *Thyroid* 1995;5:185–193.
14. Bartley G. The differential diagnosis and classification of eyelid retraction. *Ophthalmology* 1996;103,1:168–176.
15. Danesh-Meyer H, Savino P, Deramo V, et al. Intraocular pressure changes after treatment for Graves' orbitopathy. *Ophthalmology* 2001;108:145–150.
16. Nunery WR, Martin TR. The association of cigarette smoking with clinical subtypes of ophthalmic Graves' disease. *Ophthalmic Plast Reconstr Surg* 1993;9:77–82.
17. Bartley G. Evolution of classification systems for Graves' ophthalmopathy. *Ophthalmic Plast Reconstr Surg* 1995;11,4:229–237.
18. Werner SC. Modification of the classification of the eye changes of Graves' disease. *Am J Ophthalmol* 1977;83:5,725–726.
19. Van Dyck H. Orbital Graves' disease. A modification of the "NO SPECS" classification. *Ophthalmology* 1981,88:479–483.
20. Werner SC. Classification of the eye changes of Graves' disease. *J Clin Endocrinol* 1969;29:782.
21. Peyster GR. Hoover E. *Computerized Tomography in Orbital Disease and Neuro-Ophthalmology.* Chicago: Year Book Medical Publishers; 1984:97–114.
22. De Potter PV, Shields JA, Shields CL. *MRI of the Eye and Orbit.* Philadelphia: JB Lippincott; 1995.
23. Oguz V, Yolar M, Pazarli H. L'Intérêt de l'IRM dans le traitement de la myopathie de l'orbitopathie dysthyroidienne. *J Fr Ophtalmol* 2001;24:842–846.
24. Rootman, J. Graves' orbitopathy. In: Rootman J, ed. *Diseases of the Orbit.* Philadelphia: JB Lippincott; 1988:248.
25. Ossoinig, KC. The role of standardized ophthalmic echography in the management of Graves' ophthalmopathy. *Dev Ophthalmol* 1989;20:28.
26. Kennerdell, JS, Dresner, SC. The non-specific orbital inflammatory syndromes. *Surv Ophthalmol* 1984;29:97.
27. Slamovits, TL, Burde, RM. Bumpy muscles. *Surv Ophthalmol* 1988;33:189.
28. Numan AM, Günalp I. Color Doppler imaging of the orbital vasculature in Graves' disease with computed tomographic correlation. *Br J Ophthalmol* 2000;84:1027–1030.
29. Williamson TH, Harris A. Color Doppler ultrasound imaging of the eye and orbit. *Surv Ophthalmol* 1996;40:255–267.
30. Van der Pol R, Nieuewenhuis MG, Mourtis MP. Multifocal fibrosclerosis presenting as Grave's orbitopathy. Bilateral exophthalmos. *Graefe Arch Clin Exp Ophthalmol* 1999;237:256–258.
31. Lam A, Faye M, Seck CM, et al. Non-sarcomatous bilateral exophthalmos disclosing acute myeloblastic leukemia in children. *J Fr Ophtalmol* 1996;19:283–286.
32. Yazici B, Yazici Z, Gelisken O. An unusual case: bilateral orbital varices. *Acta Ophthalmol Scand* 1999;77:453–455.
33. Srivastava S, Newman J. Pseudo-pseudotumor. *Surv Ophthalmol* 2000;45:135–138.

34. Jones IS, Jakobiec FA. *Diseases of the Orbit*. New York: Harper & Row; 1979.
35. Fatourechi V. Medical treatment of Graves' ophthalmopathy. *Ophthalmol Clin North Am* 2000;13,4:683–691.
36. Marcocci C, Bartalena L, Tanda ML, et al. Comparison of the effectiveness and tolerability of intravenous or oral glucocorticoids associated with orbital radiotherapy in the management of severe Graves' ophthalmopathy: results of a prospective, single-blind randomized study. *J Clin Endocrinol Metab* 2001; 86:3562–3567.
37. Werner SC. Prednisone in emergency treatment of malignant exophthalmos. *Lancet* 1966;7:1004.
38. Bartalena L, Marocci C, Pinchera A. Treating severe Graves' ophthalmopathy. *Baillieres Clin Endocrinol Metab* 1997;11: 521–536.
39. Ebner R, et al. Tratamiento de la oftalmopatia asociada con distiroidismo con triancinolona periocular. *Arch Oftalmol Buenos Aires* 2001;76:55–66.
40. Schaefer U, Hesselmann S, Micke O, Willich N. A long-term follow-up study after retro-orbital irradiation for Graves' ophthalmopathy. *Int J Radiat Oncol Biol Phys*. 2002;52:192–197.
41. Gorman C, Garrity J, Bartley G. A prospective, randomized, double-blind placebo-controlled study of orbital radiotherapy for Graves' ophthalmopathy. *Ophthalmology* 2001;108,9: 1523–1534.
42. Meyer D. Surgical management of Graves' orbitopathy. *Curr Opin Ophthalmol* 1999;10:343–351.
43. Tarrus-Montaner S, Lucarelli J, Lemke B, Dortzbach R. The surgical treatment of Graves' orbitopathy. *Ophthalmol Clin North Am* 2000;13:693–704.
44. Goldberg RA. The evolving paradigm of orbital decompression surgery. *Arch Ophthalmol* 1998;116:95–96.
45. Nguyen VT, Park DJ, Levin L, Feldon SE. Correction of restricted extraocular muscle motility in surgical management of strabismus in Graves' ophthalmopathy. *Ophthalmology* 2002;109:384–388.
46. Harvey JT, Anderson RL. The aponeurotic approach to eyelid retraction. *Ophthalmology* 1981;88:513.

29

Mass-Forming Inflammatory Lesions of the Orbit

Zeynel A. Karcıoglu

Many inflammatory conditions, ranging from simple foreign body granuloma (Figure 29.1) to the most complex vasculitis of a collagen tissue disease, may cause proptosis owing to volume increase in the orbit.[1–3] The great majority of these disorders present with typical ocular/orbital signs and symptoms, as well as systemic manifestations, that would differentiate them from neoplastic conditions. Others, however, particularly the ones that tend to develop localized mass lesions rather than infiltrating inflammation, may simulate orbital neoplasms. This chapter summarizes the salient clinical features of the more common, mass-forming inflammatory lesions, which can be confused with orbital neoplasms; others are listed in Tables 29.1 and 29.2. Some related clinical presentations are detailed in Chapter 27 with illustrations from cases.

INFECTIONS

Tuberculosis

Ocular and adnexal tuberculosis is usually seen with typical manifestations secondary to systemic *Mycobacterium* infection, and it is rather unlikely that this entity will be confused with neoplastic disorders.[4–6] However, the clinical picture of the disease is changing, with many cases developing from atypical mycobacteria that are resistant to traditional multidrug treatment.[7,8] With the increase in the numbers of immunologically suppressed individuals secondary to viral epidemics and the wider use of immunosuppressant antimetabolites in longer surviving cancer and transplant patients, the incidence of tuberculosis has been rising steadily during the past two decades. It has been reported that individuals with HIV/AIDS have an incidence of tuberculosis 500-fold greater than that of the general population.[9]

Extrapulmonary tuberculosis, including the orbital disease, is more often seen in children and nonwhite patients.[10] Although ocular and adnexal infections due to atypical mycobacteria are rare, occasional cases presenting as dacryocystitis, endophthalmitis, localized periostitis, or periorbital and orbital mass lesions have been reported.[11,12] Orbital tuberculosis due to atypical mycobacteria may present as a well-delineated mass lesion, causing gradual displacement of the eye and extraocular motility disturbances.[13,14] The history of an antecedent penetrating injury is a well-known presentation of tuberculosis, due to atypical mycobacteria. If tuberculosis is suspected clinically, tuberculin skin testing will be helpful in differential diagnosis; but a biopsy, with or without positive cultures, is necessary for the confirmation of the disease. Histopathology of tuberculosis consists of zonal granulomatous inflammation with numerous epithelioid histiocytes surrounding a necrotic (caseating) center. Tissue diagnosis is pathognomonic only with the documentation of positive acid-fast organisms. However, it is well known that acid-fast positive mycobacteria often are not demonstrated in tuberculosis, even though cultures of orbital tissue may grow *M. tuberculosis* or atypical mycobacteria.

It should be remembered that atypical mycobacterial infections generally are resistant to routine antituberculous chemotherapy; clarithromycin, an oral macrolide antibiotic, has been reported to be an effective medication for atypical mycobacterial infections.[12]

Fungal Infections

Commonly encountered fungal infections of the orbit are mucormycosis and aspergillosis. Mucormycosis rarely produces clinical manifestations to mimic orbital tumors. The fulminant course of orbital disease with pain, massive proptosis, extensive extraocular motility disturbance, and hemorrhagic chemosis, coupled with necrotic eschars of the nasal, oropharyngeal mucosa or periorbital skin, is typical of this infection and does not leave too much room for differential diagnosis.[15] Imaging may be helpful by demonstrating a relationship between the orbital and sinus disease. T2-weighted magnetic resonance imaging (MRI) usually reveals hypointensity of fungal disease, and computed tomography (CT) shows focal calcification of the orbitosinusoidal mass.[16] However, certain cases involving the eyelids and the orbit may present with gradually de-

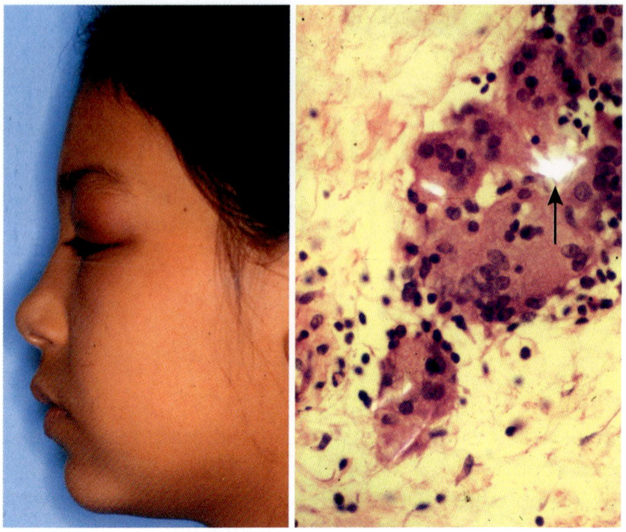

FIGURE 29.1. Foreign body granuloma of the superior orbit in a 9-year old girl. At surgery, infiltrating foreign body granuloma composed of epithelioid cells and multinucleated giant cells was identified. The nature of the foreign body (arrow) could not be determined.

veloping, localized lesions, which may be confused with rapidly growing tumors, such as rhabdomyosarcoma and Ewing's sarcoma (see Chapter 27). Diagnosis is established by documentation of typical, large mucor hyphae, which show lack of septation in tissue examination by histopathology or cytopathology.

Orbital mucormycosis is an emergency situation because it causes rapidly progressing necrotizing inflammation secondary to the propensity of the fungus to involve blood vessels. Orbital exploration should be done immediately to establish the diagnosis by identifying the broad, nonseptated hyphae and for extensive surgical debridement as well as irrigation with antifungal agents.

Orbital aspergillosis usually presents with a more insidious onset, particularly when it develops in individuals who are not immunocompromised.[17] In these cases, the disease may follow a protracted course with a well-delineated mass developing within the orbit without diagnostic features on CT or MRI.[17,18] The latter group produces a densely sclerosed, chronic inflammatory reaction with granulomatous foci. These are the cases that are difficult to diagnose and may be confused with neoplasms (Figure 29.2). The diagnosis is dependent on the confirmation of septate hyphae that branch at a typical 45° angle. The Gomori methenamine silver (GMS) technique highlights the walls of the hyphae. Although the diagnosis can easily be established by the identification of the organisms in fulminating cases, the sclerosing type may not readily reveal the causative organism in small biopsy samples. The tissue sample may show only dense fibrous tissue, without any granulomas or organisms. Although fine-needle aspiration biopsy (FNAB) has been used to diagnose fungal infections, when aspergillosis is suspected, it is better to perform incisional biopsies on the lesions. The limited sample obtained by FNAB is more likely to be nondiagnostic in sclerosing cases. The management of orbital aspergillosis includes surgical debridement and antifungal therapy. Wide surgical excision of the involved tissues is suggested in the sclerosing type, since the infection has a tendency to recur.[19,20]

Parasitic Infections

Echinococcus granulosus, otherwise known as hydatic cyst, is probably the most common parasitic disease of the orbit. Hydatid disease is most commonly encountered in the liver (60–70%) and lungs but may spread hematogenously into the systemic circulation and infect multiple extrahepatic sites. Orbital hydatid disease is rare, comprising less than 1% of all cases in the body. Once in the orbit, most lesions lie within the muscle cone in children and young adults.[21,22] The diagnosis of orbital hydatid disease is suggested by signs and symptoms of a unilateral, orbital space-occupying mass, such as gradual progressive proptosis and diminished extraocular motility. Eosinophilia is present in approximately 25% of cases. CT findings usually include a hypodense, nonenhancing, often unilocular (but occasionally multilocular) cystic lesion, well delineated by a thin capsule that may or may not show enhancement in contrast studies. MRI discloses a low intensity signal on T1-weighted images and a high-intensity signal on T2-weighted images. Microscopic examination of the cyst fluid

TABLE 29.1. Orbital Inflammations that May Cause Space-Occupying Lesions in the Orbit.

Infections	*Nonspecific inflammations*	*Specific inflammations*	*Vasculitides*	*Collagen tissue disorders*
Tuberculosis	Orbital pseudotumor	Sarcoidosis	Polyarteritis nodosa	Lupus erythematosus
Lyme disease	Foreign body granuloma	Crohn's disease	Churg–Strauss syndrome	Dermatomyositis
Dacryoadenitis	Hematic cyst/cholesteatoma	Sjögren's syndrome	Kimura's disease	Scleroderma
Mucormycosis	Mucocele	Wegener's granulomatosis	Behçet's disease	Rheumatoid arthritis
Aspergillosis				Amyloidosis
Echinococcosis				

TABLE 29.2. Vasculitis Syndromes and Collagen Tissue Disorders that May Present with Localized or Infiltrative Space-Occupying Lesions in the Orbit.

Disease	*Systemic findings*	*Ocular/Orbital manifestation*
Wegener's granulomatosis	Necrotizing vasculitis and granulomatous inflammation in upper and lower respiratory tract, kidneys and skin; C-ANCA (+) ↑ serum IgA, IgE; RF (+); anemia	Orbital granulomatosis and vasculitis with proptosis; EOM disturbance; ON vasculitis and/or compression; conjunctivitis, scleritis; choroidal ischemia
Angiolymphoid hyperplasia with eosinophilia (Kimura's disease)	Nonspecific inflammation with lymphocytes and eosinophils in the skin, upper respiratory tract, kidney; bronchial asthma; eosinophilia	Localized, poorly delineated nonspecific inflammation in the orbit causing proptosis and EOM disturbance
Polyarteritis nodosa	Systemic small and medium vessel vasculitis that may involve any organ; skin lesions; arthralgias; weight loss; peripheral neuropathy	Orbital vasculitis and soft tissue necrosis causing proptosis, EOM disturbance, scleritis and choroidal ischemia
Churg–Strauss syndrome	Small-vessel systemic vasculitis with eosinophilia; bronchial asthma	Necrotizing granulomatosis of conjunctiva and other periocular soft tissues
Lupus erythematosus	Autoimmune connective tissue disease involving skin, kidneys, joints, lungs, liver and CNS; ↑ ANA titer; anti-DNA antibody; LE prep (+); anemia, leukopenia, lymphopenia; false (+) serology for syphilis	KCS; occlusive retinopathy; conjunctivitis scleritis; ON and orbital soft tissue vasculitis causing proptosis and ophthalmoplegia
Behçet's disease	Multisystem occlusive vasculitis involving skin, mucosa, joints, urogenital, and CNS tissues *Major signs*: aphthous oral and genital ulcerations and uveitis	Uveitis; retinochoroidal vasculitis; scleritis with or without optic neuritis; extraocular myositis with EOM disturbance and proptosis
Dermatomyositis	Systemic degenerative collagen tissue disease primarily involving striated muscle, skin and mucous membranes, cardiopulmonary and GI disease secondary to muscle atrophy, myositis-specific Ab (MSAs) (+); RF (+)	Conjunctivitis; erythematous discoloration of eyelid and periorbital skin; ophthalmoplegia, ptosis and proptosis due to orbital polymyositis in cases associated with giant cell myocarditis (cadiopulmonary workup including EKG, cardiac echogram, chest x-ray, etc.)
Scleroderma	Nonspecific chronic inflammation causing tissue fibrosis; may present as localized skin (mild) or systemic (severe) disease involving heart, lungs, kidneys, and GI tract	Fibrosis of adnexal tissues causing atrophy of conjunctiva and eyelid skin; madarosis; ptosis and EOM disturbance; heterochromia iridis
Rhematoid arthritis	Common systemic autoimmune disorder with chronic polyarthritis; pulmonary, CNS and skin involvement; RF (+)	KCS with or without Sjögren's syndrome; scleritis (50% of cases) with or without scleromalasia perforans and orbital soft tissue inflammation and necrosis

Ab, antibody; ACE, angiotensin-converting enzyme; ANA, anti-nuclear antibody; C-ANCA, anti-neutrophil cytoplamic antibody; CNS, central nervous system; EOM, extraocular muscle; GI, gastrointestinal; KCS, keratoconjunctivitis sicca; MSA, major serologic antigen; LE, lupus erythematosus; LG, lacrimal gland; LN, lymph node; ON, optic nerve; RF, rheumatoid factor.

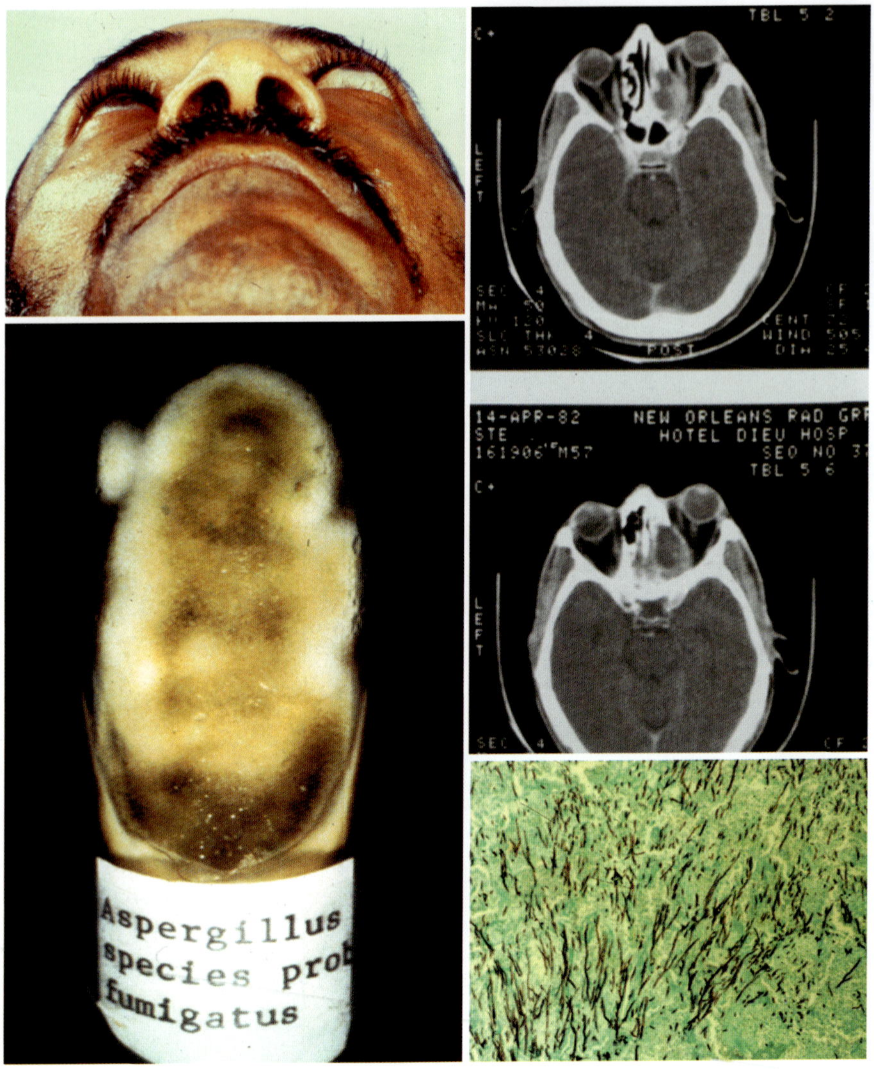

FIGURE 29.2. Aspergillosis presented in this patient as an orbitoethmoidal mass with slowly developing axial proptosis, and loss of visual acuity and visual field of the left eye. Only the third biopsy revealed the *Aspergillus* organisms, which could be demonstrated with Gomori methenamine silver and periodic acid–Schiff stains in tissue examination and were grown in culture. The first two biopsies showed only fibrous tissue and nonspecific chronic inflammation.

demonstrating daughter cysts with scoleces is diagnostic (Figure 29.3).[23–25]

Other examples of parasitic orbital infections are cysticercosis, myiasis, and trichinosis of extraocular muscles.[26–28]

NONSPECIFIC INFLAMMATIONS

Orbital Pseudotumor

Orbital pseudotumor is a nonspecific chronic inflammatory condition of unknown etiology. Although an underlying immune process is suspected, no conclusive mechanism has been established for the development of this curious entity. Clinically, the orbital pseudotumor may develop with sudden onset of painful proptosis associated with motility disturbances, eyelid swelling, redness, and chemosis.[29] It may develop as a diffuse or localized lesion, and its histopathology varies accordingly from case to case. The pseudotumor may be grouped into two main categories: diffuse and localized nonspecific orbital inflammation. The localized nonspecific inflammation is further divided according to specific sites (i.e., myositis, dacryoadenitis, periscleritis, and perineuritis). Each subgroup may present as an acute, subacute, or chronic inflammatory process in a given patient.

The histopathology of the pseudotumor usually consists of a mixed polymorphonuclear and lymphocytic infiltrate during the early phases; as the disease advances, lymphoid follicle formation and fibrous tissue proliferation dominate the picture.[30] Patchy aggregates of lymphocytes and/or lymphoid follicles are frequently seen. Occasionally the lymphoid infiltrates are confluent as in lymphoproliferative neoplasia. These cases may clinically simulate orbital lymphoma and, therefore, should be further evaluated with flow cytometry and genetic studies (see Chapter 12). In many instances, the biopsy diagnosis for the pseudotumor is not pathognomonic but must be correlated with clinical and radiologic findings. Occasionally, the

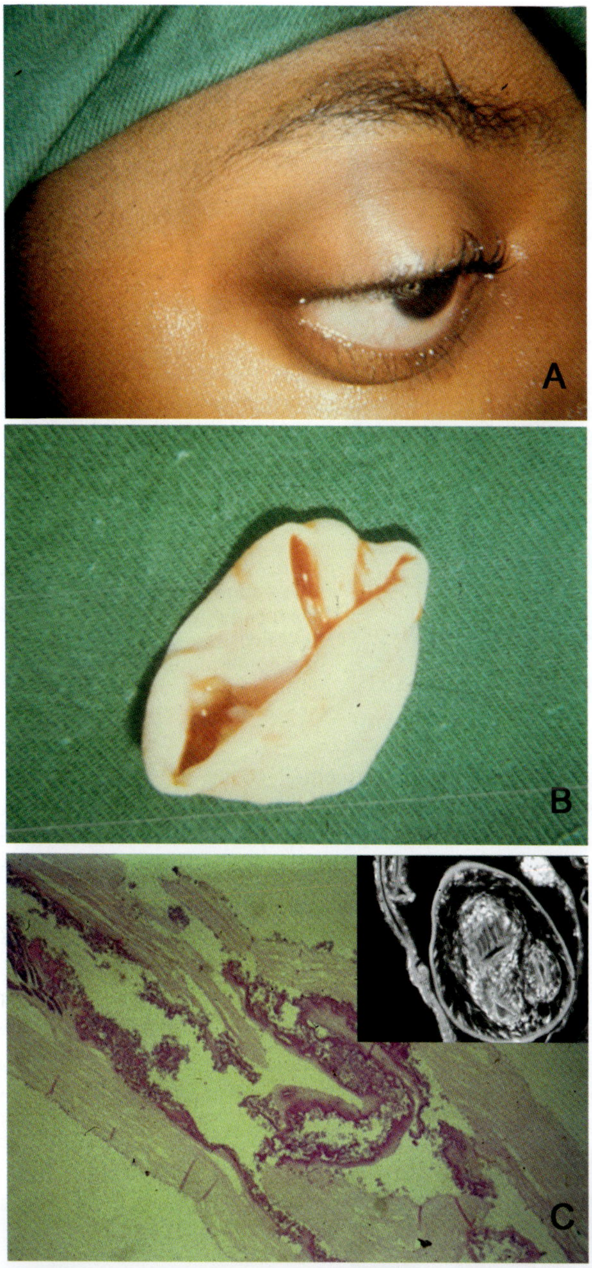

FIGURE 29.3. Echinoccocal cyst, which presented with unilateral proptosis (A). The unilocular cystic lesion shown in the gross photograph (B) was removed in toto. Histopathologic slide (C) reveals partially calcified cyst wall. *Inset*: Diagnostic scoleces recovered from the cyst fluid.

orbital pseudotumor with systemic involvement may simulate metastatic disease.[31]

CT and MRI findings of diffuse orbital pseudotumors include contrast enhancement owing to the high vascularity of inflammation, which infiltrates the fibroadipose tissues and extraocular muscle enlargement.[32] The MRI finding of hypointensity on T2-weighted images, relative to normal muscle, may be useful to differentiate pseudotumor from metastatic tumors by vascular congestion.[33] If the pseudotumor is localized with compression onto adjacent structures, including the globe, or is causing bony erosion, the differential diagnosis is difficult.[32]

The localized presentations of orbital pseudotumor, such as Tolosa–Hunt syndrome and lacrimal pseudotumor, may mimic neoplasia. Tolosa–Hunt syndrome, otherwise known as painful external ophthalmoplegia, is another orbital inflammatory process of the orbit with unknown etiology.[34,35] It is conceivable that it represents a localized form of idiopathic orbital inflammation. The clinical symptoms include a severe, deep orbital pain associated with functional deficiencies of third, fourth, fifth, and sixth cranial nerves. It is typical that the orbital pain, which presents abruptly, also responds to systemic corticosteroid treatment with the same suddenness.[36] Other symptoms of the disease, including third, fourth, and sixth cranial nerves palsies and the hypoesthesia of the periorbital skin, also respond well to corticosteroid treatment. Although bilateral cases do occur, the great majority of patients with Tolosa–Hunt syndrome present unilaterally and, therefore, their lesions should be differentiated from tumors that can involve the orbital apex area (e.g., meningioma, pituitary adenoma, neurofibroma, paraganglioma, secondary nasopharyngeal squamous cell carcinoma, metastatic tumors). Tumors of the apex, however, usually cause a gradual development of extraocular muscle dysfunction, depending on the location of the lesion, which may be accompanied by dull pain but usually not with abrupt onset of panophthalmolplegia and explosive pain.[37,38] Although the imaging studies are not specific for Tolosa–Hunt syndrome, they are helpful to rule out neoplasia. Burkitt's lymphoma has also been reported to simulate Tolosa–Hunt syndrome.[39]

Localized lacrimal fossa pseudotumor may present as an isolated mass lesion. Imaging is not very helpful to differentiate lacrimal gland masses and other anteriorly localized pseudotumors (Figure 29.4). Burkitt's lymphoma may also mimic acute-onset localized pseudotumor in the lacrimal gland fossa.[40–42] These lesions should be differentiated from lymphoma, other lacrimal gland tumors, and inflammation such as Sjögren syndrome (SS) and sarcoidosis by means of histopathologic examination (Figure 29.5).

Hematic Cyst and Cholesteatoma

Although orbital hemorrhage terminology is not very strict, *hematoma* usually refers to a localized collection of blood within soft tissues that develops secondary to trauma. Hemorrhage may occur spontaneously without any physical exertion in otherwise healthy individuals.[43] When blood collection within the orbit becomes organized and is surrounded by a thin pseudocapsule, the entity is commonly known as a hematic cyst (Figure 29.6).[44,45] Hematic cysts usually develop within 1 to 2 weeks of orbital trauma,

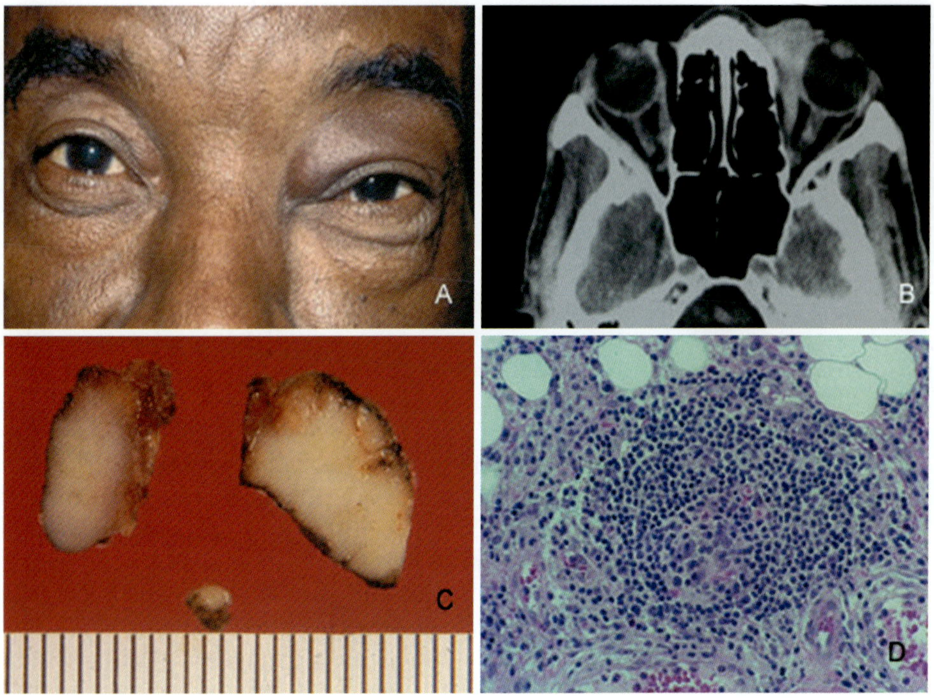

FIGURE 29.4. Pseudotumor in medial anterior orbit presented as a firm medial mass displacing the globe laterally, causing diplopia at the right gaze (A). The patient described mild pain in the past, but the lesion was not painful or tender at the time of admission. The lesion (B) was well delineated but not encapsulated; it could be peeled away from the left medial rectus muscle. The cut surface (C) was yellowish-gray and very firm. Histopathological examination (D) revealed nonspecific, chronic inflammation with occasional follicle formations.

but some cases are reported to occur up to 20 years after orbital injury.[46] These cysts may become large enough to cause proptosis, extraocular motility disturbance, or compression on the globe and optic nerve. Hematic cysts, which can be easily demonstrated with ultrasonography, CT, or MRI, are lined by fibrovascular tissue at the periphery and contain degenerated erythrocytes, protein debris, and cholesterol crystals.[47] In many instances, the thin nonepithelial lining is attached to adjacent structures by fibrous adhesions. The adhesions may be self-resolving or easily detached surgically in early cases; if the lesion persists, however, they may turn into firm fibrous bands. Hematic cysts may develop within the muscle cone or subperiosteal orbital locations.[44] If the hemorrhage develops within an existing lymphatic or vascular tumor, these lesions are known as blood cysts or chocolate cysts.

Cholesteatoma is another cystic lesion that is confined by a thicker pseudocyst wall without epithelial lining. It is conceivable that some chronic hematic cysts develop into cholesteatomas. Like chronic

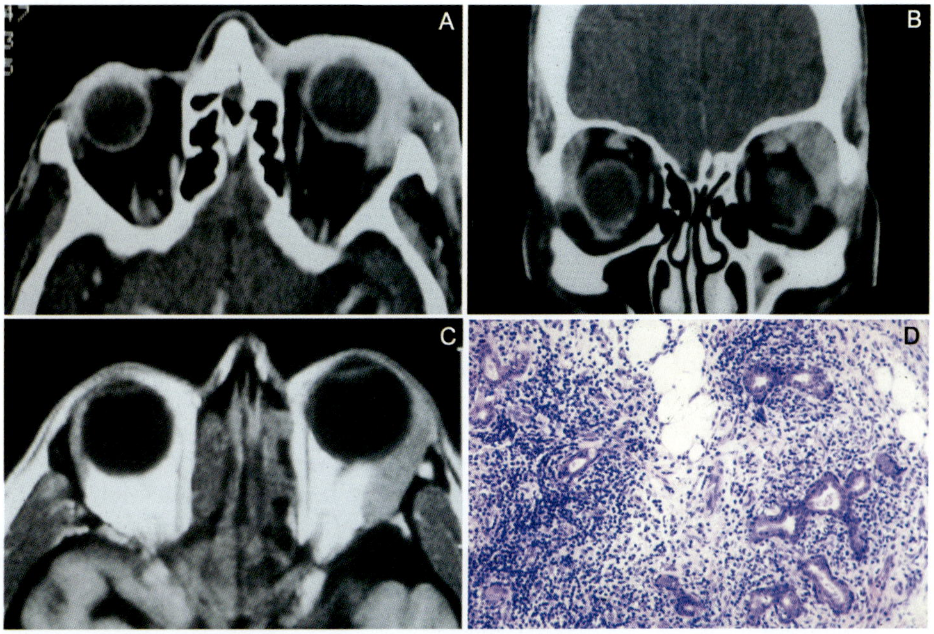

FIGURE 29.5. Lacrimal gland fossa lesions. (A) Localized pseudotumor. (B) Lymphoma. (C,D) Sjögren's syndrome. The patient presented with bilateral masses; however, the lesion in the left lacrimal gland fossa (C) was larger. (D) Histopathology revealed diffuse lymphocytic infiltrates among the atrophied acini of the lacrimal gland.

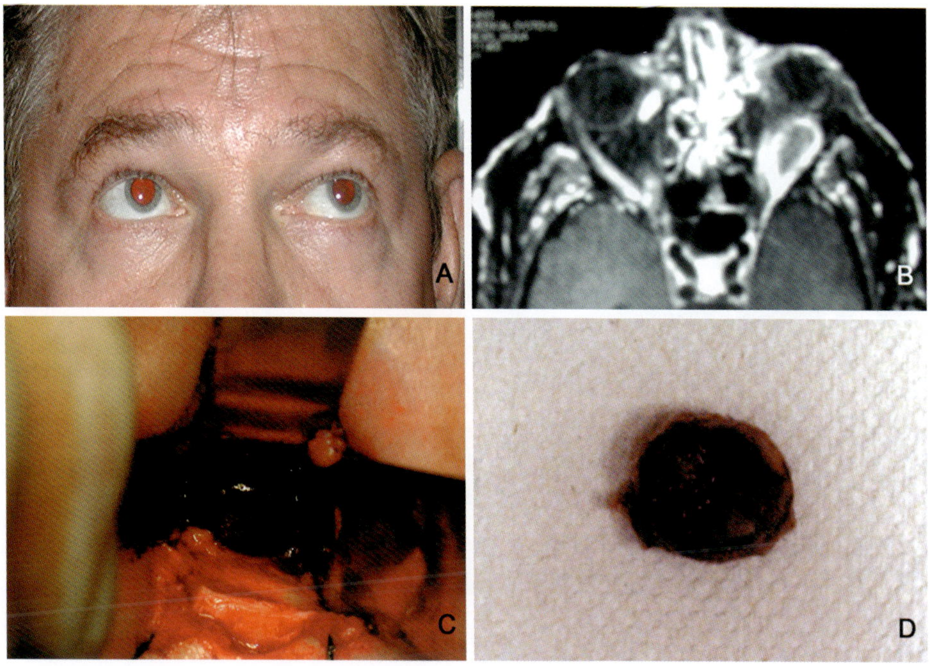

FIGURE 29.6. The patient presented with spontaneous bleeding into the orbit with minimal proptosis of the left eye and diplopia at extreme left gaze (A). MR image shows a large cystic lesion with marked enhancement in the lateral orbit (B). When the orbit was explored through a lateral orbitotomy, a dark red, spherical lesion was identified and removed with blunt dissection (C). The lesion was a totally encapsulated blood clot, which microscopically showed different degrees of organization (D).

hematic cysts, these lesions contain cholesterol crystals and other blood breakdown products that act as foreign material and trigger a fulminant granulomatous reaction.[48,49] Cholesteatomas are usually located in the superior lateral orbit within the lacrimal gland fossa. Histopathologically, the lesion is composed of cholesterol clefts, hemosiderin and hematoidin granules, other blood breakdown products, and fibrin, surrounded by a mixed lymphohistiocytic infiltrate and multinucleated foreign body giant cells (Figure 29.7). Imaging studies may show a cystic, semicystic, or solid lesion within the diploë of the bone or within the orbital soft tissues with erosion of the adjacent bone (Figure 29.8).

Although bone destruction in general may suggest malignancy, the sclerosing character of the bony destruction, which is best seen in bone window images, suggests a benign lesion. Multiple cuts of the frontal bone should be examined to rule out the possibility of intracranial extension. A recent report suggests that a preexisting bone abnormality may lead to the development of cholesteatomas at least in some cases.[50]

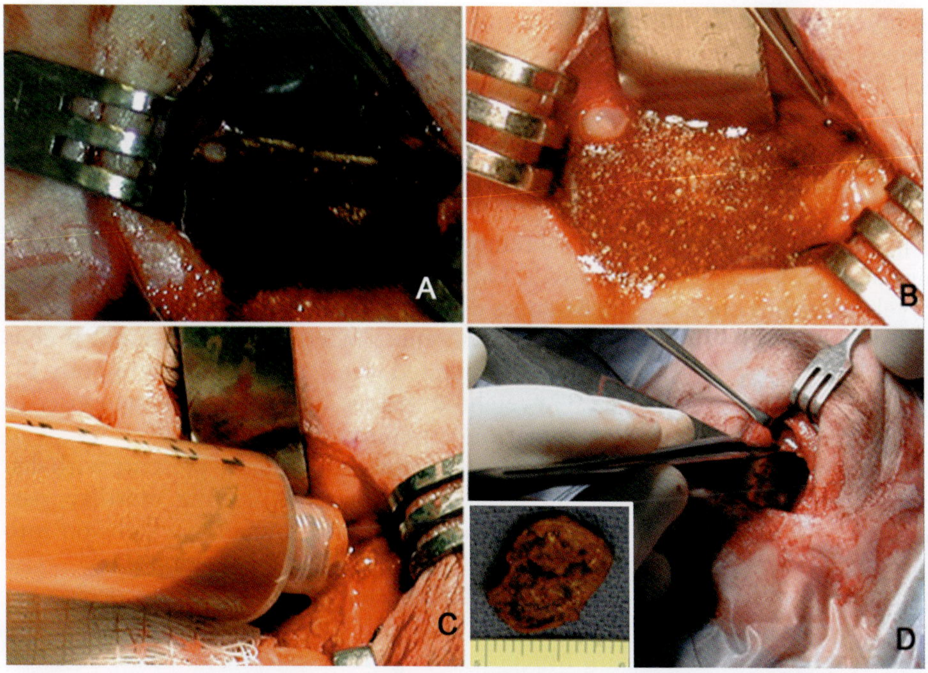

FIGURE 29.7. Lacrimal gland fossa cholesteatoma, which consisted of a very dark, red-brown pseudocyst with multiple adhesions to its surrounding soft tissues and the frontal bone (A). Sharp dissection around the lesion caused much bleeding. When the cystic structure was opened, orange-red, turbid, thick fluid containing numerous, sparkling cholesterol crystals (B,C) gushed out in copious amounts. When the dissection was complete, the erosion of the frontal bone (D) could be identified but dura was not penetrated. *Inset*: The pseudocyst wall of the cholesteatoma after the contents had been emptied.

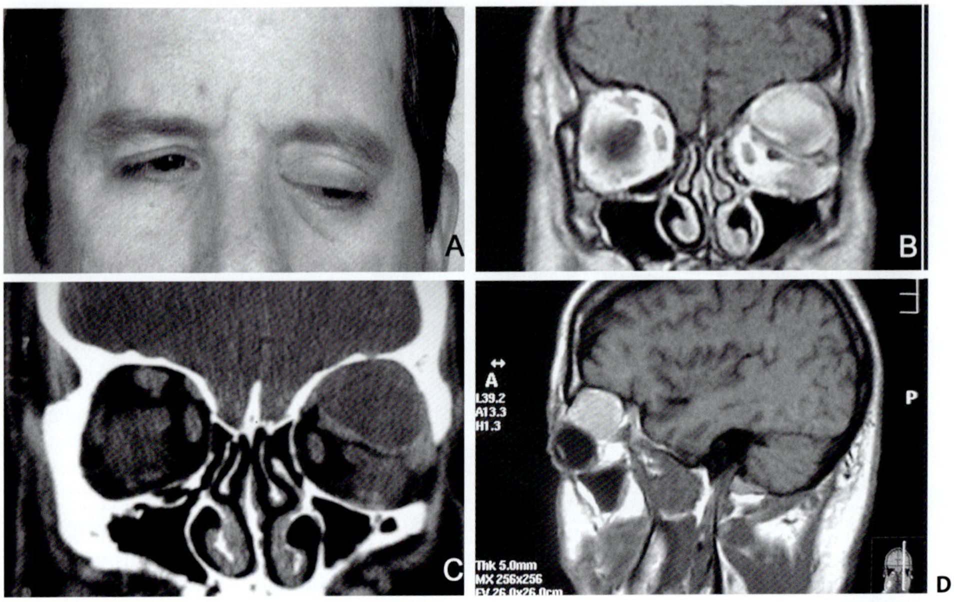

FIGURE 29.8. A cholesteatoma, located in the lacrimal gland fossa of the left orbit. (A) The patient presented with inferior proptosis, diplopia, and ptosis of the left upper eyelid. (B–D) On imaging studies, the lesion presented as a unilocular, rounded mass, causing destruction of the adjacent frontal bone.

Bone destruction makes one think along the lines of metastatic tumors, but benign lesions such as brown tumor, aneurysmal bone cyst, and ruptured or leaking dermoid[50] should also be considered.[51]

Because of the extensive foreign body reaction around the lesion, cholesteatomas usually establish many firm adhesions to the surrounding soft tissues and bone, causing destruction of these tissues. The extensive adherences make the surgical excision of these lesions difficult. Lack of capsule forces one to do sharp dissection around the lesion, which may damage vital structures such as entrapped and atrophied extraocular muscles, nerves, and blood vessels. In particular, the superior and lateral rectus muscles and the levator muscle are likely to be entrapped within the cholesteatoma and may lose their structure and function.

Osteomyelitis of the orbital bones, primarily evolving as a complication of paranasal sinusitis, is another entity that should be considered in the differential diagnosis of cholesteatoma. In osteomyelitis the bone infection extends into the soft periosteal space and beyond. Precise delineation of the lesion can be done with CT and MRI, particularly in combination with bone SPECT (single photon emission CT), a sensitive technique used to detect osteomyelitis within cranial and orbital bones.[52]

Mucocele

Although a commonly encountered space-occupying lesion in the orbit, the mucocele is technically not a neoplasm but a cyst developing as a result of inflammation or trauma. Its cavity is lined by pseudostratified respiratory epithelium prolapsing into the orbit from a paranasal sinus, most commonly the frontal sinus; ethmoid and maxillary sinuses are the other sites of mucoceles.[53] The primary mucocele develops as a result of an inflammatory obstruction of the ostium of a paranasal sinus. The histopathologic appearance of the mucocele wall, consisting of respiratory epithelium and thinned bony elements with nonspecific chronic inflammation, reflects its evolution from a chronic inflammatory process.

Secondary mucoceles, on the other hand, are most commonly seen after orbital trauma and surgery; they may also develop secondary to neoplasms of paranasal sinuses and nasal pharynx. If there is a superimposed infection, the lesions are referred to as pyocele on CT and MRI; the mucocele presents as a well-delineated cystic structure originating from a paranasal sinus. Depending on their location, secondary mucoceles may compress onto orbital structures including extraocular muscles, optic nerve, and the globe.[54]

On CT, mucoceles present as hypointense, expanding masses originating from the paranasal sinuses. Early in their development these lesions are small, mucus-containing cysts. Later in their development, they are characterized by crescent-shaped and thinned remodeling of the bony walls of the orbit and sinuses.[55] On MRI, mucocele presents with different appearances depending on the amount of free water in its luminal contents. When the intraluminal mucus becomes inspissated, the signal intensity in both T1- and T2-weighted images decreases, moving closer to that of normal air content of the sinus.[56]

Clinically, the mucocele usually presents with displacements and proptosis, extraocular motility, particularly in the direction of the sinus extension into the orbit, and other compressive symptoms.[57] The crepitant or calcified hard wall of the mucocele may be palpated underneath the superior or medial orbital rim. Mucoceles in general are rare in children; however, a unique variant, ethmoidal mucopyocele, is known to occur as a secondary space-occupying lesion in the medial canthal area, with lateral displacement of the globe.

Mucoceles of the lacrimal drainage system should not be confused with sinus lesions. Lacrimal sac mucoceles, at times, particularly in adults, may simulate lymphomas.[58]

SPECIFIC INFLAMMATIONS

Sarcoidosis

Sarcoidosis is an idiopathic multisystem disease that commonly involves the orbit and the eye. Systemically it involves the lungs and the upper respiratory tract, liver, spleen, lymphatic, and hematopoietic tissues, central nervous system, and the skin. Although there is considerable evidence that sarcoidosis is infectious, its etiopathogenesis is still unknown.[59] The typical noncaseating granulomas are made of T lymphocytes of helper and suppressor types and dendritic Langerhans cells with deoxyribose human leukocyte antigen (HLA) expression. Perivascular inflammation is characteristic of a delayed type of hypersensitivity reaction. Patients with sarcoidosis usually demonstrate the systemically deficient T-cell responses associated with T-cell lymphopenia. Although the exact significance of granuloma formation in sarcoidosis is not known, it appears that this tissue reaction is a secondary event as a result of exaggerated cellular immune response to a class of unknown antigens. The initial step in granuloma formation of sarcoidosis is considered to be triggered by the cytokine interleukin 1, which increases the proliferation of helper T lymphocytes and activates those cells. Activated helper T cells in turn secrete interleukin 2, which is a mitogen that stimulates the proliferation of helper T cells even further.[60] As a consequence, these cells aggregate at the site of the causative insult and secrete monocyte chemotactic factors that lead to the gathering of epithelioid macrophages and multinucleated giant cells to form granulomas. Sarcoidosis is also associated with abnormalities of humoral immunity manifested by polyclonal hyperglobulinemia.[61,62] Granulomas are made of epithelioid cells and multinucleated giant cells, surrounded by lymphocytes and occasional plasma cells. Many inclusion bodies have been described in the giant cells of sarcoidosis, but none of these are pathognomonic. The granulomatous response of sarcoidosis is rather typical but not unique for this entity; fungal diseases, tuberculosis, Crohn's disease, and leprosy may produce similar granulomas.[63]

Approximately one fourth of sarcoidosis patients develop ocular and orbital manifestations including anterior and posterior uveitis, chorioretinitis, conjunctival and eyelid granulomas, and orbital mass lesions (Figure 29.9). The lacrimal gland is a common site of involvement. But although autopsy studies show a high percentage of microscopic disease, only 15 to 20% of the patients present clinical symptoms. Although virtually any part of the orbit may be involved, the most common site of sarcoidosis is the lacrimal fossa. The disease in this location may be confused with chronic dacryoadenitis, Sjögren's syndrome, or space-occupying lesion (Figure 29.10).[64] Sarcoid granulomas may also extend into the orbit from adjacent sinus mucosa.[65] If other manifestations of the disease are absent, these cases may mimic secondary orbital tumors; they can be differentiated only by biopsy.

Patients with distinctive systemic manifestations

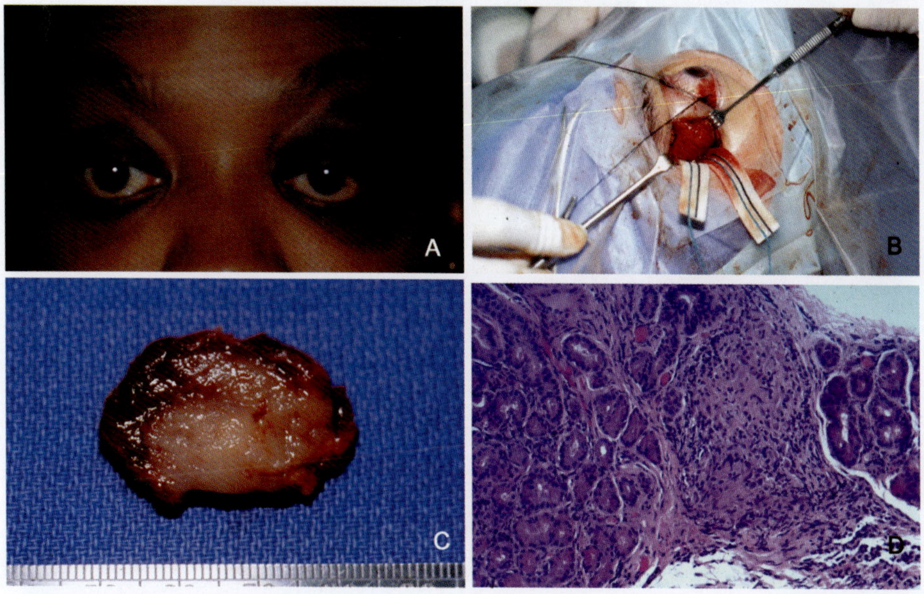

FIGURE 29.9. (A) This patient, who had no history of sarcoidosis, presented with an isolated lacrimal gland mass in the superior lacrimal fossa and the left upper eyelid; had had mild pain in 6 to 8 weeks. Although the mass was not encapsulated, it could be excised with blunt dissection (B,C). The histopathology (D) revealed extensive granulomatous inflammation consistent with sarcoidosis within the lacrimal gland and adjacent soft tissues.

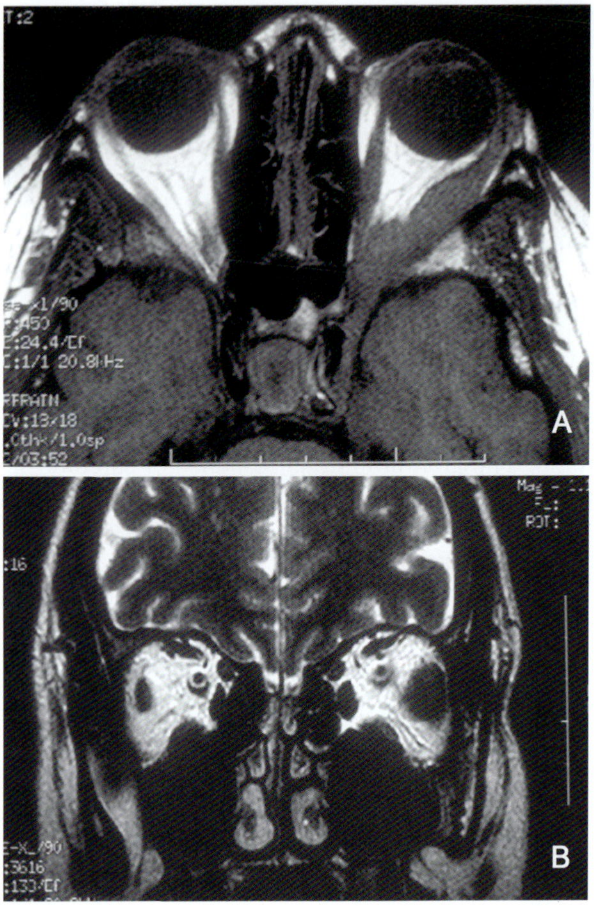

FIGURE 29.10. A large orbital mass extending to the apex and into the cavernous sinus through the optic canal in a known sarcoidosis patient. The patient was treated with oral corticosteroids and methotraxate, and the size of the orbital lesion was considerably reduced in size but persisted after 2 years of treatment.

with bilateral hilar lympadenopathy, skin lesions, uveitis, and so on, usually show increased levels of angiotensin-converting enzymes (ACEs). Serum lysozyme and calcium levels may also be increased in sarcoidosis, but neither test is specific for the disease. The ultimate diagnosis is by biopsy. Some advocate preforming biopsies only on sarcoid-suspect lesions, such as skin and conjunctival nodules in which the yield is usually rewarding. Others support random (blind) biopsy of the conjunctiva in sarcoid suspects (Figure 29.11). The yield of the random biopsy without a distinct lesion is rather low (around 25% positive). Since the conjunctival biopsy is simple to perform, has low morbidity, and can be inexpensively and quickly done in the clinic, as opposed to more invasive biopsies of transbroncheal lymph nodes, liver, and orbit, it is practical to do biopsies of the conjunctiva randomly early in the workup of a patient suspected of having sarcoidosis.[66] If the biopsy reveals granulomatous inflammation, more invasive procedures with high morbidity can be avoided.

The involvement of the optic nerve with sarcoidosis is usually an anterior process associated with typical retinal vasculitis; rarely, however, the optic nerve involvement may extend posteriorly and form a mass lesion.[67]

The treatment of sarcoidosis is directed to the systemic disease. Surgery may be necessary for purposes of biopsy or debulking orbital lesions if there is a need for histopathologic evaluation in patients with no other easily accessible biopsy sites. In a few instances, the mass forming orbital disease presents with no his-

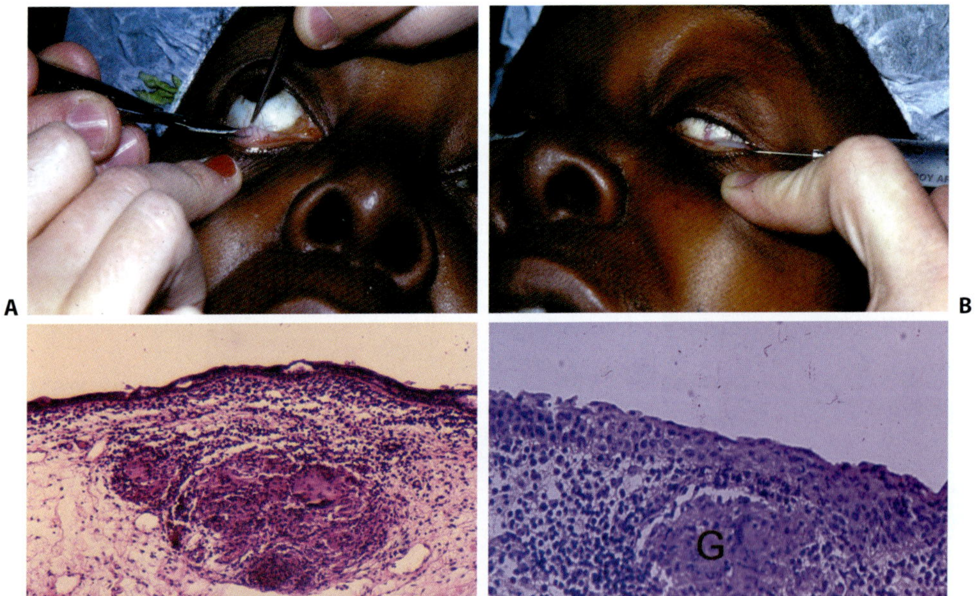

FIGURE 29.11. (A,B) Bilateral blind conjunctival biopsy procedure from lower fornices. Approximately 25% of the sarcoidosis suspects reveal subconjunctival hard granulomas (G) as shown in histopathologic slides (C) and (D).

tory or detectable symptoms of systemic sarcoidosis (Figure 29.9). The surgical removal of the orbital sarcoid lesions is usually difficult; these mass lesions do not form capsules and, therefore, need to be excised with sharp dissection, which may damage the adjacent tissues (i.e., lacrimal gland) and cause excessive bleeding. In these patients, sarcoidosis is usually a surprising diagnosis obtained from an "orbital tumor."[64] The accepted systemic treatment is the use of oral corticosteroids and antimetabolites such as methotrexate.

Crohn's Disease

Crohn's disease is a granulomatous inflammation of the bowel associated with systemic manifestations. The ocular manifestations are primarily related to uveitis, episcleritis, and scleritis; however, orbital pseudotumorlike presentations, secondary to granulomatous inflammation in the orbit has been described.[68,69] Optic neuritis has also been described in Crohn's disease.[70]

Sjögren's Syndrome

Sjögren's syndrome (SS) consists of a triad of symptoms including dry eyes (keratoconjunctivitis sicca), dry mouth (xerostomia), and "dry joints" (arthritis).[71] The primary SS is not associated with other connective tissue diseases; however, secondary SS symptoms overlap with the manifestations of systemic lupus erythematosus, polymyositis, polyarthritis nodosa, scleroderma, and rheumatoid arthritis.[72] Like many other autoimmune diseases, SS does not have a clear-cut etiology; however, it is considered to be a mononuclear inflammatory vasculopathy.[73] Many viruses, including Epstein–Barr, cytomegalovirus, hepatitis C, and HIV have been reported to have an etiologic role in SS. Immune complex formation and deposition are considered to be the physiopathology of cutaneous and ocular vasculitis.[74,75]

The histopathology of the conjunctiva as well as the lacrimal gland is nonspecific, consisting of the regular infiltrates of lymphocytic and plasma cells surrounded by eosinophilic basement membrane–like material. These units are called *epimyoepithelial islands* and are considered to be diagnostic of SS.[76,77] The lacrimal gland also reveals acinar atrophy and increased fibrosis surrounding the ductules (Figure 29.5D). The diagnosis of SS is based on minor salivary gland biopsy rather than the biopsy of the lacrimal gland, since the latter procedure is more involved surgically and carries a higher morbidity.[78]

Keratoconjunctivitis sicca is the most common presentation of SS in the eye, occurring in about 90% of patients. Diminished tear meniscus and decreased tear breakup time (BUT) with diminished tear production documented with Schirmer strips are common findings. Less commonly patients develop episcleritis/scleritis in the primary type of SS.[79] Because of peripheral and central nervous system involvement, optic neuritis and internuclear ophthalmoplegia may be seen in these patients. The asymmetrical orbital presentation of the disease may be confused with orbital lymphoma or sarcoidosis. In most cases, however, the disease presents with bilateral enlargement of the lacrimal glands and other symptomatology. Although SS is easy to diagnose, it should be kept in mind that SS patients have an increased risk of developing B-cell lymphomas in the salivary glands and cervical lymph nodes. This association has not been found to be true for the lacrimal gland. However, the orbital lymphoma that can mimic the presentation of SS should always be considered in differential diagnosis (see Chapter 13).

Wegener's Granulomatosis

Wegener's granulomatosis (WG) is an idiopathic systemic vasculitis that also causes necrotizing granulomatous inflammation.[80,81] The classic triad of the disease comprises necrotizing granulomatous vasculitis of upper and lower respiratory tracts and necrotizing glomerulonephritis. Small-vessel disease also affects the eye and orbit, leading to conjunctivitis, scleritis, uveitis, and thromboembolic phenomenon of the choroidal vessels and central retinal artery.[82–84]

Orbital involvement also results from necrotizing vasculitis (with or without granulomatous inflammation), leading to painful proptosis, eyelid and conjunctival edema, and extraocular motility disturbance. Optic nerve disease may result from the combination of vasculitis of the optic nerve and meningeal vessels and/or the compression caused by the orbital space-occupying lesion (Figure 29.12).[83] This on occasion can lead to occlusion of the central retinal artery.[85]

Although the specific idiopathogenesis of WG is unknown, there is a consensus that the disease results from an autoimmune mechanism. Unlike other forms of vasculitis, however, it does not appear to be caused by immune complex deposition.[86] It has been speculated that the vasculitis of WG is triggered by an infectious process.[87,88] As a rule, respiratory tract involvement in WG precedes renal or systemic disease; however, many atypical cases with lack of involvement of one organ system or another are well recognized.[89]

It is well known that anti-neutrophil cytoplasmic antibodies (ANCA) function to contain the inflammatory responses by proteolysis, primarily by collagenases and elastases.[90] Cytoplasmic ANCA (C-ANCA) is a very sensitive and specific serologic marker for WG, with a sensitivity increasing up to 96% for active disease.[91,92] Others hypothesize that C-ANCA is not merely a marker for the disease but in itself is pathogenic.[93] High and low C-ANCA titers

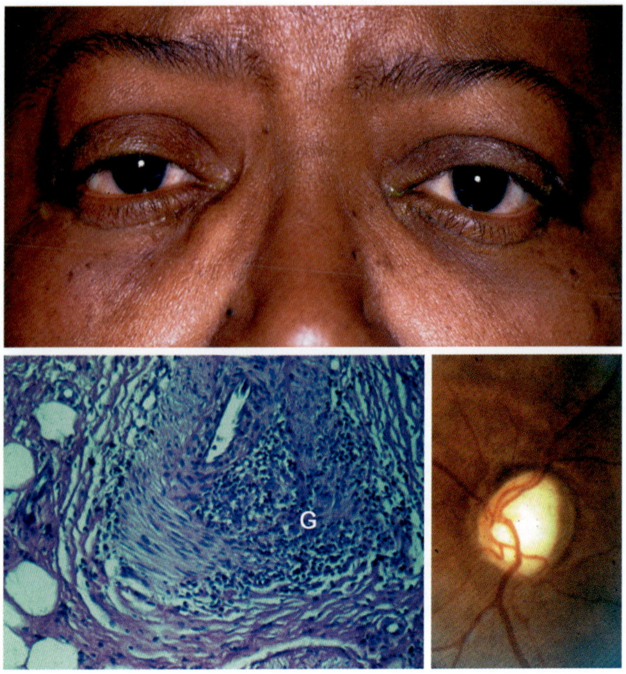

FIGURE 29.12. Recurrent Wegener's granulomatosis with minimal left proptosis but atrophy of left disk as a sequela from previous episodes of activity. The orbit biopsy material shows granulomatous (G) vasculitis.

are known to correlate well with disease activity and remission, respectively.[94] Biopsy-proven head and neck orbit WG lesions particularly are known to occur without elevated titers of C-ANCA.[95,96]

The classic histopathologic picture includes extensive necrotizing vasculitis with necrosis and granulomatous inflammation. However, considerable variability is observed in the biopsy samples obtained from different organs, and the classic appearance is not always demonstrable.[97,98] Upper respiratory tract and orbit biopsies usually show vasculitis and necrosis but rarely granulomas.[99,100] Material from lung biopsies usually shows diffuse necrotizing vasculitis of small blood vessels resembling an infectious process. Polymorphonuclear cells and eosinophils may form cuffs around blood vessels, but granulomas are rare.[101,102] Samples from kidney biopsies show necrotizing glomerulonephritis without well-formed granulomas.[103]

Samples from orbital biopsies also fail to depict the typical combination of vasculitis and granulomatous inflammation. Kalina and coworkers reported the presence of the complete triad of vasculitis, necrosis, and granulomatous inflammation in only 54% of the samples obtained from biopsies.[97]

Granulomas may also present some variability; in certain instances they are seen as typical hard granulomas made of aggregates of epithelioid cells, and giant cells surrounded by lymphocytes and occasional plasma cells. Granulomas that present within necrotic areas may present as palisading lesions containing numerous polymorphonuclear leukocytes and eosinophils.

Ophthalmic involvement of WG is best categorized in two types: focal disease that results from vasculitis and primarily affects the anterior and posterior segments of the eye and contiguous disease, seen primarily in the orbit as a result of WG extending from the nasal cavity and perinasal sinuses. Orbital disease that develops acutely with painful proptosis, eyelid and conjunctival edema, and ocular motility disturbance is the most common ocular manifestation in WG.[104,105] This presentation of WG may mimic orbital pseudotumor

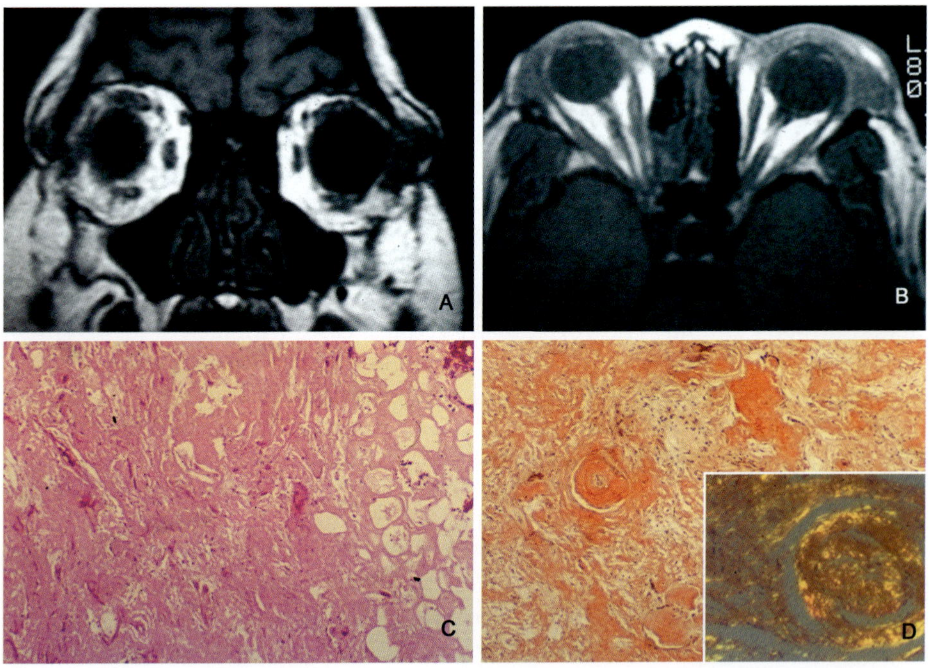

FIGURE 29.13. (A,B) Coronal and axial T1-weighted MR images showing irregular infiltrates of amyloid in the lacrimal gland fossa. (C,D) Photomicrographs showing the amorphous, acellular infiltrates of amyloid (periodic acid–Schiff and Congo red stains). *Inset*: Apple green birefringence of the amyloid deposit surrounding a blood vessel.

and infectious cellulitis as well as lymphoma and metastatic carcinoma.

Advances in the management of WG over the past 20 years have improved the survival with this disease, which in its classic form is rapidly fatal if not treated.[106] It is extremely important to establish the diagnosis of WG as early as possible, since early treatment may prevent renal failure, which is usually the cause of death. The mainstay of treatment is systemic immunosuppression with cytotoxic therapy; usually with the combination of corticosteroids and cyclophosphamide.[103] Although definitive treatment of any ophthalmic involvement is systemic immunosuppression, orbital inflammation may respond poorly to systemic cytotoxic therapy and may remain active despite the remission of the systemic disease.[103,107]

Amyloid Deposits

Amyloid deposits in orbital inflammation are a common occurrence; however, a localized mass formation of "amyloid tumor" is a very uncommon disorder.[108–110] Involvement of the lacrimal gland with amyloid deposits may mimic localized orbital pseudotumor or a neoplasm (Figure 29.13).[111] Clinically, these lesions present with painless proptosis. On imaging studies, the gland shows enlargement and molding to adjacent bones, frequently with punctate calcification. The appearance of calcification on the CT is a helpful feature, since the MRI findings are nonspecific. With MRI, amyloid deposits show hypointensity on T2-weighted images without any enhancement with contrast.[110] Lacrimal gland tumors and extramedullary plasmacytoma may simulate amyloid formations.[112,113]

Plasmacytoma is a rare type of non-Hodgkins lymphoma that primarily attacks patients after the age of 40. Diagnosis is based on the documentation of clonal plasma cell proliferation. Immunohistochemical stains should be utilized to document the light chain types (Figure 29.14). These tumors may be confused with lymphoma, localized pseudotumor, SS, and epithelial tumors of the lacrimal gland. The management of plasmacytoma is combined treatment with radiation, surgery, and chemotherapy.[114,115]

Many other vasculitides and collagen tissue disorders rarely involve the orbit and occasionally may form localized masses. These include angiolymphoid hyperplasia with eosinophilia (Kimura disease),[116–118] polyarteritis nodosa,[119,120] Churg–Strauss syndrome,[121–123] lupus erythematosus,[124–127] Behçet disease,[128,129] dermatomyositis,[130–132] scleroderma,[133–136] and rheumatoid arthritis.[137–139] Differential diagnosis of these lesions from neoplasms is usually not difficult because the disorders present with other ocular and systemic manifestations and laboratory findings. Some of these entities were summarized in Table 29.2.

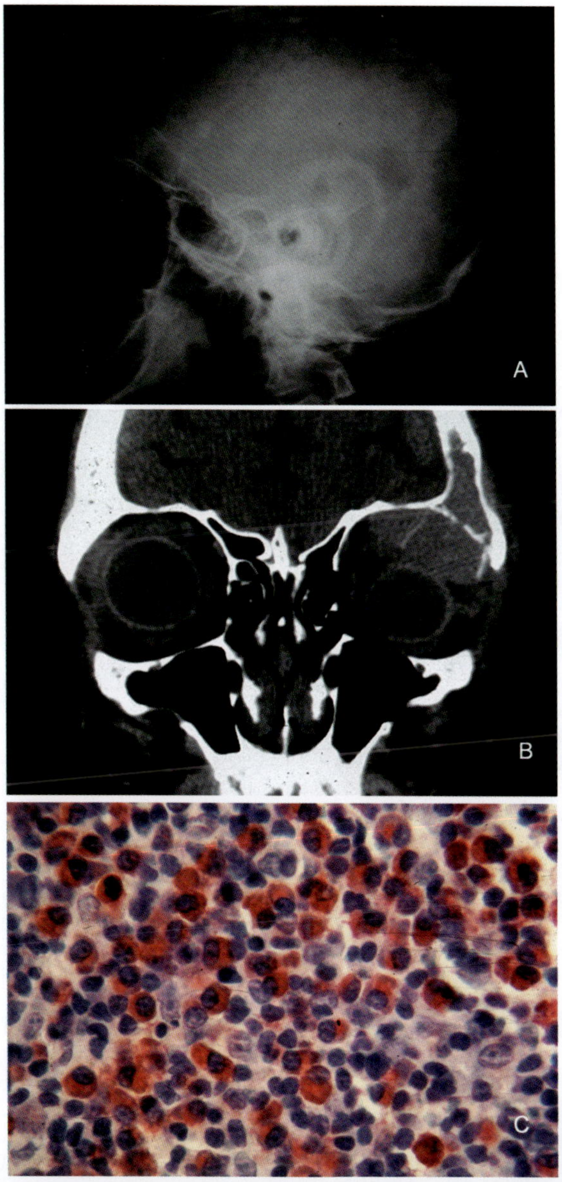

FIGURE 29.14. (A,B) Lateral view of the skull and coronal CT scan of the same patient, showing osteolytic lesions of localized plasmacytoma. The patient presented with rapidly developing proptosis and an inferior dislocation of the left eye. (C) Biopsy of the mass revealed extensive proliferation of atypical plasma cells, which were stained with κ light chains.

References

1. Unsold R, Greeven G. *Inflammatory Diseases of the Orbit*. Berlin: Springer-Verlag; 1997.
2. Shields JA. *Diagnosis and Management of Orbital Tumors*. Philadelphia: WB Saunders; 1989:67–85.
3. Rootman J, ed, *Diseases of the Orbit*. Philadelphia: JB Lippincott, 1988:143–203.
4. Mohammad AEA, Al-Hussaini MK, Karoosh SS, et al. Tuberculosis of the orbit and lacrimal gland. *Orbit* 1992;11: 199–204.
5. Sen DK. Tuberculosis of the orbit and lacrimal gland: a clinical study of 14 cases. *J Pediatr Ophthalmol Strabismus* 1980;17:232–238.
6. Khalil M, Lindley S, Matouk E. Tuberculosis of the orbit. *Ophthalmology* 1985;108:1624–1627.

7. Al-Malki FA, Issa TM, Riley F, Karcioglu ZA. Nasolacrimal tuberculosis in a patient with conjunctivodacryocystorhinostomy. *Ophthalmic Plast Reconstr Surg* 1999;15:213–216.
8. Snider DE Jr, Simone PM, Dooley SW, Bloch AB. Multi-drug resistant tuberculosis. *Sci Am Sci Med* 1994;1:16–25.
9. Barnes PF, Bloch AB, Davidson PT, Snider DE Jr. Tuberculosis in patients with human immunodeficiency virus infection [see Comments] [review]. *N Engl J Med* 1991;324:1644–1650.
10. Oakhill A, Shah KJ, Thompson AG, et al. Orbital tuberculosis in childhood. *Br J Ophthalmol* 1982;66:396–397.
11. Levine RA. Infection of the orbit by an atypical mycobacterium. *Arch Ophthalmol* 1969;82:608–610.
12. Klapper SR, Partrinely JR, Kaplan SL, Font RL. Atypical mycobacterial infection of the orbit. *Ophthalmology* 1995;102: 1536–1541.
13. Spoor TC, Harding SA. Orbital tuberculosis. *Am J Ophthalmol* 1981;91:644–647.
14. Sheridan PH, Edman JB, Starr SE. Tuberculosis presenting as an orbital mass. *Pediatrics* 1981;67:874–875.
15. Ferry AP, Abdebi S. Diagnosis and management of rhino-orbital cerebral mucormycosis (phycomycosis): a report of 16 personally observed cases. *Ophthalmology* 1983;90:1096.
16. Eustis HS, Mafee MF, Walton C, Mondonca J. MR imaging and CT of orbital infections and complications in acute rhinosinusitis. *Radiol Clin North Am* 1998;36:1165–1183.
17. Green WR, Font RL, Zimmerman LE: Aspergillosis of the orbit: report of ten cases and review of the literature. *Arch Ophthalmol* 1969;82:302.
18. Martinson FD, Alli AF, Clark BM. Aspergilloma of the ethmoid. *J Laryngol* 1977;84:857–861.
19. Harris GJ, Will BR. Orbital aspergillosis: conservative debridement and local amphotericin irrigation. *Ophthalmic Plast Reconstr Surg* 1989;5:207–211.
20. Houle TV, Ellis PP. Aspergillosis of the orbit with immunosuppressive therapy. *Surv Ophthalmol* 1975;20:35–42.
21. Morales AG, Croxatto JO, Crovetto L, Ebner R. Hydatid cysts of the orbit. A review of 35 cases. *Ophthalmology* 1988;95: 1027.
22. Awad MAN, Ray CJ, Karcioglu ZA. Echinococcus cysts of the orbit and substernum. *Am J Ophthalmol* 1994;118:676–678.
23. Betharia SM, Sharma V, Pushker N. Ultrasound findings in orbital hydatid cysts. *Am J Ophthalmol* 2003;135:568–570.
24. Kiratli H, Bilgic S, Özturkmen C, et al. Intramuscular hydatid cyst of the medial rectus muscle. *Am J Ophthalmol* 2003; 135:98–99.
25. Gökcek C, Gökcek A, Akif Bayar MN, et al. Orbital hydatid cyst: CT and MRI. *Neuroradiology* 1997;39:512–515.
26. Kersten RC, Shoukrey NM, Tabarra KF. Orbital myiasis. *Ophthalmology* 1986;93:1228.
27. Walrath JD, Lalin SC, Leib ML. Cysticercosis isolated to the orbit. *Ophthalmic Plast Reconstr Surg* 2003;19:243–244.
28. Rauniyar RK, Thakur SK, Panda A. CT in the diagnosis of isolated cysticercal infestation of extraocular muscle. *Clin Radiol* 2003;58:154–156.
29. Kennerdell JS, Dresner SC. The nonspecific orbital inflammatory syndromes. *Surv Ophthalmol* 1984;29:93–103.
30. Karcioglu ZA, Haik GB. Tissue diagnosis: orbit. In: Karcioglu ZA, ed. *Laboratory Diagnosis in Ophthalmology*. New York: Macmillan; 1987:27–29.
31. Foley MR, Moshfeghi DM, Wilson MW, et al. Orbital inflammatory syndromes with systemic involvement may mimic metastatic disease. *Ophthalmic Plast Reconstr Surg* 2003;19:324–326.
32. Flanders AE, Mafee MF, Rao VM, Choi KH. CT characteristics of orbital pseudotumors and other orbital inflammatory processes. *J Comput Assist Tomogr* 1989;13:40–47.
33. Atlas SW, Galetta SL. The orbit and visual system. In: Atlas SW, ed. *Magnetic Resonance Imaging of the Brain and Spine*. 2nd ed. Philadelphia: Lippincott-Raven; 1996:1007–1092.
34. Smith JL, Taxdal DS. Painful ophthalmoplegia. The Tolosa–Hunt syndrome. *Am J Ophthalmol* 1966;61:1466–1472.
35. Kline LB. The Tolosa–Hunt syndrome. *Surv Ophthalmol* 1982;27:79–85.
36. Forderreuther S, Straube A. The criteria of the International Headache Society for Tolosa–Hunt Syndrome need to be revised. *J Neurol* 1999;246:371–377.
37. Karcioglu ZA, Aden LB, Cruz AA, et al. Orbital invasion with prolactinoma: a clinical review of 4 patients. *Ophthalmic Plast Reconstr Surg* 2002;18:64–71.
38. Mesmer EP, Font RL, McCrary JA, et al. Epithelioid angiosarcoma of the orbit presenting as Tolosa–Hunt syndrome. *Ophthalmology* 1983;90:1414–1421.
39. Pina SC, Pascual-Castroviejo I, Fernandez, et al. Burkitt lymphoma presenting as Tolosa–Hunt syndrome. *Pediatric Neurol* 1993;9:157–158.
40. Mafee MF, Edward DP, Koeller KK, Dorodi S. Lacrimal gland tumors and simulating lesions. *Radiol Clin North Am* 1999;37:219–239.
41. Au Eong KG, Choo CT. Burkitt lymphoma manifesting as acute proptosis. *Am J Ophthalmol* 1997;123:856–858.
42. Eifrig CW, Chaudhry NA, Tse DT, et al. Lacrimal gland cyst abscess. *Ophthalmic Plast Reconstr Surg* 2001;17:131–133.
43. Law FW. Spontaneous orbital hemorrhage. *Br J Ophthalmol* 1971;55:556–558.
44. Cameron JD, Letson RD, Summers CG. Clinical significance of hematic cysts of the orbit. *Ophthalmic Plast Reconstr Surg* 1988;4:95–99.
45. Ehlinger P, Peeters L, Kockx M, et al. Hematic cyst of the orbit. *Acta Stomatol Belg* 1993;90:177–179.
46. Shapiro A, Tso MOM, Putterman AM, et al. A clinicopathologic study of hematic cysts of the orbit. *Am J Ophthalmol* 1986;102:237–241.
47. Goldberg SH, Sassani JW, Parnes RE. Traumatic intraconal hematic cysts of the orbit. *Arch Ophthalmol* 1992;110:378–380.
48. Wiot JG, Pleatman CW. Chronic hematic cysts of the orbit. *AJNR Am J Neuroradiol* 1989;10:S37–S39.
49. Parke DW, Font RL, Boniuk M, et al. Cholesteatoma of the orbit. *Arch Ophthalmol* 1982;100:612–616.
50. Selva D, Phipps SE, O'Connell JX, et al. Clinicopathological report. Pathogenesis of orbital cholesterol granuloma. *Clin Exp Ophthalmol* 2003;31:78–82.
51. Dobben GD, Fillet B, Mafee MF, et al. Orbital subperiosteal hematoma, cholesterol granuloma and infection: evaluation with MR imaging and CT. *Radiology Clin North Am* 1998; 36:1185–1200.
52. Seabold JE, Simonson TM, Weber PC, et al. Cranial osteomyelitis: diagnosis and follow-up with In-111 white blood cell and Tc-99m methylene diphosphonate bone SPECT, CT and MR imaging. *Radiology* 1995;196:779–788.
53. Ormerod LD, et al. Ophthalmic manifestations of maxillary sinus mucoceles. *Ophthalmology* 1987;94:1013.
54. Avery G, Yang RA, Close LG. Ophthalmic manifestations of mucoceles. *Ann Ophthalmol* 1983;15:734–739.
55. Friedman DP, Rao VM, Flanders AE. Lesions causing a mass in the medial canthus of the orbit: CT and MR features. *AJR Am J Roentgenol* 1993;160:1095–1099.
56. Hasso AN, Lambert D. Magnetic resonance imaging of the paranasal sinuses and nasal cavities. *Top Magn Reson Imaging* 1994;6:209–223.
57. DeSouza CE, et al. Mucoceles, proptosis, and transorbital frontoethmoidectomy. *Orbit* 1988;7:167.
58. Yip CC, McCulley TJ, Kersten RC, et al. Adult nasolacrimal duct mucocele. *Arch Ophthalmol* 2003;121:1065–1066.
59. Reich JM. What is sarcoidosis? *Chest* 2003;124:367–371.
60. Keicho N, Kitamura K, Takaku F, et al. Serum concentration of soluble interleukin-2 receptor as a sensitive parameter of disease activity in sarcoidosis. *Chest* 1990;98:112.

61. Thomas PD, Hunninghake GW. Current concepts of the pathogenesis of sarcoidosis. *Am Rev Respir Dis* 1987;135:747.
62. Kelly LD. Sarcoid disease of the skin and eye. In: Mannis MJ, Masai MS, Huntley AC, eds. *Eye and Skin Disease*. Philadelphia: Lippincott-Raven; 1996:207–218.
63. Reich JM. Deciphering histoplasmosis, systemic noncaseating granuloma, and sarcoidosis. *Chest* 1998;113:1143.
64. Jakobiec FA, Font RL. Orbit. In: Spencer WH, ed. *Ophthalmic Pathology*. Philadelphia: WB Saunders; 1986;2459–2860.
65. Bronson LJ, Fisher YL. Sarcoidosis of the paranasal sinuses with orbital extensions. *Arch Ophthalmol* 1976;94:243–244.
66. Karcioglu ZA, Brear R. Conjunctival biopsy in sarcoidosis. *Am J Ophthalmol* 1985;99:68.
67. Obenauf CD, Shaw HE, Sydnor CF, et al. Sarcoidosis and its ophthalmic manifestations. *Am J Ophthlamol* 1978;86:648–655.
68. Weinstein JM, Koch, Lane S. Orbital pseudotumor in Crohn's colitis. *Ann Ophthalmol* 1984;16:275–278.
69. Verbraeken H, Ryckaert S, Demets W. Pseudotumor of the orbit and Crohn's disease. *Bull Soc Belge Ophtalmol* 1984;210:65–72.
70. Sedwick LA, Klingele TG, Burde RM, et al. Optic neuritis in inflammatory bowel disease. *J Clin Neurophthalmol* 1984;4:3–6.
71. Talal N. Sjögren's syndrome: historical overview and clinical spectrum of disease. *Rheum Dis Clin North Am* 1992;18:507–515.
72. Callen JP, Mahl CF. Oculocutaneous manifestations observed in multisystem disorders. *Dermatol Clin* 1991;10:709–716.
73. Alexander EL. Neurologic disease in Sjögren's syndrome: mononuclear inflammatory vasculopathy affecting central/peripheral nervous system and muscle. *Rheum Dis Clin North Am* 1993;19:869–908.
74. Soter A. Cutaneous necrotizing venulitis. In: Fitzpatrick TB, Eisen AZ, Wolff K, et al, eds. *Dermatology in General Medicine*. New York: McGraw-Hill; 1993:1501–1510.
75. Provost TT, Watson R. Cutaneous manifestations of Sjögren's syndrome. *Rheum Dis Clin North Am* 1992;18:609–616.
76. Spencer WH, Zimmerman LE. Conjunctiva. In: Spencer WH, ed. *Ophthalmic Pathology*. Philadelphia: WB Saunders; 1986: 109–228.
77. Jakobiec FA, Font RL. Orbit. In: Spencer WH, ed. *Ophthalmic Pathology*. Philadelphia: WB Saunders; 1986:2459–2860.
78. Fox RI. Sjögren syndrome. In: Sullivan DA, Dartt DA, Meneray MA, eds. *Lacrimal Gland, Tear Fluid, Dry Eye Syndromes*. New York: Plenum Press; 1998:891–902.
79. Rosenbaum JT, Bennett RM. Chronic anterior and posterior uveitis and primary Sjögren's syndrome. *Am J Ophthalmol* 1987;104:346–352.
80. Wegener F. Über eine eigenartige rhinogene Granulomotose mit Besonderer. Beteiligung des Arteriensystems und der Nieren. *Beitr Pathol Anat* 1939;102:36–68.
81. Godman GC, Churg J. Wegener's granulomatosis: pathology and review of the literature. *AMA Arch Pathol* 1954;58: 533–553.
82. Robin JB, Schanzlin DJ, Meisler DM, et al. Ocular involvement in Wegener's granulomatosis. *Surv Ophthalmol* 1985; 30:127–140.
83. Bullen CL, Liesegang TJ, McDonald TJ, et al. Ocular complications of Wegener's granulomatosis. *Ophthalmology* 1983; 90:279–290.
84. Straatsma BR. Ocular manifestations of Wegener's granulomatosis. *Am J Ophthalmol* 1957;44:789–799.
85. Greenberger MH. Central retinal artery closure in Wegener's granulomatosis. *Am J Ophthalmol* 1967;63:515–516.
86. Howell SB, Epstein WV. Circulating immune complexes in Wegener's granulomatosis. *Am J Med* 1976;60:259–268.
87. Falk RJ, Jennette JC. Wegener's granulomatosis, systemic vasculitis, and anti-neutrophil cytoplasmic antibodies. *Annu Rev Med* 1991;42:459–469.
88. Fauci AS, Wolff SM. Wegener's granulomatosis: studies in 18 patients and a review of the literature. *Medicine (Baltimore)* 1973;52:535–561.
89. Coutu RE, Klein M, Lessell S, et al. Limited form of Wegener's granulomatosis. Eye involvement as a major sign. *JAMA* 1975;233:868–871.
90. Rao NV, Wehner NG, Marshall BC, et al. Characterization of proteinase 3 (PR3), a neutrophil serine protease. Structural and functional. *J Biol Chem* 1991;266:9540–9548.
91. Gans ROB, Goldschmeding R, Donker AJM, et al. Neutrophil cytoplasmic autoantibodies and Wegener's granulomatosis. *Lancet* 1989;1:269–270.
92. Cohen, Tervaert JW, Goldschmeding R, Hene RJ, et al. Neutrophil cytoplasmic autoantibodies in Wegener's granulomatosis. *Lancet* 1989;1:270.
93. Jennette JC, Ewert BH, Falk RJ. Do antineutrophil cytoplasmic autoantibodies cause Wegener's granulomatosis and other forms of necrotizing vasculitis? *Controv Clin Rheum* 1993;19:1–14.
94. Egner W, Chapel HM. Titration of antibodies against neutrophil cytoplasmic antigens is useful in monitoring disease activity in systemic vasculitides. *Clin Exp Immunol* 1990;82: 244–249.
95. Soukiasian SH, Foster CS, Niles JL, et al. Diagnostic value of antineutrophil cytoplasmic antibodies in scleritis associated with Wegener's granulomatosis. *Ophthalmology* 1992;99: 125–132.
96. Wiik A. Antineutrophil cytoplasmic antibodies in Wegener's granulomatosis. *Clin Exp Rheumatol* 1993;11:191–201.
97. Kalina PH, Lie JT, Campbell RJ, et al. Diagnostic value and limitations of orbital biopsy in Wegener's granulomatosis. *Ophthalmology* 1992;99:120–124.
98. Jordan DR, Addison DA. Wegener's granulomatosis. Eyelid and conjunctival manifestations as the presenting feature in two individuals. *Ophthalmology* 1994;101:602–607.
99. Devaney KO, Travis WD, Hoffman G, et al. Interpretation of head and neck biopsies in Wegener's granulomatosis. A pathologic study of 126 biopsies in 70 patients. *Am J Surg Pathol* 1990;14:555–564.
100. Del Buono EA, Flint A. Diagnostic usefulness of nasal biopsy in Wegener's granulomatosis. *Hum Pathol* 1991;22:107–110.
101. Travis WD, Hoffman GS, Leavitt RY, et al. Surgical pathology of the lung in Wegener's granulomatosis. Review of 87 open lung biopsies from 67 patients. *Am J Surg Pathol* 1991; 15:315–333.
102. Lombard CM, Duncan SR, Rizk NW, et al. The diagnosis of Wegener's granulomatosis from transbronchial biopsy specimens. *Hum Path* 190;21:838–842.
103. Fauci AS, Haynes BF, Katz P, et al. Wegener's granulomatosis: prospective clinical and therapeutic experience with 85 patients for 21 years. *Ann Intern Med* 1983;98:76–85.
104. Haynes BF, Fishman ML, Fauci AS, et al. The ocular manifestations of Wegener's granulomatosis. Fifteen years experience and review of the literature. *Am J Med* 1977;63:131–141.
105. Koorneef L, Melief CJM, Peterse HL, et al. Wegener's granulomatosis of the orbit. *Orbit* 1983;2:1–10.
106. Specks U, DeRemee RA. Granulomatous vasculitis. Wegener's granulomatosis and Churg–Strauss syndrome. *Rheum Clin North Am* 1990;16:377–397.
107. Foster CS. Immunosuppressive therapy in external ocular inflammatory disease. *Ophthalmology* 1980;87:140–150.
108. Levine MR, Buckman G. Primary localized orbital amyloidosis. *Ann Ophthalmol* 1986;18:165–167.
109. Murdoch IE, Sullivan TJ, Moseley I, et al. Primary localized amyloidosis of the orbit. *Br J Ophthalmol* 1996;80: 1083–1086.
110. Okamoto K, Ito J, Emura T, et al. Focal orbital amyloidosis presenting as rectus muscle enlargement: CT and MR findings. *AJNR Am J Neuroradiol* 1998;19:1799–1801.

111. Cohen MM, Lessell S. Amyloid tumor of the orbit. *Neuroradiology* 1979;18:157–159.
112. Üstün MO, Ekinci N, Payzin B. Extramedullary plasmacytoma of the parotid gland. Report of a case with extensive amyloid deposition masking the cytology and histopathologic picture. *Acta Cytol* 2001;45:449–453.
113. Uceda-Montanes A, Blanco G, Saornil MA, et al. Extramedullary plasmacytoma of the orbit. *Acta Ophthalmol Scand* 2000;78:601–603.
114. Alexiou C, Kau RJ, Dietzfelbinger H. Extramedullary plasmacytoma: tumor occurrence and therapeutic concepts. *Cancer* 1999;85:2305–2314.
115. Galieni P, Cavo M, Pulsino A, et al. Clinical outcome of extramedullary plasmacytoma. *Haematologica* 2000;85:47–51.
116. Bubbage RR, Spraul CW, Wojno TH, Grossniklaus HE. Kimura disease of the orbit and ocular adnexal. *Surv Ophthalmol* 1999;44:79–91.
117. Cook HT, Stafford ND. Angiolymphoid hyperplasia with eosinophilia involving the lacrimal gland: case report. *Br J Ophthalmol* 1988;72:710–712.
118. Francis IC, Kappagoda MB, Smith J, Kneale K. Kimura's disease of the orbit. *Ophthalmic Plast Reconstr Surg* 1988;4:235–239.
119. Ishida K, Yokota T, Wada Y, et al. Unilateral facial swelling and exophthalmos in a patient with polyarteritis nodosa. *Intern Med* 1992;31:500–503.
120. Koike R, Yamada M, Matsunaga T, et al. Polyarteritis nodosa (PN) complicated with unilateral exophthalmos. *Intern Med* 1993;32:232–236.
121. James DG. *Sarcoidosis and Other Granulomatous Disorders*. New York: Dekker; 1994.
122. Sale S, Patterson R. Recurrent Churg–Strauss vasculitis. With exophthalmos, hearing loss, nasal obstruction, amyloid deposits, hyperimmunoglobulinemia E, and circulating immune complexes. *Arch Intern Med* 1981;141:1363–1365.
123. Shields CL, Shields JA, Rosanski TI. Conjunctival involvement with Churg–Strauss syndrome. *Am J Ophthalmol* 1986;102:601–605.
124. Bankhurst AD, Carlow TJ, Reidy RW. Exophthalmos in systemic lupus erythematosus. *Ann Ophthalmol* 16:669–671.
125. Brenner E, Shock J. Proptosis secondary to systemic lupus erythematosus. *Arch Ophthalmology* 1974;91:81–82.
126. Grimson BS, Simons KB. Oribital inflammation, myositis, and systemic lupus erythematosus. *Arch Ophthalmol* 1983; 101:736–738.
127. Jabs DA, Miller NA, Neuman SA, et al. Optic neuropathy in systemic lupus erythematosus. *Arch Ophthalmol* 1986;104: 564.
128. Al-Malki AF, Hussain H, Al-Ma'ani JR, Karcioglu ZA. Extraocular myositis in Behçet's syndrome. Paper presented at: VI International Symposium on Ocular Inflammation, Istanbul, Turkey; June 2000.
129. James DG, Spiteri MA. Behçet's disease. *Ophthalmology* 1982;89:1279.
130. Ibanez HE, Bardenstein DS, Korman NJ, Reinhart WJ. Exuberant conjunctival pseudopolyposis in a patient with dermatomyositis. *Ann Ophthalmol* 1993;25:326–327.
131. Leib ML, Odel JG, Cooney MJ. Orbital polymyositis and giant cell myocarditis. *Ophthalmology* 1994;101:950–954.
132. Selva-O'Callaghan A, Mijares-Boeckh-Behrens T, Solans-Laque R, et al. Dermatomyositis and Graves' disease. *Clin Exp Rheumatol* 2001;19:595–596.
133. Anzai H, Tajima S. Systemic scleroderma associated with Graves' disease. *J Dermatol* 1996;23:896–898.
134. Horan EC. Ophthalmic manifestations of progressive systemic sclerosis. *Br J Ophthalmol* 1969;53:388–392.
135. Manschot WA. Generalized scleroderma with ocular symptoms. *Ophthalmologica* 1965;149:131–137.
136. Nicholson D, White S, Lipson A, et al. Progressive systemic sclerosis and Graves' disease. Report of three cases. *Arch Intern Med* 1986;146:2350–2352.
137. Foster CS, Sainz de la Masa M. *The Sclera*. New York: Springer-Verlag; 1994.
138. Prahalad S, Shear ES, Thompson SD, et al. Increased prevalence of familial autoimmunity in simplex and multiplex families with juvenile rheumatoid arthritis. *Arthritis Rheum* 2002;46:1851–1856.
139. Watson PG, Hazelman BL. *The Sclera and Systemic Disorders*. Philadelphia. WB Saunders; 1976.

PART SEVEN

Management of Orbital Tumors

30

Staging of Orbital Tumors

Zeynel A. Karcıoglu and Barrett G. Haik

Surgery is the most common modality of tumor treatment in the orbit, whether it is performed for total excision or for debulking or biopsy purposes.[1–4] Even in today's multimodality cancer treatment milieu, surgery remains very effective not only for diagnosis but also for treatment.[4,5] Surgical treatment is most effective in benign lesions and/or well-delineated malignant lesions. It also provides extremely useful initial information about the nature of the tumor as well as about staging, an appropriate management plan, and prognosis. In many orbital tumors, such as rhabdomyosarcoma, lymphoma, and secondary and metastatic tumors, radiation therapy alone or in combination with chemotherapy offers promising results. However, it is extremely rare that an orbital tumor patient's care does not include an initial surgical component.

Whether the objective of the therapy is cure or palliation, the management plan depends on the specific typing and staging of the neoplasm.[6,7] If the cancer is considered to be localized without evidence of spread, the tumor can be excised and the patient is cured.[8] If the cancer has spread beyond local cure, the objective is to control symptoms and maintain the maximum function of the eye and the adnexa with the best quality of life for as long as possible. Patients are generally considered to be incurable if they have distant metastasis or evidence of diffuse extension of the tumor into the cranium.[2]

The selection of the single or multimodality therapy depends on the type and the extent of the neoplasm, which is determined by staging.[1,2] For example, in general, if a neoplasm is limited to the orbit without extension into the globe, cranial cavity, and/or regional lymph nodes, the malignancy is considered curable by surgery and/or radiation. Extension of a given orbital tumor into neighboring structures including the globe, optic nerve, nose and perinasal sinuses, central nervous system, or regional lymph nodes is of great clinical importance; these features affect the staging and, therefore, the treatment of the tumor.

Three significant events determine the biological behavior of a malignant neoplasm: local tumor (T) growth, extension to lymph nodes (N), and distant metastasis (M).[6,9] These events determine the anatomic extent of the malignancy, which is more commonly known as the stage of the disease at a given time in its progression. Therefore, the letters T, N, and M represent the indicators of prognosis of the patient harboring a particular type of tumor. The type of tumor as well as the staging are determined by histopathologic examination of tissues. The TNM classification by stage grouping is possible only when based on examination of surgically excised specimens from the primary tumor, from its margins, from the regional lymph node, and from distant metastatic sites.

Clinical experience has proven that the definition of the anatomic staging varies depending on the histologic type and the anatomic site of origin. Therefore, the American Joint Committee on Cancer (AJCC) utilizes the TNM classification scheme for particular tumors of each anatomic site (Table 30.1).[9] The system is intended to provide a common language by which patient information can be shared among physicians to establish therapeutic plans and to estimate prognosis. The long-range benefit of the staging system is that it provides easy comparison of similar groups of patients when therapeutic regimens are evaluated.

In addition to the TNM classification, the histopathologic type and the grade of a given neoplasm are important therapeutic and prognostic determinants (Box 30.1). Numerical subsets that may be used for each letter, such as, T0, T1, N2, M1, etc., indicate the progression of the malignant disease, creating a shorthand notation for describing the clinical and histopathologic extent of a given malignancy. Four classifications are designed for each anatomic site:

1. Clinical classification (cTNM)
2. Pathologic classification (pTNM)
3. Retreatment classification (rTNM)
4. Autopsy classification (aTNM)

Clinical (c) classification is based on physical findings, imaging, endoscopy, and biopsy. The clinical staging is essential to make therapeutic decisions and evaluate the patient's response to that treatment.

TABLE 30.1. Definitions of TNM.

Primary tumor (T)	
TX	Primary tumor cannot be assessed
T0	No evidence of primary tumor
Tis	Carcinoma in situ
T1, T2, T3, T4	Increasing size of the primary tumor
Regional lymph nodes (N)	
NX	Regional lymph nodes cannot be assessed
N0	No regional lymph node involvement
N1, N2, N3	Increasing involvement of regional lymph nodes
Distant metastasis (M)	
MX	Distant metastasis cannot be assessed
M0	No distant metastasis
M1	Distant metastasis

BOX 30.1. Summary of Descriptors Utilized in TNM Classification

G: Histopathology grade (GX, G1–G4)
L: Lymphatic vessel invasion (LX, L0, L1)
V: Venous invasion (VX, V0, V1, V2)
R: Residual tumor (RX, R0, R1, R2)
m suffix: Presence of multiple primary tumors [e.g., pT(m)NM]
y prefix: Patients classified during or following initial therapy (e.g., ycTNM)
r prefix: Recurrent tumor after following disease-free interval (e.g., rTNM)
Histopathology grade (G) is expressed with numbers and represents the qualitative assessment of the differentiation of a given neoplasm. It ranges from most differentiated (G1) to least differentiated (G4); GX stands for a grade that cannot be assessed.

Pathologic (p) classification is based on histopathologic examination of the tissues removed by biopsy or exploratory surgery. Histopathologic evaluation provides additional data to make a management plan and estimate the prognosis.

Retreatment (r) classification is helpful to provide further management plan for a neoplasm that recurs after a disease-free interval.

Autopsy (a) classification is done in the staging of a given neoplasm not evident prior to death that is discovered by postmortem examination.

Recently, the AJCC upgraded the TNM classification for cancers of all types, including orbital neoplasms. During this upgrading of the system, the staging forms for each anatomic site were modified. The following staging forms for the malignancies of the orbit are borrowed from the current (2002) manual of the AJCC, with the written consent of the committee.

Acknowledgment Staging forms are used with the permission of the American Joint Committee on Cancer (AJCC), Chicago. The authors are grateful to AJCC and Dr. James C. Fleming, who was primarily instrumental in the development of the staging forms. The original source for this material is the AJCC *Cancer Staging Manual* (6th edition, 2002, published by Springer-Verlag New York, Inc., New York).

References

1. Morton DF. Principles of surgical oncology. In: Helens JS, Frei E, Bast RC, et al, eds. *Cancer Medicine*. 3rd ed. Philadelphia: Lea & Febiger; 1993:523—538.
2. Pollock RE, Morton DL. Principles of surgical oncology. In: Bast RC, Kufe DW, Pollock RE, et al., eds. *Cancer Medicine*. New York: BC Decker; 2000:449–558.
3. Rosenberg SA. Principles of cancer management; surgical oncology, In: Devita DT, Hellman S, Rosenberg SA, eds. *Cancer: Principles and Practice of Oncology*. Philadelphia: Lippincott-Raven; 1997.295 306.
4. Rosenberg SA. *Principles and Practice of Biologic Therapy of Cancer*. Philadelphia: Lippincott, Williams & Wilkins; 2000.
5. Niederhuber JE. Surgical therapy. In: Adeloff MD, Armitage JO, Lichter R, Niederhuber JE, eds. *Clinical Oncology*. New York: Churchill Livingston; 2000:471–481.
6. Mayer D, Davies R, Moossa AR. Investigating the oncology patient: diagnosis and staging. In: Moossa AR, Schinpff SC, Robson MC, eds. *Comprehensive Textbook of Oncology*. Baltimore: Williams & Wilkins; 1991:201.
7. Rubin P. Concepts of cancer staging. In: Caleb RE, Schuin PS, Rosenberg SA, eds. *Medical Oncology*. New York: Macmillan; 1984:157–177.
8. Schrock PR. Principles of surgical oncology. In: Carter SA, Glatstein D, Livingston RD, eds. *Principles of Cancer Treatment*. New York: McGraw-Hill; 1982:53–57.
9. American Joint Commission on Cancer. *Cancer Staging Manual*. 6th ed. New York: Springer-Verlag; 2002:349–384.

CARCINOMA OF THE LACRIMAL GLAND

Hospital Name/Address	Patient Name/Information

Type of Specimen ____________ Histopathologic Type ____________

Tumor Size ____________ Laterality: ☐ Bilateral ☐ Left ☐ Right

DEFINITIONS

Clinical	Pathologic	Primary Tumor (T)	
☐	☐	TX	Primary tumor cannot be assessed
☐	☐	T0	No evidence of primary tumor
☐	☐	T1	Tumor 2.5 cm or less in greatest dimension, limited to the lacrimal
☐	☐		gland
☐	☐	T2	Tumor more than 2.5 cm but not more than 5 cm in greatest dimension, limited to the lacrimal gland
☐	☐	T3	Tumor invades the periosteum
☐	☐	T3a	Tumor not more than 5 cm invades the periosteum of the lacrimal gland fossa
☐	☐	T3b	Tumor more than 5 cm in greatest dimension with periosteal invasion
☐	☐	T4	Tumor invades the orbital soft tissues, optic nerve, or globe with or without bone invasion; tumor extends beyond the orbit to adjacent structures, including brain

Regional Lymph Nodes (N)

Clinical	Pathologic		
☐	☐	NX	Regional lymph nodes cannot be assessed
☐	☐	N0	No regional lymph node metastasis
☐	☐	N1	Regional lymph node metastasis

Distant Metastasis (M)

Clinical	Pathologic		
☐	☐	MX	Distant metastasis cannot be assessed
☐	☐	M0	No distant metastasis
☐	☐	M1	Distant metastasis

Biopsy of metastatic site performed ..... ☐Y....... ☐N

Source of pathologic metastatic specimen ____________

Stage Grouping

No stage grouping is presently recommended.

Histologic Grade (G)

☐ GX Grade cannot be assessed
☐ G1 Well differentiated
☐ G2 Moderately differentiated: includes adenoid cystic carcinoma without basaloid (solid) pattern
☐ G3 Poorly differentiated: includes adenoid cystic carcinoma with basaloid (solid) pattern
☐ G4 Undifferentiated

Residual Tumor (R)

☐ RX Presence of residual tumor cannot be assessed
☐ R0 No residual tumor
☐ R1 Microscopic residual tumor
☐ R2 Macroscopic residual tumor

(continued)

CARCINOMA OF THE LACRIMAL GLAND *(continued)*

Additional Descriptors

For identification of special cases of TNM or pTNM classifications, the "m" suffix and "y," "r," and "a" prefixes are used. Although they do not affect the stage grouping, they indicate cases needing separate analysis.

☐ **m suffix** indicates the presence of multiple primary tumors in a single site and is recorded in parentheses: pT(m)NM.

☐ **y prefix** indicates those cases in which classification is performed during or following initial multimodality therapy. The cTNM or pTNM category is identified by a "y" prefix. The ycTNM or ypTNM categorizes the extent of tumor actually present at the time of that examination. The "y" categorization is not an estimate of tumor prior to multimodality therapy.

☐ **r prefix** indicates a recurrent tumor when staged after a disease-free interval, and is identified by the "r" prefix: rTNM.

☐ **a prefix** designates the stage determined at autopsy: aTNM.

Prognostic Indicators (if applicable)

Notes

Additional Descriptors

Lymphatic Vessel Invasion (L)

LX Lymphatic vessel invasion cannot be assessed
L0 No lymphatic vessel invasion
L1 Lymphatic vessel invasion

Venous Invasion (V)

VX Venous invasion cannot be assessed
V0 No venous invasion
V1 Microscopic venous invasion
V2 Macroscopic venous invasion

ILLUSTRATION

Indicate on diagram primary tumor and regional nodes involved.

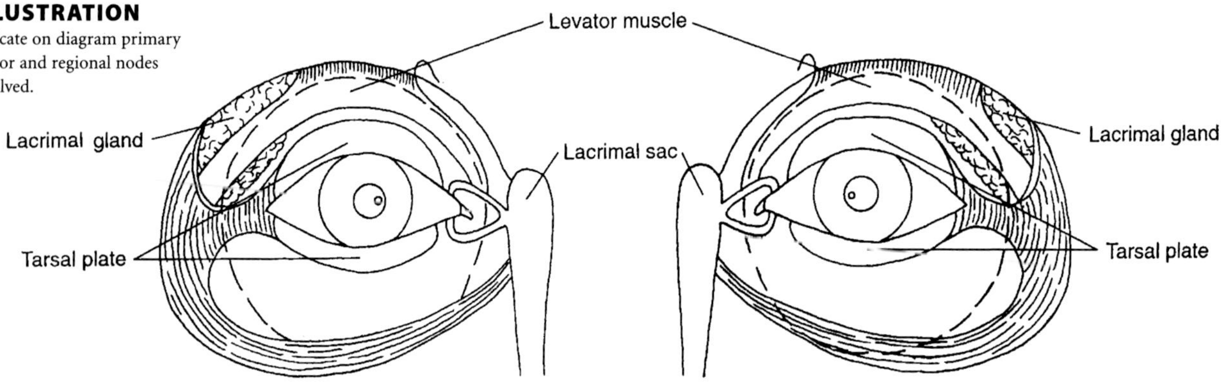

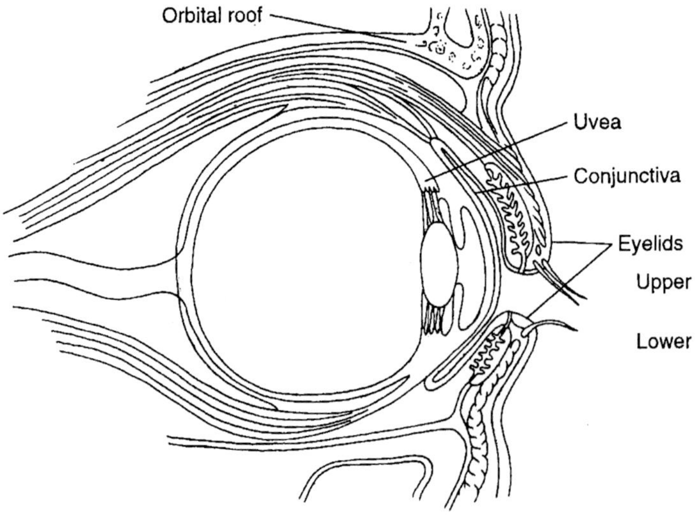

Physician's Signature ______________________ Date______________

SARCOMA OF THE ORBIT

Hospital Name/Address	Patient Name/Information

Type of Specimen ______________________

Histopathologic Type ______________________

Tumor Size ______________________

Laterality: ☐ Bilateral ☐ Left ☐ Right

DEFINITIONS

Primary Tumor (T)

Clinical	Pathologic		
☐	☐	TX	Primary tumor cannot be assessed
☐	☐	T0	No evidence of primary tumor
☐	☐	T1	Tumor 15 mm or less in greatest dimension
☐	☐	T2	Tumor more than 15 mm in greatest dimension without invasion of globe or bony wall
☐	☐	T3	Tumor of any size with invasion of orbital tissues and/or bony walls
☐	☐	T4	Tumor invasion of globe or periorbital structure, such as eyelids, temporal fossa, nasal cavity and paranasal sinuses, and/or central nervous system

Regional Lymph Nodes (N)

Clinical	Pathologic		
☐	☐	NX	Regional lymph nodes cannot be assessed
☐	☐	N0	No regional lymph node metastasis
☐	☐	N1	Regional lymph node metastasis

Distant Metastasis (M)

Clinical	Pathologic		
☐	☐	MX	Distant metastasis cannot be assessed
☐	☐	M0	No distant metastasis
☐	☐	M1	Distant metastasis

Biopsy of metastatic site performed ..... ☐Y .... ☐N

Source of pathologic metastatic specimen ______________________

Stage Grouping

No stage grouping is presently recommended.

Histologic Grade (G)

☐ GX Grade cannot be assessed
☐ G1 Well differentiated
☐ G2 Moderately differentiated
☐ G3 Poorly differentiated
☐ G4 Undifferentiated

Residual Tumor (R)

☐ RX Presence of residual tumor cannot be assessed
☐ R0 No residual tumor
☐ R1 Microscopic residual tumor
☐ R2 Macroscopic residual tumor

10

(continued)

SARCOMA OF THE ORBIT *(continued)*

Additional Descriptors

For identification of special cases of TNM or pTNM classifications, the "m" suffix and "y," "r," and "a" prefixes are used. Although they do not affect the stage grouping, they indicate cases needing separate analysis.

- ☐ **m suffix** indicates the presence of multiple primary tumors in a single site and is recorded in parentheses: pT(m)NM.
- ☐ **y prefix** indicates those cases in which classification is performed during or following initial multimodality therapy. The cTNM or pTNM category is identified by a "y" prefix. The ycTNM or ypTNM categorizes the extent of tumor actually present at the time of that examination. The "y" categorization is not an estimate of tumor prior to multimodality therapy.
- ☐ **r prefix** indicates a recurrent tumor when staged after a disease-free interval, and is identified by the "r" prefix: rTNM.
- ☐ **a prefix** designates the stage determined at autopsy: aTNM.

Prognostic Indicators (if applicable)

Notes

Additional Descriptors

Lymphatic Vessel Invasion (L)

LX Lymphatic vessel invasion cannot be assessed
L0 No lymphatic vessel invasion
L1 Lymphatic vessel invasion

Venous Invasion (V)

VX Venous invasion cannot be assessed
V0 No venous invasion
V1 Microscopic venous invasion
V2 Macroscopic venous invasion

ILLUSTRATION

Indicate on diagram primary tumor and regional nodes involved.

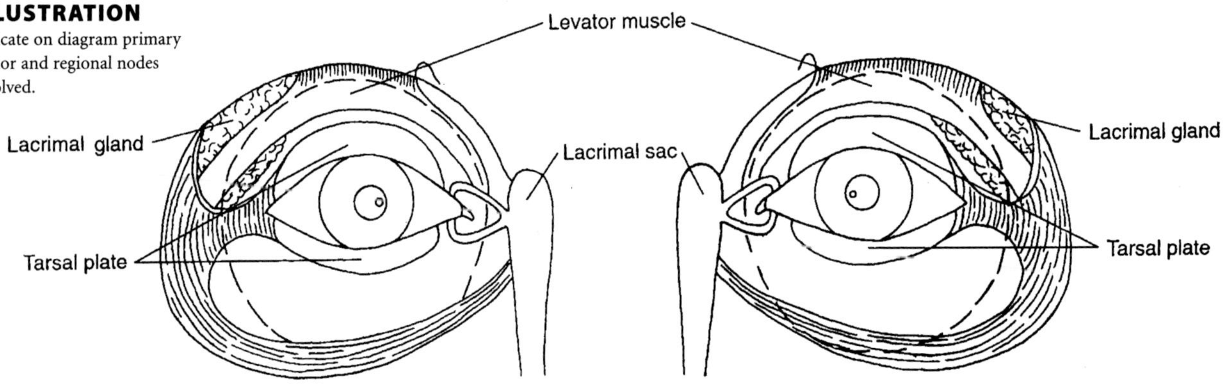

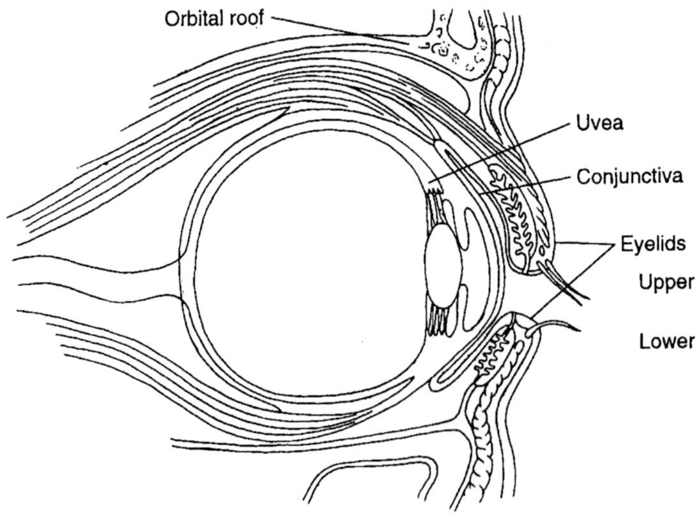

Physician's Signature ______________________ Date ______________

31

Surgical Treatment

Zeynel A. Karcıoglu

PREOPERATIVE EVALUATION

The preoperative evaluation should begin with a thorough history and physical no matter how obvious the diagnosis appears to be. The original meaning of the Greek word *historia*, from which we derive the English word history, meant "inquiry." Detailed systemic and ocular inquiry offer many useful clues for the management of the orbital tumor patient. The family history should specify any cancer, craniofacial syndrome, and other systemic familial disease such as neurofibromatosis. Particular attention should be given to the history of linking diseases as well as to other major health problems. The history of previous hospitalizations, head and neck injuries, and surgeries should be elicited. A list of the patient's medications and allergies should be obtained.

The patient's tendency toward bleeding should specifically be elicited. It is very important that the patient be instructed not to take aspirin products, other prostaglandin inhibitors, or anti–red cell and anti-platelet agents 2 weeks prior to surgery (Box 31.1). If there is any doubt regarding the bleeding status, prothrombin time (PT) and partial thromboplastin time (PTT) should be obtained prior to surgery. Younger children with questionable vascular lesions should be typed and crossed for 1 to 2 blood volumes.

The process of obtaining a detailed history and doing a thorough physical examination is an important opportunity to establish a good rapport with the patient and the family, which will strengthen their trust and confidence with the surgeon. It is absolutely essential that the patient's problem be discussed in detail at every step. One practical way to communicate with the patient is to use computed tomography (CT) and magnetic resonance (MR) to explain the problem shown on the films. Patients can understand the problem much better when they are shown images of a space-occupying lesion in an orbit compressing the eye. The orbit is a particularly good site for this approach because many times the fellow orbit can be shown as a normal comparison. Furthermore, the need for the surgical procedure and the alternative treatments should be discussed, if at all possible, on a model or a detailed diagram of the eye and the orbit. The reasons for surgery, potential benefits, as well as the complications should be detailed with the patient in a frank manner and the likelihood of complications based on the surgeon's judgment and experience should be listed.

It is important that the patient and the family, not the surgeon, decide whether to proceed with surgery. In life- and sight-threatening situations, the physician should make a clear note of his or her plan in the chart. If the advice is disregarded by the patient or family, this should also be documented in the chart. In certain situations, it may even be advisable, with the patient's agreement, to record the conversation. If the diagnosis is not certain—for example, if an orbital biopsy is required—the need of biopsy diagnosis should be clearly explained. Radiology and pathology reports, as well as visual field and other test results, should also be discussed with the patient.

The surgical complications should be explained to the patient and family, not only for consent purposes, but more important, for the patient's understanding of potential future problems. They should be told that there is a chance of infection and/or bleeding after surgery. It should also be explained that a persistent or transient visual loss, though a remote possibility, may result. Other postoperative complications include pain, a feeling of pressure, hypoesthesia or hyperesthesia, and scarring on the eyelids and the periorbital skin. It is very useful to obtain preoperative photographs and file them in the patient's chart. It also must be explained to the patient that the orbital problem may be part of a systemic disease and that better understanding of the orbital pathology may eventually help to arrive at an effective systemic treatment.

It is a sound policy to give information to the patient and the family members regarding the disease and the management plan and let them go home and think about their options. This offers them an opportunity to digest the information, check with other family members and friends, or consult other physicians. It should be clear that they can call and discuss any further concerns with the surgeon and/or with the other members of the team.

Once the history and physical exam, laboratory tests, and imaging procedures are completed, a management plan should be made. The management of a tumor patient should take into account the relation-

BOX 31.1. Partial List of the More Common Aspirin-Containing Products, Which Should Be Discontinued 2 Weeks Prior to Surgery

Advil	Empirin
Aleve	Enteric coated aspirin
Alka-Seltzer	Equagesic
Anacin	Excedrin
ASA	Fiorinal
Ascriptin	Ibuprofen products
Aspergum	Mediprin
Aspirin	Methocarbomol with ASDA
Bufferin	Midol
Cephalgesic	Motrin
Children's aspirin	Naprosyn
Cold tablets	Norgesic
Cope	Pepto-Bismol
Coricidin	Percodan
Darvon with ASA	Phenaphen
Diurex	St. Joseph Aspirin
Doan's Pills	Sine-Off Sinus Medication
Dristan	Soma Compound
Ecotrin products	Vanquish

ship of the orbital manifestations to a systemic disease, the immune status of the patient, the risk of general anesthesia, and the psychological state of the patient. Simpler plans should always be implemented before complicated ones. For example, if a fine-needle aspiration biopsy would offer information about an apical tumor, this procedure should be attempted first, no matter how small the yield, before a transcranial orbitotomy.

SURGICAL PLANNING AND PREPARATION

Imaging

Imaging has become the gold standard for the diagnosis and management of orbital lesions. All imaging procedures, including ultrasonography, CT, and MRI are helpful, not only to obtain clues for diagnosis, but also for treatment planning in adults and children.[1–3] The location, shape, internal characteristics, and relationship of a given lesion to adjacent orbital structures offer considerable clues toward diagnosis. CT and MRI, individually or together, usually provide a wealth of information on orbital lesions. Ultrasonography can be uniquely useful to reveal dynamic changes such as compressibility, multiloculation, and pulsations of cystic lesions; this kind of information cannot be obtained with other types of imaging. Furthermore, recently developing advanced techniques of imaging, such as color Doppler ultrasonography, diffusion-weighted MRI, cine-MRI, MR spectroscopy, and positron emission tomography (PET), can be useful in special situations to add information regarding the nature and behavior of space-occupying lesions within the orbit.[4–6] Because of the significance of imaging procedures for the diagnosis and management of orbital tumors, four chapters of this book are devoted to orbital imaging, offering information from the standpoint of the radiologist and the clinician, as well as covering the most recent advances and their applications to clinical practice (see Chapters 8 through 11).

Anesthesia

The great majority of orbital surgeries in adults and all the procedures in children are performed under general anesthesia. Occasional anterior orbit explorations and/or biopsies in adults can be done with local anesthesia. However, the administration of local anesthetics containing epinephrine 15 to 20 minutes prior to incision into the soft tissues of the surgical field contributes to vasoconstriction and reduces bleeding, particularly within the subcutaneous tissues. At the incision site, 1% lidocaine with epinephrine is usually injected subcutaneously. If the injection is given prior to the induction of general anesthesia, 1% lidocaine should be used because it seems to be the least painful agent. In one study, the order of local anesthetic agents, from least painful to most painful, was 1% lidocaine, 2% chloroprocaine, 1% mepivacaine, 0.5% bupivacaine, and 1% etidocaine.[7] If nasal or sinus involvement is anticipated during the orbital exploration, it may be helpful to pack the nose with a half-inch strip of gauze soaked in local anesthetic containing epinephrine or 4% cocaine solution.

Hypotensive anesthesia is useful to reduce intraoperative bleeding; it should be implemented if there are no contraindications.[8,9] The problem with this method, however, is that in some patients bleeding occurs postoperatively when the blood pressure returns to a normal level. During extubation at the end of orbital surgery, bucking of the patient should be avoided because it might lead to expulsive orbital bleeding.

GENERAL SURGICAL CONCEPTS

The best position for orbital surgery is reverse Trendelenburg, which reduces the arterial flow to the orbit as well as the venous stasis. The head should be positioned according to the planned orbitotomy. The sterile preparation usually includes the involved orbit. However, if major reconstruction is anticipated and a symmetrical appearance at the end of the procedure is of concern, both orbits should be prepared. Furthermore, if any tissue borrowing is planned from other sites (e.g., thigh, retroauricular area, fellow eyelid), graft sites should also be prepared and covered with sterile towels. If the use of microscope or endoscope is planned, the surgical team and anesthesiologist should be notified beforehand.

INCISION

Incisions for orbital surgery include the conjunctiva, skin, and bone cuts.

Skin Incisions

Skin Incisions of the eyelids and periorbital area should ideally follow the relaxed skin tension lines (RSTLs).[10] Prior to the injection with local anesthetics, the incision line should be marked with a fine-tipped surgical pen such as a Codman® marker (Figure 31.1). The skin incisions can be made with a Bard-Parker 15-C or a 3 mm, 30° sharp, disposable blade (e.g., Super Blade®). The incision should cut only the skin, not the underlying structures; it is helpful to complete the entire length of the incision in one sweep to keep blood from pooling over the incision line. In general, the skin incisions are made perpendicular to the skin surface for the eyebrow. In the eyebrow the cut is made at a 45° angle following the angulation of the hair follicles. The eyelid incisions and the lazy-S incision starting in the mid-eyelid crease are particularly useful to gain access to superior and lateral orbital space. Conjunctival incisions are preferred for an inferior orbital approach, but if one has to go through the skin, a subciliary incision in the lower lid offers easy access to the orbital floor. The most commonly used medial and superior medial skin incisions include modifications of the Lynch incision and the sub-brow incision. Although the classic Lynch incision leaves considerable scarring, it is still quite useful to provide access to lacrimal drainage system (LDS), the ethmoid sinuses, and the nasal cavity.

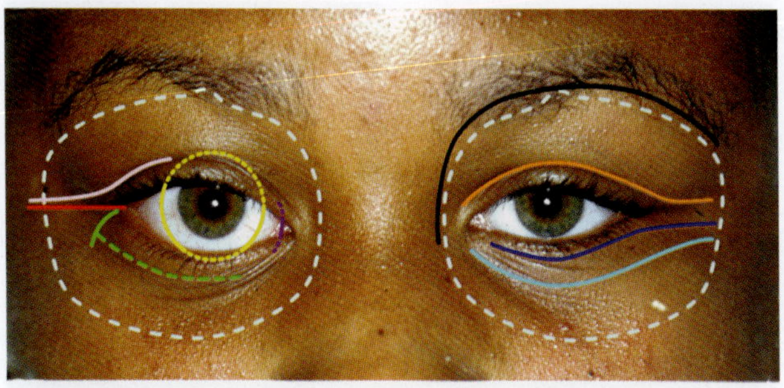

FIGURE 31.1. Skin and conjunctival incisions for orbit surgery: black: sub-brow incision in continuity with Lynch incision; orange: lid crease incision; purple: caruncular incision; red: lateral canthal incision; blue: subciliary incision; green: lateral crus incision (swinging lid incision); turquoise: lower lid incision; yellow: perilimbal incision; pink: lazy-S incision. The dotted white circle roughly corresponds to the bony margin of the orbit.

Conjunctival Incisions

In general, conjunctival incisions offer better postoperative cosmetic results. Any quadrant of the orbit can be approached through a segmental conjunctival peritomy overlying the area (Figure 31.1). Through conjunctival incisions, one can easily gain access to the intraconal space. The intraconal space is directly approached through perilimbal incisions of the conjunctiva through the sub-Tenon's space. For the extraconal space one should use forniceal incisions, which are particularly useful medially and inferiorly.[11] Superior and superior lateral fornix incisions are not ordinarily used, to avoid traumatizing the palpebral portion of the lacrimal gland and the ductules. The caruncular incision provides excellent access to the medial and posterior orbit.

Bone Incisions (Osteotomies)

Although many areas in the orbit can be accessed through skin and conjunctival incisions, the extent of the osteotomy to remove portions of the bony orbit should also be very carefully planned. It should be kept in mind that the best exposure of the orbital surgical field is accomplished through well-planned and properly executed removal of the bone.

In orbital tumor surgery, the bone is removed for two primary reasons: first, the removal of the marginal bone improves exposure, such as in lateral orbitotomy. The most common osteotomy is performed for lateral orbitotomy to allow a wide surgical field. Second, the bone is removed to control a neoplastic process in malignant orbital tumors such as adenoid cystic carcinoma.

Surgical Field

Light and Magnification

During orbital exploration, magnification and lighting are very important. A great majority of cases can be done under 3 to 5 power surgical loupes. However, at times the surgical microscope is invaluable for special purposes, such as fine dissection, with or without carbon dioxide laser, for vascular and canalicular anastomoses, and to identify tumor margins. Because of the depth of the operative field in orbit surgery, it may be preferable to use free-floating operative microscopes with variable objective focal length designed for ear, nose, and throat surgery, rather than the fixed focal microscope designed for ophthalmic surgery.

A headlight combined with surgical loupes provides the best illumination; however ceiling lights of the operating room, fiberoptic light sources, endoscopes, and the light source of the indirect ophthalmoscope may be needed occasionally.

Exposure for Exploration

The orbit is a small cavity inhospitable to the surgeon; it is crowded with vital tissues that are separated by delicate fibrous septae and fat. Orbital exploration usually begins from its anterior aspect, which commits the surgeon to a deep, three-dimensional field with poor visibility. Furthermore, changes in the anatomic relationships between structures because of the orbit's conal shape add to the difficulty of exploration. Therefore, adequate exposure of the surgical field is of utmost importance. The optimization of the exposure begins with the proper selection of skin and bone incisions and is maintained with accurate positioning of the surgical retractors and placement of traction sutures. Continuous maneuvering employed during orbital exploration to gain optimum exposure often takes more time than the actual biopsy or removal of the tumor.

Proper placement of the patient's head, positioning of the surgeon and assistants, as well as optimum lighting and magnification are the key elements of success in orbital surgery. Patience is an important virtue in orbital dissection, to maintain a bloodless surgical field and adequate exposure. Because of unanticipated shifting of the orbital fat, the surgeon should be familiar with continuous interruptions of the visibility that make the surgical field look somewhat like a Charlie Chaplin movie, but in color. The fat can be pushed away from the field, put on traction, dissected, and at times even be resected; however, all surgical maneuvers should be done atraumatically, with blunt rather than sharp dissection. The orbital surgeon should maintain a mental correlation between the imaging of the lesion and its actual position within the orbit and should approach the lesion through the appropriate planes of tissue. The importance of the definition of the plane of entry is aptly emphasized in Rootman, Stewart, and Goldberg, *Orbital Surgery: a Conceptual Approach*: "Instead of entering directly into the pathologically involved tissue planes, the surgeon should begin the dissection in the more easily distracted and pliable normal tissues adjacent to the lesion."[12] This approach allows the distinct advantage of comparing the normal tissues and the abnormal, to permit the ready identification of the pathology.

Most of the dynamic retractions throughout the procedure are done with the use of retractors. A wide range of handheld retractors, including Desmarres, Semm, and Ragnell retractors and malleable ribbon retractors (3/8 to 1 in. width) are used. In addition, rakes (Peck or Follet), muscle hooks (Graf or Jameson), and skin hooks (Joseph or Freer) function well for different levels of tissue retraction. Semipermanent retraction of the skin and subcutaneous tissues may also be accomplished with nonbarbed fishhooks attached to rubber bands at the wound edges. The advantage of the fishhooks is that they can be moved easily from one location to another; the disadvantage is that no matter how tightly they are clipped to the drapes, they tend to get loose after a while. The hooks and retractors can also be attached to self-retaining stages; however, this apparatus is usually cumbersome to operate and occupies valuable space in the surgical field (Figure 31.2).

Another method of retraction is to use sutures to retract tissues of different kinds. One common application is to use 4-0 silk for eyelids. When the suture is passed at the lid margin, it should be applied parallel to the eyelid margin with a good bite into the tarsus. This is best done with a Brown–Adson tissue forceps, sandwiching the eyelid margin and allowing the needle to be passed into the tarsus between the arms of the forceps. It is also advisable to pass a silk suture under the extraocular muscles to ensure that they can be identified during the later stages of the procedure. In particular, medial and inferior recti muscles should be anchored with sutures during orbital explorations of corresponding sites. If a considerable amount of traction is to be applied to these sutures, it is advisable that they be cuffed or replaced with silicone tubing, which may damage the underlying tissues far less when the traction is applied. Traction sutures can also be applied to the stumps of disinserted extraocular muscles. The best example of this is anchoring the stump of the medial rectus during medial orbitotomy through the conjunctival approach. It is best to run a 5-0 Vicryl or Merseline suture at the stump of the medial rectus muscle and cuff both ends of the suture with silicone tubing to avoid corneal and conjunctival damage during retraction of the globe (Figure 31.3). Corneal protection can also be accomplished by threading ocular conformers with traction sutures.

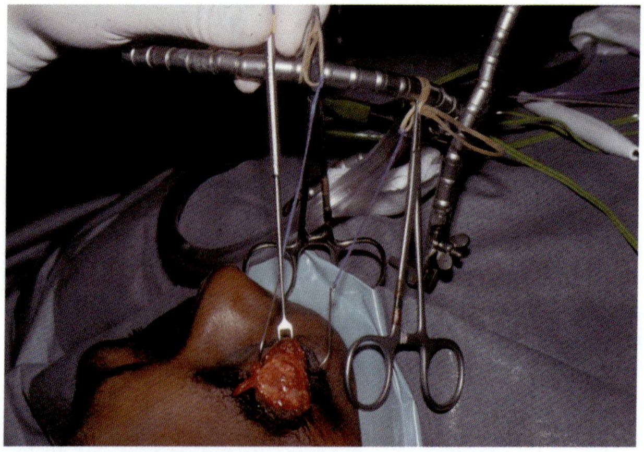

FIGURE 31.2. Self-retaining retraction apparatus with attached fishhooks. Note the crowding of the surgical field.

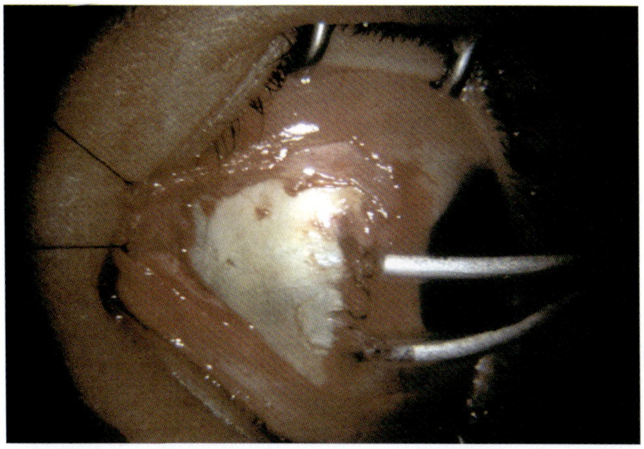

FIGURE 31.3. Silicone tubing cuffed over traction suture to protect underlying cornea and conjunctiva.

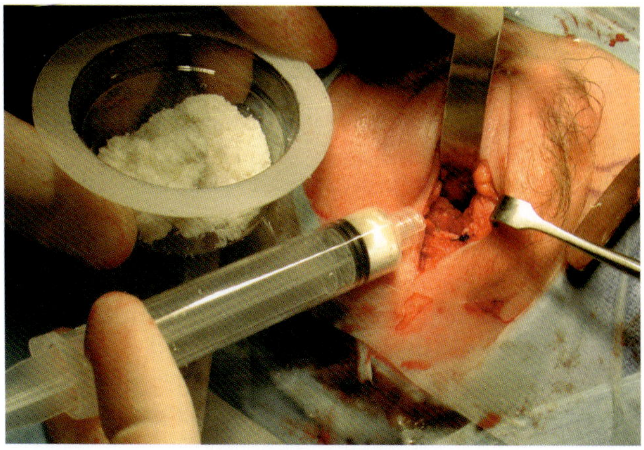

FIGURE 31.5. Delivery of powdered form of microfibrillar collagen (Avitene®) mixed with thrombin directly into the orbit to control generalized oozing of blood.

Bone can also be retracted by sutures. For example, zygomatic arche attached to the temporalis fascia/muscle can be hinged laterally and posteriorly by traction sutures passed through predrilled holes in the bone (Figure 31.4); it is best to use 2-0 Prolene for this purpose because the sharp edges of the holes might cut the finer sutures.

Hemostasis

It should be determined whether any bleeding experienced in the surgical field is due to a ruptured blood vessel or to generalized oozing. This can usually be detected by alternating gentle suction and minimal pressure. If a blood vessel is found to be responsible, it should be isolated, clamped, cauterized, or tied off before the exploration is carried on. If the bleeding is due to generalized oozing, it is beneficial to apply thrombin soaked Gelfoam or surgical cottonoids. Neurosurgical cotton paddies are preferable because they are easier to identify and remove once the oozing has stopped. Powdered Avitene® can also be packed into the surgical field or delivered by syringe (Figure 31.5). Avitene® should be irrigated gently at the end of the procedure.

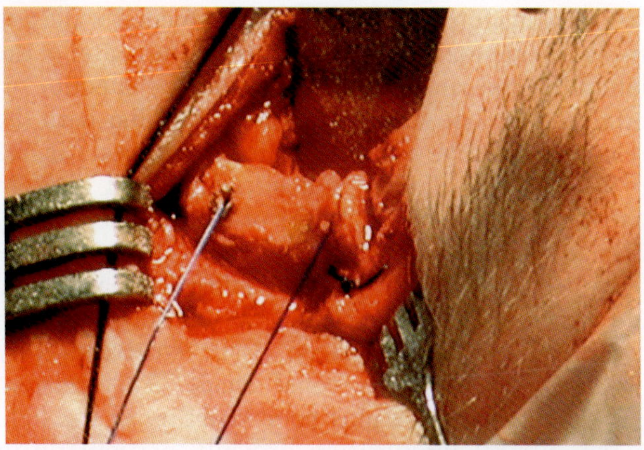

FIGURE 31.4. A 2-0 Prolene suture is used to retract the zygomatic arch laterally and maintain its position during lateral orbital exploration.

As mentioned earlier, hemostasis may be initiated by hypotensive anesthesia, as well as by injection of epinephrine-containing local anesthetics. Some authors advise the use of enfluothane (Ethrane®) anesthesia to reduce the intraoperative oozing of blood.[13] Intraoperative bleeding can be controlled with bipolar or unipolar coagulators; the fine-needle tip (Colorado tip®) is preferred. Furthermore, vascular ties, clips, and chemical adjuncts can be used to maintain hemostasis (Box 31.2).

Biopsy

Orbital biopsy is a very important procedure; more than half of tumor-related surgeries are performed just to obtain an adequate tissue sample for diagnosis. For

BOX 31.2. Hemostasis Methods During Orbital Surgery

Hypotensive general anesthesia
Reverse Trendelenburg position on the operating table
Application or injection of chemical vasoconstrictors (epinephrine, cocaine)
Application of strip gauze and/or neurosurgical paddies soaked with chemical vasoconstrictors and/or coagulators (Avitene®)
Thrombin-soaked gelatin sponge (Gelfoam®)
Oxidized regenerated cellulose (Surgicel®)
Bone wax
Cauteries (bipolar, unipolar, fine-tipped disposable)
Pressure by hand, with or without ice

proper conduct of the orbital biopsy, it is essential to establish a procedure plan. Many biopsy techniques, including FNAB, core biopsy, and excisional biopsy, are available; the biopsy procedure should be selected to fit the case.

Because of the significance of the biopsy in the diagnosis and management of orbital disease, an entire chapter is devoted to the subject. Biopsy procedures, tissue techniques, benefits of special studies, including frozen section biopsy, and sentinel lymph node biopsy, are covered in detail in Chapter 12.

Tissue Removal/Ablation

Well-delineated masses (and cysts) can be stabilized with forceps, cryoprobe, and sutures to be removed following blunt dissection around the lesion (Figure 31.6). Unlike well-encapsulated tumors, infiltrating lesions cannot be removed totally but need to be debulked. Debulking with sharp instruments causes a considerable amount of bleeding and may lead to many inaccuracies because of the obstruction of the surgical field by blood. Laser energy, on the other hand, may be a useful surgical adjunct for debulking orbital tumors. Among argon, yttrium-aluminum-garnet, dye, and carbon dioxide (CO_2) lasers, which are occasionally used in different applications of ocular plastics surgery, the CO_2 laser is the only one with substantial clinical usefulness in orbital tumor surgery. The 10,600 nm output of the CO_2 laser is strongly absorbed by tissue water. Because of this high absorption coefficient, the CO_2 laser allows great surgical precision, particularly when it is used under magnification. In skillful hands, the CO_2 laser is a precise, hemostatic, noncontact, ablation instrument for infiltrating orbital tumors. Some authors claim that it reduces postoperative pain, with improved cosmetic results.[14] Because of its precise tissue vaporization effect, it has been a useful surgical adjunct for debulking infiltrating tumors such as hemangioma, lymphangioma, plexiform neurofibroma, and Kaposi sarcoma.[15] Plexiform neurofibroma, which is otherwise known as "spaghetti tumor" because of its infiltrating character, is notoriously difficult to remove by conventional surgical means. The CO_2 laser has been proven to be a good debulking instrument for this tumor.[16] Although the debulking application of the CO_2 laser by tissue vaporization is very good, hemostasis of blood vessels larger than 0.5 mm in diameter requires defocusing of the laser beam.

Potential corneal injury with the CO_2 laser should be kept in mind, and wavelength-specific eye protection should be placed over the patient's eyes and should be mandatory for all members of the surgical team.

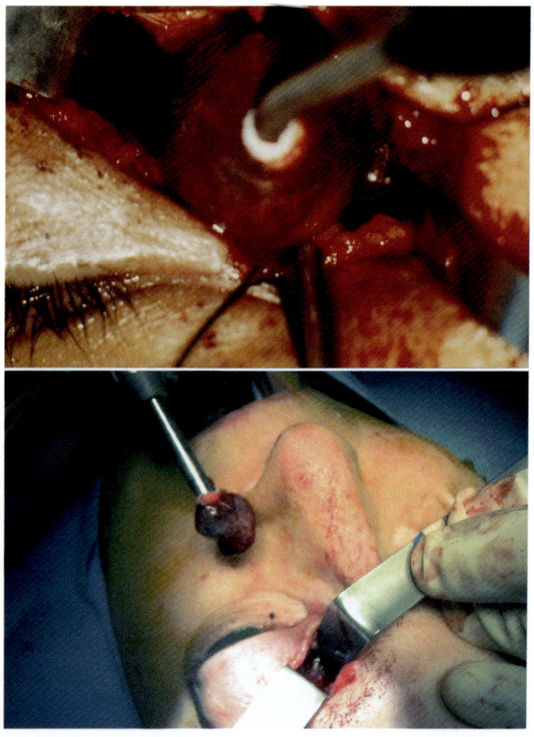

FIGURE 31.6. Use of the cryoprobe as a stabilizer during the removal of a cavernous hemangioma. The lower frame depicts a new design of a straight ("Finger probe") instrument which provides a larger zone of cryoadhesion at the tip (Courtesy of Dr. Paul Finger, New York City, NY.)

CORRELATION OF SURGICAL PROCEDURES WITH ANATOMY

The orbit is a pear-shaped bony chamber with an anterior opening measuring approximately 40 and 35 mm in horizontal and vertical diameters, respectively (Figures 31.7 and 31.8). Its volume expands approximately 1 cm posterior to the bony rim and then gradually decreases toward the apex, which consists of the optic canal at its narrowest diameter. In the axial plane, the medial wall measures approximately 45 to 50 mm from the anterior lacrimal crest to the entrance of the optic canal (Figure 31.9). In the same plane, each lateral walls forms a 45° angle to the medial walls and measures approximately 40 mm from the center of the lateral orbital rim to the opening of the superior orbital fissure. The surgeon should be familiar with the relationship of the superior and inferior orbital fissures to the superior, lateral, and inferior orbital rims. In particular, the superior aspect of the superior orbital fissure (SOF) and the inferior aspect of the inferior orbital fissure (IOF) are helpful landmarks that should not be violated during orbital exploration. The anatomic relationships between tissue structures vary because of the orbit's conal shape. This relative positional variability plus poor visibility of the field make surgical intervention difficult, particularly in the mid- and posterior orbit. A thorough knowledge of the anatomy eases this difficulty. Many elaborately

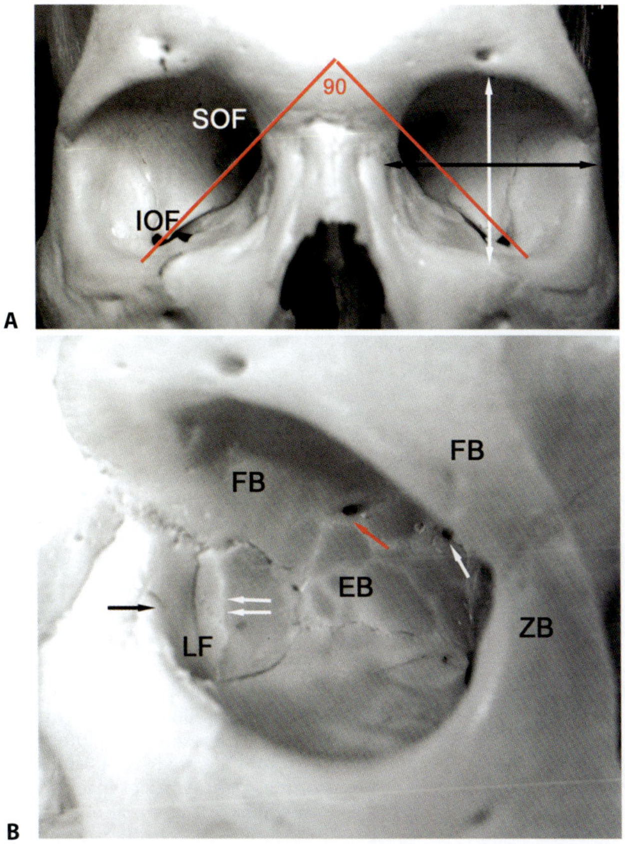

FIGURE 31.7. Parameters of orbital anatomy. (A) The vertical diameter (white arrow) is about 35 mm; the horizontal diameter (black arrow) is about 45 mm; the red lines represent the relative axis position of each orbit to the other of 90°. (B) The position of the anterior (red arrow) and posterior (white arrow) of ethmoidal foramina FB, frontal bone; ZB, zygomatic bone; EB, ethmoidal bone; LF, lacrimal fossa [bounded by anterior lacrimal crest (black arrow) and posterior lacrimal crest (double white arrows)], SOF, superior orbital fissure; IOF, interior orbital fissure.

written and illustrated textbooks and review articles exist on orbital anatomy and surgery. This chapter is not meant to be either an anatomy or surgery atlas. Only anatomic points that are pertinent to orbital tumor surgery are reviewed here; otherwise the reader is referred to detailed anatomy texts.[12,17,18]

There are three main reasons for surgery in a tumor-containing orbit: biopsy, partial excision (debulking), and total removal of the tumor. When total excision with clear margins by means of an orbitotomy is not possible because of tumor infiltration into both the globe and the soft and bony tissues of the orbit, special procedures, including enucleation, exenteration, and orbitectomy are undertaken.[19,20] Traditionally, the orbit is divided into several compartments as anterior versus posterior, extraconal versus intraconal, and superior, inferior, medial, and lateral. The surgical approach is planned according to these spaces.[21] In tumor surgery, however, the invasive and expanding nature of the pathology may force the surgeon to operate in several spaces at once.[22–24]

The most significant innovation in orbital surgery during the past decades has been the development of preoperative orbital imaging with CT and MR. The imaging not only confirms the presence of a space-occupying lesion but also shows its location relative to other orbital structures and helps immensely in surgical planning. The surgical plan for an orbital tumor is based primarily on the location of the tumor, and the incisions are done accordingly. The best exposure in the orbit is accomplished by wide bone removal; however, extensive osteotomies are known to be associated with more complications, longer procedure time, and slower postoperative recovery. Conventional planning dictates a surgical approach through the orbital wall closest to the mass lesion. Since, however, at times, more than one wall needs to be used, orientation to orbital wall anatomy is important to the surgeon. The anatomy of orbital walls and the related surgical procedures are discussed together in the following section. Capital and lowercase letters in parentheses correspond to structures shown in Figures 31.7, 31.8, and 31.9.

SURGICAL PROCEDURES

Lateral Wall and Lateral Orbitotomy

The orbital rim tapers laterally to form the thickest of all orbital walls. Although a small extension of the frontal bone is included in the superior aspect of the lateral wall of the orbit, for all practical purposes, this wall is composed of the zygomatic (ZB) and sphenoid bones. The frontosphenoid suture and superior and inferior orbital fissures limit the superior and inferior borders of the lateral orbital wall, respectively. Posteriorly, the greater wing of the sphenoid bone (gSB) separates the orbit from the middle cranial fossa.

An important superior orbital landmark, the Whitnall ligament, is the suspensory component of the levator aponeurosis. This ligament is attached to the tubercle of Whitnall, located approximately 10 mm inferior to the frontozygomatic fissure and 5 mm posterior to the lateral rim. The posterior head of the lateral canthal tendon and Lockwood's ligaments are also attached to this site. The junction between the frontal and zygomatic bones, the zygomaticofrontal (FZF) suture, is usually identified at the superior one third of the lateral orbital rim. The location of this junction to which the periosteum is firmly attached is variable, and, on occasion, it is difficult to identify during surgery.

Posteriorly, the lateral wall is bordered with the superior orbital fissure, situated between the greater and lesser (lSB) wings of the sphenoid bone. This foramen transmits the third, fourth, and sixth cranial nerves and the ophthalmic branch of the fifth cranial nerve, the superior orbital vein, and sympathetic nerves. Space-occupying lesions compressing these

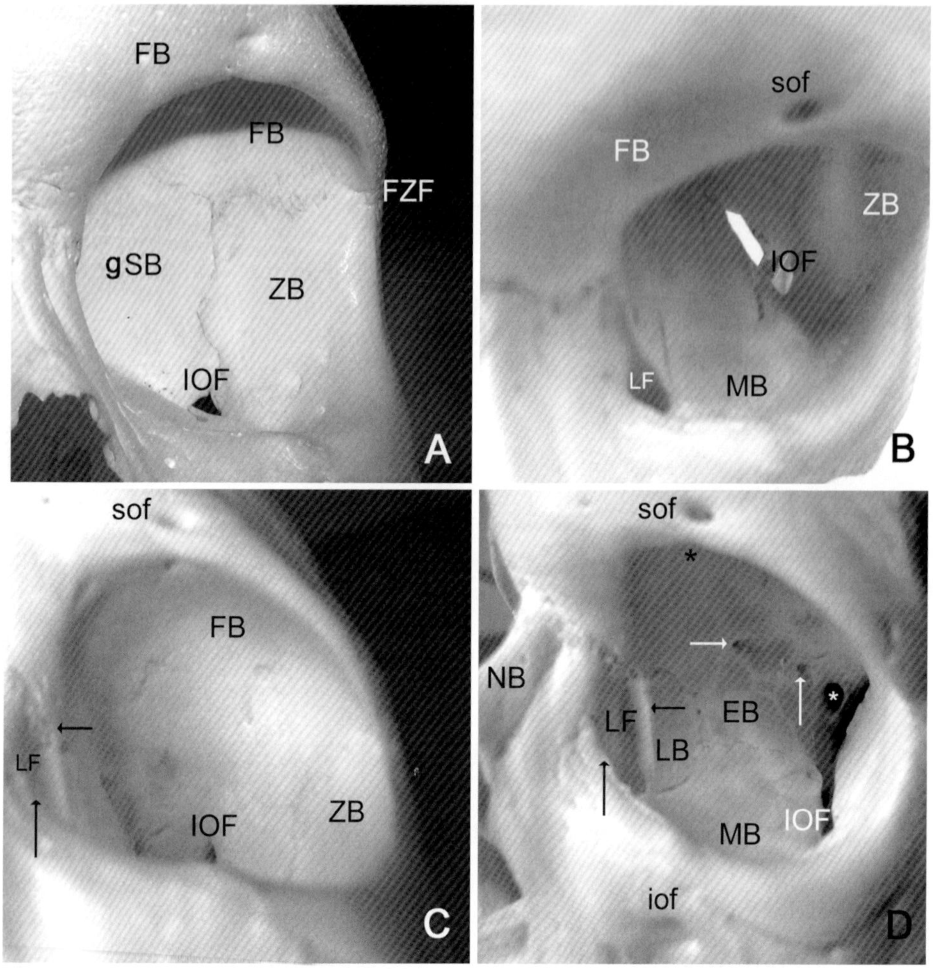

FIGURE 31.8. Anatomic landmarks of orbital walls: (A) lateral wall, (B) floor, (C) roof, and (D) medial wall. FB, frontal bone; FZF, frontozygomatic fissure; gSB, greater sphenoid bone; ZB, zygomatic bone; IOF, inferior orbital fissure; LF, lacrimal fossa; MB, maxillary bone; sof, superior orbital foramen; NB, nasal bone; EB, ethmoidal bone; LB, lacrimal bone; iof, inferior orbital foramen; horizontal black arrow: posterior lacrimal crest; vertical black arrow: anterior lacrimal crest; horizontal white arrow; anterior ethmoidal foramen; vertical white arrow; posterior ethmoidal foramen; black asterisk; superior orbital notch; white asterisk; optic canal.

structures or originating from them present with signs and symptoms of ocular motor palsies related to these cranial nerves.

The lateral orbitotomy is considered the best approach to gain access to the mid- and posterior orbit. Kronlein's original technique, which was described in the late 1800s, has been modified on numerous occasions, by Berke, Reese, Wright, and others.[20,25–28] In practice, all who utilize lateral orbitotomy come up with minor modifications until the technique suits them well.[29]

Numerous skin approaches to lateral orbitotomy exist: superotemporal lazy S in the eyebrow, superonasal lazy S in the lid crease, lateral canthal incision, inferotemporal lid incision for the "swinging" eyelid approach, and scalp incision for coronal approach (Figure 31.1). Most of these skin incisions allow access to the bony and soft tissue structures of the lateral, superiolateral, and inferolateral orbit. Therefore, the incision preference of the surgeon is based on minimizing the amount of postoperative scarring and the operative time, as well as staying away from important eyelid structures.

Although bone removal is occasionally performed in orbitotomies of other types, in lateral orbitotomy bone excision is a routine part of the procedure. It is important to realize that maximum exposure in the field of surgery targeted by the surgeon is governed by the amount of bone excision rather than the skin incision. This concept is succinctly expressed by Rootman, Stewart, and Goldberg: "Careful preoperative evaluation should determine whether or not the lesion will require more than the standard bone removal because virtually *all* of the anterior walls can be removed from the region, lateral to the superior orbital notch (SON) and posteriorly as far as the superior orbital fissure (SOF)."[12] If additional access is needed inferiorly, a portion of the inferior rim and the floor as far medially as the inferior orbital fissure can be excised (Figure 31.10).

Before the skin incision is made, a 4-0 silk traction suture is placed under the lateral rectus muscle to tag the muscle during the procedure. The author feels most comfortable with the lazy-S incision through the lid crease as the routine approach for lateral orbitotomy. Prior to injection, the incision is drawn with a microsurgical marker and made in one sweep for its entire length. The subcutaneous tissues and muscle may be cut with a fine-tip (Colorado® tip) unipolar cautery, or, if one is concerned about the heat effect on the underlying

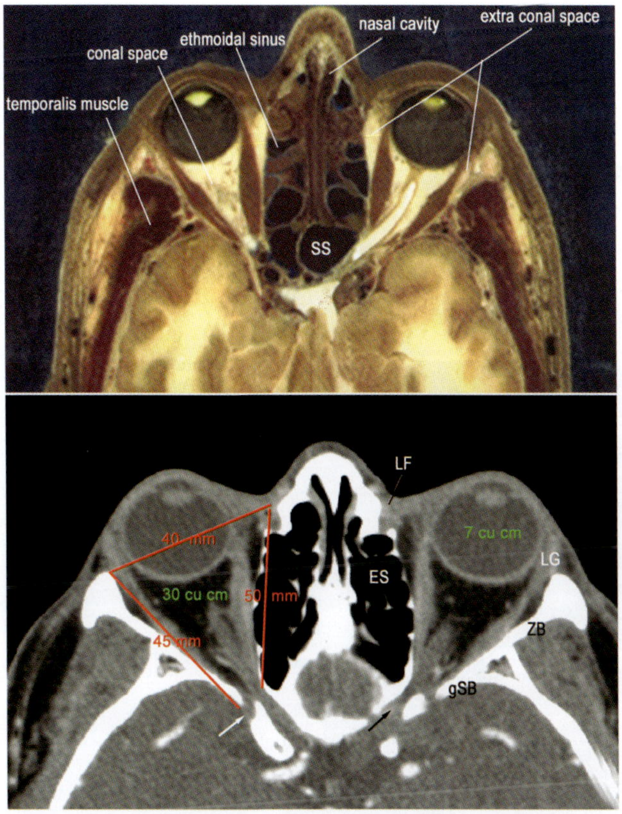

FIGURE 31.9. Corresponding planes of anatomic specimen and axial CT scan at midglobe level. Superior orbital fissure (white arrow); optic canal (black arrow). ES, ethmoidal sinus; gSB, greater wing of sphenoid bone; LG, lacrimal gland; LF, lacrimal fossa; SS, sphenoid sinus; ZB, zygomatic bone.

lesion, the subcutaneous tissues can be dissected bluntly with a curved hemostat or Stevens scissors.

The skin incision starts from the middle of the eyelid crease and extends laterally over the frontozygomatic process about 4 mm superior to the lateral canthal tendon. The incision should not go more than 30 mm or so beyond the frontozygomatic suture (Figure 31.11). It is helpful to identify the frontozygomatic process prior to the marking the skin incision. Subcutaneous tissues are bluntly dissected or gently cauterized over the temporalis muscle fascia to minimize the damage to the branches of the seventh nerve. The blunt dissection may be facilitated if two (superior and inferior) 4-0 silk traction sutures are placed into the subcutaneous tissues to retract the open wound and expose the lateral orbital rim. These sutures should be placed into the subcutaneous tissue with a wide, horizontal bite to avoid the "cheese-wiring" of the skin during traction. The extent of immobilization of the overlying tissues should be customized according to the planned extent of the osteotomy. When the orbital rim has been visualized, the periosteum is incised with a curvilinear cut approximately 2 mm posterior to the lateral orbital rim and extended superiorly and inferiorly as much as is necessary. A horizontal relaxing incision is made in the middle, and then the periosteum of the zygoma is separated from the bone with a sharp periosteal elevator. The periosteum is stripped over the zygomatic arch in all directions; however, the temporalis muscle attachment from the bone is not completely severed inferiorly with this technique.

Once the orbital rim has been exposed as bare bone, the osteotomy sites are marked with the unipolar cautery and then the vertical bony incisions are made with an oscillating saw, under irrigation to avoid extensive heating. Suction is applied to the area of bone incisions to collect small fragments of bone and bone marrow, which could disseminate and cause inflammation later. The bone incisions are usually made at the superior lateral margin of the orbit a few millimeters above the zygomaticofrontal suture and inferiorly through the zygomatic bone just above the junction of the inferior orbital rim. The extent of the osteotomy should be tailored to the size, location, and the nature of the tumor. Therefore, more extensive osteotomies can be designed to include superior, inferior, and posterior orbital bones (Figure 31.10). When the horizontal bone incisions are completed, their anterior edges are extended into the orbit and the horizontal incisions are connected with a vertical one, following the contour of the lateral orbital wall (Figure 31.11). The vertical cut is best created by gently tapping on a sharp, curved osteotome with a mallet about 15 to 20 mm posterior to lateral rim. Even a very shallow horizontal cut connecting the superior and inferior bony incisions leads to a clean break, controls the posterior extent of the osteotomy much better, and usually avoids the additional removal of the bones with rongeur or burrs. If one chooses to burr additional bone, it should be remembered that on the other side of the bone in this area lies the middle cranial fossa.

Most surgeons prefer to drill holes on either side of the bone incisions prior to the osteotomies because it is much easier to drill while the bone is stable. Par-

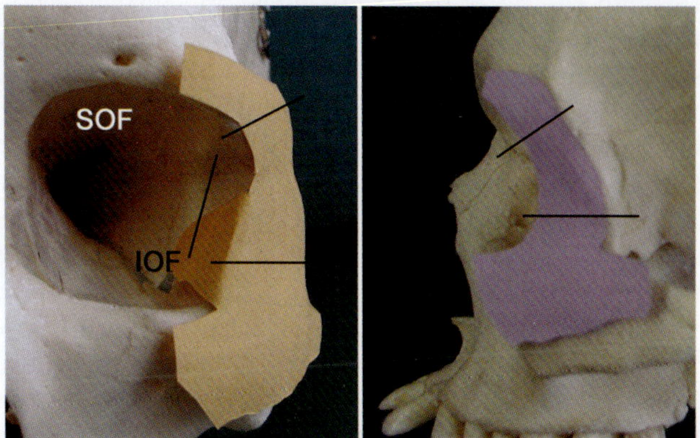

FIGURE 31.10. Depiction of the extent of bony removal on frontal and lateral views of the human skull. The black lines delineate the margins of bone removal for conventional lateral orbitotomy. SOF, superior orbital fissure; IOF, inferior orbital fissure.

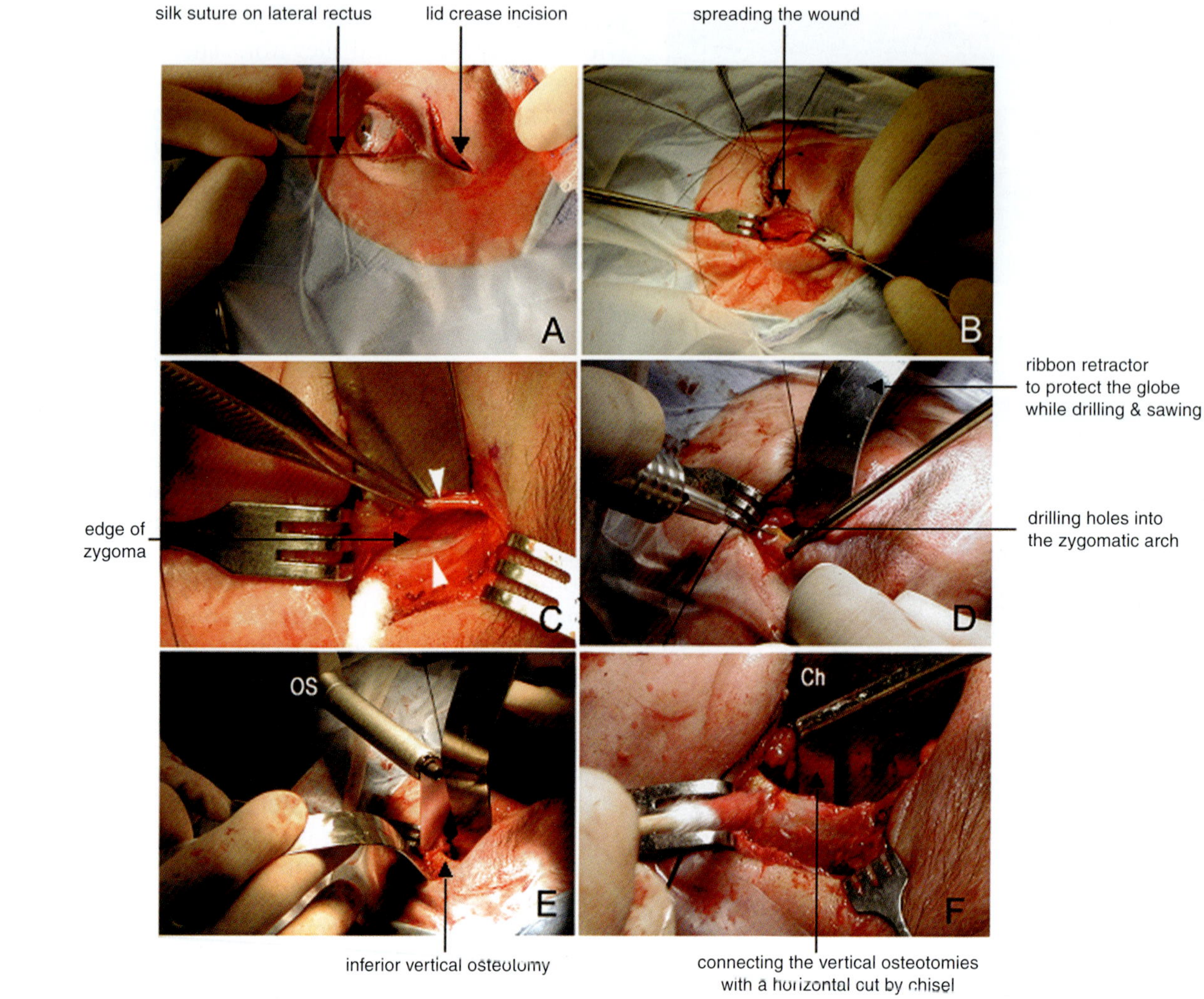

FIGURE 31.11. Lateral orbitotomy procedure. (A) Anchoring the lateral rectus muscle with a silk traction suture; a note lazy-S lid crease incision. (B) Spreading the wound with sharp and blunt dissection to reach to the underlying bone. (C) Cutting the periosteum and undermining the edges (arrowheads) to expose the bone. (D) Drilling holes into the zygomatic bone. (E) Cutting the zygomatic bone with an oscillating saw (OS). (F) Cutting the posterior aspect of the zygomatic bone with a chisel (Ch).

ticularly if the zygomatic arch is going to be left attached to the temporalis muscle, drilling of the bone just prior to repositioning may be cumbersome. Furthermore, a 3-0 Prolene traction suture can be passed through the holes of the cut piece and retracted posteriorly to keep the bone–muscle flap away from the surgical field (Figure 31.11). After all horizontal and vertical bone cuts have been completed, a large, front-biting bone rongeur is placed on the zygomatic arch and the lateral orbital wall is out-fractured by bending the rongeur laterally and posteriorly. If there is resistance, the surgeon should extend the bony incisions rather than applying excessive force onto the bone, which may lead to irregular cracks into the orbit. The lateral rim of the orbit is cut but not totally removed from the surgical field; it is hinged laterally with a traction suture while it is still attached to the temporalis muscle. In a great majority of cases, this maneuver provides enough exposure of the surgical field.

Once the bone flap is out of the way and the surgeon is satisfied with the full exposure of the orbit, periorbita is incised, generally, with one vertical cut. Periorbita should be cut with extreme care. It usually helps to hold it with a 0.5 or 0.9 forceps and make a shallow nick into it with a sickle-shaped no. 12 Bard-Parker blade. When this has been accomplished, one blade of the blunt Stevens scissors is inserted under the periorbita and it is carefully cut. The initial placement of the nick with the scalpel should not be directly over the lateral rectus muscle.

Alternatively, the initial nick of the scalpel blade can be slightly enlarged with a small curved hemostat, which is then inserted underneath the periorbita for blunt dissection of the underlying fat and attachments. When this has been accomplished, the hemostat is pulled up to tent the periorbita, away from the lateral rectus muscle, which then can be cut safely with blunt Stevens scissors. The edges of periorbita may be tagged with silk sutures to facilitate its approximation at the closure. With the orbital surgical field exposed to the surgeon's satisfaction, the exploration is carried out with the use of narrow ribbon retractors, blunt microsurgical dissectors, small curved hemostats, and cotton tip applicators. At times a dual cotton tip holder may be positioned on each side of a tumor and by pushing this instrument posteriorly, one may break the adhesions to the lesion, whereupon the tumor may eventually come forward without too much damage to the surrounding tissues. This simple instrument (Figure 31.12D) is also very handy to stabilize the optic nerve during the sheath fenestration procedure.[30] If the anterolateral presentation of the tumor does not happen readily, a fine-toothed Adson forceps or a retinal cryoprobe may be applied to the surface of the tumor capsule (or pseudocapsule) and with rotating and rocking motions can allow the mass to be pulled out (Figure 31.6). In rare instances, traction sutures may also be applied to the tumor for manipulation. The suturing of cystic tumor mass may be a mixed blessing. Oozing of luminal contents or blood from a cystic mass may reduce the size of the tumor and expedite the removal. On the other hand, once the cyst has collapsed, the surgeon loses the advantage of the force it applies to the adjacent tissues, and the mass does not easily push itself out of the orbit. This may be a particular disadvantage if there are strong tissue adhesions to the posterior surface of the mass. A right-angled vascular clamp may be a handy instrument to place behind the mass to break the adhesions.

If the purpose of the orbital exploration is not the removal of a tumor in toto but rather to perform an incisional biopsy or tumor debulking procedure, more bleeding should be expected in the field following the initial cut of the tumor. Therefore, the surgeon should make every effort to expose a large area of the tumor for the initial biopsy and excise as much tissue as possible during the first pass. This may be accomplished as a wedge biopsy with the use of a long scalpel blade and an Adson forceps. At times, a disposable skin punch or a small-diameter corneal trephine attached to the tip of a straight hemostat can be used to core out a tumor biopsy sample to be cut with an angled knife. For the posteriorly located or apical lesions, where the exposure is difficult, a core biopsy can be done with a Jamshidi bone marrow needle or with the fine-needle aspiration technique (see Chapter 12). If the lesion to be sampled is very small and confined to the apex, ultrasound guidance or a stereotactic image guidance system may be used (see Chapter 32).

At the end of the exploration, one must ensure that the bleeding is adequately controlled. After this, the periorbita is carefully approximated and closed by means of interrupted 5-0 Vicryl sutures and then the bone muscle flap is moved to its original position to be reinserted and secured with 2-0 nylon sutures using the preplaced drilled holes. The periosteum can then be closed over the bone with several interrupted 5-0 Vicryl sutures, and the same type of suturing can be applied to the overlying temporalis fascia if it was detached from the bone; if the bone–muscle flap has been left intact, this is not necessary. A drain should be inserted during the closure.

The skin wound is closed with 6-0 nylon sutures on a bolster in a continuous or subcuticular fashion. The placement of the suture with a bolster expedites

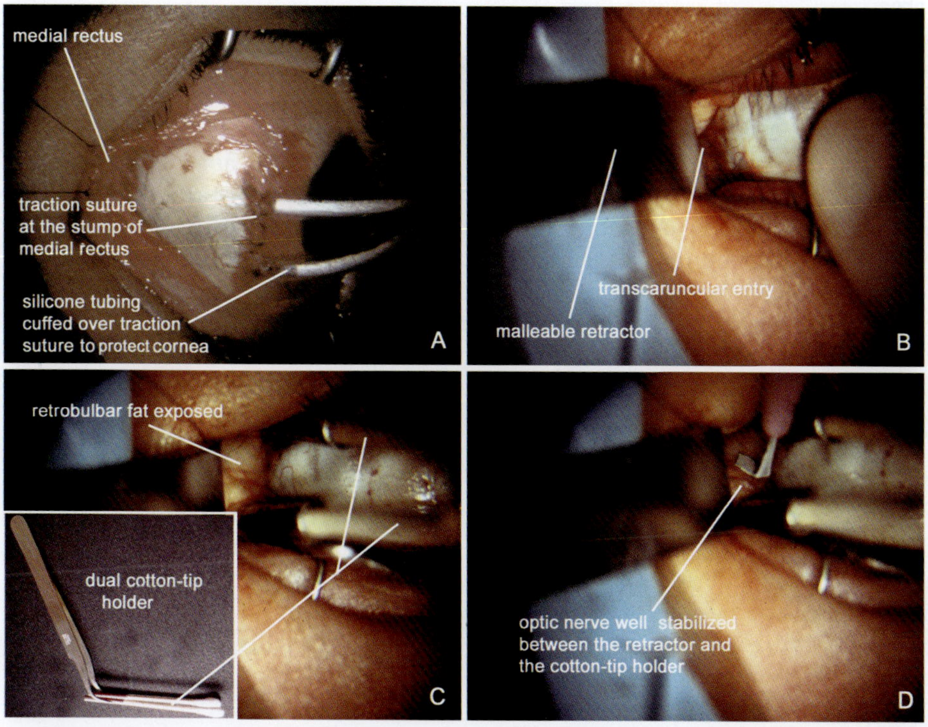

FIGURE 31.12. Transcaruncular medial orbitotomy procedure. Medial rectus muscle is disinserted and anchored with double-armed 6-0 Vicryl suture following a mid-conjunctival peritomy. (A) A 5-0 Mersilene traction suture was placed at the medial rectus stump in a running fashion and cuffed with silicone tubing to protect the underlying cornea during retraction of the globe. The incision was extended toward the caruncule, and Horner's muscle is cut to reach the underlying medial conal space with down and lateral displacement of the globe. (B,C) Exploration of the medial and retrobulbar conal space with a malleable ribbon retractor and cotton tip holder. (D) Stabilization of the optic nerve with a cotton tip holder and the incision into the optic nerve sheath with an angled disposable blade.

the removal. After skin closure, the traction sutures and the anchoring suture of the lateral rectus muscle are removed and the conjunctiva is closed with bipolar cautery or with one or two absorbable sutures. Following this, the conjunctival sac is irrigated with a small amount of buffered saline solution, and Maxitrol ophthalmic ointment is instilled; the ointment is also applied to the wound and to the drain site. During the surgery, antibiotics and corticosteroids are given intravenously. It is important that the extubation of the patient at the end of surgery be done gently, without bucking of the patient.

Inferior Wall (Floor) and Inferior Orbitotomy

The triangular orbital floor primarily consists of the maxillary bone (MB) and the greater wing of the sphenoid bone; between these two bones is the inferior orbital fissure. The IOF connects the orbit with the pterygopalatine fossa. The inferior orbital nerve and the veins that drain the inferior orbit transmit through the IOF. The inferior orbital nerve enters a bony groove of the floor approximately 25-mm posterior to the rim and travels forward to enter the fascial tissues through the inferior orbital foramen. The dissection for extraperiosteal orbitotomy should, therefore, be done posterior to the exit of this nerve. However, it should be kept in mind that the nerve may lie rather superficially under the bone, and one should be aware of its actual location. Damage to the nerve would lead to numbness in the lower lid and inferior periorbital region, cheek and upper lip. Rarely are tumors found in the inferior orbit. However, lymphoid lesions, peripheral nerve tumors, and metastatic tumors are occasionally encountered in this area.

For inferior orbitotomy there are two basic approaches. If the pathology is located anterior to the septum, a subciliary incision allows the surgeon to gain easy access to the lesion. The same incision can also be used to access the inferior orbital space through the septum. The direct cutaneous incision approximately 25 mm inferior to the lid margin would allow one to get into the orbit by avoiding the lower lid retractors and the inferior oblique muscle and does not interfere with the lower lid function postoperatively. Since, however, the scar of this incision may be unsightly, in cutting one should follow the relaxed skin tensions lines.

From the cosmetic standpoint, the preferred approach is transconjunctival through the inferior fornix; this approach also offers access to the midorbit.[31,32] This is best accomplished by doing a canthotomy incision by scalpel blade over the inferior crus of the lateral canthal tendon.[33] Once the lateral canthal tendon is cut, the lower lid is stabilized with a forceps and pulled down, exposing the conjunctiva of the lower fornix. The lower fornix conjunctiva may be incised with curved Stevens scissors or by fine-tipped (Colorado tip) unipolar cautery. During this incision, by passing a traction suture under the inferior rectus muscle to rotate the eye upward and resting the scissors on the bone of the inferior orbital rim, one can easily become oriented to the anatomy. On the other hand, the advantage of the cautery incision is that the underlying lower lid retractors can also be cut with a minimal amount of bleeding. When the lower lid retractors have been cut at their point of attachment to Lockwood's ligament, one enters the inferior space anterior to the inferior oblique muscle. An incision along this line causes minimum trauma to the lower lid retractors. The advantages of this "swinging eyelid" or "hinged eyelid" technique include good exposure of the infraorbital space, quick closure, and minimal postoperative complications and scarring (Figure 31.13). The inferior fornix incision should be closed with a few interrupted 6-0 Vicryl sutures, which can also be used for the reattachment of the inferior crus of the lateral canthal tendon to its disinsertion point. Conjunctiva can be closed with a 6-0 or 7-0 chromic running suture. If the infraorbital orbitotomy extends toward the medial aspect of the orbit, one should be aware of the anatomy of the lower canaliculus and lacrimal sac. During surgery, the canaliculus may be probed and isolated; care should be taken at the closure to avoid symblepheron formation of the conjunctiva, which may lead to epiphora and ectropion of the eyelid after surgery.

Medial Wall and Medial Orbitotomy

Most of the medial wall consists of the thin lamina papyracea separating the orbit from the neighboring ethmoid sinus. Lamina papyracea is primarily made of ethmoidal bone (EB) with neighboring frontal bone (FB) superiorly, lacrimal bone (LB) anteriorly, and maxillary (MB) bone inferiorly. Anterior and posterior ethmoidal neurovascular bundles usually lie at the suture line between the ethmoid and frontal bones (Figure 31.8). This is a critical landmark because it helps identify the roof of the ethmoid sinus, and the disruption of the bone above this level may damage the dura of the frontal lobe (Figure 9.2). A useful mnemonic to remember the approximate positions of the ethmoidal neurovascular bundles relative to anterior lacrimal crest is "24-12-6." The numbers indicate that the distance from the lacrimal crest to the anterior ethmoid foramen is 24 mm; there is 12 mm from the anterior to the posterior ethmoid foramen; and the measurement from the posterior ethmoid foramen to the anterior osteum of the optic canal is 6 mm. If one is well oriented with the anatomy, the anterior and posterior

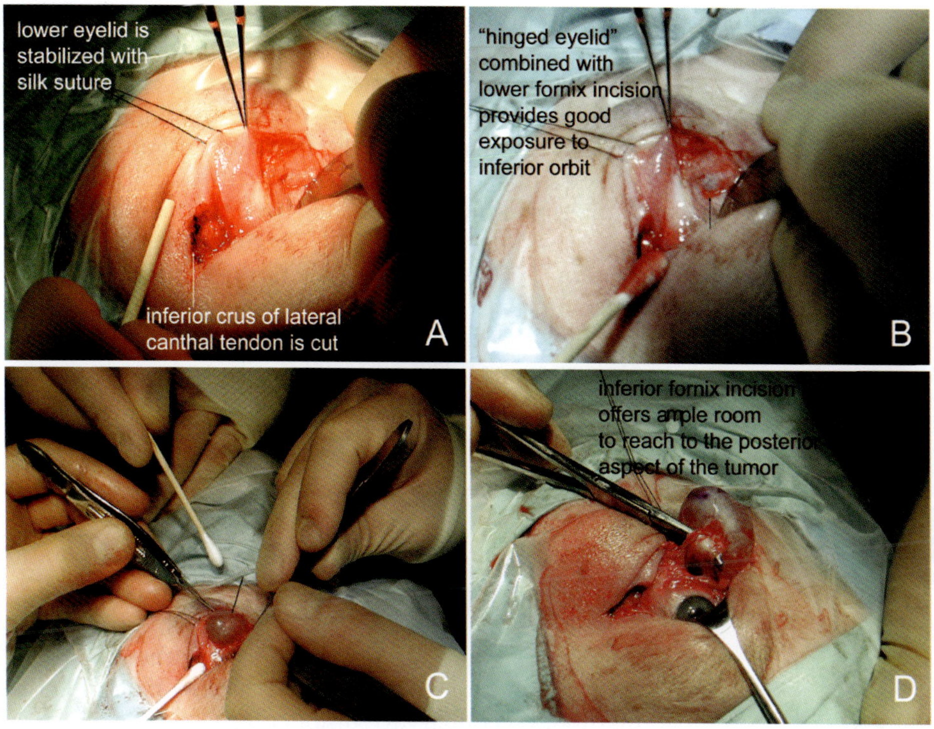

FIGURE 31.13. Transconjunctival inferior orbitomy with "hinged-eyelid" technique. (A) The incision of the inferior crus of the lateral canthal tendon and the stabilization of the lower eyelid, exposing the inferior fornix, which is medially incised. (B) Further dissection into the inferior medial orbit, exposing the tip of a cystic tumor (arrow). (C) The cystic tumor (arrow) is further dissected. (D) Easy access to the posterior aspect of the cystic tumor through the inferior fornix incision. A thick fibroadipose band on the posterior surface of the tumor is undermined with a hemostat. The closure of this type of orbitotomy is fast, and postoperative cosmetic results are excellent.

ethmoidal arteries can easily be identified and tied, clipped, or cauterized to maintain a bloodless field during medial wall exploration.

Lacrimal drainage system anatomy should also be kept in mind during medial orbitotomy. The lacrimal sac and the superior portion of the nasolacrimal duct lie within a shallow bony fossa, bordered anteriorly by the anterior lacrimal crest, which is made of an ascending extension of the maxillary bone (Figures 31.7 and 31.8). The lacrimal sac fossa is limited posteriorly by the lacrimal crest of the lacrimal bone. The anterior and posterior limbs of the medial canthal tendon insert onto the anterior and posterior lacrimal crests, respectively.

Another important landmark in medial orbital exploration is the sphenoethmoid junction, where the ethmoidal bone meets the sphenoid bone posteriorly. The location of this junction is variable but usually is at the level of the anterior osteum of the optic canal. In this posterior location, the exposure is practically nil, even in bloodless, well-illuminated fields. One very useful technique for orienting the surgeon to the anatomy is image-guided stereotactic surgery, in which the identifying probe is placed on apical structures that can be seen on the monitor with the help of the image guidance system (see Chapter 32). Although this procedure is primarily useful to identify the posterior ethmoidal cells and to perform decompression surgery, it can also be helpful to identify apical tumors. Blind dissection is likely to damage the vital structures of the orbit going through the optic canal and the superior orbital fissure. At best, the lesions in this area, such as meningiomas and other posteriorly located nerve tumors, can be biopsied with the help of the image guidance system,[34] ultrasonography, or CT during the biopsy procedure.

Medial orbitotomy can be done through a cutaneous approach or a transconjunctival (transcaruncular) approach. The skin approach is best accomplished by direct or modified Lynch incision, which is a slightly curved cut, starting from mid-eyebrow and extending downward and medially toward the lateral surface of the nose (Figure 31.1). It is best to keep the skin cut shallow and to do the subcutaneous dissection carefully, since the superomedial orbit contains several important structures. The beginning of the Lynch incision is usually initiated at the level of the superior orbital rim or a few millimeters above it. In this area, one should be careful not to damage the nerves of the superior orbital bundle (sof in Figure 31.8). As the incision makes a bend inferiorly, it overlies the trochlea, which is a small cartilaginous structure located in a bony fossa in the superomedial orbit 5 to 7 mm posterior to the rim.[35] If a mass lesion within the medial fat pad does not directly involve the trochlea, the blunt dissection should be done posterior to this structure to avoid any damage. In most cases, the superior oblique muscle tendon can easily be retracted away from the exploration field. However, if the removal of the trochlea is mandatory, it should be done with care. The trochlea is a U-shaped ring with its opening firmly attached toward the medial wall periosteum (Figure 31.14). The superior oblique muscle tendon passes between the periosteum and the cartilaginous flange of the trochlea and turns posteriorly to form its reflected arm.[36] When the trochlea is removed from the underlying bone, it is advisable to leave a stump of periosteum attached to the trochlea, which is marked with a silk suture for accuracy during reattachment. The reattachment suturing should be done from periosteum to periosteum. No suture should be passed into the medial aspect of the trochlea, since this can easily scar the superior oblique tendon and may lead to a postoperative superior oblique restriction (acquired Brown's syndrome).

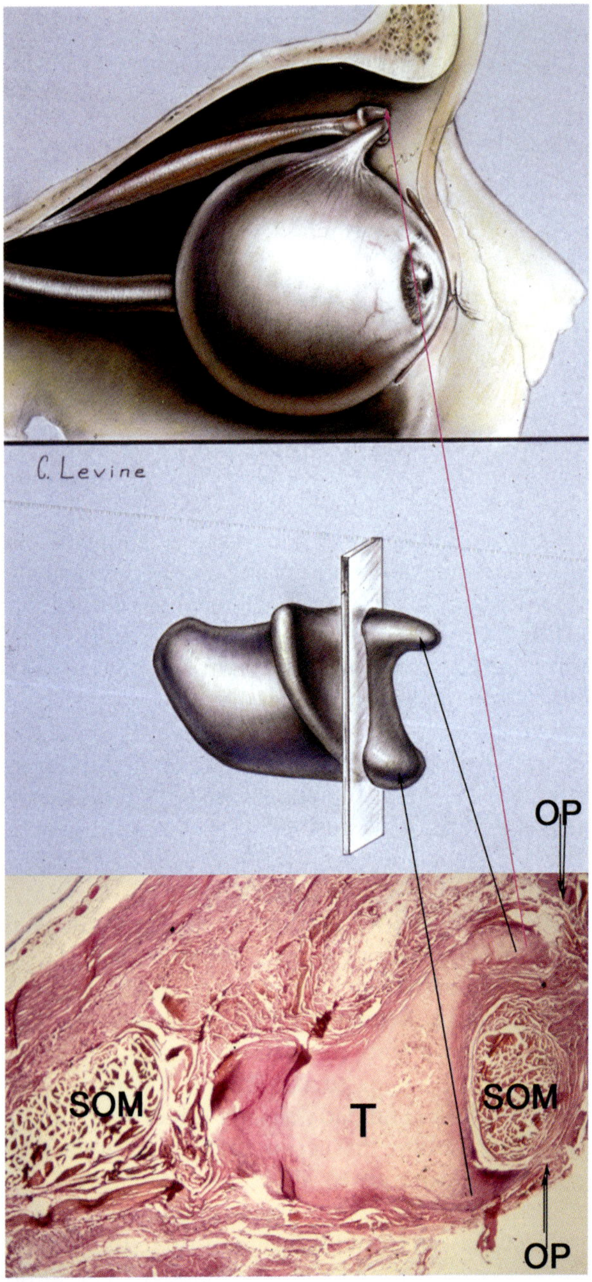

FIGURE 31.14. Diagram of the anatomy of the trochlea combined with the histologic section going through a vertical plane. T, trochlea; SOM, superior oblique muscle; OP, orbital periosteum. (Courtesy of Dr. Joel Sacks of New Orleans, Louisiana.)

As the Lynch incision curves down to follow the inferior orbital rim, it may overlie the angular artery and vein and approach the upper canaliculus and the underlying medial canthal tendon (MCT). If the lower limb of the incision extends over the medial canthal area, the surgeon should be aware of the level of the tendon (MCT) and the underlying lacrimal sac.[37,38] The anterior limb of the MCT, which can be palpated through the skin, may be visualized after a shallow skin incision. The anterior limb under which the lacrimal sac lies originates from the anterior lacrimal crest (Figure 31.7). The MCT cannot be retracted easily for dissection. If wide exposure is needed in this area (e.g., lacrimal sac tumors), the MCT should be disinserted from the periosteum and reattached in its proper position after the exploration.

One may choose to probe the canaliculi during the dissection in this area; it is also advisable to irrigate the lacrimal drainage system following the medial orbital exploration to ensure its patency. If the LDS is disrupted secondary to tumor compression, every possible effort should be made to repair the damage; on the other hand, if the system is infiltrated with a malignancy, it must be sacrificed during dissection. The anatomy of the proximal LDS may be maintained after the removal of benign, well-encapsulated lesions. If this cannot be managed, dacryocystorhinostomy (DCR) may be performed during the same session and silicone stents passed into the nose. Same-session DCR is advisable only if the tumor is benign and the surgeon does not anticipate any further surgery. If, however, postoperative external beam radiation therapy (EBRT) is anticipated, silicone intubation may prove advantageous to minimize radiation scarring of the drainage system. If the canaliculi are intact but the sac or the nasolacrimal duct is damaged beyond repair, the same approach is advised. However, if the canaliculi cannot be salvaged because of extensive tissue loss, it is best to reconstruct the eyelid and the canthus as well as possible and to leave the lacrimal bypass surgery for a future session after the scarring of the area is stabilized.[38]

The medial orbit can also be explored through a transcaruncular incision.[39–42] During transcaruncular medial orbitotomy, a crescent-shaped incision is made through the posterior limb of the medial canthal tendon to which the deep head of pretarsal orbicularis muscle attaches to reach the underlying bone.[39] About 10 to 15 mm posterior to the caruncle, the deep head of the pretarsal orbicularis muscle (Horner's muscle) becomes visible. When this muscle is cut, the orbital fat presents itself; upon retracting the fat with a thin ribbon retractor, one can easily identify the posterior lacrimal crest. At this point the periosteum may be cut and elevated and the dissection may be carried posteriorly below the periosteum with periosteal elevators and malleable retractors. On the other hand, one may choose to stay within the periorbita to explore retrobulbar tumors located in midorbit. This approach is also a direct route to the optic nerve and is preferred by many surgeons for optic nerve sheath decompression. The optic nerve can be reached through the transcaruncular approach without disinserting the medial rectus muscle. However, the exposure, which may be good for the removal of small tumors and for biopsy purposes, does not offer the best surgical field to operate on the optic nerve sheath. For this purpose it is best to do a 120° peritomy a few millimeters anterior to the insertion of the medial rectus muscle and to isolate the medial rectus muscle with a double-armed 6-0 Vicryl suture. Then a 5-0 Merseline suture on a spatula needle is passed through the stump of the tendon of the medial rectus muscle in a running fashion. Both ends of the Merseline suture are threaded with silicone tubing to protect the cornea while retracting the globe laterally (Figure 31.14). The next maneuver is to push the globe down gently while retracting the silicon tubing laterally as the assistant retracts the medial rectus complex medially with a malleable retractor. This affords a quick and easy access to the midconal space; however, visibility is obscured by retrobulbar fat. When the retrobulbar fat has been bluntly dissected with cotton tip applicators, the posterior ciliary arteries and the optic nerve come into view. If the orbitotomy is being performed for optic nerve sheath fenestration procedure, a cotton tip applicator holder may be useful to push the fat posteriorly on both sides of the optic nerve and isolate the dura (Figure 31.14). The cotton tip applicator holder is particularly helpful if one is doing the procedure alone because it will stand up on its own while the surgeon is handling other instruments. When the dura is exposed, it is picked up with microsurgical forceps (the author prefers the Belushi forceps, a microforceps for middle ear surgery) toward the edge of the optic nerve and a vertical incision is made into the dura with a no. 75 blade. At the time of this cut, it is common to see cerebrospinal fluid gushing through the incision. Next, a cut parallel to the first one can be made and a rectangular window removed with microscissors. Or a small muscle hook can be inserted through the first incision, whereupon the subarachnoid trabeculae are broken away from the overlying nerve sheath, and a small amount of Healon® is injected to balloon the dura. When enough room has been created, the glaucoma punch (Katena®) is inserted underneath the dura and a round hole is punched out in the optic nerve sheath. This may be difficult to do in deep orbits because of the limited length of the punch instrument. Following the establishment of the opening, the medial rectus muscle is reinserted and the conjunctival peritomy is closed.[43]

The most commonly encountered space-occupying lesions in the medial orbit are mucoceles, bone and peripheral nerve tumors, and hemangiopericytomas. Small mucoceles may be removed in toto, but in most instances these lesions extend into the sinuses (Figure 31.15). In these cases, the bony shell can be removed partially and the mucosa of the cyst is stripped off completely or as much as possible. If some of the mucosal lining cannot be removed, it is best to cauterize the leftover mucosa and establish an opening between the mucocele and the adjacent sinuses.

Combined Medial–Lateral Orbitotomy

If the lesion is medially located but close to the apex, exposure is not possible laterally and may also be limited through a medial caruncular approach. In this situation, a combination of medial and lateral orbitotomies may be performed. This approach is also useful when the tumor to be removed is too large for the exposed surgical field. First, lateral orbitotomy is done and the medial rectus muscle is disinserted so that the globe can be retracted laterally, allowing more room for tumor dissection in the medial orbit. With the medial rectus muscle disinserted, the globe can be displaced temporally, offering a better exposure of the medial apex area (Figure 31.16).[44] This combination approach is useful for small, apical tumors. Larger lesions, particularly the infiltrative lesions, however, cause considerable anatomic distortion, and therefore, a transfrontal craniotomy may be needed to provide wide exposure of the posterior orbit.[45]

Superior Wall (Roof) and Superior Orbitotomy

Superiorly the rim is most protuberant. The supraorbital notch is located at the medial third of the rim. This notch provides a safe landmark to identify the supraorbital neurovascular bundle, which harbors the superior orbital branch of the frontal nerve and blood vessels. The trunks of the supraorbital and supratrochlear nerves are important sensory branches of the ophthalmic nerve (CN V-I). The trauma to the supraorbital nerve should be minimized during superior orbitotomy and transcoronal orbital approach. Often one can chisel out a small rectangular bony piece of the superior rim around the nerve, which allows the nerve to be moved away from the surgical field, but if there is an infiltrating lesion this may not be possible. During a subperiosteal approach, one should look for the trunk exiting the superior orbital foramen because variations may happen. The posterior dissection of the periosteum should be made cautiously because, in some cases, the supraorbital nerve leaves the bone posterior to its usual location. The orbital roof primarily consists of the frontal bone and the lesser wing of the sphenoid bone. The anterior cranial fossa and the

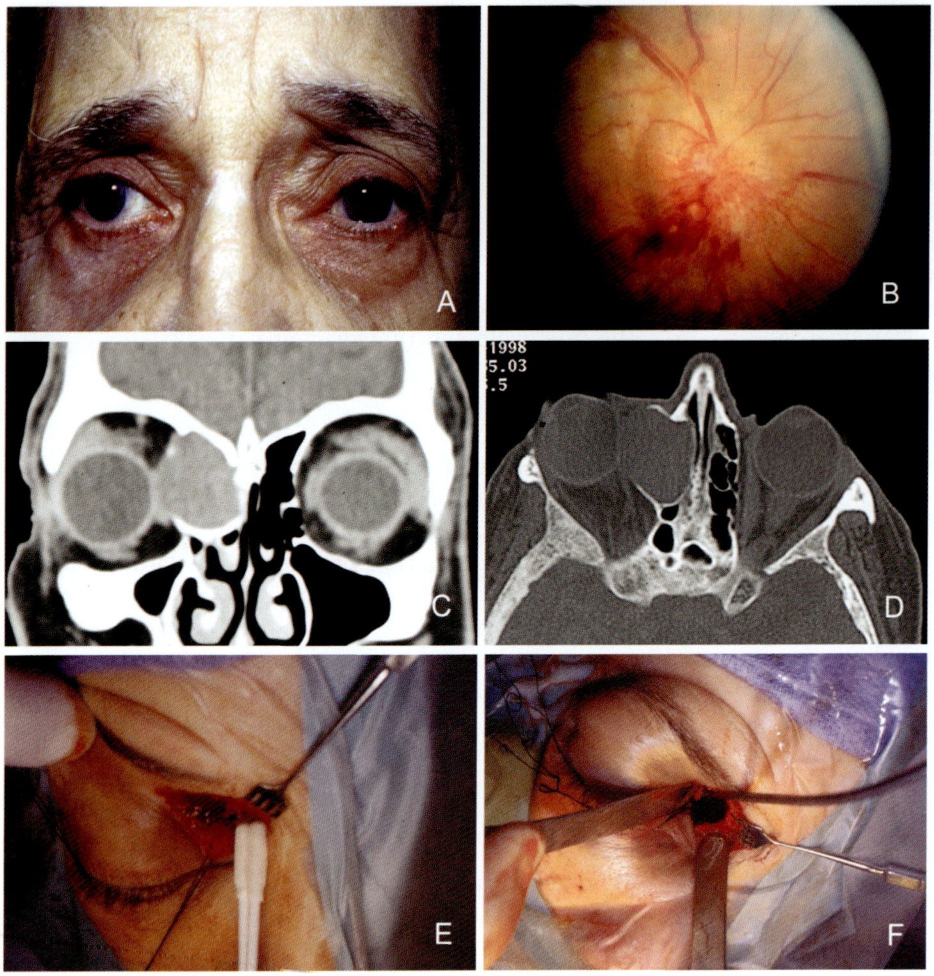

FIGURE 31.15. (A,B) Facial photograph of patient in whom a frontoethmoidal mucocele of the right orbit was causing proptosis. In addition, there was lateral dislocation of the globe, extraocular motility disturbance, and compressive optic neuropathy. (C,D) Coronal and axial (bone window) CT scans delineate the lesion accurately. (E) Superior medial orbitotomy is initiated through a Lynch incision and the mucocele is exposed. Note that the mucocele luminal contents are being cultured at this stage. (F) Later the mucocele cavity was fully exposed by removing mucosal and bone elements of its wall.

frontal sinus are located above the orbital roof, and, therefore, one should be familiar with the anterior margin of the cranial fossa to limit the superior orbital osteotomy. Since both the anterior extent of the cranial fossa and the aeration of the frontal sinus vary from case to case, it is best to determine these relationships to the superior orbit prior to the exploration, by a thorough inspection of the CT scan. Recurrent benign and malignant tumors (e.g., lacrimal gland lesions) may easily violate the frontal sinus and cranial bone, distorting the anatomy and extending into the sinus or cranial fossa (Figure 31.17).

One should keep in mind that even the small tumors developing in this region such as dermoids (particularly leaking dermoids, which cause secondary inflammation), cholesteatomas, or mucoceles may easily disturb the anatomy and function of the trochlear apparatus. Therefore, this region should be dissected carefully, particularly in the presence of pathology. The superior ophthalmic vein originates within the same superior medial fat pad and runs posteriorly, leaving the orbit through the superior orbital fissure above the annulus of Zinn.

Orbital Apex

In adults, the optic canal is approximately 10 mm long and varies from 5 to 6 mm in diameter at its orbital osteum.[46] It is located at the posterior-most extension of the orbital apex between the lateral, medial, and superior walls of the orbit within the lesser wing of the sphenoid bone. It transmits optic nerve, ophthalmic artery, and sympathetic fibers from the orbital cavity to cavernous sinus.[47] The optic nerve, surrounded by the meninges, enters the canal on the medial aspect of the posterior orbit. In the adult, the nerve measures approximately 25 mm from the posterior sclera to the entry of the optic canal; however, the posterior sclera is only about 18 mm anterior to the canal. This 7 mm infero-temporal slack on the nerve allows the globe to move to all gazes freely without applying tension on the nerve. Gradual loss of visual acuity and visual field are generally due to optic nerve compression secondary to apical tumors. Nerve appearance and function can be monitored with color vision testing, afferent pupillary light reflex, visual perimetery, visual evoke response (VER), or ophthalmoscopy, depending on the clinical setting (See Chapter 7).

pathology is located posteriorly, such as a choroidal melanoma, extending into the orbit secondarily, there is no reason to remove the eyelids, and the procedure can be done as a lid-sparing exenteration. Individualization of exenteration cases should take into account the location, size, and aggressiveness of the pathology as well as the reconstruction plan. A recent report of 25 exenterations revealed that subtotal procedures would offer improved functional and aesthetic results, while being comparable to total exenteration procedures in terms of eradication of the disease.[85]

If the bones of the orbit are involved with malignancy, bone resection should be performed at the time of initial orbitotomy, even if that procedure is not an exenteration.[20] In recurrent or advanced cases, the extent of the bone invasion should be mapped carefully with preoperative CT scans. At the time of exenteration, the bone should be removed well beyond the margins of the tumor depicted by CT, provided the part of the orbital wall is made of expendable bone. Wider margins are advisable in bone resection because frozen section monitoring cannot be done in bony tissue. Most of the orbital bone, except for the roof of the orbit and the orbital apex, can be removed after the exenteration. There are no standard techniques for bone resection; in most cases, the removal depends on the extent and the location of the bony invasion. In most areas of the orbit, it is preferable to deeply incise the bone with an oscillating saw along the predetermined limits of resection and then attempt to break the bone en bloc with a strong rongeur. In some areas, this may not be difficult; in other sites, a sharp osteotome and a mallet may be needed to remove pathologic bone in layers (see Chapter 16; Figure 16.8).

Wide excision of the bone from the lateral wall of the orbit is usually indicated in cases of malignant epithelial tumors of the lacrimal gland. Long-term survival has been reported following this type of surgery.[86,87] The removed pieces of bone should be properly oriented and labeled for permanent histopathologic examination to determine the extent of tumor. This may be a tedious procedure; however, it is a rewarding one to help decide whether the patient needs further treatment.

In total exenteration, the eyelids are secured in closed position with two silk sutures and a circumferential skin incision overlying the orbital rim is done (Figure 31.21). When the underlying soft tissues have been reached, the incision is continued with the use of unipolar cautery with a fine needle tip (Colorado

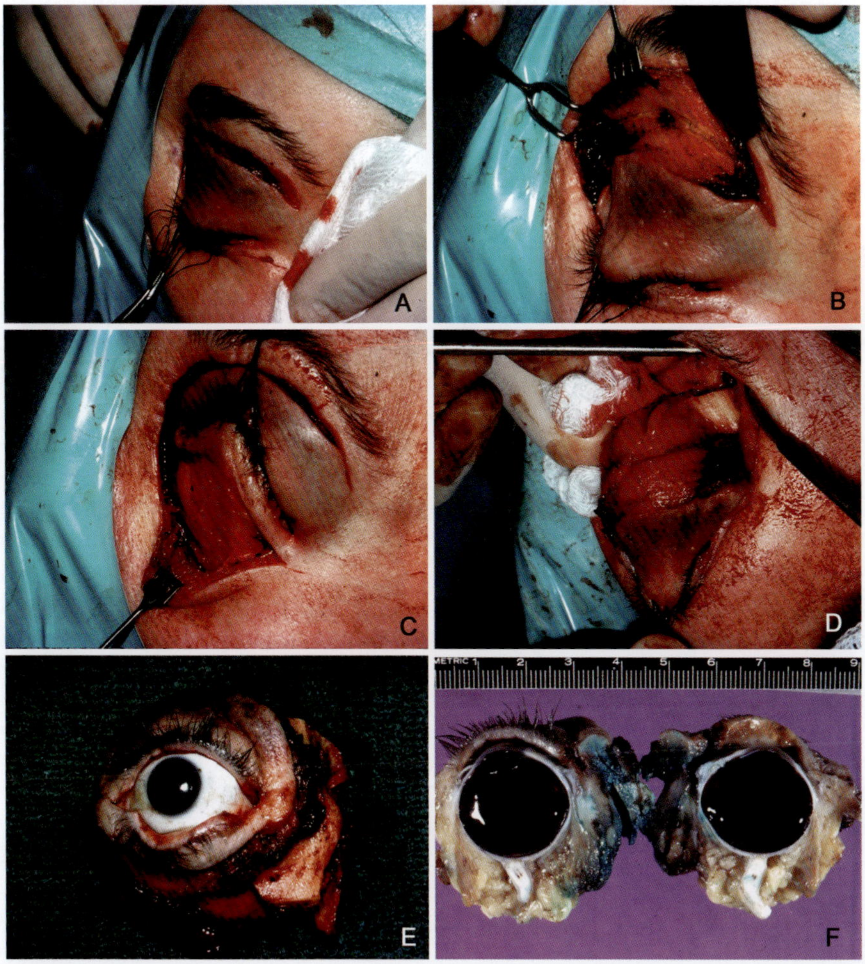

FIGURE 31.21. Exenteration procedure: total exenteration (A–D) and bone removal (E) from the lateral wall for adenoid cystic carcinoma (F).

tip). From the standpoint of minimizing the bleeding, we prefer to begin the incision in the upper quadrant, around 12 o'clock, and proceed clockwise, postponing the dissection of the vascular nasal quadrant to the end of the procedure. Then the periorbita is elevated with a sharp-tipped periosteal elevator and further dissected with malleable retractors. When the periosteum of the orbital rim is reached, the periosteum is elevated and the dissection is swiftly continued beyond the rim into the orbit, to complete the procedure as quickly as possible. During dissection, which is done while the blood is suctioned, bleeding is ignored unless hemorrhage is so profuse that it interferes with the view of the surgical field. When the soft tissue dissection is complete, hemostasis with cautery and other means is addressed. Once the dissection toward the apex is completed 360°, one reaches posteriorly to the apical bundle of soft tissues, including extraocular muscles, blood vessels, and nerves. These abundant tissues at the tip of the orbital cone cannot be clamped or cut with one move. We approach this bundle from its nasal aspect, place a strong, curved hemostat, and cut the pedicle with unipolar cautery above the hemostat; then the same maneuver is repeated laterally and inferiorly to free the apex from orbital soft tissues. To cut the apical tissues with unipolar cautery reduces the hemorrhage somewhat, but the bleeding sources in the apex should be identified and clamped and tied after the removal of the bulk of the soft tissue. Application of electrocautery at the apex too much and too long may create damage in the remaining portion of the optic nerve, which may extend into the chiasm.

Alternatively, others approach the procedure with tedious attention to hemostasis throughout the dissection. The author's preference, however, is the first approach, which shortens the procedure time; with today's suction and cautery equipment, the total soft tissue excision can be done in less than 15 minutes without any significant blood loss. Most of the bleeding originates from the supraorbital and infraorbital bundles, the anterior and posterior ethmoidal arteries, and the ophthalmic artery, as the dissection reaches the apex. Although the posterior bleeding is the most significant, it is easier to control, since by the time one reaches the apex of the orbit, all soft tissues have been freed and the surgeon maintains better visibility. After the major bleeding sites are controlled by tying the vessels or cauterization, smaller bleeding sites are addressed by cautery, bone wax, or simply by pressing thrombin-soaked Gelfoam onto the sites of oozing; Avitene® may also be used to control bleeding.

Cerebrospinal fluid (CSF) leak is not a very common complication of orbital surgery in general.[88] However, when leakage takes place during surgery or postoperatively, the procedure and/or hospitalization are prolonged and prognsosis may worsen. Since orbital exenteration is an extensive procedure, one expects CSF leak to occur more often. In a series of 39 exenteration cases reported by Bonovolonta and deConcilis, CSF leak was experienced approximately 18% of the time, and majority of patients had invasive secondary tumors from conjunctiva, eyelids, and globe.[89] In 26 out of 39 cases, one or more orbital wall was removed, and, therefore, the dural exposure and the CSF leak incidence were higher.

When CSF leak takes place during surgery, the conventional treatment is to suture the dura whenever possible; when this is out of the question, the area is packed with temporalis muscle, fascia, or fibroadipose tissue. The successful use of cyanoacrylate adhesive for CSF leaks during orbital surgery has been reported.[90] At times, particularly in CSF leaks that happen after surgery or ones that do not respond to repair and continue to leak intraoperatively, lumbar puncture to lower the CSF pressure may help.

In eyelid-sparing exenteration, one may need to spare either the entire eyelid structure or just the eyelid skin. If the eyelid skin is to be spared, the skin incision is placed approximately 2 to 3 mm above and below the lash lines in upper and lower eyelid, respectively. Then the skin is dissected superiorly and inferiorly until the orbital rim is reached; the periosteum outside 2 mm of the orbital rim is cut 360° to carry on the rest of the exenteration procedure. If the entire eyelid anatomy will be preserved, the operation is similar to an extended enucleation in which the eye with the bulbar conjunctival lining and the rest of the orbital tissues are removed en bloc. Eyelid-sparing subtotal exenteration offers significant advantages in terms of reconstruction of the orbit and cosmesis. The simplest approach to cosmetic rehabilitation is to pack the orbit with iodine gauze and let the socket granulate by itself.

When the eyelids are entirely removed, the free skin margin is tacked to the orbital rim with interrupted silk sutures for 360° and the socket is lined with antibiotic-soaked Vaseline or Xeroform gauze. Then more gauze is packed into the orbit, compressing the initial gauze strip lining firmly over the concavity of the orbital bones. Maxitrol ointment is then instilled to the edges of the wound, the exenteration cavity is covered with dry gauze squares, and a firm dressing is applied. In some instances, the interrupted 5-0 silk sutures at the skin margin may be left long and tied over the socket gauze pack (Figure 31.22). The initial dressing is removed 7 days postoperatively, and from then on the site should be irrigated frequently with 2% hydrogen peroxide solution. The initial debridement of the socket can be done at the clinic every other day or on third-day visits. After 2 weeks, the irrigation can be done with running water from a showerhead by the patient at home. The entire granulation process may take 8 to 10 weeks to complete (Figure

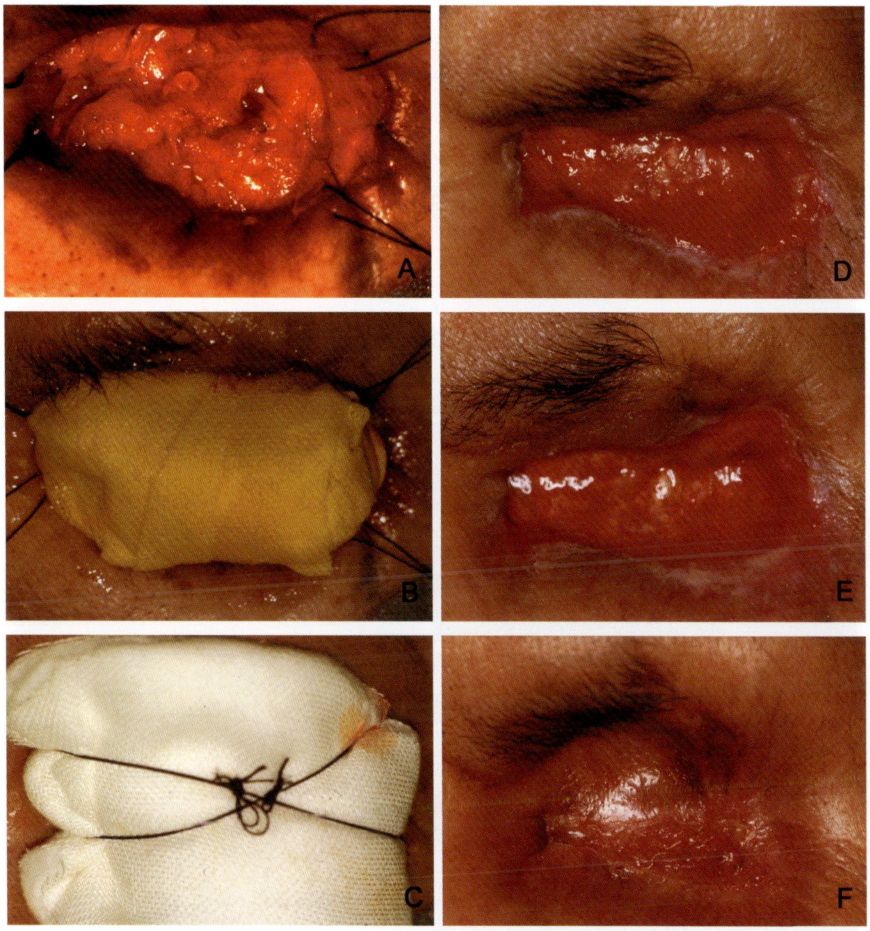

FIGURE 31.22. (A) Dressing of the exenteration cavity at the end of surgery. (B) Packing of the cavity with Xeroform gauze. (C) Tying the marginal skin sutures over the socket gauze pack. The gradual healing process of an exenteration socket at 4 weeks (D), 6 weeks (E), and 11 weeks (F).

31.22). By the time the granulation is complete, the orbit is covered with a very thin layer, which has the advantage of allowing the detection of recurrent tumor at an early stage. The resulting cavity is deep but can usually be fitted well with a silicone oculofacial prosthesis (Figure 31.23). The cosmetic results of the prosthesis are acceptable, particularly with shaded glasses (Figure 31.24).

Alternatively, the socket may be lined immediately at the completion of the exenteration procedure with split-thickness skin graft. The recommended thickness for the graft varies, but it should be free of hair follicles. A graft measuring approximately 10 cm × 5 cm in greatest dimensions would be sufficient to cover the orbital cavity. A graft of this size can easily be obtained from the front surface of the thigh. When the skin graft has been fitted into the orbit, one should ensure close approximation, preferably contact, of the graft to the recipient bony orbit. It is positioned and sutured to the marginal edges of the skin with interrupted absorbable sutures, and the orbit is packed with Xeroform gauze as a mold to provide firm apposition of the graft to the recipient area. Maxitrol ointment is applied to the edges of the skin, and a firm dressing is applied to keep the packing gauze in position for 10 days.[91] Some surgeons perforate the graft with small slits, which may make the fitting of the graft easier and allow an evacuation route for early postoperative bleeding, avoiding the accumulation of blood under the graft. Blood under the graft delays healing and may become a site of infection.

Although the orbits that are covered by skin grafts heal a few weeks faster than the uncovered ones, the grafted cavities have the disadvantage of not developing fibrosis to reduce the depth of the orbital cavity, which is commonly observed in the sockets that granulate on their own. Most surgeons agree that the orbits heal in a more uniform fashion without the skin graft; but the rehabilitation of the socket with numerous hospital visits for uncomfortable debridement and redressing of the socket makes this option rather unappealing for many patients.

To facilitate the healing of the exenteration socket, we use vacuum-assisted closure (VAC) in selected cases (Figure 31.25). The premise of this method is to apply controlled subatmospheric pressures to the wound to remove the edema, increase the localized blood flood, and enhance the formation of granulation tissue.[90,92,93] The VAC technique entails placing an open-cell foam dressing into the exenteration cavity

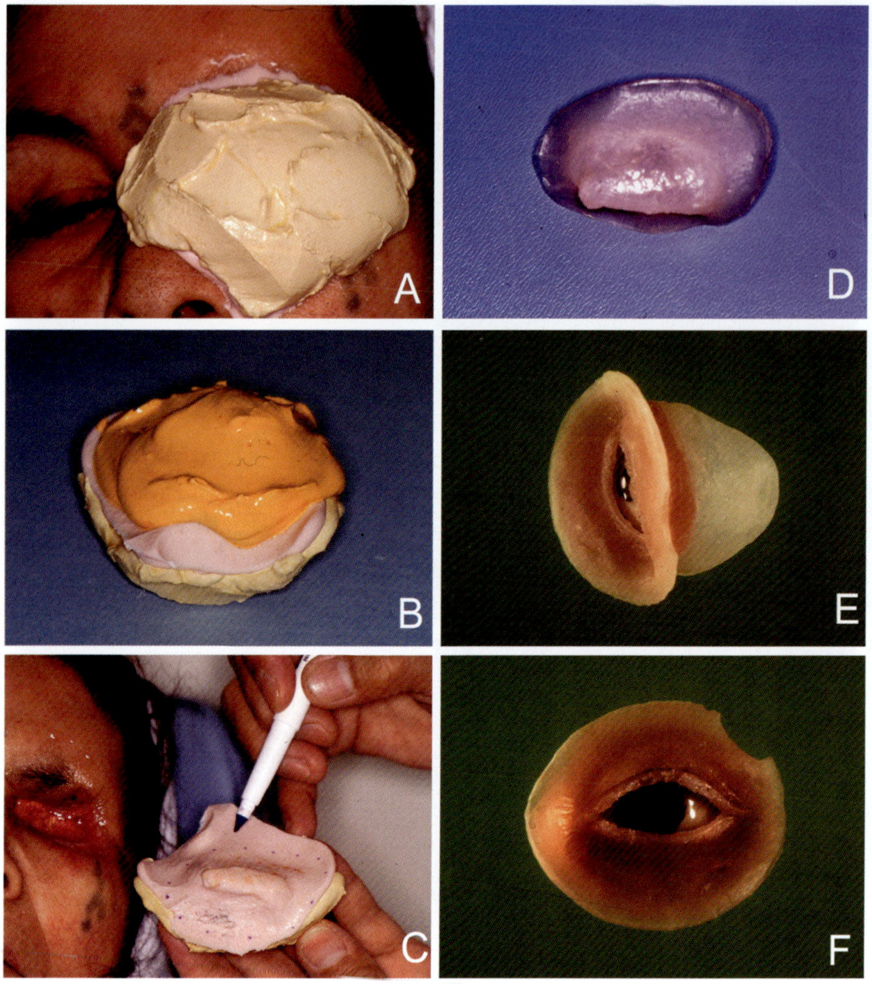

FIGURE 31.23. Molding of the socket (A–C) for the preparation of an orbitofacial prosthesis with an artificial eye (D–F).

at the end of surgery and sealing the socket with an adhesive plastic drape so that intermittent subatmospheric pressures can be applied to the socket during the next 2 to 3 days. The sterile foam dressing should be trimmed to fit into the socket and to allow the evacuation tube to sit centrally from the orbit (Figure 31.25). Cyclic intermittent negative pressures of 75 to 100 mmHg are used for 3 days while the patient is still in the hospital. Although the patient remains attached to the VAC pump during the hospitalization, the negative pressure does not seem to cause discomfort, and the procedure is well tolerated. The granulation of the orbit is markedly expedited and the socket heals well within 4 to 5 weeks as opposed to the usual 8 to 10 weeks of the granulation process. The removal of the sponge from the socket may create some dis-

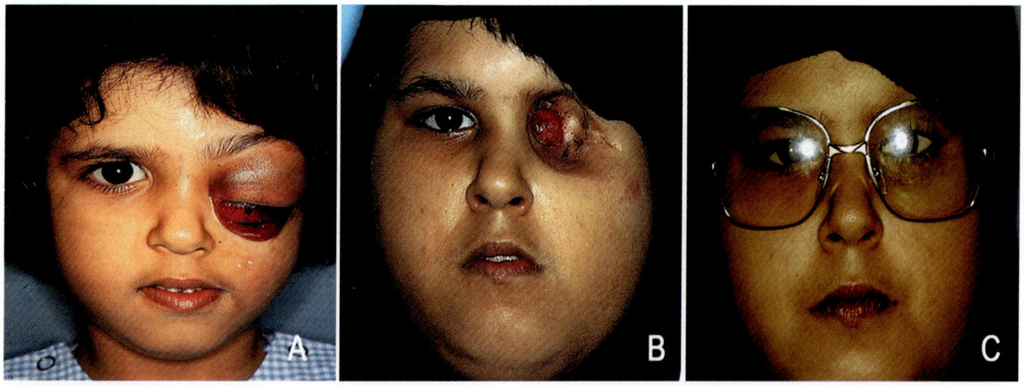

FIGURE 31.24. Facial prosthesis with glasses fitted to a patient following exenteration due to hemangiopericytoma. Patient is shown at the ages of 4 (A), 12 (B), and 15 (C) years. (Courtesy of Dr. Amin M. Nasr, Beirut, Lebanon.)

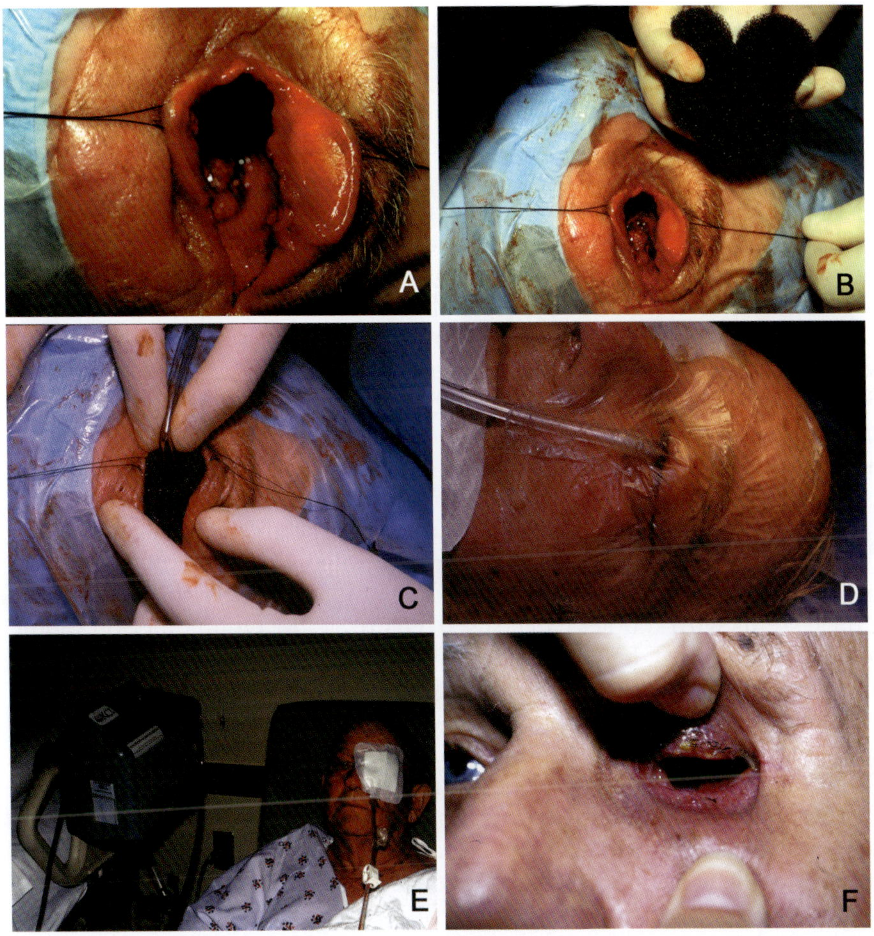

FIGURE 31.25. (A) Partial lid-sparing exenteration procedure was performed because of the extension of a choroidal melanoma into the orbit. (B,C) The placement of the cell foam sponge into the socket. (D) The draping of the socket with an adhesive plastic in a watertight fashion. (E) The patient is attached to VAC pump during hospitalization. (F) The appearance of the well-granulated socket only 4 weeks postoperatively.

comfort, particularly in eyelid-preserved exenterations. It is advisable for the patient to be sedated when the sponge is removed at the bedside. Skillman and coworkers reported the utilization of the VAC for improved healing of split-thickness skin grafting in exenteration cavities.[94,95]

In certain cases in which the orbital tumor is extensive, an orbitocraniofacial approach may facilitate the exenteration.[96,97]

No matter what approach is used and how limited exenteration may be, it is still extensive surgery and requires considerable reconstruction work. The primary objectives of reconstruction are to reach an optimal aesthetic result by restoring the boundaries between the orbit and surrounding cavities while allowing enough visibility for follow-up examinations to detect recurrent disease. In many cases, allografts cannot be used extensively because of concern about recurrent tumor, and most surgeons prefer to let the exenterated orbit heal by secondary intention.[91] Although this approach is not aesthetically ideal, the socket heals with a very thin layer of tissue, which allows early detection of recurrent tumor.

Regional surgical solutions, including transfer of the temporalis muscle and fascia and other regional pedicle flaps, as well as myocutaneous flaps with microvascular anastomosis, offer better cosmetic results. However, these procedures should not be performed unless one is absolutely sure that the malignant process has been totally cured. In some instances, early placed flaps and free grafts cover the recurrent disease and delay its diagnosis. When it is confirmed that there is no recurrent malignancy at the site of surgery, regional flaps or vascular myocutaneous flaps may be used for cosmetic rehabilitation. A common procedure is to borrow a portion of the temporalis muscle from its anterior half, pass it through the lateral wall, and fill the orbital cavity with the bulk of this graft. Skin graft can later be positioned over the muscle flap; in most instances this procedure effectively makes the exenteration cavity shallow.[98] Many patients are satisfied simply by wearing a black "pirate's patch" over the defect; others prefer the use of oculofacial prostheses. Early reconstruction during the exenteration procedure with myocutaneous and other flaps may be considered in children, since the tissue transfer will allow much easier postoperative wound care than split-thickness skin grafting and primary intention healing. Primary reconstruction may be recommended for very old patients as well as young children who require orbital exenteration but cannot tolerate the traditional postoperative debridement process.[99]

WOUND CLOSURE AND POSTOPERATIVE CARE

Wound closure is the last step of any surgical procedure. Although the techniques vary from one surgeon to another, certain basic principles should be followed. When the surgeon is ready to close the wound, layers of the exploration should be inspected, to ensure that the deep and superficial tissues are in optimal condition to be closed. All tissues, including bone, periosteum, orbital soft tissues, and skin/conjunctiva, should be properly approximated to their original anatomic planes as much as possible to minimize the functional deficit and postoperative scarring.

The bone is usually closed with heavy nylon or Prolene sutures; wires and bone fixation systems with metal plates and screws should be avoided. Although bioabsorbable bone fixation systems can be used, these devices are hardly necessary to reattach bone after tumor surgery. Alternatively, the bone may be repositioned in its original site without suturing and the periosteum may be pulled over to secure the underlying bone. For this purpose, the periosteum should be undermined. Another helpful point is to mark the edges of the periosteum with silk sutures at the time of incision; when the time of closure is reached, the periosteal layers are then easy to identify and reattach. The closure of the periosteum is usually accomplished with interrupted 5-0 or 6-0 Vicryl sutures.

The deep soft tissues of the orbit can be aligned and closed with 5-0 or 6-0 Vicryl sutures on a reverse cutting or spatula needle. It is best to close the subcutaneous tissues with an inverted suturing technique so that the knot will be hidden at the base of the closure, rather than being positioned immediately under the skin. Proper placement of deep sutures not only orients the tissues to their anatomic layers to minimize postoperative scarring but also avoids the "dead space" in between tissue recesses. "Dead space" between tissue planes leads to inaccurate wound closure and delays the wound healing; it also creates room for postoperative blood accumulation, which, in turn, may lead to infection. Then the overlying subcutaneous tissue and skin are closed with silk, nylon, or fast-absorbing gut sutures. In most tumor surgery cases, the margins of the skin are straight and clean as opposed to the ragged skin edges of trauma and infectious cases. Skin edges should be accurately positioned and sutured at two or three cardinal positions to ensure correct approximation. Then, interrupted sutures are placed between the initial cardinal sutures and tied with gentle eversion of the wound edges.

McCord and coworkers emphasize the proper eversion of the skin edges in closure to minimize postoperative functional deficit and scar formation.[41,44] Larger skin wounds may be closed with horizontal mattress and "near-far/far-near" suturing techniques in which more uniform tension is applied to the wound. Although these techniques minimize postoperative scarring, they are hardly ever necessary for orbitotomy incisions. Subcuticular running 6-0 nylon suture may also be used for skin closure. It is helpful to place the running suture on a bolster for easy removal in the clinic. For eyelid incisions, where the skin is thin, subcutaneous closure is not necessary, and the skin is directly closed with interrupted 7-0 nylon sutures.

The drain should be placed carefully to ensure the best surgical results. The author's preference is to insert a vacuum drain through an ab externo site. A Hemovac® drain or a 21-gauge butterfly tubing with cut holes can be used (Figure 31.26). Drain function should be checked by applying gentle suction, and the tubing of the drain should be anchored to the skin to avoid accidental displacement during the postoperative period. For lateral and superior orbitotomies, it is preferable to position the drain immediately adjacent to the lateral edge of the eyebrow in which the scar can be hidden. Incorporating the drain into the initial skin incision may increase the postoperative scar formation, particularly in black patients. Suturing the eyelids together after (or during) orbital surgery is bad practice because of its pressure effect on the eye and also because it does not allow the eye to be observed during the immediate postoperative period.

At the end of the orbitotomy, a red top laboratory tube is attached to the drain to evacuate the initial blood and residual fluids from the surgical site; the tube is replaced with a new one before the patient is sent to the recovery area. The vacuum tube should ideally be positioned inferior to the surgical site, where it can be taped onto the skin in a

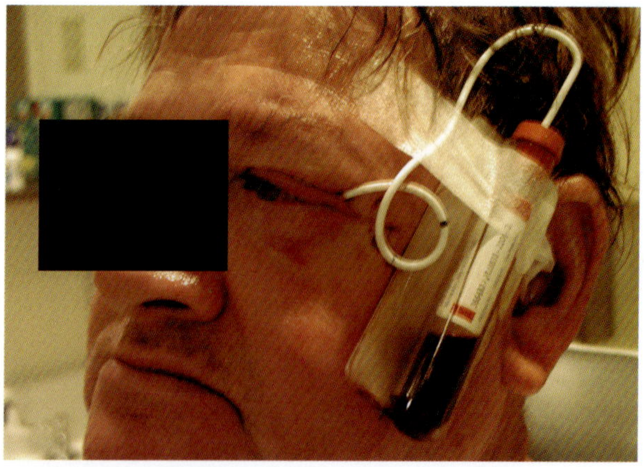

FIGURE 31.26. Hemovac® drain in place one day after lateral orbitotomy.

vertical fashion. After application of ophthalmic ointment (Maxitrol or Tobrex), a light dressing with one or two eye pads should be applied to the wound, using the fewest possible tapes to hold the dressing in position without putting too much pressure on the suture line. This point is important because if postoperative, intraorbital hemorrhage occurs, the nonpressure dressing will not contribute to the increased intraorbital/intraocular pressure, which could lead to a number of serious problems, including increased intraocular pressure and an arterial or venous thromboembolic phenomenon.

Following the dressing, the orbit should be covered with a few layers of clean gauze and an icepack should be applied immediately, preferably before the patient leaves the operating room, and continued during the first 24 to 48 hours of the postoperative period. Ice is extremely useful to reduce the postoperative edema and may also be helpful in reducing the chances of a postoperative intraorbital hemorrhage. On the other hand, if there is no concern for complications related to the globe, such as in enucleation–exenteration cases, pressure dressing can be applied to keep postoperative edema to a minimum. For the pressure dressing, two or three pads are applied to the closed eyelids and covered with tight Elastoplast taping.

Application of Benzoin is useful to increase the stickiness of the tape to the skin. However, when Benzoin is applied to the periorbital area, care should be taken that it not spill into the eye. If Elastoplast dressing does not stick well, a gauze head roll may be used. The pressure dressing is not left in place more than 3 days, even when there is no underlying globe to worry about. In some exenteration cases, the pressure dressing may stay in place longer, up to one week. The nylon and Prolene sutures are generally removed in 5 to 7 days; $^{1}/_{8}$ in. SteriStrips may be applied to the wound after the removal of the skin sutures and left in place for another 7 days.

Postoperative antibiotics and corticosteroids, including 500 mg of oral Keflex every 8 hours and 60 to 80 mg of prednisone per day for 2 days, are given. Keflex is continued for 7 to 10 days.

COMPLICATIONS

Intraoperative Complications

The most serious complication during surgery is the laceration of a vital structure such as a nerve, a muscle, a blood vessel, or the globe. Although this kind of injury is rare, the damage should be repaired before the procedure is continued. Scleral lacerations are extremely rare and should be treated as an open globe. Vascular lacerations are difficult if not impossible to repair because of the small size of the blood vessels and the difficulty in locating the ends. It should be ensured that the violated blood vessel is tied or cauterized to avoid postoperative hemorrhage. If a major peripheral nerve is cut accidentally, it is ideal to anastomose the nerve under high magnification (preferably with the microscope) with 9-0 nylon suture from perineurium to perineurium after the cut ends of the nerve have been aligned. If anastomosis is not possible, the nerve edges should be approximated to facilitate healing. If an extraocular muscle is cut inadvertently, it should be approximated and sutured with a 6-0 Vicryl suture.

Lacerations to the nasolacrimal drainage system may also cause postoperative problems. Here, as well, every attempt should be made to repair the laceration, and canalicular silicone tubing should be placed in position to maintain the patency of the LDS. If the damage is limited at the canaliculus level, both ends of the cut canaliculus should be aligned and repaired with fine sutures under the operating microscope. If the damage is serious at the lacrimal sac or nasolacrimal duct level and judged to be irreparable, a DCR may be the choice of treatment at the end of the orbital exploration or at a later date.

If dural laceration is suspected during surgery, it should be identified to rule out CSF leak. Although small lacerations can be repaired with direct suturing, the visualization is usually not good enough to allow this procedure. The best way to repair the dural rents is to apply free grafts from temporalis fascia or muscle, which can be applied with tissue adhesives.[100] If the CSF leak cannot be controlled, neurosurgical consultation should be sought intraoperatively. A lumbar puncture may be of some help to reduce the CSF pressure and thereby allowing the surgeon to control the leak better.

Intraoperative hemorrhage due to vascular laceration or generalized oozing is the most detested part of orbital surgery because it interferes with direct visualization and disrupts the procedure. Therefore, intraoperative bleeding during orbit surgery should be addressed methodically until hemostasis is regained; without the control of bleeding, surgery cannot proceed. The first objective should be the identification of the bleeding source. Suction and pressure by hand may accomplish this. If any obvious bleeding from blood vessels is detected, these should be cauterized or tied off. If no direct source can be seen, generalized pressure with epinephrine-soaked gauze or thrombin-soaked Gelfoam can be applied with gentle pressure. Bleeding from the bone is best controlled with generous application of unipolar cautery. If this is not successful, bone wax may be applied. Excess bone wax should be carefully removed because it could cause foreign body reaction.[101]

Postoperative Complications

The most dreaded postoperative complication in orbital surgery is hemorrhage, which can happen overnight or weeks after surgery but generally occurs in the 4 to 6 days following the procedure. Because the orbit is small and closed, any size hematoma may be of significance, depending on its location. Generous application of ice and elevation of the head of the bed during the first 24 to 48 hours of the postoperative period reduce the likelihood of orbital bleeding; however, postoperative hemorrhage may happen even in patients without risk factors such as hypertension or hypocoagulability. Physician's orders should be clearly written to alert the nursing staff to recognize symptoms of postoperative hemorrhage, including loss of vision, pain, and rapidly increasing proptosis. Small postoperative hematomas that produce some proptosis and chemosis but no pain or afferent pupillary defect can be observed under conservative treatment and usually get better within days. If a large postoperative hematoma is suspected, the eye should be examined immediately by checking the visual acuity, intraocular pressure, and the pupillary light reflex. Imaging studies, preferably MRI, should be obtained immediately. Even if an obvious nerve compression is not identified in the MRI image, but the clinical symptoms warrant an acute increase in intraorbital pressure, the patient should be managed urgently.

An acute rise in the pressure of the orbit may cause compressive optic neuropathy as well as hypoperfusion to the optic nerve and retina.[13] If the patient complains of visual loss in the presence of rapidly developing painful proptosis, one should check orbital pressure. One can assess increased orbital pressure by digital palpation, by observation of pulsating retinal vessels, and by increased intraocular pressure. If the orbit is tense while the patient is still carrying a drain, the position of the drain tubing should be manipulated while it is placed on suction. Because of the fibrous septae and the fibrin loculations during the orbital surgery, the hematomas, which may be localized, can be evacuated with position change of the drain. A great majority of patients are on steroids and antibiotics after orbital surgery; however, addition of Manitol and Acetazolamide should be considered to lower the pressure. Acute increase in orbital pressure is an emergency, and if the high pressure persists it should be relieved surgically. The simplest and the most effective way of relieving the orbital pressure is a lateral canthotomy. This can easily be done with the lyses of the inferior crus of the lateral canthal tendon. If the pressure is not relieved, the superior crus is cut in the same fashion. When the canthotomy is done, the lids may not cover the cornea; the cornea should be protected with ointment, collagen shield, bandage contact lens, or light patching.

Imaging may reveal the localization of the blood, which sometimes can be evacuated with a 20-gauge needle (Figure 31.27). Subperiosteal hematomas are the easiest ones to tap with a needle. This maneuver can also be done under CT guidance. B-scan ultrasonography may also be useful to guide a needle into anteriorly located hematomas.

If all these maneuvers fail, and the increased orbital pressure cannot be relieved, the patient should be taken back to the operating room so that the wound can be opened to evacuate the blood. If bleeders are observed, hemostasis should be accomplished and new drains should be placed before reclosure.

The best protection against postoperative increase of intraorbital pressure, due to hematoma or infection, is the meticulous performance of orbital surgery. The chances of postoperative hemorrhage can be decreased with complete hemostasis before closing the orbital cavity and with proper placement of a drain. The patient should be extubated carefully without developing Valsalva maneuvers, and the blood pressure should slowly rise in cases of hypotensive anesthesia. Tight pressure dressings should be avoided; ice should immediately be applied to the orbit. A certain degree of hemorrhagic chemosis cannot be avoided after orbit surgery; this can be managed with ophthalmic oint-

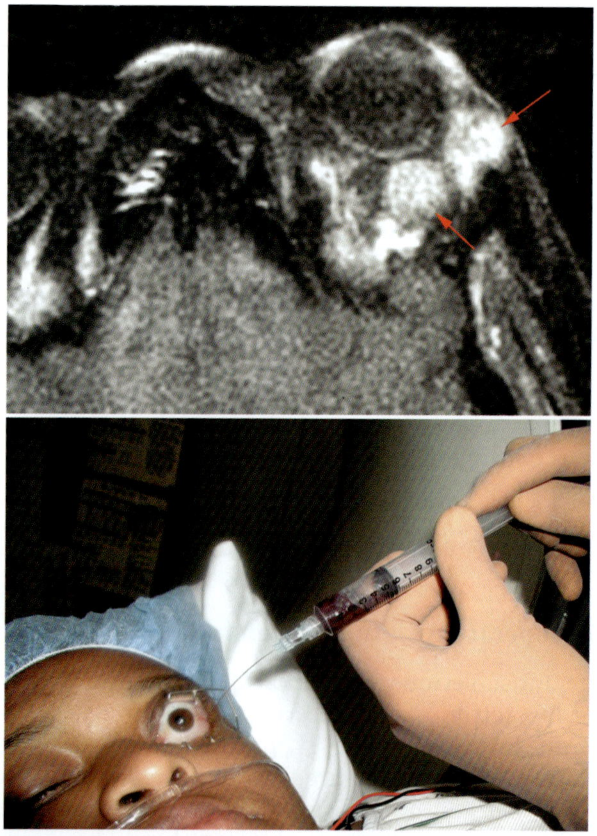

FIGURE 31.27. Evacuation of blood (red arrows on MRI) from orbit with a 21-gauge catheter.

ments. On occasion, the chemosis in the inferior fornix becomes semisolid and persistent. In these cases, a roll of gauze soaked in Vaseline can be placed into the inferior fornix with pressure patching on the eye. This can be left in place for 24 hours.

Excessive traction or blind dissection of the orbital tissues may damage the nerves, causing postoperative sensory and motor complications. For example, abduction weakness after lateral orbitotomy is a common occurrence, but this usually subsides without any interference. One hundred fifty-two patients who underwent surgery for orbital tumors during a 7-year period were reviewed for surgical complications. The highest number of complications was recorded in lateral orbitotomies (35%).[102] Ninety-seven anterior orbitotomies revealed minor problems in only 3% of the surgeries.

The complications of lateral orbitotomies included extraocular motility problems, particularly abduction deficit (17.5%) and loss of pupillary reflex (10%). Occasional cases of ptosis, neurotrophic keratitis, and intraorbital hemorrhage were also seen. The most significant risk factor was found to be the intraconal location of the tumor. The majority of the complications were associated with the lateral approach to excise intraconal tumors; tumor type did not appear to be a factor. Ptosis may also be a problem following lateral and superior orbitotomies. During these procedures it is common to have hemorrhages into the levator muscle with subsequent ptosis. Again, this is not usually persistent; it usually resolves in weeks to months. Damage to the superior division of the third nerve and injury in the orbital apex can also produce long-term ptosis.[103] If ptosis is secondary to nerve laceration, the repair may take a long time; these patients should be observed for up to a year. Overzealous dissection may injure the ciliary ganglion in lateral orbitotomies, particularly after removal of intraconal lesions, and the patient may develop dilated, nonreactive pupil, postoperatively. Again, it may take up to 6 months for the repair process. In superior medial orbitotomies, if the trochlea is injured, the patient may develop acquired Brown's syndrome, postoperatively. This usually resolves during observation. In superior lateral orbitotomies, the lacrimal gland or its connecting ductules may be damaged, resulting in dry eye in many patients. This is usually a permanent problem and should be managed with artificial tears, ointments, and punctal plugs.

Postoperative emphysema may occur in small amounts and in localized fashion following the orbitotomy, owing to established passages from the sinuses and nasal cavity to the orbit. Small localized pockets of air are benign and usually resolve within days. On the other hand, if the volume of air entrapped in the orbit is large enough to increase intraorbital pressure and compromise the optic nerve, evacuation should be performed, preferably with a 20-gauge needle under ultrasonographic control.

Wound infection and dehiscence as well as orbital cellulitis are unusual postoperative complications following tumor surgery. However, if the patient develops signs and symptoms of an infection, broad-spectrum antibiotics are given and cultures obtained from the wound or from the drainage fluid. Warm compresses should be applied. Imaging procedures, preferably MRI, should be done to identify localized abscess formation. If the patient fails to respond to medical treatment, the abscess should be evacuated in the operating room.

Another long-term complication in any surgical procedure is scar formation, which in general can be minimized with strict attention to precise surgical technique. The surgical approach for tumor patients is usually well planned and accomplished with relatively small skin incisions. Therefore, scars are seen less often after orbital tumor surgery than following treatment for other orbital problems, such as trauma and inflammation. On the other hand, conjunctival scarring and focal symblepharon formation can be seen after surgery and postoperative radiation. In certain cases, particularly in darkly pigmented individuals, there may be scarring of the periorbital skin at the incision site or at the site of the drain insertion. Contraction of the scar is the last phase of wound healing and may take a long time, extending over many weeks to months.[104] Therefore, even if medical or surgical treatment is contemplated to revise a scar, this should not be undertaken until the area has stabilized, usually after several months. Some of the hypertrophic scars and keloids may respond to steroid ointments or intradermal injection of steroids or low-dose radiation. For example, 0.1 mL of triamcinolone (Kenalog) may be directly injected into the scar with a 27- or 30-gauge needle; the injections may be repeated every 2 weeks. Darkly pigmented individuals may experience depigmentation. A certain degree of response is obtained in hypertrophic scars, but keloids usually recur.[105] If there is severe contracture and irregularity of the skin, excision of the scar (scar revision) and/or skin grafting may be indicated; scar revision surgery is rarely needed after planned orbitotomies. More significantly, scarring may take place within the underlying soft tissues of the wound owing to excessive dissection, cauterization, hemorrhage, or improper closure of the soft tissues and periosteum. Scar formation around the extraocular muscles and peripheral nerves may result in the malfunction of the involved structures; most commonly leading to postoperative diplopia.[103] In most cases, diplopia also resolves over the coming months; if it does not, in the absence of recurrent tumor, the possibility of strabismus surgery should be entertained.

Conjunctival scarring and symblepharon may also occur occasionally, but these scars are usually small and do not interfere with lid function. If surgical repair is needed, it is best to wait 4 to 6 months, to allow the reparative process to stabilize.

References

1. Mafee MF. Imaging in ophthalmology. *Radiol Clin North Am* 1987;25:509–528.
2. Müller-Forell WS. *Imaging of Orbital & Visual Pathway Pathology*. Berlin: Springer-Verlag; 2002.
3. Hopper KD, Sherman JL, Boal DKB. Abnormalities of the orbit and its contents in children: CT and MR imaging findings. *Am J Radiol* 1991;156:1219–1224.
4. Trobe JD, Gebarski SS. Looking behind the eyes. The proper use of modern imaging. *Arch Ophthalmol* 1993;111:18:1185–1186.
5. Williamson TH, Harris A. Color Doppler ultrasound image of the eye and orbit. *Surv Ophthalmol* 1996;40:255–267.
6. Lieb WE, Flaharty PM, Ho A, Sergott RC. Color Doppler imaging of the eye and orbit: a synopsis of 400 case experiences. *Acta Ophthalmol* 1992;204(suppl):50–54.
7. Morris R, McKay W, Mushlin P. Comparison of pain associated with intradermal and subcutaneous infiltration with various local anesthetic agents. *Anesth Analg* 1987;66:1180–1182.
8. Bilyk JR, Sutula FC. Anesthesia for ophthalmic plastic surgery In: Stewart WB, ed. *Surgery of the Eyelid, Orbit and Lacrimal System*. San Francisco: AAO Ophthalmic Monographs; 1993;26–57.
9. Smith GB. Anesthesia for orbital surgery: observed changes in the visually evoked response at low blood pressures. *Mod Probl Ophthalmol* 1975;14:457.
10. Borges AF. Relaxed skin tension lines (RSTL) versus other skin lines. *Plast Reconstr Surg* 1984:73:144–150.
11. Appling WD, Patrinely JR, Saizer TA. Transconjunctival approach vs subciliary skin–muscle flap approach for orbital fracture repair. *Arch Otolaryngol Head Neck Surg* 1993;119:1000–1007.
12. Rootman J, Stewart B, Goldberg RA. *Orbital Surgery: a Conceptual Approach*. Philadelphia: Lippincott-Raven; 1995.
13. McCord CD. Complications of orbital surgery. *Otolaryngol Clin North Am* 1988;21:183–188.
14. Kaplan I, Kott I, Giler S. Carbon dioxide laser in treatment of lesions of the eyelids and periorbital region. *J Clin Laser Med Surg* 1996;14:185–187.
15. Kennerdell JS, Maroon JC, Garrity JA, et al. Surgical management of orbital lymphangioma with the carbon dioxide laser. *Am J Ophthalmol* 1986;102:308–314.
16. Dailey RA, Sullivan SA, Wobig JL. Surgical debulking of eyelid and anterior orbital plexiform neurofibromas by means of carbon dioxide laser. *Am J Ophthalmol* 2000;130:117–119.
17. Dutton JJ. *Atlas of Clinical and Surgical Orbital Anatomy*. Philadelphia: WB Saunders; 1994;256.
18. Zide BM, Jelks GW. *Surgical Anatomy of the Orbit*. New York: Raven Press; 1985:88.
19. Kennerdell JS, Maroon JC, Malton ML. Surgical approaches to orbital tumors. *Clin Plast Surg* 1988;15:273–282.
20. Henderson JW, Farrow GM. *Orbital Tumors*. 2nd ed. New York: BC Decker; 1980:580–584.
21. Osuthorpe JD. Surgical access to primary orbital tumors. *Otolaryngol Clin North Am* 1988;21:135–153.
22. Leone CR. Surgical approaches to the orbit. *Ophthalmology* 1979;86:930–941.
23. McCord CD Jr. Surgical approaches to orbital disease. In: McCord CD, Tanenbaum M, eds: *Oculoplastic Surgery*. New York: Raven Press;1987:257–278.
24. Nowinski T, Anderson RL. Advances in orbital surgery. *Ophthalmic Plast Reconstr Surg* 1985;1:211–217.
25. Berke RM. A modified Kronlein operation. *Arch Ophthalmol*. 1954;51:6096–6132.
26. Wright JE. Surgery of the orbit. In: Miller S, ed. *Operative Surgery*. 3rd ed. London: Butterworth; 1976.
27. Callahan A. Wright's lateral orbitotomy. In: Jakobiec FA, ed. *Ocular and Adnexal Tumors*. Birmingham, AL: Aesculapius Publishing; 1978:843–897.
28. Wright JE, Stewart WV. Orbital surgery. *Int Ophthalmol Clin* 1978;1:149–167.
29. Stallard HB. A plea for lateral orbitotomy with certain modifications. *Br J Ophthalmol* 1960;44:718.
30. Karcioglu ZA. Optic nerve sheath decompression. Paper presented at: 13th European Congress of Ophthalmology. Istanbul, Turkey; June 2001.
31. Goldberg RA, Lessner AM, Shorr N, Baylis HI. The transconjunctival approach to the orbital floor and orbital fat: a prospective study. *Ophthalmic Plast Reconstr Surg* 1990;6:241–246.
32. Nowinski T, Anderson RL. Advances in orbital surgery. *Ophthalmic Plast Surg* 1985;1:211–217.
33. McCord CD, Moses JL. Exposure of the inferior orbit with fornix incision and lateral canthotomy. *Ophthalmic Surg* 1979;10:59–63.
34. Mascott CR. The magnetic system. In: Germano I. ed. *Contemporary Image-Guided Surgery*. Stuttgart: G. Thieme; 2002.
35. Helveston EM, Merriam WW, Ellis FD, et al. The trochlea. A study of the anatomy and physiology. *Ophthalmology* 1982;89:124–133.
36. Sacks JG. The shape of the trochlea. *Arch Ophthalmol* 1984;102:932–933.
37. Anderson RL. Medial canthal tendon branches out. *Arch Ophthalmol* 1977;95:2051–2052.
38. Hurwitz JJ. *The Lacrimal System*. Philadelphia: Lippincott-Raven; 1996:218–219.
39. Graham SM, Thomas RD, Carter KD, Nerad JA. The transcaruncular approach to the medial orbital wall. *Laryngoscope* 2002;112:986–989.
40. Lai PC, Liao SL, Jou JR, et al. Transcaruncular approach for the management of frontoethmoid mucoceles. *Br J Ophthalmol* 2003;87:699–703.
41. Frante RG, Elner VM. Transcaruncular approach to medial canthal tendon plication for lower eyelid laxity. *Ophthalmic Plast Reconstr Surg* 2001;17:16–27.
42. Shorr N, Baylis HI, Goldberg RA, et al. Transcaruncular approach to the medial orbit and orbital apex. *Ophthalmology* 2000;107:1459–1463.
43. Bourman MD, Spoor TC, Ramocki JM. Optic nerve sheath decompression for pseudotumor cerebri. *Arch Ophthalmol* 1988;106:1378–1383.
44. McCord CD, Cole HP. Surgical approaches to the orbit. In: McCord CD, Tannenbaum M, Nunery WR, eds. *Oculoplastic Surgery*. 3rd ed. New York: Raven Press; 1995:504–507.
45. Blacklock JB, Webber RS, Lee YY, Goepfert H. Transcranial resection of tumors of the paranasal sinuses and nasal cavity. *J Neurosurg* 1989;71:10–15.
46. Goldberg RA, Hannanai K, Toga AW. Microanatomy of the orbital apex: computed tomography and microcryoplaning of soft and hard tissue. *Ophthalmology* 1992;99:1447–1452.
47. Housepian EM. Microsurgical anatomy of the orbital apex and principles of transcranial orbital exploration. *Clin Neurosurg* 1978;25:556–573.
48. Catalano PJ, Laidlow D, Sen C. Globe sparing exenteration. *Otolaryngol Head Neck Surg* 2001;125:379–384.
49. Polito E, Leccisotti A. Recurrent conjunctival melanomas. *Orbit* 1992;11:93–98.
50. Paridaens AD, McCartney AC, Minassian DC, et al. Orbital exenteration in 95 cases of primary conjunctival malignant melanoma. *Br J Ophthalmol* 1994;78:520–528.

51. Shields JA, Shields CL, Gündüz K, et al. Clinical features predictive of orbital exenteration for conjunctival melanoma. *Ophthalmic Plast Reconstr Surg* 2000;16:173–178.
52. Shields JA, Shields CL, Freire JE, et al. Plaque radiotherapy in the management of selected orbital malignancies: preliminary observations: the 2002 Montgomery Lecture, part 2. *Ophthalmic Plast Reconstr Surg* 2003;19:91–95.
53. Shields JA, Shields CL. Orbital malignant melanoma. *Ophthalmic Plast Reconstr Surg* 2003;19:262–299.
54. Cha SB, Shields JA, Shields CL, Wang MX. Squamous cell carcinoma of the conjunctiva [review]. *Int Ophthalmol Clin* 1993;33:19–24.
55. Karcioglu ZA, Toth J. Relation between *p53* over-expression and clinical behavior of ocular/orbital invasion of conjunctival squamous cell carcinoma. *Ophthalmic Plast Reconstr Surg* 2000;16:443–449.
56. Lee GA, Hirst LW. Ocular surface squamous neoplasia [review]. *Surv Ophthalmol* 1995;39:429–450.
57. Liarikos S, Rapidis AD, Roumeliotis A, et al. Secondary orbital melanomas: analysis of 15 cases. *J Craniomaxillofac Surg* 2000;28:148–152.
58. Affeldt JC, Minckler DS, Azen SP, et al. Prognosis in uveal melanoma with extrascleral extension. *Arch Ophthalmol* 1980;98:1975–1979.
59. Shields JA, Shields CL. Massive orbital extension of posterior uveal melanoma. *Ophthalmic Plast Reconstr Surg* 1991;7:238–251.
60. Shields JA, Augsburger JJ, Corwin S, et al. The management of uveal melanomas with extrascleral extension. *Orbit* 1986;6:31–37.
61. De Potter P, Shields JA, Shields CL, et al. Modified enucleation via lateral orbitotomy for choroidal melanomas with massive orbital extension. *Ophthalmic Plast Reconstr Surg* 1992;8:109–113.
62. Shields JA, Shields CL, Demirci H, et al. Experience with eyelid-sparing orbital exenteration: the 2000 Tullos O. Coston Lecture. *Ophthalmic Plast Reconstr Surg* 2001;17:355–361.
63. Shields JA, Shields CL, Suvarnamani C, et al. Orbital exenteration with eyelid sparing: indications, technique, and results. *Ophthalmic Surg* 1991;22:292–297.
64. Hopping W, Waubke TN, Sack H. Orbital involvement in retinoblastoma. *Mod Probl Ophthalmol* 1975;14:382–387.
65. Finger PT, Harbour JW, Karcioglu ZA. Risk factors for metastasis in retinoblastoma. *Surv Ophthalmol* 2002;47:1–16.
66. Kopelman JE, McLean IW, Rosenberg SH. Multivariate analysis of risk factors for metastasis in retinoblastoma treated by enucleation. *Ophthalmology* 1987;94:371–377.
67. Svedberg H, Al-Mesfer SA, Riley FC. Survival trends of retinoblastoma patients with extraocular extension. *Cong Eur Soc Ophthalmol.* Abstract:502;1999.
68. Kiratli H, Bilgic S, Ozerdem U. Management of massive orbital involvement in intraocular retinoblastoma. *Ophthalmology* 1988;105:322–326.
69. Moshfeghi DM, Moshfeghi AA, Finger PT. Enucleation. *Surv Ophthalmol* 2000:44:277–301.
70. Soll DB. Enucleation surgery: a new technique. *Arch Ophthalmol* 1972;87:196–197.
71. Schaefer DP, DellaRocca RC. Enucleation In: DellaRocca RC, Nesi FA, Lisman RD, eds. *Ophthalmic Plastic Reconstructive Surgery*. St Louis: CV Mosby; 1987:1278–1299.
72. La Piana FG. Modified enucleation. *Adv Ophthalmic Plast Reconstr Surg* 1990;8:73–74.
73. Karcioglu, ZA, Al-Mesfer SA, Mullaney PB. Porous polyethylene orbital implant in patients with retinoblastoma. *Ophthalmology* 1998;105:1311–1316.
74. Karesh JW, Dresner SC. High-density porous polyethylene (Medpor) as a successful anophthalmic socket implant. *Ophthalmology* 1994;101:1688–1695.
75. Migliori ME, Putterman AM. The domed dermis-fat graft orbital implant. *Ophthalmic Plast Reconstr Surg* 1991;7:23–30.
76. Hornblass A, Biesman BS, Eviatar JA. Current techniques of enucleation: a survey of 5,439 intraorbital implants and a review of the literature. *Ophthalmic Plast Reconstr Surg* 1995;11:77–86.
77. Jordan DR, Munro SM, Brownstein S, et al. A synthetic hydroxyapatite implant: the so-called counterfeit implant. *Ophthalmic Plast Reconstr Surg* 1998;14:244–249.
78. Karcioglu ZA, Al-Ghamdi H, Al-Bateri A, Rostem A. Radiation absorption properties of orbital implants. *Orbit* 1998;17:161–167.
79. Arora V, Weeks K, Halperin C, et al. Influence of coraline hydroxyapatite used as an ocular implant on the dose distribution of external beam photon radiation therapy. *Ophthalmology* 1992;99:380–382.
80. Levin PS, Dutton JJ. A 20 year series of orbital exenteration. *Am J Ophthalmol* 1991;112:496–501.
81. Bartley GB, Garrity JA, Waller RR, et al. Orbital exenteration at the Mayo Clinic. *Ophthalmology* 1989;96:468–474.
82. Schwartz JN, Donnelly EH, Klintworth GK. Ocular and orbital phycomycosis. *Surv Ophthalmol* 1977;22:3–28.
83. Naquin HA. Exenteration of the orbit. *Arch Ophthalmol* 1954;51:850–862.
84. Rathbun JE, Beard C, Quickert MH. Evaluation of 48 cases of orbital exenteration. *Am J Ophthalmol* 1971;72:191–199.
85. Goldberg RA, Kim JW, Shorr N. Orbital exenteration: results of individualized approach. *Ophthalmic Plast Reconstr Surg* 2003;19:229–236.
86. Reese AB, Jones IS. Bone resection in the excision of epithelial tumors of lacrimal gland. *Arch Ophthalmol* 1964;71:382–385.
87. Marsh JL, et al. Lacrimal gland adenoid cystic carcinoma: intracranial and extracranial *en bloc* resection. *Plast Reconstr Surg* 1981;68:577.
88. Bonavolonta G. Ocular complications following conservative orbital surgery. *Orbit* 1982;1:214.
89. Bonavolonta G, DeConciliis C. Incidence and treatment of dural exposure and CSF leak during orbital exenteration. *Ophthalmic Plast Reconstr Surg* 1987;3:61–64.
90. Tse DT, Panje WR, Anderson RM. Cyanoacrylate adhesive used to stop CSF leaks during orbital surgery. *Arch Ophthalmol* 1984;102:1337–1339.
91. Levin PS, Ellis DS, Stewart WB, et al. Orbital exenteration: the reconstructive letter. *Ophthalmic Plast Reconst Surg* 1991;7:84–92.
92. Argenta LC, Mor YK, Mas MJ. Vacuum-assisted closure: a new method for wound control and treatment: clinical experience *Ann Plast Surg* 1997;38:563–576.
93. Joseph E, Hamori CA, Bergmen S, et al. A prospective randomized trial of VAC versus standard therapy of chronic nonhealing wounds. *Wounds* 2000;12:60–67.
94. Skillman J, Kirkpatrick N, Coombes C, et al. Vacuum assisted closure (VAC) dressing for skin graft application following exenteration of the orbit [abstract]. Paper presented at: ESOPRS meeting Münster, Germany; 2002.
95. Lafuente H. Exenteration of the orbit in selected cases of severe orbital contracture. *Ophthalmology* 1983;90:236–238.
96. Maroon JC, Kennerdell JS. Surgical approaches to the orbit: indications and techniques. *J Neurosurg* 1984;60:1226–1235.
97. Terz JJ, Young HF, Lawrence W. Combined craniofacial resection for locally advanced carcinoma of the head and neck, tumor of skin and soft tissues. *Am J Surg* 1980;140:613–617.
98. Ellis DS, Toth BA, Stewart WB. Temporal parietal facial flaps for orbit and eyelid reconstruction. *Ophthalmic Plast Reconstr Surg* 1992;89:606–612.
99. Uusitalo MM, Ibarra M, Fulton L, et al. Reconstruction with

rectus abdominus myocutaneous free flap after orbital exenteration in children. *Arch Ophthalmol* 2001;119:1705–1709.

100. Tse DT, Panje WR, Anderson RL. Cyanoacrylate adhesive used to stop CSF leaks during orbital surgery. *Arch Ophthalmol* 1984;102:1337–1339.
101. Karcioglu ZA, Nasr AM. Diagnosis and management of orbital inflammation and infections secondary to foreign bodies: a clinical review. *Orbit* 1998;17:247–267.
102. Purgason PA, Hornblass A. Complications of surgery for orbital tumors. *Ophthalmic Plast Reconstr Surg* 1992;8:88–93.
103. Krohel GB. Blepharoptosis following traumatic third nerve palsies. *Am J Ophthalmol* 1979;88:598.
104. Peacock EE, Van Winkle W. *Wound Repair*. 2nd ed., Philadelphia: WB Saunders, 1976.
105. Ketchum LD, Robinson DW, Masters FW: Follow-up on treatment of hypertrophic scars and keloids with triamcinolone. *Plast Reconstr Surg* 1971;48:256

32

Computer Image Guidance and Skull-Base Strategies

Christopher R. Mascott and Zeynel A. Karcıoglu

As in many areas of medicine, computerized imaging modalities (CT and MRI in particular) have also revolutionized the diagnosis of orbital tumors. The therapeutic impact of these imaging techniques has only recently been explored in select cases of orbital tumors. Computer image guidance has seen remarkable development in other specialties, notably in neurosurgery.[1,2] It is therefore not surprising that the initial experience with this technology in the surgery of orbital tumors has entailed tumors with intracranial extension, requiring a multidisciplinary approach of ophthalmological and neurological surgeons. In addition to image guidance, a standard craniotomy to expose the orbital roof and areas of intracranial tumor extension can be supplemented by a skull-base approach in select cases with minimal to no additional morbidity. Other treatment modalities include radiosurgery (computer image-guided stereotactic radiation).[3] A limiting factor for radiosurgery both for intraorbital and intracranial treatment is the risk of functional damage to the optic pathways. In this chapter, we discuss our multidisciplinary approach to select orbital tumors with special reference to emerging technologies and surgical approaches.

COMPUTER IMAGE GUIDANCE

In recent years, systems that permit computer-guided navigation during surgery using preoperatively acquired computer-based imaging have seen exponential development in neurosurgery and to a lesser degree in the ear, nose, and throat field. The fundamental principle of surgical navigation is to acquire computed tomography (CT) or magnetic resonance (MR) as a volumetric data set, usually implying image acquisition in the form of an elevated number of parallel slices with no intervening gaps between slices. Such a data set can then be reconstructed into a volume, which can be reformatted in any plane. The volumetric study can also be reconstructed to define three-dimensional renderings of the head, the orbit, the eye, the optic nerves, and the brain, as well as of tumors. These three-dimensional models are thus defined in "image space."

To use imaging data for intraoperative real-time navigation, the three-dimensional structures in image space must be correlated with the real anatomic structures in the "surgical space" of the actual patient. To accomplish this, surgical space must be defined so that exact coordinates can be determined for areas of interest at surgery. In neurosurgery, the traditional frame of reference has been a stereotactic frame rigidly affixed to the skull prior to imaging and maintained during surgery. Computer image guidance with a frame was pioneered by Kelly et al.[4] Over the past 10 years, there has been an accelerated development of "frameless" image guidance systems, in which the rigid frame has been replaced by using the reconstructed three-dimensional rendering of the head. The position of the head, which needs to be rigidly immobilized only at the time of surgery (using a standard three-point headholder), needs to be referenced in space by means of a mechanical, ultrasonic, optical, or magnetic system.[5–11] Ultrasonic referencing has fallen from favor for lack of reliability, and mechanical systems are seen less frequently because of their cumbersome nature. The most common systems presently available use infrared light or ambient light to define the position of probes during surgery. There is growing interest in using a magnetic field as a frame of reference for defining space, since this methodology interferes least with surgical procedures.[12]

Regardless of the methodology used, the principles of frameless image guidance remain the same. Several landmarks must be chosen on the three-dimensional head rendering (in image space) and the corresponding landmarks on the patient (surgical space) are correlated at the time of surgery by detecting and tracking the position of a probe with regard to a reference (e.g., by two cameras for optical tracking, by a magnetic receiver attached to the probe for magnetic tracking). The procedure of correlating selected points in image space with their homologues in surgical space is known as *registration* and is performed by touching the designated points with a nonsterile tracked probe and recording them (Figure 32.1). The accuracy of image guidance at surgery (using a sterile probe) depends greatly on the quality of registration. It must also be kept in mind that following registration, the computer usually gives an estimate of calculated accuracy (should be less than 3 mm), but this number may or may not correspond to the true surgical accuracy (also termed *application accuracy*) during surgery. Overall, it is therefore necessary to know the principles and limitations of this technology and to evaluate the true accuracy intraoperatively against recognizable surgical landmarks. To facilitate registration, many surgeons apply special adhesive skin markers prior to imaging. The presence of these additional landmarks adds accuracy to registration, provided they are applied to areas of skin or scalp that are unlikely to move during imaging or surgical positioning. In selected cases, where high accuracy is paramount, optimal accuracy can be obtained by MRI/CT markers attached to small titanium screws implanted in the skull under local anesthesia prior to imaging and kept in place until surgery to permit registration.[12,13]

TECHNIQUES AND SETUP

We have been fortunate to have two different image guidance systems at our disposal. The StealthStation (Medtronics Surgical Navigation Technologies, Louisville, CO) is an optical referencing and tracking system. The Cygnus-PFS (Compass International, Rochester, MN) is a magnetic referencing and tracking system. Since we have a research interest in image guidance, we have used both systems simultaneously in over 70 cases, including in orbital tumors.[12] This has allowed us to compare systems and evaluate accuracy.

Preoperative images are acquired according to volumetric protocols, so that the data sets can be imported and reconstructed by the image guidance workstations. Transfer is accomplished either by network or via a variety of digital media (optical disk, DAT tape, recordable CD, etc.). We usually place adherent markers around the head prior to imaging to facilitate point-to-point registration (Figure 32.1). If imaging is done the day before surgery, the markers can be left overnight and a marking pen used to highlight their position, should they move before surgery. If surgery is to occur several days after imaging, we usually try to align the markers with birthmarks, angiomas, or scars on the scalp to find the correct points at surgery. A small cruciate scratch will also last several days. When accuracy is paramount, we implant small titanium screws (Stryker-Leibinger, Freiburg, Germany) under local anesthesia and attach MRI/CT markers to these (Figure 32.1). The screws can remain in place for days (or weeks) after the markers have been removed.

The optical system employs a large workstation and a dual infrared camera mounted on a pole. To define the position of the head in space during registration, an optical reference arc is attached to the headholder when the head has been immobilized at surgery (Figure 32.1). This nonsterile arc is then replaced by a sterile one after draping (Figure 32.2). The magnetic system runs on a laptop, and there are no cameras. The system is therefore minimally obtrusive. A magnet is attached to the headholder at the time of surgery, and this remains under the drapes. The nonsterile probe is exchanged for a sterile probe after draping (Figure 32.2).

WHY USE IMAGE GUIDANCE IN ORBITAL TUMORS?

Computer image guidance systems have found applications in neurosurgery for brain tumors and other procedures requiring surgical navigation inside the brain. What can a surgical navigation system contribute to surgery of orbital tumors? Unlike surgery of the brain, finding a tumor within the relatively narrow confines of the orbit and its surroundings is not a great challenge. For this reason, the application of image guidance for the orbit is not frequently reported.[14,15]

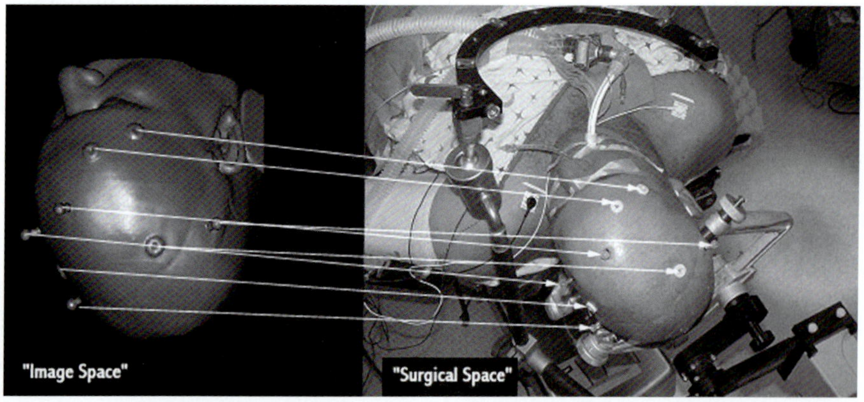

FIGURE 32.1. *Registration* consists of the mathematical matching of defined points in image space with their homologues in surgical space. This is accomplished by touching the predetermined locations at the time of surgery with a probe that is referenced and tracked in space. An optical reference arc is seen near the top of the image and is attached to the head-holder. This defines the location of the head with respect to the cameras (not shown). The magnetic system, which was used in parallel, uses a magnetic field as a reference. The magnet generating this field can be seen attached to the head holder in the lower right-hand corner of the surgical space photo.

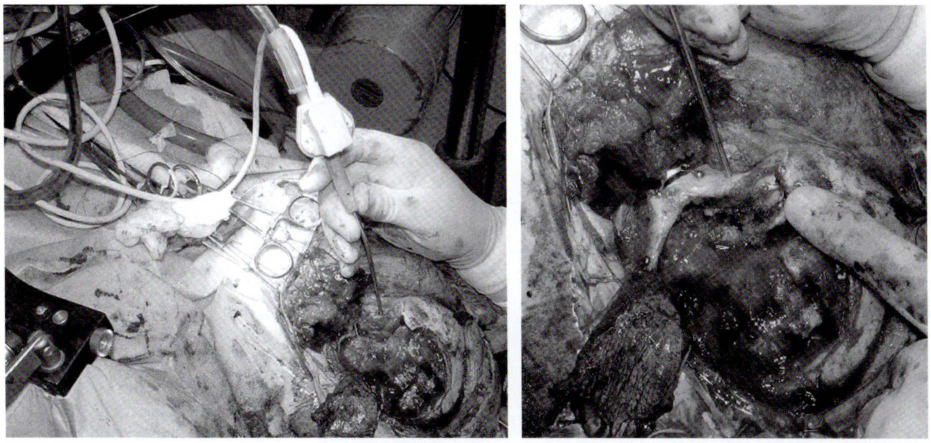

FIGURE 32.2. Image-guided orbitofrontozygomatic craniotomy. The sterile reference arc for the optical system can be seen on the left. The suction is attached to a receiver for the magnetic system. In this situation, the tip of the suction is shown as crosshairs on a multiplanar computer display. The probe for the optical system (not shown) has infrared light-emitting diodes. *Left*: The suction tip is on periorbital tissues after removal of the lateral orbital rim and zygoma. *Right*: Reconstruction of the orbital rim and zygoma with microplates (Stryker-Leibinger, Freiburg, Germany).

On the other hand, some of the more sophisticated offshoots of image guidance can be quite invaluable. All current image guidance systems are capable of "fusing" or "correlating" a second data set with complementary information. It is thus possible to "fuse" a volumetric CT study with a contrast-enhanced MRI, which permits optimal visualization of bone erosion on CT and soft tissue tumor invasion on MRI. With intraoperative guidance, it is then possible to locate these specific areas at surgery, even if tumor infiltration is not clearly seen under the surgical microscope.

IMAGE FUSION FOR ORBITAL TUMORS

CT/MRI SPGR (T1-Type Weighting)

We have found a number of image fusion strategies to be particularly useful in skull-base surgery including that of orbital tumors with extraorbital invasion. The most common fusion we employed was that described earlier: merged CT and MRI with contrast. Figure 32.3 illustrates surgical image guidance using CT/MRI fusion. The patient had a middle fossa meningioma invading the orbit on the left. The skull renderings show a previous craniotomy site in which the tumor had been subtotally excised. Tumor is best seen on MRI, yet bone erosion is well visualized only on CT.

CT/MRI FLAIR, MRI SPGR/MRI FLAIR

Fluid-attenuated inversion recovery (FLAIR) MR imaging, introduced by Hajnal et al. in 1992, is an imaging sequence based on the suppression or reduction of the water signal with the use of an inversion recovery pulse sequence employing a long T1 (inversion time).[16] This sequence has the potential to highlight pathologic changes including tumor infiltration with great sensitivity. We have fused FLAIR sequences, acquired in 3 mm slices (no gaps) with either T1-type MRI (SPGR: radiofrequency-**sp**oiled **gr**adient-**R**ecalled) or CT volumetric studies and have used the FLAIR-bright imaging to determine tumor margins or presence of tumor infiltration of soft tissues.[17] A good illustration of the benefits of importing FLAIR images can be seen in Figures 32.4 and 32.5. The patient was a 14-year-old black female with a large optic nerve glioma of the right orbit that had been followed in clinic over many years. The optic nerve glioma was diagnosed at the age of 3 and was treated with exter-

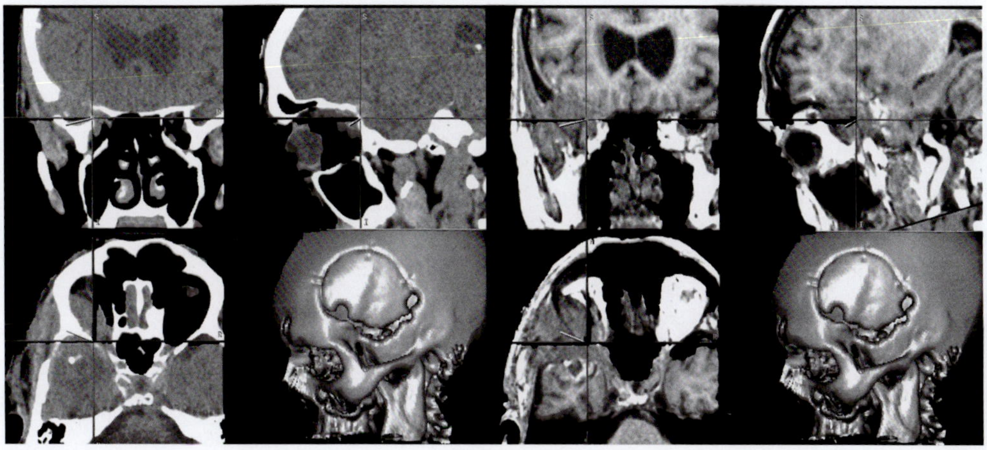

FIGURE 32.3. Image fusion between CT and MRI (here performed by "ImMerge"™ StealthStation). The crosshairs show the same point localized on CT and MRI.

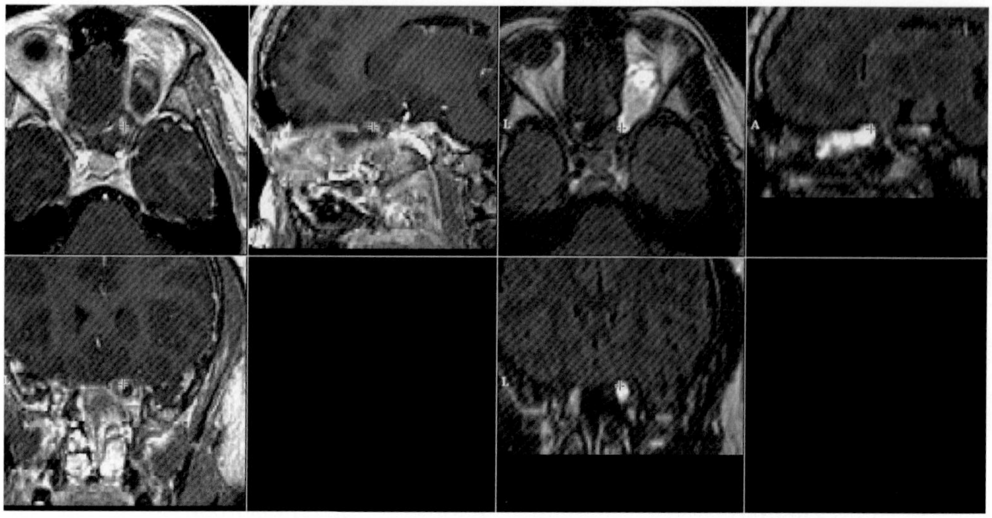

FIGURE 32.4. The posterior limits of this optic nerve glioma are best seen on MRI FLAIR sequences (the three images on the right) and are less well defined on the MRI SPGR with contrast (on the left). This image fusion between two data sets was accomplished using Image Correlation (Cygnus-PFS).

nal beam radiation therapy at the age of 6. Subsequently, the tumor continued to grow within the orbit and extended into the chiasm. Hertel exophthalmometry of the right eye revealed a 2 mm proptosis with a 2+ afferent pupillary defect (APD). Extraocular motility was full, and visual acuity in the right eye was sufficient for the patient to count fingers at 1 foot and 20/20 in the left eye. The right optic disk was pale with total atrophy. The left optic disk was within normal limits. The MRI study with oblique images revealed that the tumor extended into the nerve posteriorly, approaching the chiasm, with increased tumor size in comparison to an MRI performed approximately a year earlier. At this point, the Goldmann visual field of the left eye was performed and found to be normal, and it was decided that the tumor should be excised surgically because of the possibility of extension into the chiasm and the increased risk of visual loss in the good eye.

The patient underwent a craniotomy and superior orbitotomy through the roof of the orbit, and the optic nerve glioma was excised. Both anterior and posterior margins of the tumor were confirmed with image guidance. The anterior margin of the tumor was easy to resect. Posteriorly, however, the tumor was extensively adherent to the surrounding tissues within the optic canal that had to be dissected and cauterized following the unroofing of the canal. The image-guided system was particularly useful to determine the posterior extent of the tumor into the chiasm, especially on FLAIR sequences (Figures 32.4 and 32.5). By importing images from the MRI FLAIR sequence into the image guidance systems and fusing these with the MR SPGR sequence (Figure 32.4), or with volumetric CT (Figure 32.5), it was possible to determine the posterior margin of the tumor and to section the nerve just beyond the tumor without undue endangerment of the chiasm. Histopathologic examination of the tumor specimen confirmed tumor-free anterior and posterior resection margins.

Both CT/SPGR and SPGR/ FLAIR fusion were employed in a 43-year-old man presenting with a recurrent benign mixed lacrimal gland tumor. The initial diagnosis of the tumor was made at the age of 14 when the patient was undergoing a ptosis procedure. The lesion was partially excised and histopathologically di-

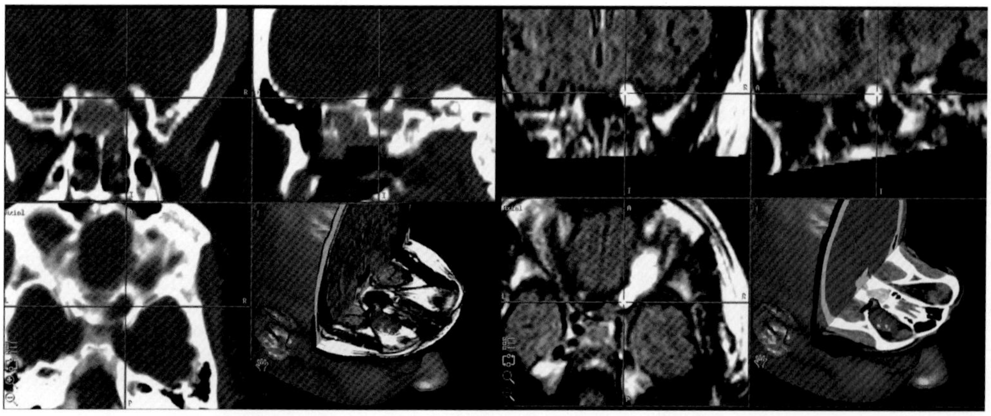

FIGURE 32.5. A CT/MRI FLAIR fusion in the patient whose images are shown in Figure 32.3 ("ImMerge" StealthStation).

agnosed to be a pleomorphic adenoma (benign mixed tumor). The patient subsequently underwent three other surgical procedures for tumor recurrence. At the last recurrence, a superior medial mass was identified; the lesion was firm with an irregular surface and extended into the superior orbit. The patient's best corrected visual acuities were 20/20 and 20/40 − 2 for the right and left eye, respectively. The left superior eyelid had mechanical ptosis, and the extraocular motility was severely limited at all gazes. Pupils were equal, round, and equally reactive to light; color vision testing was within normal limits. On the CT and MRI examinations, a large superior orbital mass was identified extending into the roof of the orbit and the frontal sinus (Figure 32.6). CT showed irregular bony invasion, and on MRI the mass revealed increased intensity in T2-weighted images and presented a rather homogeneous appearance.

On several cuts of the coronal CT scans, the tumor was seen to involve the bone with questionable extension into the cranial cavity.

At surgery, the tumor was very difficult to distinguish owing to an abundance of scar tissue from the prior operations. Image guidance was particularly useful in this context for indicating areas of contrast enhancement or FLAIR hyperintensity that correlated well with the presence of the tumor within the scar tissue.

On histopathologic examination, the tumor was diagnosed as a recurrent pleomorphic adenoma with focal intraepithelial carcinoma; no invasive malignancy was seen. Two years after surgery, no recurrent disease was present.

EXTENDED CRANIOTOMY APPROACHES AND THE ORBIT

Of extended craniotomy approaches in neurosurgery, the one that most obviously applies to orbital tumors is the orbitofrontozygomatic craniotomy. This skull-base approach does add time to surgery but adds very little in terms of morbidity. This technique has become more routine in the neurosurgical repertoire over recent years.[18–20] It consists of an extension of a frontotemporal craniotomy by removing the zygomatic arch along with the roof of the orbit. This is accomplished by performing osteotomies from the inferior orbital fissure through the orbitozygomatic process anteriorly, transecting the root of the zygoma posteriorly, and cutting and mobilizing the orbital rim along with the orbital roof. This craniotomy can be performed in one piece or in two pieces, as illustrated in Figure 32.7.

This approach not only provides wide exposure to the contents of the orbit but also provides extraordinary exposure to the lateral orbital and periorbital structures by the complete mobilization of the temporalis muscle (Figure 32.8). The approach is illustrated by the case of a 75-year-old man with a residual left middle fossa atypical meningioma invading the orbit (Figure 32.3). Surgery had been performed 3 months earlier by a neurosurgeon at another institution. Initial surgery had not been radical and had not extended to the orbit. At the time of our initial assessment, the patient's vision was 20/30 and 20/60 in the right and left eye, respectively. A firm, irregular

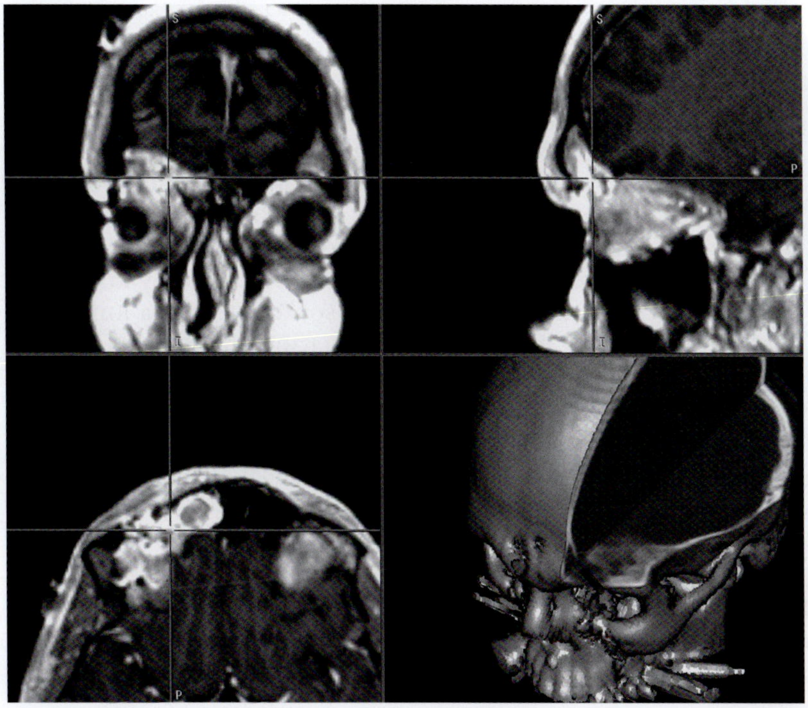

FIGURE 32.6. Frontal sinus invasion in a pleomorphic adenoma of the lacrimal gland represented by means of fusion of CT/MRI SPGR and MRI/FLAIR. Tumor-infiltrated tissues were indistinguishable from scar tissue at surgery. A high correlation between suspected tumor infiltration on image guidance and serial biopsies was found.

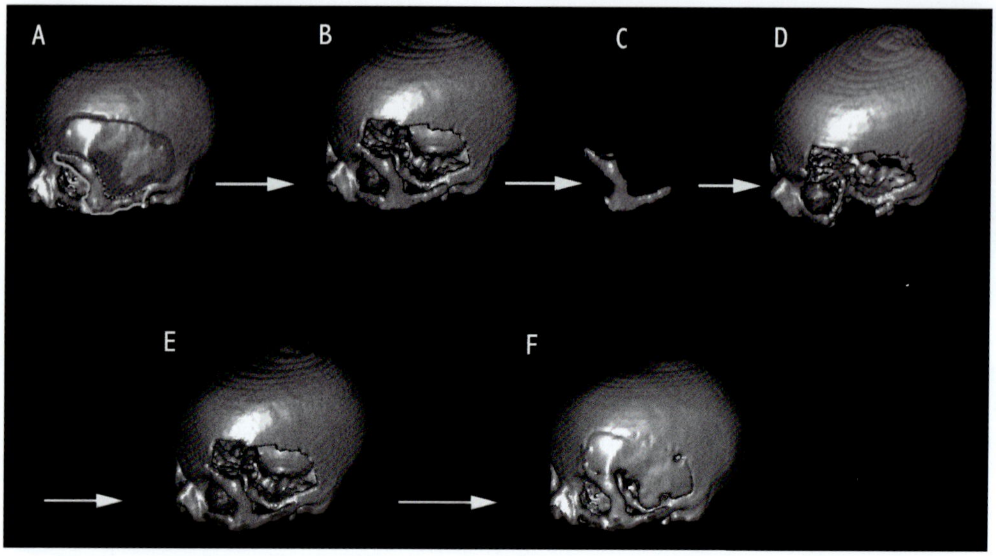

FIGURE 32.7. Left orbitofrontozygomatic craniotomy and subsequent closure. The orbitozygomatic osteotomy is shown as a separate procedure. The bone can also be removed in one piece.

mass was palpable in the left superior lateral orbit, causing a 3 mm proptosis and restriction of horizontal and vertical eye movements. The patient complained of diplopia at all gazes except the primary gaze. The left upper eyelid had ptosis. The left pupil revealed a 2+ APD, but no disk edema or atrophy was detected. Goldmann perimetry revealed a large blind spot and arcuate field defect superiorly in the left eye. The ocular and systemic examinations were otherwise unremarkable.

The patient underwent an orbitofrontozygomatic craniotomy and superiolateral orbitotomy under the computer-assisted image guidance (Figure 32.2). The orbitofrontozygomatic osteotomy was mobilized, and the lateral roof of the orbit and the zygomatic process were removed in one piece. The area just under the lacrimal "keyhole" was suspect for tumor infiltration. The extent of tumor into this area was identified with the help of image guidance. Meningioma was identified in the dura of the middle fossa, the skull base, lateral orbital wall, and extending into the lateral periorbita. Tumor margins of the orbital wall and periorbita were also monitored by image guidance and were confirmed by frozen sections during resection. Although the periorbita was involved, the orbital soft tissues were free of tumor. Ten months after surgery, the patient's visual acuity in the left eye was 20/25 + 1 and he was free of diplopia at all gazes with 1 mm proptosis.

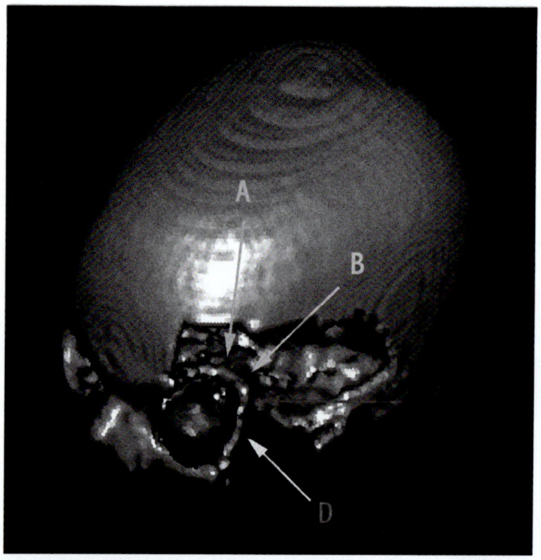

FIGURE 32.8. Exposure of orbital structures by an orbitofrontozygomatic craniotomy.

RADIOSURGERY

Stereotactic delivery of single fraction radiation has been available for many years and has on some occasions been employed in orbital tumors, or more commonly, in tumors extending into extraorbital areas such as the cavernous sinus. Radiosurgery requires the precise targeting of a tumor by many convergent linear radiation sources (gamma knife) or a single moving linear radiation source (LINAC: linear accelerator).[21–23] At present, most of these systems still require the application of a rigid stereotactic frame, but more systems could develop "frameless" options in the near future. The major limitation in using this form of tumor treatment in or near the orbit is the known sensitivity of the visual pathways to radiation damage. Although we have radiosurgery systems at our disposal, we have little personal experience with radiosurgery of orbital tumors.

BIOPSIES AND MINIMALLY INVASIVE APPROACHES

There are many advantages of image-guided surgery in the orbit. It can be particularly useful during minimally invasive approaches to pathologically altered orbital anatomy, especially deep in the orbit (i.e., small lesions in the posterior orbit). Even with larger, direct exposure, distorted anatomy from tumors, congenital anomalies and trauma can be confusing. We have already illustrated that image-guidance is also helpful in defining the extent of tumor infiltration in order to obtain tumor-free margins in combination with serial biopsies and pathological analysis. A further advantage of the technology in tumor surgery is the superimposition of CT and MRI images during the operation, since MRI offers greater soft tissue detail, but CT has better bone delineation. One of the potential uses of frameless stereotaxis for the orbital surgeon is to obtain biopsy material from the depth of the orbit without major surgery. Probes can easily reach the orbital apex and be guided to any lesion with accuracy. With a filter-type catching device at the end of a stereotactic suction, sufficient histological/cytological can be obtained. With the availability of Cytospin and/or frozen section capability, the material can be evaluated in 15 to 20 minutes during surgery. This technique can save a considerable amount of time over orbitotomy and is far less invasive. This is particularly useful in posteriorly located small lesions. Although Cygnus has a biopsy kit, we are developing one intended to better preserve orbital biopsy material. Image-guidance has also been reported as an adjunct to posterior orbital foreign body removal.[14]

CONCLUSIONS

We have presented some of the advantages of computer image guidance in the orbit and its surrounding structures. As with any technology, it is important to be familiar with the basic principles and limitations involved. We have also discussed both extended and minimally invasive approaches to tumors of the orbit.

References

1. Gildenberg PL, Tasker RR, eds. *Textbook of Stereotactic and Functional Neurosurgery*. New York: McGraw-Hill; 1998.
2. Germano, IM, eds. *Advanced Techniques in Image-Guided Brain and Spine Surgery*. Stuttgart: G Thieme; 2002.
3. Thompson TP, Lunsford LD, Flickinger JC. Radiosurgery for hemangiomas of the cavernous sinus and orbit: technical case report. *Neurosurgery* 2000;47:778–783.
4. Kelly PJ, Goerss SJ, Kall BA. Evolution of contemporary instrumentation for computer assisted stereotactic surgery. *Surg Neurol* 1988;30:204–215.
5. Roberts DW, Strohbein JW, Hatch JF, et al. A frameless stereotactic integration of computerized tomographic imaging and the operating microscope. *J Neurosurg* 1986;65:545–549.
6. Reinhardt H, Meyer H, Amrein E. A computer-assisted device for the intraoperative CT-correlated localization of brain tumors. *Eur Surg Res* 1988;20:51–58.
7. Watanabe E, Watanabe T, Manaka S, et al. Three-dimensional digitizer (neuronavigator): new equipment for CT-guided stereotactic surgery. *Surg Neurol* 1987;27:543–547.
8. Bucholz RD, Smith KR. A comparison of sonic digitizers versus light emitting diode-based localization. In: Maciunas RJ, ed. *Interactive Image-Guided Neurosurgery*. Park Ridge, IL: American Association of Neurological Surgeons; 1993: 715–720.
9. Gumprecht HK, Widenka DC, Lumenta CB. BrainLab Vector Vision Neuronavigation system: technology and clinical experience in 131 cases. *Neurosurgery* 1999;44:97–105.
10. Kato A, Yoshimine T, Hayakawa T, et al. A frameless, armless navigational system for computer assisted tomography. *J Neurosurg* 1991;74:845–849.
11. Mascott CR. The Compass Cygnus-PFS image-guided system. *Neurosurgery* 2000;46:235–238.
12. Mascott CR. The magnetic system. In: Germano IM, ed. *Advanced Techniques in Image-Guided Brain and Spine Surgery*. Stuttgart: G Thieme; 2002.
13. Maurer CR, Fitzpatrick JM, Wang MY. Registration of head volume images using implantable fiducial markers. *Trans Med Imaging* 1997;16:447–462.
14. Klapan I, Barbir A, Simicic R, et al. Dynamic 3D computer-assisted reconstruction of a metallic retrobulbar foreign body for diagnostic and surgical purposes. *Orbit* 2001;20:35–49.
15. Srivastava SK, Reichman OS, Lambert SR. The use of an image guidance system in retrieving lost medial rectus muscles. *JAAPOS* 2002;6:309–314.
16. Hajnal JV, De Coene B, Lewis PD, et al. High signal regions in normal white matter shown by heavily T2-weighted CSF nulled IR sequences. *J Comput Assist Tomogr* 1992;16: 506–513.
17. Mascott CR, Summers L. Image-fusion of fluid-attenuated inversion recovery (FLAIR) MRI sequences for surgical image-guidance. *Neurosurgery*. In press.
18. Tew JM, van Loveren HR. *Atlas of Operative Microsurgery*. Vol 1. *Aneurysms and Arteriovenous Malformations*. Philadelphia: WB Saunders; 1994:16–23.
19. Sindou M, Emery E, Acevedo G, Ben-David U. Respective indications for orbital rim, zygomatic arch and orbito-zygomatic osteotomies in the surgical approach to central skull base lesions. Critical, retrospective review in 146 cases. *Acta Neurochir (Wien)* 2001;143:967–975.
20. Akiyama H, Kondoh T, Suzuki H, et al. Usefulness of fronto-orbito-zygomatic approach for intraorbital tumors: report of 31 cases [in Japanese]. *No Shinkei Geka* 1997;25:913–917.
21. Mueller AJ, Talies S, Schaller UC, et al. Stereotactic radiosurgery of large uveal melanomas with the gamma-knife. *Ophthalmology* 2000;107:1381–1387; discussion 1387–1388.
22. Bellmann C, Fuss M, Holz FG, et al. Stereotactic radiation therapy for malignant choroidal tumors: preliminary, short-term results. *Ophthalmology* 2000;107:358–365.
23. Ertl A, Zehetmayer M, Schoggl A, et al. Dosimetry studies with TLDs for stereotactic radiation techniques for intraocular tumours. *Phys Med Biol* 1997;42:2137–2145.

33

Radiation Treatment

Paul T. Finger

The anatomy of the orbit provides unique challenges for radiation therapy. By definition, orbital tumors occur in the space between the eyeball and bony orbital walls. While the bones, muscle, and fat within the orbit can tolerate a relatively high radiation dose, components of the eye and lacrimal system are more radiation sensitive. Side effects such as dry eye, eyelash loss, cataract, neovascular glaucoma, radiation retinopathy, and optic neuropathy are all potential complications of orbital radiation therapy.[1–3, 4–9] Therefore, though tumor control is the primary goal, when possible treatment plans are shaped to avoid the retina, lacrimal system, and natural lens. Radiation therapy continues to play an integral role in the treatment of both malignant and benign orbital tumors.

TECHNIQUES

External beam radiation therapy (EBRT) is currently delivered utilizing photons (γ-rays or x-rays), or particles (e.g., protons and neutrons) with linear accelerators doing the bulk of the work.[10–21] The linear accelerator creates energetic photons by using high-frequency electromagnetic waves to accelerate electrons through a microwave accelerator structure. The high-energy electron beam can be used either by itself to treat superficial tumors or to strike a high-Z target to produce a bremsstrahlung x-ray beam (for treating deep-seated tumors).[21–24]

Charged particles (e.g., protons) have also been used in the treatment of orbital tumors.[12,25,26] The absorption characteristics of charged particles allow radiation treatment with dose distributions that are highly conformal with target-volume shapes. It is important to note that protons travel relatively straight paths through tissue, slowing as a result of contacts with surrounding electrons and owing to occasional nuclear interactions. There is a fairly constant dose over the entry "plateau" followed by a sharp Bragg peak in dose at the end of the particles' path. Dose at the peak is typically four times that at the plateau in laboratory situations. In clinical practice, techniques that spread out each Bragg peak to cover a tumor target volume reduce the plateau-to-peak ratio (increase the entry dose).[3,22,23]

Neutron beam radiation therapy is being investigated in the treatment of orbital tumors refractory to current radiation modalities.[13,27] Modern neutron therapy machines produce neutron beams with depth–dose characteristics equivalent to 6 MV x-rays.[11] Fission neutrons, although suitable for neutron capture therapy, cannot be used for teletherapy because of their low energy and poor penetration. Therefore, the proton Berylium (pBe) reaction is the most commonly used in modern isocentric neutron therapy machines.[22,23]

ORBITAL DISEASES

Vascular Tumors

Infantile hemangiomas can occur in the eyelids and orbit (Figure 33.1). When they occur in the eyelids, they can cover the visual axis, deviate the eye, and induce amblyopia. When posterior to the eye, these tumors can also produce proptosis, corneal exposure, and optic nerve compression. Though capillary hemangiomas are radiation sensitive (5–7.5 Gy in two to three fractions), those not causing optic nerve compression, amblyopia, or strabismus can be watched over 3 to 4 years for spontaneous regression or treated with intralesional steroids.[28–32] Because of concerns about secondary carcinogenesis and long-term effects of irradiation, we consider radiotherapy for infantile hemangiomas only when other treatments have failed.[31,32]

In contrast, radiation therapy for Kaposi sarcoma is very effective.[33] Here radiation is typically given to older patients for localized disease (vs systemic chemotherapy for systemic manifestations). Typically, electron beam radiation is used to limit penetration.[33]

Lymphoid Tumors

Lymphoid tumors can present in the orbit, eyelids, and conjunctiva (see Chapter 13). They can be divided into atypical lymphoid hyperplasia (pseudolymphoma), and lymphomas (Figure 33.2). Observation, resection, steroid therapy, antibiotics, and radiation therapy have been employed for local control. Each lesion is treated differently, but all have been noted to be relatively

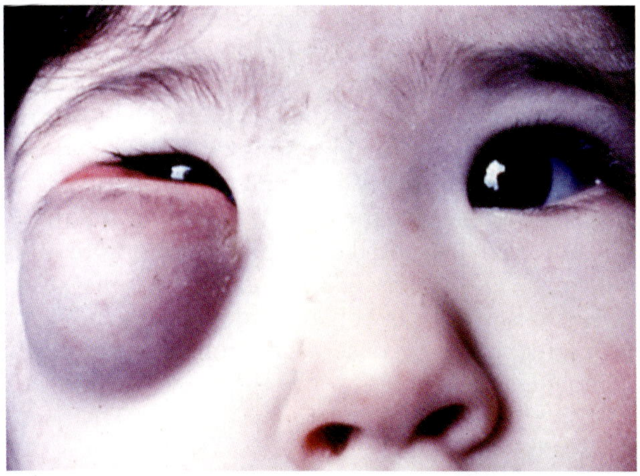

FIGURE 33.1. Orbital hemangioma of childhood involving the eyelids and orbit. (Courtesy of Dr. Barrett Haik, Memphis, Tennessee.)

radiation sensitive. In general, the more benign-appearing tumors tend to respond less dramatically than malignant lesions.[10,15,34,35]

Radiation therapy has been reported to consist of a single exposure of 8 Gy through an anterior portal, to a more typical 20 to 25 Gy (in 10 to 14 daily fractions) for MALTomas and benign lymphoid hyperplasia. Malignant lymphomas have been treated to as much as 35 to 45 Gy (in 18–24 fractions). Bolek et al. reported a 95% local control rate (at a median 25 Gy external beam radiation therapy).[10,36]

Thyroid-Related Ophthalmopathy

Thyroid-related "Graves" ophthalmopathy can occur in hyperthyroid, euthyroid, and hypothyroid patients. Indications for radiation include progressive exophthalmos, corneal exposure, and optic nerve compression (typically with vasculopathy). In practice, steroid therapy is typically a first-line treatment followed by radiation or surgery as needed. Radiation is typically applied via a single lateral portal to a dose of 20 Gy in 10 to 12 fractions.[16,37] Electrons (12–15 MeV) may be preferred in that they minimize treatment of the fellow eye and orbit, although the dose to the involved orbit is less homogeneous. Sandler and associates reported that 71% of patients receiving doses in this range required no further steroid treatment or surgical decompression.[38] The main prognostic factor for failure was radiation at less than 6 months from the time of onset of ophthalmopathy. There is now controversy about the efficacy of radiation for thyroid-related orbitopathy.[39,40]

Conjunctival, Eyelid, and Sinus Tumors

Eyelid, adnexal, and sinus tumors can invade the orbit, making local resection difficult or impossible.[41–45] In these cases, adjuvant radiation therapy can be used to treat the nonresectable margins.[41,45] Radiation is typically done with photon-based external beam therapy. Adjuvant chemoreduction of orbital tumors prior to radiation has also been tried.[41,46] The doses required for treatment of basal cell, squamous cell, and malignant melanoma typically exceeds the tolerance of the eye and lacrimal system (45–60 Gy).[47–49] Therefore, techniques utilizing protective eye shields, intensity-modulated radiation therapy, and brachytherapy boosts have been employed.[48] External beam radiation is also used for presumed residual microscopic disease (after resection of the primary tumor).

Sebaceous Carcinoma of the Meibomian Gland

Though it occurs in less than 5% of eyelid tumors, sebaceous carcinoma has been reported to carry a significant mortality rate. This is thought to result from its tendency toward pagetoid spread and multifocality. Radiation therapy has been used in treatment of selected cases when surgery has failed or when negative surgical margins are not obtainable.[50] Sebaceous carcinoma is a relatively radiation resistant tumor, and doses in excess of 60 to 65 Gy (in 2 Gy daily fractions) are required. Pardo et al. reported a large series of patients treated for nonresectable orbital sebaceous carcinoma or for palliation.[51,52]

Meningiomas

Orbital meningiomas may arise from the intracranial cavity, optic nerve, paranasal sinuses, or (rarely) the orbital soft tissues.[53,54] These slow-growing tumors tend to present by compression or displacement of orbital tissues. Intracranial meningiomas are most likely to cause bilateral vision loss, while optic nerve sheath

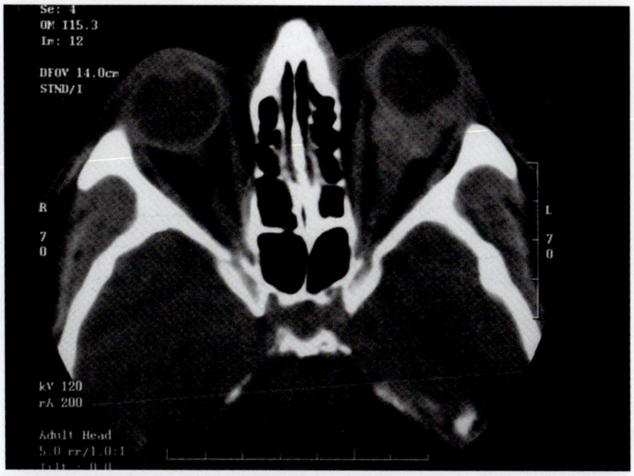

FIGURE 33.2. This case of biopsy proven bilateral orbital lymphoma was treated with external beam radiation therapy (40 Gy) to both orbits. Axial CT image demonstrates bilateral soft tissue densities centered posterior to each globe.

meningiomas more typically present early with compressive optic neuropathy. Most intracranial meningiomas that affect the orbit arise from the dura of the sphenoid bone.[54]

Total surgical excision is recommended after progression has been documented.[55] Radiation therapy is typically employed when surgical margins are not possible, when the tumor is recurrent, or when the remaining sighted eye is affected (vision has been lost in the fellow eye).[54,56–61] When radiation is used as an adjuvant to resection, postoperative doses of 50 to 54 Gy over 5 to 6 weeks are typical. Conformal fields are used to avoid normal brain tissue. As primary treatment, doses of 60 Gy in 33 fractions can be employed.[62] At these levels, the long-term prognosis for vision is poor.

Orbital Metastasis

The incidence of orbital metastasis is difficult to quantify. Typically the goals of treatment for orbital metastasis are palliative (to improve the patient's quality of life by salvaging vision and the cosmetic use of the globe). We treat to avoid the development of a blind and painful eye that may require enucleation or exenteration. Treatment options include observation, systemic drug therapy, EBRT, brachytherapy, exenteration, and stereotactic radiosurgery.

For decades, EBRT has been employed in the treatment of orbital tumors.[63–66] Typically palliative, techniques vary depending on the proximity of radiation-sensitive structures to the orbital tumor (Figure 33.3). Normal tissue tolerance and a patient's long-term prognosis will often guide the selection of technique, dose, and dose rate.

Patients with orbital metastasis may have a slightly prolonged median survival. Therefore, it is reasonable to select from among such lens-sparing techniques as right-angled wedged fields, direct lateral field posterior to the lens (where the anterior margin is positioned at the temporal canthus, posterior to the lens), oblique lateral field with lens shielding, and anterior field with lens block. Rectangular field sizes typically range from 3 to 5 cm. Typical energies range from 4 to 16 MeV for electrons or 4 to 15 MeV for photons. Higher energy photons are used to generate greater depth within the orbit, sinuses, or brain.

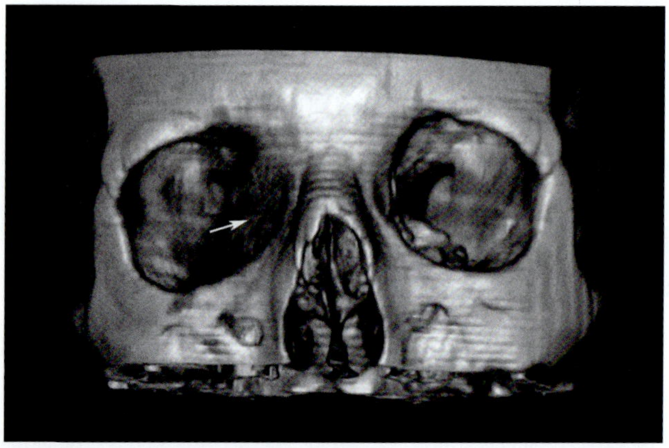

FIGURE 33.3. A three-dimensional reconstruction of a computed radiographic tomogram reveals the position of a metastatic adenocarcinoma in the medial portion of the right orbit (arrow).

Commonly accepted doses range from 30 to 40 Gy (typically delivered in 2–3 Gy daily fractions) over 2 to 4 weeks. There is considerable controversy about the correct dose. A dose escalation study would be invaluable.

Optic Glioma

Optic nerve glioma typically affects children under 15 years of age and occurs as only 1% of all central nervous system tumors. There may be a genetic component with a higher incidence in patients with neurofibromatosis and in females. Optic nerve gliomas grow slowly, are initially asymptomatic, and involve the optic chiasm in 50% of cases.[67] When symptoms occur, they include exophthalmos, visual field defects, nystagmus, optic atrophy, and intracranial signs (with hypothalamic involvement).[68]

Treatment should include complete surgical excision (when possible); positive margins are treated aggressively.[26] Radiation is used when intracranial or progressive symptoms are evident. Multiport beam arrangements are typically used to minimize the entry dose and concentrate the radiation within the targeted zone.[12,69] Orbital tumors are typically treated with a wedged-pair external (photon beam) technique. Doses of 45 to 50 Gy (in daily fractions of 1.8–2.0 Gy) are typically employed.[26,70] To avoid the side effects of radiation in young children, chemotherapy is considered to be an alternative.[68]

Numerous reports document the value of radiation for patients with optic glioma. Long-term survival rates have been reported to be as high as 80 to 100%. Khafaga et al. reported on 50 children with optic glioma.[71] Sixteen were treated with primary radiation therapy to a median dose of 50 Gy. The overall 10-year, relapse-free survival was as high as 87.5% at 5 years and 75% at 10 years. Overall, patients with tumors affecting the anterior visual pathway fared better than those with posterior tumors.[71]

Rhabdomyosarcoma

Rhabdomyosarcoma is the most common primary malignancy of the orbit in children. Parents might first notice ptosis followed by rapid progressive proptosis. Most tumors are located in the superonasal orbit, with imaging showing a tumor adjacent or attached to one of the ocular muscles. When the tumor has metastasized to the brain or lung, prognosis is poor. But for

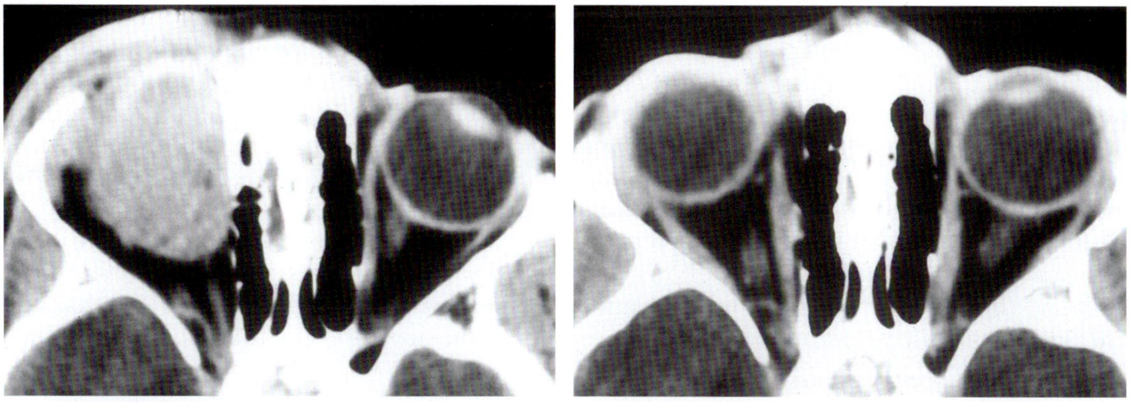

A B

FIGURE 33.4. (A) Computed radiographic tomogram of orbital rhabdomyosarcoma. (B) After treatment with a combination of chemotherapy and external beam irradiation, the tumor demonstrated complete regression and long-term local control. (Courtesy of Dr. Aaron Rausen of New York City.)

lesions localized to the orbit, a combination of biopsy, chemotherapy, and irradiation currently offers a 90% survival rate (Figure 33.4).[72,73]

Sagerman et al. and Schulla et al. have suggested that a minimum tumor dose should be 45 to 50 Gy over 5 to 7 weeks.[17,18] Lens blocks are typically placed to protect the anterior segment (when possible). Though survival has been excellent, doses in this range typically develop late radiation side effects.[5]

Lacrimal Gland Tumors

The high mortality associated with lacrimal gland tumors is associated with the difficulty of obtaining negative surgical margins and the tendency of certain tumors (e.g., adenoid cystic carcinoma of the lacrimal gland) to invade surrounding tissues.[74]

Adenoid cystic carcinoma is considered to be radiation resistant. Most believe that the orbit should be irradiated only after resection, to reduce the incidence of postoperative recurrences.[25,43,75–77] If the tumor is removed within a well-defined capsule, recurrence is uncommon and postoperative radiation may be deferred. Many such tumors have been subjected to biopsy or extend outside the capsule prior to surgery. In these cases, orbital exenteration with secondary EBRT is employed.

Recent investigations of brachytherapy boosts to the tumor bed together with complete irradiation of the orbit has allowed for organ (eye) preservation. Others advocate neutron radiation therapy for adenoid cystic carcinoma of the lacrimal gland (Figure 33.5). Other orbital tumors of the lacrimal fossa include benign mixed tumor, adenocarcinoma, sarcoidosis of the lacrimal gland, and inflammatory diseases.

Orbital Pseudotumor

Inflammatory tumors of the orbit can mimic neoplasia and are termed "orbital pseudotumor." Typically,

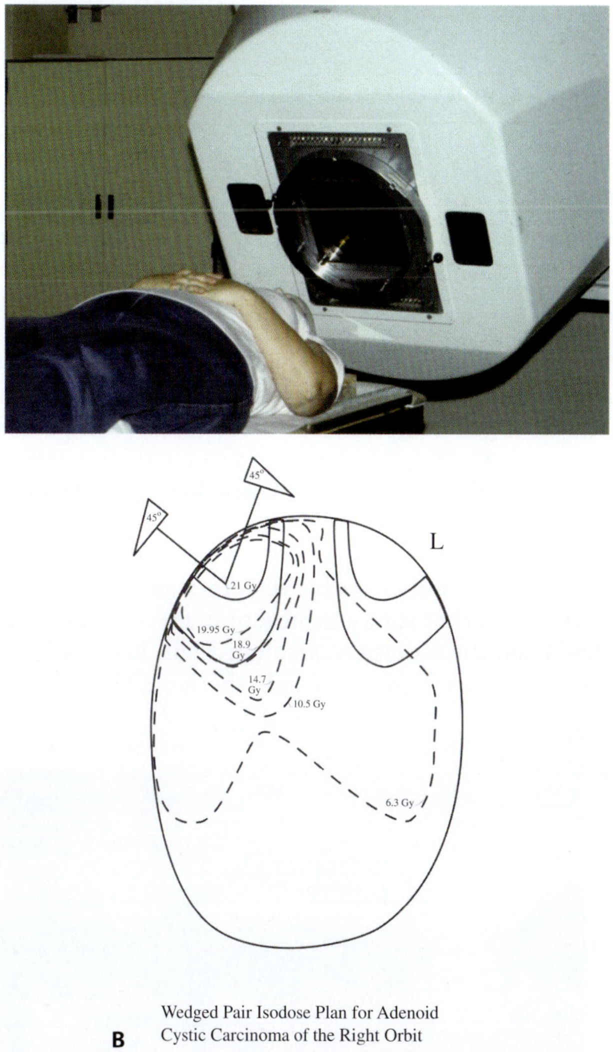

A B

FIGURE 33.5. (A) A patient with adenoid cystic carcinoma of the lacrimal gland being treated at the University of Washington Fast Neutron Radiotherapy facility. (Courtesy of Dr. George E. Laramore, Seattle.) The isocentric gantry and multileaf collimator make it possible to use angled, shaped fields that spare the optic chiasm and contralateral eye. (B) An isodose curve for a 66 MeV fast neutron beam in treatment of an adenoid cystic carcinoma of the lacrimal gland. (Courtesy of Fermilab Visual Media Services and Dr. Arlene Lennox.)

biopsy samples are removed from these orbits to establish the diagnosis. Blood tests and radiographic images are obtained to rule out known infectious, inflammatory, and neoplastic tumors.[78,79]

Most patients found to have idiopathic orbital pseudotumor are treated with systemic steroids or immunosuppressive or cytotoxic-immunosuppressive agents.[46] Radiation is also employed to suppress the immune reaction and secondary fibrosis.[80–85] The author has found the subset of fibrosing pseudotumors to be less radiation sensitive (Figure 33.6). They occasionally require exenteration surgery to prevent extension into the cavernous sinus.

INTRAOCULAR TUMORS THAT REQUIRE ORBITAL RADIATION THERAPY

Uveal Metastasis

The most common intraocular cancer, uveal metastasis, can be treated with EBRT.[86] Although these metastases are mostly derived from breast cancer in women and from lung cancer in men, other common primary sites include the colon, kidney, prostate, and thyroid.[87,88] Most intraocular metastases are asymptomatic, go undiagnosed, and are left untreated.

In clinical practice, most patients are examined when they develop involvement of the macular retina and/or visual symptoms. In these cases, prompt treatment with EBRT (25–40 Gy in 2–3 Gy daily fractions) typically offers the best chance for preservation of vision.[89,90]

It is important to have the ophthalmic oncologist determine whether both eyes are affected and to ascertain whether tumor is present in the anterior chamber. Then the radiation oncologist will know whether to treat one or both eyes and whether a shield can be placed to spare the lens. Uveal metastases should not be treated until the primary or cell type is known. In some cases, the intraocular tumor may be the only source of tissue to indicate the source of cancer. In practice, most patients with uveal metastasis are found to have multiorgan disease or a history of metastatic cancer.

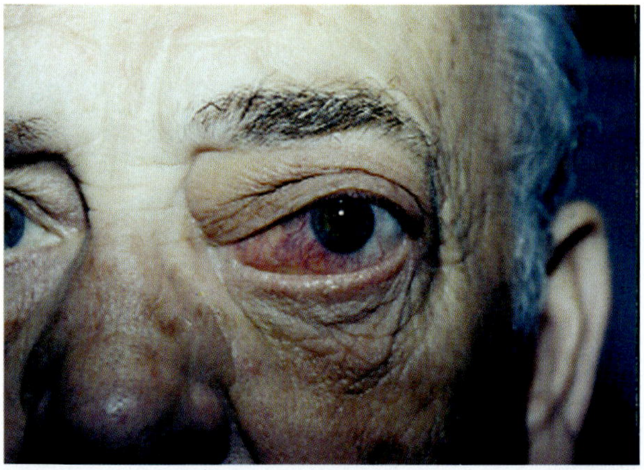

FIGURE 33.6. This patient with fibrosing orbital pseudotumor with secondary proptosis failed to exhibit any response to EBRT (20 Gy) delivered in 11 fractions after a surgical debulking procedure.

Since both breast and lung cancer are radiation sensitive, most patients with uveal metastasis can be treated with relatively low-dose external beam radiation therapy.[89–92] Ophthalmic plaque irradiation or enucleations are occasionally required for radiation resistant tumors (e.g., renal metastasis) and for uncontrollable glaucoma secondary to anterior segment metastasis.[20,87,88,93]

The author has noted that current improvements in survival among patients with uveal metastases have been accompanied by an increase in the incidence of secondary radiation retinopathy and local tumor recurrence. Though rare, both are becoming more common, which suggests divergent needs to lower the dose (or dose volume) to protect against radiation retinopathy and to increase the dose to prevent tumor recurrence.

Extrascleral Extension of Choroidal Melanoma

Gross extrascleral extension of uveal melanoma is rare, but microscopic evidence of intrascleral tumor and invasion of emissary veins has been found in as many as 50% of enucleated specimens.[94] Studies suggest that when there is "gross" or visible evidence of extraocular tumor extension, patients have a worse prognosis for survival.[95] On the other hand, massive extrascleral melanomatous extension with orbital invasion is often treated by exenteration with or without adjuvant radiation therapy.[3,20]

External beam radiotherapy is an alternative to exenteration for patients with extrascleral (orbital) extension of their uveal melanoma. Hykin studied 17 patients enucleated for choroidal melanoma with localized extrascleral extension whose tumor had not visibly extended into orbital tissues.[95] In this study, patients received 50 Gy in 22 fractions within 2 months of enucleation. The actuarial melanoma-related survival rate was 51% at 5 years with one local orbital recurrence.[95] Though this survival rate is comparable to that of patients with large melanomas treated by enucleation alone, orbital tumor margins are often difficult or impossible to obtain, and radiotherapy offers a treatment for residual microscopic melanoma cells. Clearly, most patients would prefer to undergo some form of treatment for their residual melanoma.

I typically offer postenucleation 50 Gy (in 1.8–2 Gy daily fractions) adjuvant external beam radiotherapy for patients noted to have encapsulated or well-defined nodules of extrascleral extension present after enucleation surgery. When there are large areas of extrascleral spread, removal of all pigmented tissue followed by external beam radiotherapy for presumed microscopic orbital melanoma is prescribed (as a reasonable approach to obtaining definable treated-tumor margins). Such an approach offers a method to decrease the rate of recurrence with a result that is more cosmetically acceptable than orbital exenteration.

Retinoblastoma

Despite concerns of secondary carcinogenesis, EBRT continues to play an important role in the treatment of extrascleral and intraneural extension of retinoblastoma (Figure 33.7).[46,96] Residual and recurrent orbital retinoblastoma is a significant risk factor for metastasis and typically is treated by a combination of systemic chemotherapy and external beam irradiation.[46,97]

The most common complication (with the lens-sparing technique) of external beam irradiation for retinoblastoma is radiation retinopathy.[7,98] First described by Stallard (following radon seed application for treatment of retinoblastoma), radiation retinopathy is characterized by retinal capillary microaneurysms, cotton-wool spots, retinal neovascularization, and vitreous hemorrhage.[99] Other radiation complications include ischemic optic neuropathy and neovascular glaucoma.[100] Less common complications include dry eye and eyelash loss.[2,100,101]

In general, with schedules of 2 Gy daily fractions and long-term follow-up, radiation retinopathy has been reported to occur in as many as 10% of eyes dosed to 35 Gy (EBRT), in 66% of eyes treated to 45 Gy, and 100% of eyes given 80 Gy or more.[2,7,98,101–103] On a histopathologic basis, the retinal vessels have been shown to develop hyalinized walls, and the lumen may be partially or completely obliterated. Narrowing of the central retinal and ciliary arteries has also been observed.

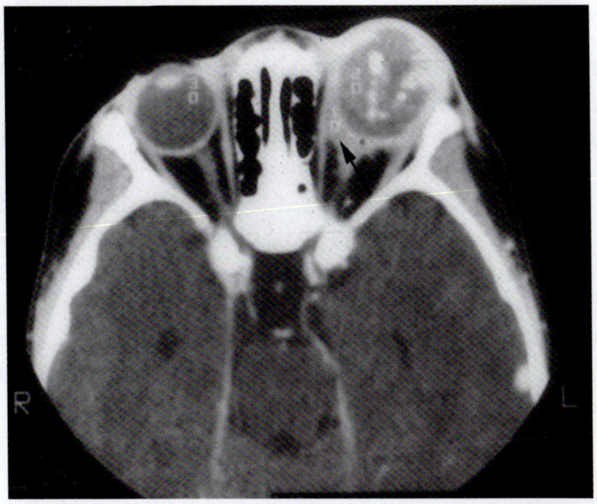

FIGURE 33.7. Extrascleral extension of retinoblastoma (arrow) is a significant risk factor for metastasis and is treated by EBRT to the orbit after enucleation surgery.

Radiation optic neuropathy has been reported after high-dose EBRT and ophthalmic plaque radiation therapy. It is believed to be secondary to radiation vasculopathy.[7,100,103]

Growth retardation of irradiated orbital bones can result in significant facial malformations.[100,104] Modern authors believe that the incidence of bony dysgenesis is less with modern megavoltage radiation techniques (in comparison to the older orthovoltage machines).[6,7,98,106–108] In addition, doses for treatment of retinoblastoma have been reduced to 35 to 45 Gy.

Postlaminar optic nerve and orbital extension of retinoblastoma are known risk factors for metastasis and are typically treated with radiation therapy.[97] In addition, the chemotherapeutic agents cisplatinum, etoposide, vincristine, and cyclophosphamide are often employed.[46,96] Some centers add intrathecal methotrexate or craniospinal irradiation.[46] Pradhan et al. treated 28 eyes with EBRT to the orbit for retinoblastoma extension. Nineteen patients were also given chemotherapy. Local control was maintained in 71% for a mean follow-up of 22.6 months.[103]

Sagerman et al. described a dose–response relationship demonstrating an increased risk of second malignant tumors with increasing radiation dose.[101,109,110] This was confirmed by Alberti et al., who showed a 47.5% incidence at 16 years for second tumors within the radiation field in patients treated to 55 Gy or more versus a 5% incidence in those treated with smaller doses ($p = 0.0006$).[7,101]

SIDE EFFECTS OF ORBITAL RADIATION THERAPY

It was not long after the discovery of the x-ray that Chalupecky published his study on its effect on the eye.[111] The eye was noted to be relatively radiation sensitive by Birch-Hirshfeld and Ammon, who reported the first radiation-induced cataract.[112,113] Sagerman and Alberti have provided a relatively current review of the management of radiation effects on the eye and orbit.[114]

Eyelids

Skin changes associated with radiation therapy include acute erythema, depigmentation, atrophy, telangiectasias, hair loss, and ectropion or entropion of the eyelid.[33,115,116] Radiation typically travels through the skin of the eyelids on its way to treat orbital tumors. Eyelid skin reacts like skin of other sites, but it is thinner and has less integument. The first reaction is erythema (typically 2–4 weeks after starting treatment), followed by dry and moist desquamation (and rarely necrosis). Erythema is usually transient and disappears rapidly. Silver sulfadiazine cream can be helpful to treat the acute reaction and to prevent secondary infection.

Moist desquamation is more common after doses of 50 to 60 Gy (in 1.8–2.2 Gy daily fractions) over 5 to 6 weeks and also more common where superficial lesions break the skin. Healing is typically slow and may take up to 4 weeks. There is usually no resultant radiation-related scar unless high dose rates are used or secondary infection occurs.[114]

Cicatricial scarring can result in entropion or ectropion of the eyelids. Slowly progressive skin changes (which may appear over subsequent years) include thinning of the skin, depigmentation, and telangiectasias.[114]

Eyelash loss may be incomplete or complete depending on the dose and dose rate. It may occur with as little as 10 Gy but can be permanent with as little as 30 Gy. At more than 50 Gy, radiation has been used to produce permanent epilation in patients with trichiasis and secondary corneal disease. The tarsus and meibomian glands appear to tolerate doses in the range of 40 to 50 Gy.[114]

Lacrimal Apparatus and Dry Eye

The lacrimal gland, accessory lacrimal glands, punctum, and lacrimal sac make up the lacrimal apparatus. Radiation damage to the lacrimal glands can produce irreversible dry eye. Published studies indicate that doses in the range of 30 to 40 Gy can be delivered to the entire orbit without long-term keratitis sicca. Evidence of histopathologic atrophy of the lacrimal gland has been reported with single doses of 20 Gy and after 50 to 60 Gy given over a 6-week period.[15] Parsons has reported symptomatic dry eye in 0% of patients treated with less than 30 Gy and in 100% of patients treated with more than 57 Gy (in standard fractions).[114,117]

Cornea, Lens, and Conjunctiva

Though direct corneal injury can result from high-dose irradiation, most acute corneal toxicity results from loss of the tear film with secondary keratitis sicca. Fairly high doses of brachytherapy have been delivered to the cornea with no long-term sequelae.[3,93,118,119]

Cataracts are common complications of radiation therapy (Figure 33.8).[120] Merriam and Focht have shown that as little as 2 Gy in a single fraction or 8 Gy in multiple fractions can induce cataract.[9,121–123] Because cataracts are common in the elderly, studies on children with retinoblastoma are particularly telling. Schipper et al. delivered 45 Gy to the retina in 15 fractions in 5 weeks to 73 eyes of 39 children with retinoblastoma.[7,19,98] Cataracts developed in 18 eyes (where Schipper noted that more than 1 mm of the posterior lens was included in the field). In this study, 8 Gy in 15 fractions was the minimum cataractogenic dose.

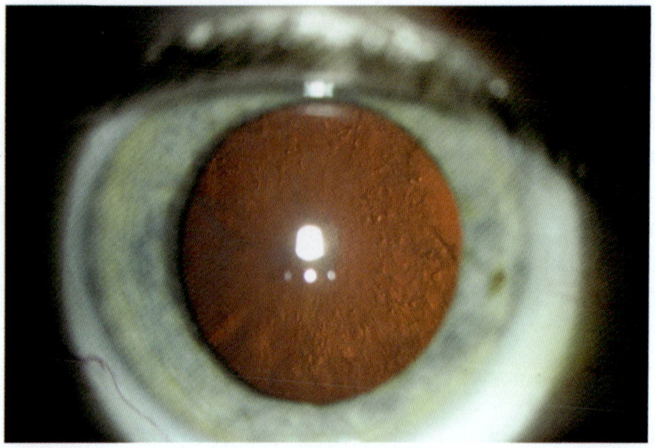

FIGURE 33.8. A posterior subcapsular (PSC) "radiation" cataract. Though PSC cataracts are most commonly associated with radiation, the author has also observed anterior subcapsular and progression of nuclear sclerotic cataracts immediately after irradiation.

Sclera

The sclera is particularly resistant to radiation (like the cornea).[119] No scleral radiation damage has been reported after external beam radiation doses of 60 Gy.[114] In contrast, it has been my experience that the relatively high scleral brachytherapy doses (e.g., >600 Gy) can cause melting of the sclera.[3] In practice, strontium-90 (^{90}Sr) and ruthenium-106 (^{106}Ru) are more likely to deliver much higher scleral doses than iodine-125 (^{125}I) or palladium-103 (^{103}Pd) during plaque radiation therapy of intraocular tumors.[3,124]

Iris

Iritis has been reported with a single dose of 10 to 20 Gy, but more severe anterior uveitis has been observed with doses of 30 to 40 Gy (in 10 Gy fractions) and after 70 to 80 Gy (over 6–8 weeks).[114,116] Radiation therapy can cause a dry eye–related corneal ulceration that can exacerbate iritis and iris neovascularization. Secondary glaucoma can also be related to iritis or iris neovascularization. Localized iris atrophy has been noted after plaque radiation therapy for iridociliary melanomas but not after external beam radiation therapy for orbital tumors.[80,93,119,125]

Retina, Choroid, and Optic Nerve

Radiation-related chorioretinal changes have generally been attributed to external beam radiation doses of 45 to 60 Gy. In the author's experience, doses as low as 18 Gy can induce radiation retinopathy in patients with compromised chorioretinal circulation (e.g., due to diabetes) and those on chemotherapy (Figure 33.9). Patients receiving 35 to 50 Gy carry a moderate risk, and those getting more than 50 Gy will eventually develop some form of the disease.[102] Radiation retinopathy is characterized by closure of small retinal capillaries, microinfarctions of the retina (cotton-wool spots), intraretinal hemorrhages, and neovascularization.[114,126] Radiation retinopathy in the macula causes vision loss and blindness.

In addition, radiation can cause closure of the blood vessels within the optic nerve (radiation optic neuropathy).[49,127] Parsons et al. described radiation optic neuropathy in 12 patients out of 131 whose optic nerves had been irradiated. No optic nerve that received less than 59 Gy developed optic neuropathy. Among optic nerves that received greater than 60 Gy, the 15-year actuarial risk of optic neuropathy was 11% when fraction size was less than 1.9 Gy per day and 47% with larger fractions.[102]

Hypothalamus and Pituitary Dysfunction

Hypothalamic and pituitary dysfunction is most often seen in children who have been irradiated for optic nerve glioma.[26,68,71,128] Brauner et al. described the effect of optic nerve glioma and its radiation therapy in 21 patients treated with intracranial radiation to 55 Gy. Growth hormone deficiency was present in 1 patient before irradiation and in 21 afterward. Height loss was also noted.[129] Clearly, patients irradiated for optic nerve gliomas should be monitored for hypothalamic and pituitary dysfunction.

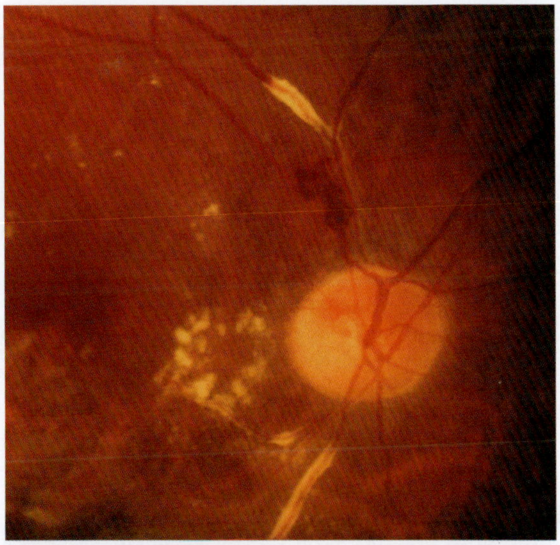

FIGURE 33.9. Fundus photograph of radiation retinopathy. Note the vascular sheathing, ghost vessels, intraretinal exudation, intraretinal microangiopathy, and optic neuropathy.

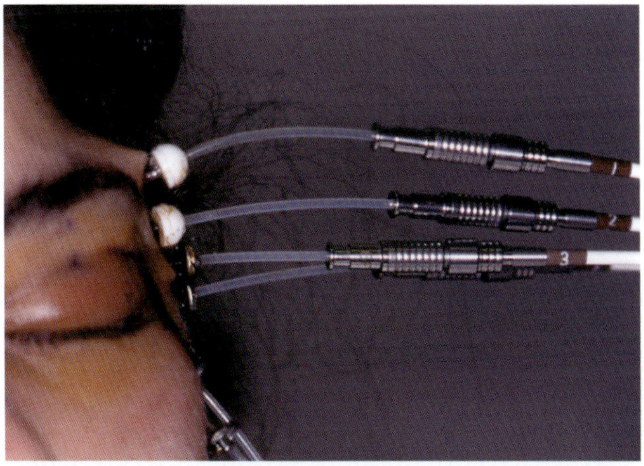

FIGURE 33.10. For a brachytherapy boost, surgically placed catheters are afterloaded with radiation sources placed in an array within the orbit and tumor bed (after resection of an adenoid cystic carcinoma of the orbit).

NEW FRONTIERS IN ORBITAL RADIATION THERAPY

Stereotactic Radiosurgery and the "Gamma Knife"

Stereotactic techniques were developed to deliver relatively high radiation doses to small fixed targets.[14,53,69] This is accomplished by creating multiple small entry beams that intersect within a three-dimensional target volume. Gamma knife and stereotactic radiosurgery treatments are typically given in a single or a few large fractions using either a linear accelerator or a cobalt source (gamma knife). Using multiple entry beams, the "entry dose" radiation is divided among several locations outside the target zone. This technique was initially used in the treatment of intracranial malignancies, arteriovenous malformations, and acoustic neuromas.[69] To date, no evidence-based results suggest that stereotactic radiosurgery is better than standard external beam techniques to prevent local recurrence or side effects related to radiation therapy of orbital tumors.

Brachytherapy Boost Technique

A new multidisciplinary approach to orbital radiation therapy is emerging to spare patients from exenteration surgery. Instead of removing the eyelids and orbital tissue as is done in exenteration, the bulk of the tumor is removed and a pattern of radiation (seeds or afterloaded sources) is placed temporarily (for several days) in the tumor bed (Figure 33.10). The seeds deposit a bolus of radiation where residual microscopic tumor cells are most likely to have escaped resection. Then, an additional (reduced) external beam radiation dose is delivered to the entire orbit including the tumor bed (boost volume). This overlay of radiation is given to provide an additional margin of safety. The reduced external beam dose is still high, leaving the patient with a high probability of both ocular complications and organ preservation.

Indications for the brachytherapy boost technique are as follows:

1. When the standard EBRT dose would likely result in a blind and painful eye owing to radiation retinopathy, keratopathy, and/or neovascular glaucoma
2. When exenteration of the orbit is the only option but offers historically poor local control rates (e.g., adenoid cystic carcinoma)
3. When a recurrent tumor has already received maximal EBRT
4. When a patient refuses exenteration surgery

Our local control rates have been over 75% using this brachytherapy boost technique for selected cases of adenoid cystic carcinoma, orbital basal cell, and sebaceous carcinoma and hemangiopericytoma of the orbit.

Abramson et al. have used orbital brachytherapy in a case of recurrent orbital rhabdomyosarcoma.[130] Tijl et al. used it for a recurrent hemangiopericytoma, and Sealy and Stannard have used it as an alternative to external beam irradiation of the orbit in retinoblastoma.[131–133] Bacskulin and Kim have developed applicators specifically for treating the orbit after enucleation or exenteration.[134,135]

CONCLUSIONS

Radiation therapy has played an important role in the management of benign and malignant orbital tumors, as well as sinus, intraocular, and adnexal tumors with orbital extension. Research on neutron therapy, stereotactic radiosurgery, and brachytherapy boost techniques appears promising for the goals of increasing local control and decreasing secondary radiation complications.

Acknowledgments This work was supported by The EyeCare Foundation, Inc., New York City.

The author thanks Drs. Anthony Berson and Madhavi Kurli for reviewing this chapter.

References

1. Rosenblatt E, Brook OR, Erlich N, et al. Late visual and auditory toxicity of radiotherapy for nasopharyngeal carcinoma. *Tumori* 2003;89:68–74.
2. Alberti W. Acute and late side effects of radiotherapy for ocular disease: an overview. *Front Radiat Ther Oncol* 1997;30:281–286.
3. Finger PT. Radiation therapy for choroidal melanoma. *Surv Ophthalmol* 1997;42:215–232.
4. Hungerford JL, Foss AJ, Whelahan I, et al. Side effects of photon and proton radiotherapy for ocular melanoma. *Front Radiat Ther Oncol* 1997;30:287–293.
5. Fiorillo A, Migliorati R, Vassallo P, et al. Radiation late effects in children treated for orbital rhabdomyosarcoma. *Radiother Oncol* 1999;53:143–148.
6. Imhof SM, Mourits MP, Hofman P, et al. Quantification of orbital and mid-facial growth retardation after megavoltage external beam irradiation in children with retinoblastoma. *Ophthalmology* 1996;103:263–268.
7. Schipper J, Alberti W. Late effects of radiation on surviving retinoblastoma patients. *Ophthalmology* 1985;92:60A–63A.
8. Merriam GR Jr, Focht EF. A clinical study of radiation cataracts and the relationship to dose. *AJR Am J Roentgenol Radium Ther Nucl Med* 1957;77:759–785.
9. Merriam GR Jr, Focht EF. Radiation dose to the lens in treatment of tumors of the eye and adjacent structures: possibilities of cataract formation. *Radiology* 1958;71:357–369.
10. Bolek TW, Moyses HM, Marcus RB Jr, et al. Radiotherapy in the management of orbital lymphoma. *Int J Radiat Oncol Biol Phys* 1999;44:31–36.
11. Huber PE, Debus J, Latz D, et al. Radiotherapy for advanced adenoid cystic carcinoma: neutrons, photons or mixed beam? *Radiother Oncol* 2001;59:161–167.
12. Fuss M, Hug EB, Schaefer RA, et al. Proton radiation therapy (PRT) for pediatric optic pathway gliomas: comparison with 3D planned conventional photons and a standard photon technique. *Int J Radiat Oncol Biol Phys* 1999;45:1117–1126.
13. Sidrys LA, Fritz KJ, Variakojis D. Fast neutron therapy for orbital adenoid cystic carcinoma. *Ann Ophthalmol* 1982;14:42–45.
14. Ahn YC, Lee KC, Kim DY, et al. Fractionated stereotactic radiation therapy for extracranial head and neck tumors. *Int J Radiat Oncol Biol Phys* 2000;48:501–505.
15. Kennerdell JS, Flores NE, Hartsock RJ. Low-dose radiotherapy for lymphoid lesions of the orbit and ocular adnexa. *Ophthalmic Plast Reconstr Surg* 1999;15:129–133.
16. Marcocci C, Bartalena L, Rocchi R, et al. Long-term safety of orbital radiotherapy for Graves' ophthalmopathy. *J Clin Endocrinol Metab* 2003;88:3561–3566.
17. Sagerman RH, Cassady JR, Tretter P. Radiation therapy for rhabdomyosarcoma of the orbit. *Trans Am Acad Ophthalmol Otolaryngol* 1968;72:849–854.
18. Schuller DE, Lawrence TL, Newton WA, Jr. Childhood rhabdomyosarcomas of the head and neck. *Arch Otolaryngol* 1979;105:689–694.
19. Schipper J. An accurate and simple method for megavoltage radiation therapy of retinoblastoma. *Radiother Oncol* 1983;1:31–41.
20. Moshfeghi DM, Moshfeghi AA, Finger PT. Enucleation. *Surv Ophthalmol* 2000;44:277–301.
21. Brady LW, Simpson LD, Day JL, Tapley ND. Clinical applications of electron beam therapy. In: Perez CA, Brady LW, eds. *Principles and Practice of Radiation Oncology*. 3rd ed. Philadelphia: Lippincott-Raven; 1997.
22. Purdy JA. Advances in three-dimensional treatment planning and conformal dose delivery. *Semin Oncol* 1997;24:655–671.
23. Purdy JA. Principles of radiologic physics, dosimetry, and treatment planning. In: Perez CA, Brady LW, eds. *Principles and Practice of Radiation Oncology*. 3rd ed. Philadelphia: Lippincott-Raven; 1997.
24. Purdy JA, Klein EE. External photon beam dosimetry and treatment planning. In: Perez CA, Brady LW, eds. *Principles and Practice of Radiation Oncology*. 3rd ed. Philadephia: Lippincott-Raven; 1997.

25. Hug EB, Adams J, Fitzek M, et al. Fractionated, three-dimensional, planning-assisted proton-radiation therapy for orbital rhabdomyosarcoma: a novel technique. *Int J Radiat Oncol Biol Phys* 2000;47:979–984.
26. Kortmann RD, Timmermann B, Taylor RE, et al. Current and future strategies in radiotherapy of childhood low-grade glioma of the brain. I. Treatment modalities of radiation therapy. *Strahlenther Onkol* 2003;179:509–520.
27. Stelzer KJ, Laramore GE, Griffin TW, et al. Fast neutron radiotherapy. The University of Washington experience. *Acta Oncol* 1994;33:275–280.
28. Plowman PN, Harnett AN. Radiotherapy in benign orbital disease. I. Complicated ocular angiomas. *Br J Ophthalmol* 1988;72:286–288.
29. Steahly LP, Almquist HT. Steroid treatment of an orbital or periocular hemangioma. *J Pediatr Ophthalmol* 1977;14:35–37.
30. Vainshtein ES, Burdianskaia EI, Podliashuk EL. [Late results of the x-ray therapy of angiomas of the orbital area and adjacent portions of the face in children]. *Oftalmol Zh* 1982;37:71–75.
31. Wilde G, Sjöstrand J. A clinical study of radiation cataract formation in adult life following gamma irradiation of the lens in early childhood. *Br J Ophthalmol* 1997;81:261–266.
32. Wisnicki JL. Hemangiomas and vascular malformations. *Ann Plast Surg* 1984;12:41–59.
33. Shuler JD, Holland GN, Miles SA, et al. Kaposi sarcoma of the conjunctiva and eyelids associated with the acquired immunodeficiency syndrome. *Arch Ophthalmol* 1989;107:858–862.
34. Moshfeghi DM, Finger PT, Cohen RB, et al. Visual recovery after radiation therapy of orbital lymphoma. *Am J Ophthalmol* 1992;114:645–646.
35. Tsang RW, Gospodarowicz MK, Pintilie M, et al. Stage I and II MALT lymphoma: results of treatment with radiotherapy. *Int J Radiat Oncol Biol Phys* 2001;50:1258–1264.
36. Stafford SL, Kozelsky TF, Garrity JA, et al. Orbital lymphoma: radiotherapy outcome and complications. *Radiother Oncol* 2001;59:139–144.
37. van Ouwerkerk BM, Wijngaarde R, Hennemann G, et al. Radiotherapy of severe ophthalmic Graves' disease. *J Endocrinol Invest* 1985;8:241–247.
38. Sandler HM, Rubenstein JH, Fowble BL, et al. Results of radiotherapy for thyroid ophthalmopathy. *Int J Radiat Oncol Biol Phys* 1989;17:823–827.
39. Bartalena L, Marcocci C, Gorman CA, et al. Orbital radiotherapy for Graves' ophthalmopathy: useful or useless? Safe or dangerous? *J Endocrinol Invest* 2003;26:5–16.
40. Gorman CA, Garrity JA, Fatourechi V, et al. A prospective, randomized, double-blind, placebo-controlled study of orbital radiotherapy for Graves' ophthalmopathy. *Ophthalmology* 2001;108:1523–1534.
41. Morley M, Finger PT, Perlin M, et al. *cis*-Platinum chemotherapy for ocular basal cell carcinoma. *Br J Ophthalmol* 1991;75(7):407–410.
42. Ellingwood KE, Million RR. Cancer of the nasal cavity and ethmoid/sphenoid sinuses. *Cancer* 1979;43:1517–1526.
43. Katz TS, Mendenhall WM, Morris CG, et al. Malignant tumors of the nasal cavity and paranasal sinuses. *Head Neck* 2002;24(9):821–829.
44. Johnson TE, Tabbara KF, Weatherhead RG, et al. Secondary squamous cell carcinoma of the orbit. *Arch Ophthalmol* 1997;115:75–78.
45. Amdur RJ, Kalbaugh KJ, Ewald LM, et al. Radiation therapy for skin cancer near the eye: kilovoltage x-rays versus electrons. *Int J Radiat Oncol Biol Phys* 1992;23:769–779.
46. Wilson MW, Czechonska G, Finger PT, et al. Chemotherapy for eye cancer. *Surv Ophthalmol* 2001;45:416–444.
47. Rodriguez JM, Deutsch GP. The treatment of periocular basal cell carcinomas by radiotherapy. *Br J Ophthalmol* 1992;76:195–197.
48. Bowyer JD, Sullivan TJ, Whitehead KJ, et al. The management of perineural spread of squamous cell carcinoma to the ocular adnexae. *Ophthalmic Plast Reconstr Surg* 2003;19:275–281.
49. Nakissa N, Rubin P, Strohl R, Keys H. Ocular and orbital complications following radiation therapy of paranasal sinus malignancies and review of literature. *Cancer* 1983;51:980–986.
50. Perlman E, McMahon RT. Sebaceous gland carcinoma of the eyelid. *Am J Ophthalmol* 1978;86:699–703.
51. Pardo FS, Borodic G. Long-term follow-up of patients undergoing definitive radiation therapy for sebaceous carcinoma of the ocular adnexae. *Int J Radiat Oncol Biol Phys* 1996;34:1189–1190.
52. Pardo FS, Wang CC, Albert D, Stracher MA. Sebaceous carcinoma of the ocular adnexa: radiotherapeutic management. *Int J Radiat Oncol Biol Phys* 1989;17:643–647.
53. Swain RE Jr, Kingdom TT, DelGaudio JM, et al. Meningiomas of the paranasal sinuses. *Am J Rhinol* 2001;15:27–30.
54. Rootman J. Tumors: neurogenic tumors. In: Rootman J, ed. *Diseases of the Orbit*. Vol 1. Philadelphia: JB Lippincott, 1988.
55. Gaillard S, Lejeune JP, Pellerin P, et al. Long-term results of the surgical treatment of spheno-orbital osteomeningioma. [in French]. *Neurochirurgie* 1995;41:391–397.
56. Maroon JC, Kennerdell JS, Vidovich DV, et al. Recurrent spheno-orbital meningioma. *J Neurosurg* 1994;80:202–208.
57. Mirimanoff RO, Dosoretz DE, Linggood RM, et al. Meningioma: analysis of recurrence and progression following neurosurgical resection. *J Neurosurg* 1985;62:18–24.
58. Paulus WM, Brandt T, Kuhne D, et al. Therapy of orbital and retroorbital space occupying processes with optic nerve compression [in German]. *Nervenarzt* 1985;56:519–534.
59. Perilongo G, Sutton LN, Goldwein JW, et al. Childhood meningiomas. Experience in the modern imaging era. *Pediatr Neurosurg* 1992;18:16–23.
60. Sheikh BY, Siqueira E, Dayel F. Meningioma in children: a report of nine cases and a review of the literature. *Surg Neurol* 1996;45:328–335.
61. Walther E, Gloor B. [Radiotherapy of malignant tumours of the orbit (author's transl)] in German. *Klin Monatsbl Augenheilkd* 1979;174:959–968.
62. Wara MW, Bauman GS, Sneed PK, et al. Brain, brain stem, and cerebellum. In: Perez CA, Brady LW, eds. *Principles and Practice of Radiation Oncology*. 3rd ed. Philadelphia: Lippincott-Raven; 1997.
63. Zografos L, Ducrey N, Beati D, et al. Metastatic melanoma in the eye and orbit. *Ophthalmology* 2003;110:2245–2256.
64. Kokufu I, Tanei T, Taniguchi H, et al. Two cases of effective weekly paclitaxel administration and concurrent radiation for metastatic breast cancer [in Japanese]. *Gan To Kagaku Ryoho* 2003;30:111–114.
65. Ratanatharathorn V, Powers WE, Grimm J, et al. Eye metastasis from carcinoma of the breast: diagnosis, radiation treatment and results. *Cancer Treat Rev* 1991;18:261–276.
66. Amichetti M, Caffo O, Minatel E, et al. Ocular metastases from breast carcinoma: a multicentric retrospective study. *Oncol Rep* 2000;7:761–765.
67. Cohen ME, Duffner PK. Optic pathway tumors. *Neurol Clin* 1991;9:467–477.
68. Grabenbauer GG, Schuchardt U, Buchfelder M, et al. Radiation therapy of optico-hypothalamic gliomas (OHG)—radiographic response, vision and late toxicity. *Radiother Oncol* 2000;54:239–245.
69. Lim YJ, Leem W. Two cases of gamma knife radiosurgery for low-grade optic chiasm glioma. *Stereotact Funct Neurosurg* 1996;66(suppl 1):174–183.

70. Regueiro CA, Ruiz MV, Millan I, et al. Prognostic factors and results of radiation therapy in optic pathway tumors. *Tumori* 1996;82:353–359.
71. Khafaga Y, Hassounah M, Kandil A, et al. Optic gliomas: a retrospective analysis of 50 cases. *Int J Radiat Oncol Biol Phys* 2003;56:807–812.
72. Haik BG, Jereb B, Smith ME, et al. Radiation and chemotherapy of parameningeal rhabdomyosarcoma involving the orbit. *Ophthalmology* 1986;93:1001–1009.
73. Raney RB Jr, Donaldson MH, Sutow WW, et al. Special considerations related to primary site in rhabdomyosarcoma: experience of the Intergroup Rhabdomyosarcoma Study, 1972–76. *Natl Cancer Inst Monogr* 1981;56:69–74.
74. Marsh JL, Wise DM, Smith M, Schwartz H. Lacrimal gland adenoid cystic carcinoma: intracranial and extracranial en bloc resection. *Plast Reconstr Surg* 1981;68:577–585.
75. Lederman M. Radiotherapy of primary malignant tumours of the orbit. *Mod Probl Ophthalmol* 1975;14:170–176.
76. Osguthorpe JD, Weisman RA, Tapert MJ. Management of lacrimal fossa masses. *Arch Otolaryngol Head Neck Surg* 1986;112:164–167.
77. Uzura S, Matsumura K, Watanabe K, Matsuda M. Adenoid cystic carcinoma of the lacrimal gland: report of a case [in Japanese]. *Nippon Geka Hokan* 1990;59:272–277.
78. Grossniklaus HE, Lass JH, Abramowsky CR, Levine MR. Childhood orbital pseudotumor. *Ann Ophthalmol* 1985;17: 372–377.
79. Fujii H, Fujisada H, Kondo T, et al. Orbital pseudotumor: histopathological classification and treatment. *Ophthalmologica* 1985;190:230–242.
80. Smitt MC, Donaldson SS. Radiation therapy for benign disease of the orbit. *Semin Radiat Oncol* 1999;9:179–189.
81. Zurlo A, Sancesario G, Bernardi G, Loasses A. Orbital pseudotumor: case report and literature review. *Tumori* 1999;85:68–70.
82. Donaldson SS, McDougall IR, Egbert PR, et al. Treatment of orbital pseudotumor (idiopathic orbital inflammation) by radiation therapy. *Int J Radiat Oncol Biol Phys* 1980;6:79–86.
83. Lanciano R, Fowble B, Sergott RC, et al. The results of radiotherapy for orbital pseudotumor. *Int J Radiat Oncol Biol Phys* 1990;18:407–411.
84. Noble SC, Chandler WF, Lloyd RV. Intracranial extension of orbital pseudotumor: a case report. *Neurosurgery* 1986;18(6): 798–801.
85. Weissler MC, Miller E, Fortune MA. Sclerosing orbital pseudotumor: a unique clinicopathologic entity. *Ann Otol Rhinol Laryngol* 1989;98(7 pt 1):496–501.
86. Wiegel T, Bottke D, Kreusel KM, et al. External beam radiotherapy of choroidal metastases—final results of a prospective study of the German Cancer Society (ARO 95–108). *Radiother Oncol* 2002;64:13–18.
87. Finger PT, Warren FA, Gelman YP, McCormick SA. Adult Wilms' tumor metastatic to the choroid of the eye. *Ophthalmology* 2002;109:2134–2136.
88. Finger PT, Marin JP, Berson AM, et al. Choroidal metastasis from adenoid cystic carcinoma of the lung. *Am J Ophthalmol* 2003;135:239–241.
89. Rosset A, Zografos L, Coucke P, et al. Radiotherapy of choroidal metastases. *Radiother Oncol* 1998;46:263–268.
90. Maor M, Chan RC, Young SE. Radiotherapy of choroidal metastases: breast cancer as primary site. *Cancer* 1977;40: 2081–2086.
91. Rudoler SB, Corn BW, Shields CL, et al. External beam irradiation for choroid metastases: identification of factors predisposing to long-term sequelae. *Int J Radiat Oncol Biol Phys* 1997;38:251–256.
92. Thatcher N, Thomas PR. Choroidal metastases from breast carcinoma: a survey of 42 patients and the use of radiation therapy. *Clin Radiol* 1975;26:549–553.
93. Marigo FA, Finger PT. Anterior segment tumors: current concepts and innovations. *Surv Ophthalmol* 2003;48(6):569–593.
94. Robertson DM, Campbell RJ, Weaver DT. Residual intrascleral and intraretinal melanoma: a concern with lamellar sclerouvectomy for uveal melanoma. *Am J Ophthalmol* 1991;112:590–593.
95. Hykin PG, McCartney AC, Plowman PN, Hungerford JL. Postenucleation orbital radiotherapy for the treatment of malignant melanoma of the choroid with extrascleral extension. *Br J Ophthalmol* 1990;74:36–39.
96. Finger PT, Czechonska G, Demirci H, Rausen A. Chemotherapy for retinoblastoma: a current topic. *Drugs* 1999;58: 983–996.
97. Finger PT, Harbour JW, Karcioglu ZA. Risk factors for metastasis in retinoblastoma. *Surv Ophthalmol* 2002;47:1–16.
98. Schipper J. Retinoblastoma. A medical and experimental study. Thesis, University of Utrecht, Rotterdam. 1980.
99. Stallard H. Radiant energy as (a) a pathogenic (b) a therapeutic agent in ophthalmic disorders. *Br J Ophthalmol* 1933; Monogr suppl 6.
100. Anteby I, Ramu N, Gradstein L, et al. Ocular and orbital complications following the treatment of retinoblastoma. *Eur J Ophthalmol* 1998;8:106–111.
101. Sagerman RH, Alberti WE. Diagnosis and management of retinoblastoma. In: Sagerman RH, Alberti WE, eds. *Radiotherapy of Intraocular and Orbital Tumors.* Vol 2. Berlin: Springer-Verlag; 2003.
102. Parsons JT, Bova FJ, Fitzgerald CR, et al. Radiation retinopathy after external-beam irradiation: analysis of time–dose factors. *Int J Radiat Oncol Biol Phys* 1994;30:765–773.
103. Pradhan DG, Sandridge AL, Mullaney P, et al. Radiation therapy for retinoblastoma: a retrospective review of 120 patients. *Int J Radiat Oncol Biol Phys* 1997;39:3–13.
104. Yue NC, Benson ML. The hourglass facial deformity as a consequence of orbital irradiation for bilateral retinoblastoma. *Pediatr Radiol* 1996;26:421–423.
105. Reese AB, Merriam GR Jr, Martin HE. Treatment of bilateral retinoblastoma by irradiation and surgery. *Am J Ophthalmol* 1949;32:175–190.
106. Reese AB, Hyman GA, Merriam GR Jr, Forrest AW. The treatment of retinoblastoma by radiation and triethylene melamine. *Am J Ophthalmol* 1957;43:865–872.
107. Fountain TR, Goldberg RS, Murphree AL. Orbital development after enucleation in early childhood. *Ophthalmic Plast Reconstr Surg* 1999;15:32–36.
108. Kaste SC, Chen G, Fontanesi J, et al. Orbital development in long-term survivors of retinoblastoma. *J Clin Oncol* 1997;15: 1183–1189.
109. Sagerman RH, Cassady JR, Tretter P, Ellsworth RM. Radiation induced neoplasia following external beam therapy for children with retinoblastoma. *AJR Am J Roentgenol Radium Ther Nucl Med* 1969;105:529–535.
110. Cassady JR, Sagerman RH, Tretter P, Ellsworth RM. Radiation therapy in retinoblastoma. An analysis of 230 cases. *Radiology* 1969;93:405–409.
111. Chalupecky H. Über die Wirkung der Röntgenstrahlen auf das Auge und die Haut. *Zentralbl Augenheilkd* 1897(21):234.
112. Birch-Hirschfeld A. Die Wirkung der Roentgen- und Radiumstrahlen auf das Auge. *Graefes Arch Clin Exp Ophthalmol* 1904;59:229–310.
113. Amman E. Zur Wirkung der Roentgenstrahlen auf das menschliche Auge. Korrespondenz-Blett fur Schweizer, Arzte 15.
114. Sagerman RH, Alberti WE. Radiosensitivity of ocular and orbital structures. In: Sagerman RH, Alberti WE, eds. *Radiotherapy of Intraocular and Orbital Tumors.* Vol 2. New York: Springer-Verlag; 2003.
115. Macfaul PA, Bedford MA. Ocular complications after therapeutic irradiation. *Br J Ophthalmol* 1970;54:237–247.

116. Servodidio CA, Abramson DH. Acute and long-term effects of radiation therapy to the eye in children. *Cancer Nurs* 1993; 16:371–381.
117. Parsons JT, Bova FJ, Fitzgerald CR, et al. Severe dry-eye syndrome following external beam irradiation. *Int J Radiat Oncol Biol Phys* 1994;30:775–780.
118. Reminick LR, Finger PT, Ritch R, et al. Ultrasound biomicroscopy in the diagnosis and management of anterior segment tumors. *J Am Optom Assoc* 1998;69:575–582.
119. Finger PT. Plaque radiation therapy for malignant melanoma of the iris and ciliary body. *Am J Ophthalmol* 2001;132: 328–335.
120. Finger PT. Tumour location affects the incidence of cataract and retinopathy after ophthalmic plaque radiation therapy. *Br J Ophthalmol* 2000;84:1068–1070.
121. Merriam GR Jr, Worgul BV, Medvedovsky C, et al. Accelerated heavy particles and the lens. I. Cataractogenic potential. *Radiat Res* 1984;98:129–140.
122. Merriam GR Jr, Worgul BV. Experimental radiation cataract—its clinical relevance. *Bull N Y Acad Med* 1983;59:372–392.
123. Merriam GR Jr, Focht EF. A clinical and experimental study of the effect of single and divided doses of radiation on cataract production. *Trans Am Ophthalmol Soc* 1962; 60:35–52.
124. Bacin F, Amara S, Kemeny JL, et al. [Comparative study of beta irradiation (106Ru/106Rh) and gamma irradiation (125I) on the rabbit eye.] *Ophthalmologica* 1998;212:429–438.
125. Smith RA, Dzugan SA, Kosko P. Postoperative beta irradiation for control of pterygium. *J Miss State Med Assoc* 2001;42:167–169.
126. Guyer DR, Mukai S, Egan KM, et al. Radiation maculopathy after proton beam irradiation for choroidal melanoma. *Ophthalmology* 1992;99:1278–1285.
127. Jiang GL, Tucker SL, Guttenberger R, et al. Radiation-induced injury to the visual pathway. *Radiother Oncol* 1994;30:17–25.
128. Brauner R, Rappaport R, Prevot C, et al. A prospective study of the development of growth hormone deficiency in children given cranial irradiation, and its relation to statural growth. *J Clin Endocrinol Metab* 1989;68:346–351.
129. Brauner R, Malandry F, Rappaport R, et al. Growth and endocrine disorders in optic glioma. *Eur J Pediatr* 1990;149: 825–828.
130. Abramson DH, Fass D, McCormick B, et al. Implant brachytherapy: a novel treatment for recurrent orbital rhabdomyosarcoma. *J MOPS* 1997;1:154–157.
131. Tijl JW, Koornneef L, Blank LE. Recurrent hemangiopericytoma and brachytherapy. *Doc Ophthalmol* 1992;82:103–107.
132. Stannard C, Sealy R, Hering E, et al. Postenucleation orbits in retinoblastoma: treatment with ^{125}I brachytherapy. *Int J Radiat Oncol Biol Phys* 2002;54:1446–1454.
133. Sealy R, Stannard C, Shackleton D. Improved cosmesis in retinoblastoma patients treated with iodine-125 orbital irradiation. *Ophthalmic Paediatr Genet* 1987;8:95–99.
134. Bacskulin A, Ehrhardt M, Strietzel M, et al. An adjuvant afterloading brachytherapy device for use after orbital exenteration in patients with orbital malignancies. *Ger J Ophthalmol* 1996;5:484–488.
135. Kim TH, Gerbi BJ, Deibel FC, et al. An afterloading brachytherapy device utilizing thermoplastic material. *Radiother Oncol* 1989;15:341–344.

34

Chemotherapy for Childhood Tumors

Marta K. Rozans

TREATMENT OF CHILDREN

Malignancy in childhood is relatively rare, compared with that in adults; only about one child in 300 will develop any form of cancer,[1] and only a tiny minority of children with any malignancy will have orbital involvement. Furthermore, only a small number of orbital lesions are malignant. Of 241 orbital lesions in children aged 0 to 20 years, only 17 (7.1%) were reported to be malignant.[2] Shields et al.[3] reported on 250 consecutive biopsies of orbital masses in children 18 years of age or younger. They found a total of 23 malignant tumors (9.2%). However, they caution that this figure may be an underestimate, since many children have malignant orbital disease within the context of metastatic disease, and the diagnoses are made from elsewhere.

Nevertheless, it is clear that pediatric orbital malignancy is a rare event, and understanding and improvement in outcome will come about only with a cooperative, multidisciplinary approach within the context of large group trials.

PRIMARY MALIGNANT ORBITAL TUMORS

Orbital Rhabdomyosarcoma

Rhabdomyosarcoma is a rare tumor with an annual incidence of 4.3 per million children.[4] The orbit is the primary site in about 10% of these tumors.[5] Each year, about 350 new rhabdomyosarcomas are diagnosed in children in this country; thus only about 35 cases of orbital rhabdomyosarcoma are diagnosed each year in the United States.[6]

Prior to the 1960s, the standard of care for treatment of rhabdomyosarcoma was to attempt complete resection of the tumor.[7,8] For orbital primaries, this meant enucleation and possible exenteration of the orbit. Radiation therapy was sometimes used,[9–12] but chemotherapy was generally reserved for patients with recurrent or disseminated disease. Outcomes were poor, and many children had recurrence of localized or distant disease.

In the mid-1960s, higher doses of local radiation began to be used, and local surgical control was not uniformly attempted. In addition, chemotherapy was sometimes used for local control. These approaches seemed beneficial, but the number of children studied in any systematic way was very small.

In the early 1970s, the Intergroup Rhabdomyosarcoma Study (IRS) Group was formed, with the goal of studying large numbers of children with rhabdomyosarcoma in a short period of time, thus answering important questions as rapidly as possible.

In the first IRS study (IRS-I), all patients were treated with chemotherapy. Patients with group I disease (localized disease that is completely excised) were randomized to treatment with vincristine, actinomycin D, and cyclophosphamide (VAC) with or without radiation therapy; patients with group II disease (microscopic residual or completely resected regional disease with lymph node positive) all received vincristine–actinomycin D (VA) and radiation therapy with or without cyclophosphamide; and patients with groups III (gross residual) and IV (metastatic) disease all received VAC and radiation therapy with or without doxorubicin.[13,14] Cyclophosphamide was given orally in all groups.

Of the 56 patients with primary disease of the eye and orbit (including the eyelid), 16 were in group II (microscopic residual) and 39 patients had group III disease (gross residual disease). One patient had group IV disease (distant metastases) at presentation.[14]

One of the most remarkable findings of this large study was that patients with localized orbit primaries did well regardless of the extent of initial resection (group II or III). Fifteen of 16 (94%) patients with group II disease and 33 of 39 (85%) patients with group III disease survived 6 to 12 years from diagnosis.[14] At the final report, the 5-year overall survival for all patients with orbital primary disease was 89%.[15]

Because of the excellent outcome in patients with group II and group III disease, an initial attempt at complete or gross total excision of orbital rhabdomyosarcoma ceased to be the standard of care.[13,14]

Importantly, of the six deaths that occurred within the first 3 years, two were due to infection and one was related to a secondary leukemia.[14] The other three early deaths and both late deaths were related to recurrent disease.

The second IRS study (IRS-II) ran from 1978 to 1984. Patients with group I disease were treated with VA or VAC (and no radiation). Patients with group II disease all received local radiation and intensive VA with or without cyclophosphamide, and patients with group III disease received radiation and intensive VAC with or without Adriamycin. There was no improvement in any of the more intensive arms, over those receiving the less intensive regimen. However, all arms did better than the comparable group on the IRS-I protocol. When the patients with orbital disease from IRS-I and IRS-II are combined, local control was achieved in 93% of patients who did not undergo exenteration. However, 11% of patients with group III disease in the IRS-II study had local failure.[16] Following local recurrence, many of the patients could still be salvaged.

Long-term complications were common. Infectious complications were more likely in patients who had had initial exenteration, and most patients developed some degree of unilateral visual loss—primarily owing to cataract formation related to local radiation therapy.[14] In addition, patients with second malignancies were beginning to be described, some of whom may have had a genetic predisposition to malignancy.[17] Thus, there was a strong incentive to decrease therapy in patients who had a good prognosis, to spare them secondary complications.

In the third study (IRS-III), the number of patients with orbital group II and III tumors was not expected to be sufficient to merit the design of a randomized study powerful enough to answer a question; this is due to the tremendously good response seen by the end of the IRS-II study—the better the outcome, the more patients needed to demonstrate a difference between two groups. Therefore, all group II and III patients with orbital rhabdomyosarcoma were treated with VA and local radiation for only one year; these patients were then compared with patients in IRS-II. There was no statistically significant difference in outcome between the patients treated in IRS-III and IRS-II.[18]

The fourth study (IRS-IV) enrolled patients from 1991 to 1997 and continued the use of vincristine and actinomycin for all group I and II orbital primaries. Conventional radiation therapy was given to patients with group II disease. Patients with group III disease were randomized between VAC, vincristine, actinomycin D, and ifosfamide (VAI), and vincristine, ifosfamide, and etoposide (VIE). In addition, these patients were randomized to receive either conventional radiation therapy or hyperfractionated radiation therapy at a higher dose (presumed equitoxic dose). For 22 patients with group I and II orbital disease, the 3-year failure-free survival (FFS) is 91%, and the 3-year overall survival (OS) is 100%. This represents no change from IRS-III, as would be expected. For the 59 patients with group III disease, the 3-year FFS was 94% and the OS was 98%. There was no difference between the three chemotherapy groups or two radiation groups. Compared with the FFS on IRS-III (80% for the group III orbit primaries), however, patients with group III primary tumors benefited more from three drugs than from vincristine and actinomycin D only.[19]

The staging for rhabdomyosarcoma became much more complicated upon recognition that outcome is very highly influenced by primary tumor *site*, in addition to more conventional factors (size, nodal involvement, etc.). The details of the current staging classification are not presented here, except to say that all orbit primaries are stage I unless there is dissemination of disease at the time of diagnosis, which is stage IV. Since most orbital tumors are subjected to biopsy without attempt at resection, there is gross residual disease (group III); thus, most orbital rhabdomyosarcomas are stage I/ group III, a minority are stage I/group I or II, and, rarely, a primary orbital rhabdomyosarcoma is stage IV.

Considering the concerns about complications associated with alkylating agents (cyclophosphamide and ifosfamide) and etoposide, there seems to be a push to decrease the use of these drugs. However, replacing them with radiation therapy leads to the localized side effects of radiation.

The current (IRS-V) study uses standard doses of actinomycin D and vincristine, combined with a decreased dose of radiation therapy (4500 cGy vs 5000 cGy) for patients with low risk rhabdomyosarcoma, including group III orbital disease. This study is ongoing.

Lymphoma

Pediatric orbital lymphomas are quite rare and have not generally been studied as a separate entity. Instead, therapeutic studies have focused on the pathology and the extent of the lymphoma, rather than the specific site of primary or disseminated disease.

Pediatric non-Hodgkin's lymphoma is typically considered to be a systemic disease; thus, even "localized" non-Hodgkin's lymphoma is treated with chemotherapy. This is extremely important for the ophthalmologist to keep in mind, since aggressive surgical intervention is neither required nor necessarily helpful. In the case of localized orbital lymphoma, the surgeon is certainly needed to make the diagnosis. However, in the event of disseminated or multifocal disease, the diagnosis may best be made from another tissue site.

Unlike the adult lymphomas, which are low and intermediate grade, pediatric non-Hodgkin's lymphomas are typically high grade, and these comments are confined to the most common ones: Burkitt's and Burkitt's-like/small noncleaved-cell, B-large cell, anaplastic large cell, and lymphoblastic lymphomas.

For the purposes of treatment, the pediatric non-Hodgkin's lymphomas can be classified as low risk and high risk. Patients with high-risk features include all stage III and stage IV disease, as well as patients with lower stage disease but extensive mediastinal or gastrointestinal primaries. Some groups have used lactate dehydrogenase level at diagnosis to help classify some of the lymphomas as low or high risk. Patients with low-risk disease include those with stage I or stage II diseases, excluding the special groups already mentioned. Patients with stages I and II lymphoblastic lymphoma fall somewhere in between the low- and high-risk groups. All patients with central nervous system (CNS) involvement are considered to be at high risk.

Many studies have been done, and a detailed discussion of them is beyond the scope of this chapter. However, certain conclusions and principles can be derived. Most children with non-Hodgkin's lymphoma of any histology or stage can expect to be cured. Thus, these children may have 50 years or more in which to develop long-term side effects, including second malignancies and gonadal failure. Thus, there has been a major effort to reduce exposure to agents that may lead to these devastating outcomes. Since most pediatric patients with lymphoma can be expected to have a long-term disease-free survival (cure) regardless of the presenting stage, the terms "high" and "low" risk have more to do with the treatment strategy than with prognosis.

Burkitt's lymphoma (small noncleaved, Burkitt's-like lymphoma) is an extremely rapidly growing tumor. Rapid diagnosis is key to the successful treatment of this disease, since death may otherwise occur within days or weeks of presentation with symptoms. This disease has such a rapid turnover that patients who relapse will do so very early. Conversely, a patient who remains in remission for 12 to 24 months from diagnosis is generally considered to be cured.

For low-stage Burkitt's and B-large-cell lymphoma, a relatively short course of systemic chemotherapy is successful at leading to long-term disease-free survival (cure) in 80 to 100% of the patients. Studies comparing 6 vs 18 months[20] of therapy and 4 vs 7 months[21] of therapy failed to demonstrate any added benefit to longer treatment regimens for children with nonlymphoblastic low-stage lymphoma. Recent trials have utilized as little as 9 weeks of cyclophosphamide, doxorubicin, vincristine, and prednisone (CHOP),[22,23] whereas others have omitted the cyclophosphamide, in an attempt to decrease exposure to alkylating agents even further.

Radiation therapy has also been directly evaluated. In patients who have low-risk disease but are at high risk of CNS relapse, which includes patients with head and neck primary tumors, radiation therapy has been demonstrated to be unnecessary as long as adequate systemic and intrathecal chemotherapy are given. Involved field radiation therapy was demonstrated to offer no disease-free survival benefit.[24] Thus, radiation therapy has been completely eliminated from a number of recent trials targeting pediatric patients with low-risk lymphomas.

Multiagent, intensive chemotherapy has been demonstrated to greatly improve the outcome of children who have high-stage small noncleaved lymphoma. In 1977 the Children's Cancer Group (CCG) demonstrated that children with nonlymphoblastic lymphoma had improved survival with cyclophosphamide, vincristine, methotrexate, and prednisone (COMP) over children who had received the LSA_2L_2 (cyclophosphamide, vincristine, methotrexate, daunomycin, prednisone, cytarabine, thioguanine, L-asparaginase, carmustine, hydroxyurea), with 2-year disease-free survivals of 57 and 29%, respectively.[25,26]

The French Society for Pediatric Oncology noted that patients with CNS disease did worse than those without CNS involvement.[27] This finding was substantiated by all the early major lymphoma studies. Patients without CNS involvement were subsequently treated with either 7 or 4 months of therapy; there was no added benefit to the longer treatment. Decreasing the duration of treatment resulted in decreased toxicity and a long-term disease-free survival improved to greater than 80%.[21] The CCG likewise found that 6 months of treatment in patients with nonlymphoblastic non-Hodgkin's lymphoma was comparable to 18 months of treatment. This study included patients with Burkitt's, Burkitt's-like and large-cell lymphomas.[20]

CCG compared the French protocol with another successful but less toxic regimen. The U.S. researchers found a lower toxic mortality but the same disease-free survival in patients with lower stage disease who were treated on the less toxic "orange" arm. However, for patients with high-risk disease, disease-free survival was improved on the more toxic "French" arm.

The Pediatric Oncology Group (POG) demonstrated that intrathecal chemotherapy could replace cranial radiation as prophylaxis against CNS relapse in patients without initial CNS disease.[28]

It is now reasonable to anticipate a long-term disease-free survival (cure) for children with all stages of small noncleaved cell (Burkitt's) and B-large-cell lymphomas of 80 to 90% or better. Recent studies have moved toward maintaining this excellent response rate while decreasing the short- and long-term morbidity. Thus, it remains critical that children with these diseases continue to be entered in large multi-institutional studies.

Lymphoblastic lymphomas are typically of T-cell origin. They may be considered to be a solid, lower grade version of T-cell lymphoblastic leukemia, a relatively common childhood acute leukemia. Stage IV lymphoblastic lymphoma and T-cell leukemia may differ only slightly, or the difference may be purely academic. Biologically, they react in the same fashion and require the same therapy.

Patients with low-stage lymphoblastic lymphoma, especially including the mediastinum, have shown more resistance to successful treatment than have the low-stage B-cell lymphomas. This population has required either more agents or longer treatment or both.[20,23,29] However, even in this group of children, involved field radiation therapy has been shown to confer no added benefit over no radiation therapy. These patients may be treated for 6 months to 2 years, depending on the specific protocol.

Patients with high-stage lymphoblastic lymphoma were shown to have an inferior outcome when treated with COMP chemotherapy instead of the more aggressive LSA_2L_2 treatment.[24,25] The LSA_2L_2 regimen has been modified several times, including high doses of methotrexate, for improved outcome in treatment of lymphoblastic lymphoma.[29]

Anaplastic large-cell lymphoma comprises a heterogeneous group of lymphomas that may be of T- or B-cell origin that includes Ki-1 positive lymphomas. Some of these lymphomas have been difficult to distinguish from Hodgkin's disease, and thus, interpretation of prior studies must be done with caution. Various intergroup studies have differing requirements, and some of the studies, including several mentioned earlier, include treatment of the anaplastic large-cell lymphomas along with the B-large-cell lymphomas, or with the lymphoblastic lymphomas. In addition, the anaplastic large-cell lymphomas have also been treated like Hodgkin's disease. All these approaches have some merit, and the optimal treatment strategy remains to be defined.

Granulocytic Sarcoma

The entity described as a solid mass of myeloid leukemia, found outside the bone marrow (medullary) space, is variably known as extramedullary leukemia, granulocytic sarcoma, chloroma, and reticulin cell sarcoma.[30] For simplicity, "granulocytic sarcoma" is used in this section.

Granulocytic sarcoma is a relatively uncommon presentation for acute nonlymphoblastic leukemia (ANLL) and may present simultaneously with, or prior to, bone marrow involvement with leukemia. One of the most common sites of granulocytic sarcoma seems to be the orbit.[31] In certain areas of the world, as many as 30% of granulocytic sarcomas will be in the orbit,[32–34] though the incidence in Europe and the United States seems to be lower.

Initial misdiagnosis is relatively common,[30,31] especially when there is no initial bone marrow involvement. When granulocytic sarcoma presents as an isolated finding, however, it is a preleukemic finding, since if local therapy only is offered, bone marrow "relapse" invariably follows.[31]

Byrd et al. reviewed all reports of extramedullary leukemia published between 1965 and 1995. In that 30-year period, they found reference to 154 cases of primary extramedullary leukemia—that is, there was no concurrent bone marrow disease.[31] Thirteen of these 154 cases were found in the orbit; 72 were initially misdiagnosed. Thirty patients received local therapy only, and 29 of 30 experienced relapse in the bone marrow between 1 and 25 months after presentation. Only a single patient remained disease free at 5 years. On the other hand, of 29 patients initially treated with the therapy typically prescribed for acute myelogenous leukemia (AML), only 33% ever went on to develop AML. Of the nine children in this subgroup, four had primary extramedullary leukemia of the orbit.

The Byrd series also looked specifically at children 16 years of age and younger who presented with AML and extramedullary leukemia. The most common site of extramedullary leukemia in this group was found to be the orbit, though most cases were reported from Turkey and India. In these regions of the world, orbital granulocytic sarcoma may present in as many as 30% of the pediatric patients with AML.[32,33]

In a limited institution retrospective review in South Africa, 15 of 88 children with AML had granulocytic sarcoma at presentation; 2 of the 15 were diagnosed with primary extramedullary leukemia. The orbit was the site of extramedullary disease in 9 of 15 cases. All of the patients were treated for systemic AML on BFM (Berlin–Frankfurt–Münster), POG, or CCSG protocols. Overall, 8 patients had long-term disease-free survival, and 5 of the 9 patients with orbital presentations were long-term disease-free survivors. These numbers were significantly better than the disease-free survival seen in patients who had AML without granulocytic sarcoma, which was about 30%.[34]

As long as patients with granulocytic sarcoma are treated with appropriate AML-type therapy, the presence of extramedullary disease does not seem to adversely affect outcome and may confer an advantage.[35] The exact role of local irradiation, however, remains somewhat controversial. Since AML therapy in pediatrics is constantly being refined, specific recommendations cannot be made. These patients deserve the full benefit of large multi-institutional controlled clinical trials and should be immediately referred to a pediatric oncologist.

MALIGNANT TUMORS WITH DISTANT ORBIT METASTASES

Neuroblastoma

The majority of children with neuroblastoma present with stage IV disease, with bone and bone marrow being the most common sites of distant spread. Neuroblastoma has a peculiar predilection for facial bones, and initial presentation with "raccoon eyes," bilateral or unilateral periorbital ecchymoses, is fairly common. The ecchymoses are due to hemorrhage related to tumor invading the orbital bones. Neuroblastoma is the most common metastatic tumor of this age group to invade the orbit and cause proptosis and other findings of a space-occupying lesion. The tumor may extend into the intracranial vault.

These stage IV patients have a fairly grim prognosis, with long-term disease-free survivals reportedly between 10 and 40%. Interestingly, however, neuroblastoma is one of the lesions most responsive to chemotherapy, and even very large tumors may "melt" in the face of appropriate chemotherapy. Most stage IV patients will actually enter complete remission, only to subsequently relapse and die from the disease.

The major strategy for treatment of this disease has been (1) treatment with intensive chemotherapy, (2) local control with both surgery and radiation, (3) high-dose chemotherapy with autologous stem cell transplantation, and (4) biotherapy, especially with *cis*-retinoic acid. More recently immunotherapy has begun to make an impact on the outcome of neuroblastoma.

One of the primary goals of chemotherapy is to reduce the tumor burden, which may be considerable. In addition, initial chemotherapy may render resectable an initially unresectable tumor. Finally, since bone marrow is so commonly involved in patients with neuroblastoma, the initial chemotherapy may lead to improvement of or resolution of bone marrow involvement, thus making harvesting of either bone marrow or peripheral blood stem cells feasible.

Local control refers not only to the primary tumor site but also to metastatic sites, including the orbits. While intra-abdominal sites are typically resected (and irradiated), the orbital bony disease is not amenable to this approach, and radiation therapy is the preferred method of control. Neuroblastoma not only is sensitive to a variety of chemotherapeutic agents, it is also quite radiosensitive, and doses in the order of 2100 to 2400 cGy are typically used.

High-dose chemotherapy with autologous stem cell transplant has been shown by some, but not all studies, to lead to improved long-term disease-free survival. In a well-conceived and well-executed phase III trial by the CCG, children with stage IV neuroblastoma (and certain other high-risk neuroblastoma patients) were randomly assigned to either ongoing chemotherapy or high-dose chemotherapy with autologous stem cell rescue. Patients randomized to transplant did better, with a 3-year event-free survival of 34% vs 22%, on an intent-to-treat basis.[36]

In the same CCG study, patients were also randomized between posttreatment *cis*-retinoic acid and no *cis*-retinoic acid. Patients received either ongoing chemotherapy and no *cis*-retinoic acid, ongoing chemotherapy with *cis*-retinoic acid, transplant and no *cis*-retinoic acid, or transplant with *cis*-retinoic acid. Patients who received *cis*-retinoic acid did better than those who were not thus treated, and patients treated with stem cell transplant and *cis*-retinoic acid fared the best.

cis-Retinoic acid can induce neuroblastoma cells to differentiate. Another retinoid, fenretinoid, has been shown to induce apoptosis in neuroblastoma cells and may provide a more effective therapy than *cis*-retinoic acid.

Current studies are evaluating the relative roles of (1) rapid vs slower remission induction, (2) purged vs nonpurged autologous stem cells prior to transplant, (3) newer chemotherapeutic agents, (4) immune modulation and tumor vaccines, and (5) tandem stem cell transplants.

Ewing Tumors

The Ewing family of tumors includes Ewing's sarcoma, peripheral primitive neuroectodermal tumor (PPNET), and Askins tumor of the chest wall. The primary difference between Ewing's sarcoma and PPNET is the degree of histologic differentiation, with Ewing's sarcoma being very poorly differentiated and PPNET demonstrating some neural differentiation. These two tumors share a common translocation t(11;22). Rare alternative splicing sites that join with the 22q12 (*EWS* gene) have been described, especially t(21;22). These tumors seem to behave similarly to chemotherapy, though there have been fewer studies of PPNETs than of Ewing's.

Orbital Ewing's or PPNET may present as primary disease, though this is very rare. More commonly, if the orbit is involved, it is within the context of metastatic or relapsed disease.

In general, Ewing's/PPNET is a systemic disease, and chemotherapy is a cornerstone of treatment. Chemotherapy regimens that incorporate multiple drugs are the standard. Agents that have been particularly helpful include vincristine, doxorubicin, cyclophosphamide, etoposide, ifosfamide, and actinomycin D. High-dose chemotherapy with stem cell rescue has had some modest success in patients with relapsed disease.

Control of the local disease is essential. In children, surgical resection with appropriate margins is encouraged because radiation therapy has so many side effects in growing children. However, this tumor is radiosensitive, and local high-dose radiation is considered adequate and appropriate for local control.

Wilms Tumor

Wilms tumor is one of the most common tumors of childhood. In the past 35 years, the outlook in children having this tumor has improved from 60% long-term disease-free survival to 90% of children expected to be cured of this disease. Metastases are typically to the lung, to the liver, or via contiguous spread. The orbit is a distinctly rare site of metastatic Wilms tumor.[37–39]

There are no studies at all addressing the orbit as a specific site of disease in Wilms tumor. However, agents active in other sites include vincristine, actinomycin D, and doxorubicin. Etoposide, carboplatin, and ifosfamide are the most frequently used agents used for refractory or relapsed disease. Radiation therapy plays a major role in the complete management of metastatic Wilms tumor.

MALIGNANT TUMORS WITH SECONDARY INVASION OF THE ORBIT

Retinoblastoma

Most retinoblastomas in the United States are diagnosed while still contained within the globe, and treatment of intraocular retinoblastoma is not discussed in this chapter. Orbital retinoblastoma may be primary (present at diagnosis) or secondary (present at relapse). Historically, the presence of orbital retinoblastoma was a very poor prognostic feature, with 20 to 25% long-term disease-free survival.[40,41]

In a very small series of patients from St. Jude's, single-agent chemotherapy with cyclophosphamide or ifosfamide (or other single agents) in relapsed or primary orbital retinoblastoma was shown to have minimal effect on tumor growth, whereas combination chemotherapy with vincristine and cyclophosphamide was more effective.[42]

A 1990 report from the United Kingdom noted that 5 children with orbital recurrence of retinoblastoma remained disease-free at 8 months to 7 years after combined treatment with surgery, local radiation therapy, and vincristine plus cyclophosphamide or vincristine, cisplatin, etoposide, and cyclophosphamide (OPEC).[43] These 5 patients are compared with another group of 9 patients treated with surgery and radiation therapy, all of whom failed with distant and/or local recurrence.

In India, 8 patients with advanced primary or relapsed retinoblastoma (including 6 with orbital involvement) were treated with combination cyclophosphamide, Adriamycin, cisplatin, and etoposide for two or three 75-day cycles. All patients had a complete response after the first cycle, though 3 patients subsequently relapsed, 2 died of toxicity, and 3 were still on treatment at the time of publication.[44]

French investigators reported a 17-year experience with chemotherapy and orbital disease.[45] They treated 33 patients between 1977 and 1991 with various combinations of chemotherapy with and without radiation therapy, and with and without surgery. From 1977 to 1985, the chemotherapeutic agents included cyclophosphamide, vincristine, dactinomycin, doxorubicin, teniposide, lomustine, and procarbazine. After 1985, therapy included combinations of cyclophosphamide, doxorubicin, and vincristine (CADO), cisplatin and teniposide (PE), and carboplatin and etoposide. Some patients were treated with intrathecal chemotherapy, and 7 patients went on for high-dose chemotherapy with autologous bone marrow transplantation. Twelve of 33 patients remain disease-free 2 months to 11.5 years after treatment. The authors note an improvement in outcome in patients treated after 1985. Dose intensity increased after 1985, and the authors suggest that this accounts for the improved outcome. Consistent with this notion, 5 of 6 patients treated with a uniform bone marrow transplant regimen (carboplatin, etoposide, and cyclophosphamide) were long-term disease-free survivors.

In Argentina, Schvartzman and coworkers treated patients with retinoblastoma based upon stage. This included 29 patients with orbital involvement. Patients were treated with cyclophosphamide (20 mg/kg), vincristine (0.05 mg/kg), and doxorubicin (0.67 mg/kg) every 3 weeks for eight courses. In the induction course there was a higher dose of cyclophosphamide (40 mg/kg). After the eight courses, cyclophosphamide (30 mg/kg) and vincristine (0.05 mg/kg) were continued every 3 weeks for another 12 courses. In addition, patients had initial surgery, local radiation, and intrathecal chemotherapy, if appropriate. Twenty-five of 29 patients so treated were long-term disease-free survivors, with all events occurring within the first 12 months.[46]

The combination of etoposide (160 mg/m^2/day for 5 days) and carboplatin (160 mg/m^2 for 5 days) was piloted in a phase II trial in France for patients with extraocular retinoblastoma. Seventeen of 20 patients had a complete or partial remission. All patients subsequently went on to receive additional chemotherapy, including bone marrow transplantation in 14 of the patients. Of 6 patients with orbit disease, 4 had an initial partial remission, and 4 had no evidence of disease at 10 to 50 months of follow-up.[47]

Idarubicin is an anthracycline [like doxorubicin (Adriamycin)] with improved CNS penetration and a prolonged half-life. Idarubicin was used in a phase II window in patients with extraocular retinoblastoma. The initial dose of 15 mg/m^2/day for 2 days was found to be too toxic, and subsequent courses used 10 mg/m^2/day for 2 days. Following two 2-day courses, 6 of 10 patients had complete or partial remission.[48]

Chantada et al. updated the Argentina series in 2003.[49] The patients treated after 1994 received alternating courses of cyclophosphamide (65 mg/kg), vincristine (0.05 mg/kg), and idarubicin (10 mg/m^2) with carboplatin (18.7 mg/kg) twice and etoposide (3.3 mg/kg) three times. Each course was given four times, for a total of eight courses of chemotherapy. Including patients treated both before[46] and after[49] 1994, the researchers found an 84% 5-year event-free survival for patients with orbital or orbital and preauricular nodal involvement (no CNS or other metastatic involvement). The number of patients was too small to permit the evaluation of the relative merits of the two treatment regimens.

Patients with hereditary, bilateral retinoblastoma represent a special population (see Chapter 5). These children have a constitutional absence—either a mutation[50] or deletion[51–53]—of one of the copies of the *Rb1* gene. This gene encodes for a tumor suppressor, pRB, and loss of functioning pRB protein has been implicated in growth of a number of tumor types[54–57] in addition to retinoblastoma. The incidence of multiple primary malignancies in patients who survived childhood hereditary retinoblastoma has been measured to be between about 4 and 25% at 10 to 30 years, respectively, after retinoblastoma treatment.[58–63] The increase in second malignant neoplasms is greatest for those with hereditary (bilateral) retinoblastoma who have received radiation therapy.[64,65]

A reasonable concern might arise regarding the risk of second malignant neoplasms in survivors of hereditary retinoblastoma who are treated with chemotherapy. Are they also at increased risk of second malignancies in the same way as those treated with radiation therapy? Children with intraocular retinoblastoma who have been treated with chemotherapy as primary therapy have been followed for development of second malignant neoplasms. Thus far, their risk seems to be *decreased* compared with patients treated with primary enucleation and radiation therapy.[66] However, the final answer to this intriguing question is not yet in.

In summary, the child with orbital extension of retinoblastoma presents a challenge to the ophthalmologist, as well as to the pediatric oncologist. Multimodality therapy seems to be the most promising course, though further refinement is needed. While all children who have had orbital retinoblastoma require careful ocular and oncologic follow-up, this is especially true for the child with bilateral, hereditary retinoblastoma.

Optic Nerve Glioma

Optic nerve glioma is commonly associated with neurofibromatosis type 1 (see Chapters 7 and 17). This tumor may grow very slowly over many years. Thus, in the absence of visual compromise, observation without therapy is the rule. Treatment is generally reserved for children with evidence of progression of disease or those for whom vision is felt to be threatened if the tumor enlarges at all. In the absence of vision, the tumor and affected optic nerve may be resected, rather than attempting either radiation or chemotherapy. Older children may be treated with definitive radiation therapy, but since radiation is so detrimental to the developing central nervous system, chemotherapy is typically the initial treatment modality in small children with progressing optic nerve glioma. The goal is to slow growth of the tumor, to preserve vision, and to delay radiation therapy as long as possible—ideally until the child is older than 5 years.

In 1991 Petronio et al. reported a small study of 18 patients with progressive optic nerve glioma who were treated with a five-drug regimen consisting of vincristine, CCNU, [*N*-(2-chloroethyl)-*N*′-cyclohexyl-*N*-nitrosourea], 6-thioguanine, procarbazine, and dibromodulcitol. Vision stabilized or improved in 16 of 18 patients.[67] Packer et al. subsequently showed that the combination of carboplatin and vincristine could effectively stabilize disease in young children with progressive optic nerve glioma.[68] The POG treated children younger than 5 years of age who had progressive optic nerve glioma with repeated courses of carboplatin. Thirty-nine of 50 children (78%) had stabilization or improvement in their disease.[69]

Esthesioneuroblastoma

Esthesioneuroblastoma is an exceedingly rare malignant tumor of the nasal sinuses and olfactory tract.[70] This entity is also known as olfactory neuroblastoma or olfactory neuroepithelioma. The tumor may extend locally to invade the orbit. There have been no randomized controlled studies to evaluate the relative merits of various chemotherapy regimens in the treatment of esthesioneuroblastoma, and at least one author believes that this sort of trial may never take place owing to the rarity of this disease.[71] Several groups have combined surgery and radiation therapy with cisplatin plus etoposide with some success.[72,73]

In a retrospective review of the Mayo Clinic experience, 10 patients with advanced esthesioneuroblastoma were treated with various chemotherapy regimens over a 25-year period. The authors noted that patients with high-grade tumors were more likely to respond to chemotherapy than those with low-grade tumors. However, survival was better for those with low-grade tumors.[74]

In patients with relapsed metastatic esthesioneuroblastoma, Chamberlain noted a modest response to treatment with combination radiation therapy and vincristine, carboplatin, and lomustine. Four of 6 patients had partial responses lasting a median of 9 months.[75]

In a study of 34 patients with esthesioneuroblastoma treated at the University of Virginia over an 18-year period, 16 patients received neoadjuvant chemotherapy consisting mostly of cyclophosphamide and vincristine. The authors noted an apparent improved survival for patients with disease that was chemotherapy sensitive, compared with those who had no decrease in tumor size with chemotherapy.[76]

The usefulness of chemotherapy in the overall management of esthesioneuroblastoma, however, has not clearly been established.[77] Perhaps the best use of chemotherapy will be within the context of appropriate radiation therapy and surgery. It seems likely that the only way to answer these questions appropriately will be within the context of a large cooperative group study.

NONMALIGNANT TUMORS

Hemangioma

Hemangiomas are a very common neoplasm in childhood, occurring in about 12% of children by the age of one year.[78] Typically, the tumors are small (or even absent) at birth, enlarge for the first 1 to 2 years, and then regress over the next 5 to 8 years.[79] Hemangiomas are especially common in the head and neck, and orbital involvement may lead to nerve impingement, ocular displacement, or visual obstruction and amblyopia.

Steroids have long been the mainstay of treatment. The steroids may be given systemically, injected intralesionally, or applied topically. Systemic steroids have been used at various doses. Sadan and Wolach treated 60 infants with either 3 or 5 mg/kg/day of prednisone. They noted that there were significantly more "excellent" responses in the high-dose group than in the lower dose group.[80] Both lower and higher doses of various corticosteroids have been reported.[81,82]

Intralesional corticosteroid injections have been used with significant success[83,84] and may be combined with systemic steroid administration.[85] Even topical steroid therapy has been used, though the response may not be rapid enough to eliminate visual sequellae.[86,87]

Many anecdotal reports of the use of interferon alfa-2a were followed by a series of 20 children with threatening hemangiomas, including three that were in the periorbital region.[88] Overall, 18 of 20 patients did well, including 2 of 3 patients with periorbital lesions. The dose of interferon was 1 million to 3 million U/m^2/day given subcutaneously.

Fifteen children with head and neck hemangiomas were treated with recombinant interferon alfa-2b at the University of Minnesota.[89] Six of the children had involvement of the orbit or eyelid. Patients were eligible for study if they had hemangiomas leading to deleterious physiologic effects, functional compromise, or severe cosmetic disfigurement. Patients received 3 million U/m^2/day of interferon alfa-2b (dosing was twice a day if the patient had severe thrombocytopenia or bleeding disorder). After 6 months, the dose was decreased to 3 times a week, and after another 6 months the drug was stopped unless there were ongoing symptoms. Major or partial responses were seen in 12 of 15 patients, and 10 patients were able to come off treatment without recurrence. Side effects were mild and self-limiting.

Hastings et al. studied 40 children with orbit or eyelid hemangiomas that were unresponsive to systemic steroid therapy.[90] These children received 3 million U/m^2 of interferon alfa-2b daily for 3 months and then tapered as tolerated. All lesions demonstrated significant reduction in size. Five of 15 patients had moderate amblyopia, though those patients were treated at a relatively later age than patients with no visual sequelae.

Chemotherapy[82,91,92] and radiation[82] therapy have been used for life-threatening hemangiomas with some success but cannot be recommended as frontline therapy.

Histiocytosis

Langerhans cell histiocytosis (LCH) may present either focally or diffusely or with multiple organ involvement. The orbit may be involved as a single site or as one of several sites (see Chapter 15). If the lesion is not causing any loss in function, observation may be warranted, and spontaneous regression may occur. In the event of orbital involvement, however, there is concern that vision may be compromised. While there are numerous case reports[93–95] and some small series, there are no formal studies of treatment for orbital histiocytosis.

Moore et al. noted 18 of 76 (24%) children with histiocytosis X had orbital involvement.[96] Several of the patients had spontaneous regression of their disease, though most were treated with some form of chemotherapy.

In a larger series of patients reported by Kilpatrick et al.,[97] 18 of 172 pediatric patients with LCH of bone had proptosis. Interestingly, within the entire group of 172 pediatric patients, 14 died of disease, and 6 of these had proptosis, suggesting that orbital involvement may be indicative of relatively aggressive disease. It is not clear how many of these patients also had more disseminated disease, since the entity known as Hand–Schuller–Christian disease (osteolytic lesions, diabetes insipidis, and exophthalmos) is only rarely fatal.

There is no single standard medical therapy for the treatment of Langerhans cell histiocytosis. A number of agents have been used with varying degrees of success, including systemic steroids, intralesional steroids,[98] vinblastine,[99] etoposide,[99,100] local irradiation,[101,102] 2-chlorodeoxyadenosine (cladribine, 2-CdA), other chemotherapies,[103] or various combinations of these agents.

Maarten Egeler et al.[104] reported 18 patients with either recurrent multifocal or extensive/systemic LCH that required treatment. They treated their patients with cytosine arabinoside, prednisolone, and vincristine. Of the 18 patients, two died of their disease despite aggressive therapy; both patients who died had systemic involvement with organ involvement.

Ceci et al. reported the results of a large, multicenter cooperative trial for the treatment of children with LCH.[105] This trial utilized a sequential approach: good-prognosis patients were successively treated with immunotherapy ("thymic extract") followed by vinblastine, doxorubicin, then etoposide. Each new agent was begun only if the patient did not respond to the previous agent. Poor-prognosis patients were treated with combination chemotherapy (prednisone, vincristine, cyclophosphamide, and doxorubicin) up front. Of the good-prognosis patients, only 10% of those treated with immunotherapy had a complete response, whereas 63% of those treated with vinblastine and 88% of those treated with etoposide had a complete response. Results with doxorubicin were intermediate. Only 18% of patients with poor prognosis responded to the multiagent regimen. This group concluded that etoposide resulted in the best response rate, but that the best therapy for LCH was not known.

More recently, the Histiocyte Society directly compared etoposide with vinblastine for the treatment of LCH.[106] One hundred forty-three children were treated with high-dose methylprednisolone, along with either etoposide (150 mg/m^2 for 3 days every 3 weeks) or vinblastine (6 mg/m^2 weekly). Both groups were treated for 24 weeks. Overall, 62% of the children had a response to therapy with no significant differences between the groups. This outcome was felt to be remarkably good, considering that many of these children had multisystem disease with organ dysfunction and were believed likely to have a poor prognosis without multiagent therapy. Also of note, patients with a rapid early response had a better outcome than did those with poor early response. The follow-up study, LCH-II, is comparing initial treatment with two versus three agents.

In summary, the manifestations of Langerhans cell histiocytosis remain protean, with orbital involvement seen in a significant percentage of patients. The correct therapy remains elusive, and a number of agents have been used with some success. Progress has been made; however, real improvement will come only with time and a concerted effort to enter children with this rare disease in cooperative trials.

CONCLUSIONS

Orbital tumors are rare events in children. The treatments for many, if not all of these tumors are works in progress, and conclusions that are true today may not hold up, even in the near future. The standard of care for children with cancer is to be treated as part of a clinical study whenever possible. Therefore, when a child presents to the ophthalmologist with a potential malignancy, it is crucial that the pediatric oncologist be notified as soon as possible. Coordination of sample collection, pathologic evaluation, staging, and treatment is a team effort. This team approach has produced fantastic progress in both ocular outcome and overall survival in merely the past 40 years. As we continue to work together, the outlook for children with orbital tumors can only improve.

References

1. Smith MA, Gloeckler Reis LA. In: Pizzo PA, Poplack DG, eds. *Principles and Practices of Pediatric Oncology*. 4th ed. Philadelphia: Lippincott, Williams & Wilkins; 2002.
2. Rootman J. In: Rootman J, ed. *Diseases of the Orbit: A Multidisciplinary Approach*. Philadelphia: JB Lippincott; 1988: 124.
3. Shields JA, Blakewell B, Augsburger JJ, et al. Space-occupying orbital masses in children. A review of 250 consecutive biopsies. *Ophthalmology* 1986;93:379–384.
4. Gurney JG, Young JL Jr, Roffers SD, et al. Soft tissue sarcomas. In: Ries LAG, Smith MA, Gurney JG, et al, eds. *Cancer Incidence and Survival Among Children and Adolescents: United States SEER Program 1975–1995. National Cancer Institute SEER Program.* National Institutes of Health Publication No 99-4649. Bethesda, MD: NIH; 1999:111.
5. Mauer HM, Gehan EA, et al. The Intergroup Rhabdomyosarcoma Study—II. *Cancer* 1993;71:1904–1922.
6. Wexler LH, Crist WM, Helman LJ. Rhabdomyosarcoma and the undifferentiated sarcomas. In: Pero PA, Poplack DG, eds. *Principles and Practices of Pediatric Oncology*. 4th ed. Philadelphia: Lippincott, Williams & Wilkins; 2002:939–971.
7. Jones IS, Reese AB, Krout J. Orbital rhabdomyosarcoma: an analysis of sixty-two cases. *Trans Am Ophthalmol Soc* 1965; 63:223–255.
8. Frayer WC, Enterline HT. Embryonal rhabdomyosarcoma of the orbit in children and young adults. *Arch Ophthalmol* 1959;62:203.
9. Sagerman RH, Cassady JR, Tretter P. Radiation therapy for rhabdomyosarcoma of the orbit. *Trans Am Acad Ophthalmol Otol* 1968;72:849–854.
10. Aviles E. Rhabdomyosarcoma of the orbit. *Int Surg* 1974; 59:297–299.
11. Abramson DH, Ellsworth RM, Tretter P., et al. The treatment of orbital rhabdomyosarcoma with irradiation and chemotherapy. *Ophthalmology*, 1979;86:1330–1335.
12. Jereb B, Haik BG, et al. Parameningeal rhabdomyosarcoma (including the orbit): results of orbital irradiation. *Int J Radiat Oncol Biol Phys* 1985;11:2057–2065.
13. Sutow WW, Lindberg RD, Gehan EA, et al. Three-year relapse-free survival rates in childhood rhabdomyosarcoma of the head and neck. Report from the Intergroup Rhabdomyosarcoma Study. *Cancer* 1982;49:2217.
14. Heyn R, Ragab A, Raney B, et al. Late effects of therapy in orbital rhabdomyosarcoma in children. A report from the Intergroup Rhabdomyosarcoma Study. *Cancer* 1986;57:1738.
15. Maurer HM, Beltangady M, Gehan EA, et al. The Intergroup Rhabdomyosarcoma Study—I. A final report. *Cancer* 1988; 61:209.

16. Wharan MD, Hanfelt JJ, Tefft MC, et al. Radiation therapy for rhabdomyosarcoma: local failure risk for clinical group III patients on Intergroup Rhabdomyosarcoma Study II. *Int J Radiat Oncol Biol Phys* 1997;4:797.
17. Heyn R, Haeberlen V, Newton WA, et al. Second malignant neoplasms in children treated for rhabdomyosarcoma. *J Clin Oncol* 1993;11:262.
18. Crist W, Gehan EA, Ragab AH, et al. The Third Intergroup Rhabdomyosarcoma Study. *J Clin Oncol* 1995;13:610.
19. Crist WM, Anderson JR, Meza JL, et al. Intergroup Rhabdomyosarcoma Study IV: results on patients with nonmetastatic disease. *J Clin Oncol* 2001;19:3091.
20. Meadows AT, Sposto R, et al. Similar efficacy of 6 and 18 months of therapy with four drugs (COMP) for localized non-Hodgkin's lymphoma of children: a report from the Children's Cancer Study Group. *J Clin Oncol* 1989;7:92–99.
21. Patte C, Philip T, et al. High survival rate in advanced stage B cell lymphomas and leukemias without CNS involvement with a short intensive polychemotherapy. Results of a randomized trial from the French Pediatric Oncology Society (SFOP) on 216 children. *J Clin Oncol* 1991;9:123.
22. Suryanarayan K, Schuster JJ, et al. Treatment of localized primary non-Hodgkin's lymphoma of bone in children: a Pediatric Oncology Group study. *J Clin Oncol* 1999;17: 456–459.
24. Link MP, Schuster JJ, et al. Treatment of children and young adults with early stage non-Hodgkin's lymphoma. *N Engl J Med* 1997;337:1259–1266.
24. Link MP, Donaldson SS, et al. Results of treatment of childhood localized non-Hodgkin's lymphoma with combination chemotherapy with or without radiotherapy. *N Engl J Med* 1990;322:1169–1174.
25. Anderson J, Wilson J, et al. Childhood non-Hodgkin's lymphoma. The results of a randomized therapeutic trial comparing a 4-drug regimen (COMP) with a 10-drug regimen (LSA_2L_2). *N Engl J Med* 1983;308:559.
26. Anderson J, Jenkin D, et al. Long-term follow-up of patients treated with COMP or LSA_2L_2 therapy for childhood non-Hodgkin's lymphoma: a report of CCG-551 from the Children's Cancer Group. *J Clin Oncol* 1993;11:1024.
27. Patte C, Philip T, et al. Improved survival rate in children with stage III and IV B cell NHL and leukemia using a multiagent chemotherapy: results of a study of 114 children from SFOP. *J Clin Oncol* 1986;4:1219.
28. Sullivan MP, Ramirez I. Curability of Burkitt's lymphoma with high dose cyclophosphamide, high dose methotrexate therapy and intrathecal chemoprophylaxis. *J Clin Oncol* 1985;3:627.
29. Patte C, Kalifa C, et al. Results of the LMT81 protocol, a modified LSA_2L_2 protocol with high dose methotrexate, on 84 children with non-B-cell (lymphoblastic) lymphoma. *Med Pediatr Oncol* 1992;20:105.
30. Menasce LP, Banerjee SS, et al. Extra-medullary myeloid tumor (granulocytic sarcoma) is often misdiagnosed: a study of 26 cases. *Histopathology* 1999;34:391–398.
31. Byrd JC, Edenfield J, et al. Extramedullary myeloid cell tumors in acute nonlymphoblastic leukemia: a clinical review. *J Clin Oncol* 1995;13:1800.
32. Cavdar AO, Babacan E, Grözdasoglu S, et al. High risk subgroup of acute myelomonocytic leukemia with orbito-ocular granulocytic sarcoma in Turkish children. *Acta Haematol* 1989;81:80–85.
33. Shome DK, Gupta NK, Prajapati NC, et al. Orbital granulocytic sarcomas in acute nonlymphoblastic leukemia. *Cancer* 1992;70:2298–2301.
34. Schwyer R, Sherman GG, et al. Granulocytic sarcoma in children with acute myeloblastic leukemia and t(8;21). *Med Pediatr Oncol* 1998;31:144.
35. Felice MS, Zubizarreta PA, et al. Good outcome of children with acute myeloid leukemia and t(8;21)(q22;q22), even when associated with granulocytic sarcoma. A report from a single institution in Argentina. *Cancer* 2000;88:1939–1944.
36. Matthay KK, Villablanca JG, et al. Treatment of high risk neuroblastoma with intensive chemotherapy, radiotherapy, autologous bone marrow transplant and 13-*cis*-retinoic acid. A Children's Cancer Group Study. *N Engl J Med* 1999;341:1165.
37. Apple DJ. Wilms' tumor metastatic to the orbit. *Arch Ophthalmol* 1968;80:480.
38. Fratkin JD, Purcell JJ, et al. Wilms' tumor metastatic to the orbit. *JAMA* 1977;238:1841.
39. Rowe S, Siegel S, Benedict W. Ophthalmologic manifestations of genitourinary diseases. *Urology* 1992;39:523.
40. Ellsworth RM. Treatment of retinoblastoma. *Am J Ophthalmol* 1968;66:49.
41. Hyman GA, Ellsworth RM, et al. Combination therapy in retinoblastoma. A 15-year summary of methods and results. *Arch Ophthalmol* 1968;80:744.
42. Pratt CB, Crom DB, Howarth C. The use of chemotherapy for extraocular retinoblastoma. *Med Pediatr Oncol* 1985;13: 330–333.
43. Goble RR, McKenzie J, et al. Orbital recurrence of retinoblastoma successfully treated by combined therapy. *Br J Ophthalmol* 1990;74:97–98.
44. Advani SH, Rao SR, et al. Pilot study of sequential combination chemotherapy in advanced and recurrent retinoblastoma. *Med Pediatr Oncol* 1994;22:125–128.
45. Doz F, Khelfaoui F, et al. The role of chemotherapy in orbital involvement of retinoblastoma. The experience of a single institution with 33 patients. *Cancer* 1994;74:722–732.
46. Schvartzman E, Chantada G, et al. Results of a stage-based protocol for the treatment of retinoblastoma. *J Clin Oncol* 1996;14:1532–1536.
47. Doz F, Neuenschwandwer S, et al. Etoposide and carboplatin in extraocular retinoblastoma: a study by the Société Française d'Oncologie Pédiatrique. *J Clin Oncol* 1995;13:902–909.
48. Chantada GL, Fandino A, et al. Phase II window of idarubicin in children with extraocular retinoblastoma. *J Clin Oncol* 1999;17:1847–1850.
49. Chantada G, Fandino A, et al. Treatment of overt extraocular retinoblastoma. *Med Pediatr Oncol* 2003;40:158–161.
50. Harbour JW. Overview of RB gene mutations in patients with retinoblastoma. Implications for clinical genetic screening. *Ophthalmology* 1998;105:1442–1447.
51. Ward P, Packman S, Loughman W, et al. Location of the retinoblastoma susceptibility gene(s) and the human esterase D locus. *J Med Genet* 1984;21:92–95.
52. Francke U. Retinoblastoma and chromosome 13. *Cytogenet Cell Genet* 1976;16:131–134.
53. Squire J, Gallie BL, Phillips RA. A detailed analysis of chromosomal changes in heritable and nonheritable retinoblastoma. *Hum Genet* 1985;70:291–301.
54. Eng C, Li FP, Abramson DH, et al. Mortality from second tumors among long-term survivors of retinoblastoma. *J Nat Cancer Inst* 1993;85:1121–1128.
55. Hansen MF, Koufos A, Gallie BL, et al. Osteosarcoma and retinoblastoma: a shared chromosomal mechanism revealing recessive predisposition. *Proc Natl Acad Sci U S A* 1985;82: 6216–6220.
56. Harbour JW, Lai S-L, Whang-Peng J, et al. Abnormalities in structure and expression of the human retinoblastoma gene in SCLC. *Science* 1988;241:353–357.
57. T'ang A, Varley JM, Chakraborty S, et al. Structural rearrangement of the retinoblastoma gene in human breast carcinoma. *Science* 1988;242:263–266.
58. DerKinderen DJ, Koten JW, Nagelkerke NJ, et al. Non-ocular cancer in patients with hereditary retinoblastoma and their relatives. *Int J Cancer* 1988;41:499–504.

59. Draper GJ, Sanders BM, Kingston JE, et al. Second primary neoplasms in patients with retinoblastoma. *Br J Cancer* 1986;53:661–671.
60. Leuder GT, Judisch F, O'Gorman TW. Second nonocular tumors in survivors of heritable retinoblastoma. *Arch Ophthalmol* 1986;104:372–373.
61. Desjardins L, Haye C, Schlienger P, et al. Second non-ocular tumors in survivors of bilateral retinoblastoma. A 30-year follow-up. *Ophthalmic Pediatr Genet* 1991;12:145–148.
62. Roarty JD, McLean IW, Zimmerman LE. Incidence of second neoplasms in patients with bilateral retinoblastoma. *Ophthalmology* 1988;95:1583–1587.
63. Karcioglu ZA, Al-Rasheed W, Gray AJ. Second malignant neoplasms in retinoblastoma. *Mid East J Ophthalmol* 1997;5:99–104.
64. Abramson DH, Ellsworth RM, Kitchin FD, et al. Second nonocular tumors in retinoblastoma survivors. Are they radiation induced? *Ophthalmology* 1984;91:1351–1355.
65. DeSutter E, Mesmer E, Hoepping H. Retinoblastoma: importance of time interval in onset of second tumors. *Bull Soc Belge Ophtalmol* 1986;213:27–40.
66. Shields CA, Shields JA, and Meadows AT. Chemoreduction for retinoblastoma may prevent trilateral retinoblastoma [letter]. *J Clin Oncol* 2000;18:236–237.
67. Petronio J, Edwards MS, et al. Management of chiasmal and hypothalamic gliomas of infancy and childhood with chemotherapy. *J Neurosurg* 1991;74:701.
68. Packer RJ, Ater J, et al. Carboplatin and vincristine chemotherapy for children with newly diagnosed progressive low-grade gliomas. *J Neurosurg* 1997;86:747.
69. Mahoney DH, Cohen ME, et al. Carboplatin is effective therapy for young children with progressive optic pathway tumors: a Pediatric Oncology Group phase II study. *Neurooncology* 2000;2:213.
70. Morita A, Ebersold MJ, Olsen KD, et al. Esthesioneuroblastoma: prognosis and management. *Neurosurgery* 1993;32:706–715.
71. Sheehan JM, Sheehan JP, Jane JA, et al. Chemotherapy for esthesioneuroblastomas. *Neurosurg Clin North Am* 2000;11:693–701.
72. Bhattacharyya N, Thornton AF, Joseph MP, et al. Successful treatment of esthesioneuroblastoma and neuroendocrine carcinoma with combined chemotherapy and proton radiation: results in 9 cases. *Arch Otolaryngol Head Neck Surg* 1997;123:34–40.
73. Resto VA, Eisele DW, Forastiere A, et al. Esthesioneuroblastoma: the Johns Hopkins experience. *Head Neck* 2000;22:550–558.
74. McElroy EA, Buckner JC, Lewis JE. Chemotherapy for advanced esthesioneuroblastoma: the Mayo Clinic experience. *Neurosurgery* 1998;42:1023–1027.
75. Chamberlain C. Treatment of intracranial metastatic esthesioneuroblastoma. *J Clin Oncol* 2002;20:357–358.
76. Polin RS, Sheehan JP, Chenelle AG, et al. The role of preoperative adjuvant treatment in the management of esthesioneuroblastoma: the University of Virginia experience. *Neurosurgery* 1998;42:1029–1037.
77. Dulguerov P, Allal AS, Calcaterra TC. Esthesioneuroblastoma: a meta-analysis and review. *Lancet Oncol* 2001;2:683–690.
78. Soumekh B, Adams GA, Shapiro RS. Treatment of head and neck hemangiomas with recombinant interferon alpha 2. *Ann Otol Rhinol Laryngol* 1996;105:201–206.
79. Mulliken JP. Diagnosis and natural history of hemangiomas. In: Mulliken JB, Young AE, eds. *Vascular Birthmarks: Hemangiomas and Malformations*. Philadelphia: WB Saunders; 1988:41–62.
80. Sadan N, Wolach B. Treatment of hemangiomas of infants with high doses of prednisone. *J Pediatr* 1996;128:141–146.
81. Ozsoylu S. Megadose methylprednisolone therapy for Kasabach–Merritt syndrome [letter]. *J Pediatr* 1996;129:947.
82. Stanley P, Geer GD, et al. Infantile hepatic hemangiomas. Clinical features, radiologic investigations, and treatment of 20 patients. *Cancer* 1989;64:936–949.
83. Kushner BJ. Intralesional corticosteroid injection for infantile adnexal hemangioma. *Am J Ophthalmol* 1982;93:496–506.
84. Kushner BJ. The treatment of periorbital infantile hemangioma with intralesional corticosteroid. *Plast Reconstr Surg* 1985;76:517–526.
85. Iwanaka T, Tsuchida Y, et al. Intralesional corticosteroid injection with short-term oral prednisolone for infantile hemangiomas of the eyelid and orbit. *J Pediatr Surg* 1994;29:482–486.
86. Elsas FJ, Lewis AR. Topical treatment of periocular capillary hemangioma. *J Pediatr Ophthalmol Strabismus* 1994;31:153–156.
87. Cruz OA, Zarnegar SR, et al. Treatment of periocular capillary hemangioma with topical clobetasol propionate. *Ophthalmology* 1995;102:2012–2015.
88. Ezekowitz RAB, Mullikin JB, Folkman J. Interferon alfa-2a therapy for life-threatening hemangiomas of infancy. *N Engl J Med* 1992;326:1456–1463.
89. Soumekh B, Adams GL, Shapiro RS. Treatment of head and neck hemangiomas with recombinant interferon alpha 2B. *Ann Otol Rhinol Laryngol* 1996;105:201–206.
90. Hastings MM, MJ Barsoum-Homsey, et al. Recombinant interferon alfa-2b in the treatment of vision-threatening capillary hemangiomas in childhood. *J Am Assoc Pediatr Ophthalmol Strabismus* 1997;1:226–230.
91. Payarols JP, Masferrer JP, Gomez C. Treatment of life-threatening infantile hemangiomas with vincristine [correspondence]. *New Engl J Med* 1995;333:69.
92. Hurvitz CH, Alkalay AL, et al. Cyclophosphamide therapy in life-threatening vascular tumors. *J Pediatr* 1986;109:360–363.
93. Stromberg JS, Wang AM, Huang TE, et al. Langerhans cell histiocytosis involving the sphenoid sinus and superior orbital fissure. *AJNR Am J Neuroradiol* 1995;16:964–967.
94. LaBorwit SE, Karesh JW, Hirschbein MJ, et al. Multifocal Langerhans cell histiocytosis involving the orbit. *J Pediatr Ophthalmol Strabismus* 1998;35:234–236.
95. Erly WK, Carmody RF, Dryden RM. Orbital histiocytosis X. *AJNR Am J Neuroradiol* 1995;16:1258–1261.
96. Moore AT, Pritchard J, Taylor DSI. Histiocytosis X: an ophthalmological review. *Br J Ophthalmol* 1985;69:7–14.
97. Kilpatrick SE, Wenger DE, Gilchrist GS, et al. Langerhans cell histiocytosis (histiocytosis X) of the bone. A clinicopathologic analysis of 263 pediatric and adult cases. *Cancer* 1995;76:2471–2484.
98. Egeler RM, Thompson RC. Intralesional infiltration of corticosteroids in localized Langerhans cell histiocytosis. *J Pediatr Orthop* 1992;12:811.
99. Ladisch S, Gadner H, et al. LCA-I: a randomized trial of etoposide vs. vinblastine in disseminated Langerhans cell histiocytosis. *Med Pediatr Oncol* 1994;23:107.
100. Ceci A, DeTerlizzi M, Colella R, et al. Etoposide in recurrent childhood Langerhans cell histiocytosis: an Italian cooperative study. *Cancer* 1988;62:2528–2531.
101. Gramatovici R, D'Angio GJ. Radiation therapy in soft tissue lesions in histiocytosis X (Langerhans cell histiocytosis). *Med Pediatr Oncol* 1988;16:259.
102. Selch MT, Parker RG. Radiation therapy in the management of Langerhans cell histiocytosis. *Med Pediatr Oncol* 1990;18:97.
103. Donadieu J, Thomas C, Brugueres L, et al, for the French Langerhans Cell Study Group. A multicenter retrospective

survey of Langerhans cell histiocytosis: 348 cases observed between 1983 and 1993. *Arch Dis Child* 1996;75:17–24.

104. Maarten Egeler R, de Kraker J, Voute PA. Cytosine-arabinoside, vincristine, and prednisolone in the treatment of children with disseminated Langerhans cell histiocytosis with organ dysfunction: experience at a single institution. *Med Ped Oncol* 1993;21:265–270.

105. Ceci A, de Terlizzi M, Colella R, et al. Langerhans cell histiocytosis in childhood: results from the Italian Cooperative AIEOP-CNR-H.X '83 study. *Med Pediatr Oncol* 1993;21:259–264.

106. Gadner H, Grois N, Arico M, et al. A randomized trial of treatment for multisystem Langerhans cell histiocytosis. *J Pediatr* 2001;138:728–734.

35

Chemotherapy for Adult Tumors

Matthew W. Wilson and Carlos Galindo-Rodriquez

The orbit contains a variety of tissues, including bone, striated and smooth muscles, peripheral and cranial nerves, fibrovascular adipose tissue and cartilage. The walls of the orbit are composed of seven bones, which lie adjacent to the paranasal sinuses and cranial cavity. Given its unique composition and location, the orbit may manifest a wide spectrum of disease that may be of primary origin, secondarily invasive, or a part of a more extensive systemic and inflammatory disorder. Comprehensive reviews of orbital diseases have been published.[1–6] Primary neoplasms and systemic and inflammatory disorders each account for roughly 30% of all orbital diseases, while secondary neoplasms and metastases account for roughly 10 and 4%, respectively.[1] This vast range of possible tumors lends itself to multimodality therapy. Radiation and surgery, where possible, are the mainstays of treatment; however, some diseases, such as those that are systemic and inflammatory, are best managed with chemotherapy. This chapter reviews the chemotherapeutic agents and their indications for usage in the treatment of orbital tumors as well as other diseases. The side effects and toxicities of each agent are reviewed at the end of the chapter. Because the literature contains numerous isolated case reports citing individual patients' responses to novel regimens, the focus is on representative established chemotherapeutic protocols.

INFLAMMATORY AND LYMPHOPROLIFERATIVE DISORDERS

Thyroid Eye Disease (Graves Disease)

Graves disease (GD) is an autoimmune disorder most commonly associated with hyperthyroidism but has been associated with both euthyroid and hypothyroid states. Lymphocytes infiltrate the orbit leading to deposition of mucopolysaccharides, glycosaminoglycans, and collagen. The resultant signs and symptoms of lid lag, exophthalmos, strabismus, and visual loss are well recognized. Management may include systemic immunosuppression, external beam radiation, and/or surgical decompression of the orbit. Strabismus and eyelid surgery may follow once the disease has become quiescent.[7]

Indications for immunosuppression vary, and it should be noted that owing to differences between the acute and the chronic phases of inflammation, not all patients with GD show a significant response. Patients with an acute lymphocytic infiltrate will respond to immunosuppression, whereas those with chronic fibrotic changes will not.[7] Thus, an accurate assessment of disease activity is needed.

Systemic corticosteroids are the most common immunosuppressants used in the treatment of GD. The exact mechanism by which these drugs decrease the orbital inflammation remains unclear; however, it most likely involves inhibiting the activity of T- and B-cell lymphocytes through a reduction in the recruitment of neutrophils, monocytes, and macrophages and subsequent reduction in the release of inflammatory mediators such as cytokines. This sequence ultimately would decrease the deposition of glycoaminoglycans by orbital fibroblasts.[8,9]

Patients who present with severe orbital inflammation and congestion with or without compressive optic neuropathy should be considered for corticosteroids. Oral prednisone (1.0–1.5 mg/kg) should be started for 7 to 10 days and subsequently tapered. In cases of severe visual loss, intravenous pulse methylprednisolone can be administered. Rapid improvement of signs and symptoms should occur; however, complete resolution is uncommon. Rebound of symptoms should be expected as the steroids are tapered and the dosage adjusted accordingly. Definitive therapy may ultimately be needed with orbital radiation and/or surgical decompression.[10,11]

Numerous side effects have been associated with prolonged use of corticosteroids. Most notably these include avascular necrosis of the hip, cataracts, cushingoid features, diabetes, glaucoma, hypertension, increased appetite, mood disturbances, osteoporosis, and gastric ulcers. Corticosteroid use should be limited to a few months. Agents that protect against osteoporosis and gastric irritation should be considered.

In addition to corticosteroids, cyclosporine, cyclophosphamide, and azathioprine have been used in patients who are resistant to or intolerant of steroids.[8] Of these, cyclosporine has been the most extensively

TABLE 35.1. Summary of Chemotherapeutic Agents Used in Orbital Disease.

Class	*Type of agent*	*Other names*	*Orbital disease*	*Clinical toxicity*
Alkylating agents	Nitrogen mustards	Cyclophosphamide (Cytoxan)	Thyroid eye disease Lymphoma Adenoid cystic carcinoma Sarcomas, Osteosarcoma	Nausea, vomiting, sterility; leukopenia; alopecia
		Ifosfamide	Sarcomas/Osteosarcoma Lymphoma	Nausea, vomiting, anorexia, leukopenia, nephrotoxicity, CNS disturbances
		Melphalan (L-phenylalanine)	Hepatatic metastases for uveal melanoma	Hematological toxicity
		Chlorambucil	Pseudotumor Lymphoma	Myelosuppressive activity
	Ethylenimines	Thiotepa	Conjunctival or corneal epithelial neoplasia	Myelosuppression, mucositis
	Nitrosoureas	Carmustine (BCNU)	Lymphoma Malignant melanoma	Delayed hematopoietic depression, nausea, vomiting, late renal and pulmonary effects
	Triazenes	Dacarbazine (DTIC)	Malignant melanoma Sarcomas/Osteosarcoma	Nausea, vomiting
Antimetabolites	Folic acid analogues	Methotrexate	Pseudotumor Rosai–Dorfman Osteosarcoma	Mucositis, myelosuppression, thrombocytopenia
	Pyrimidine analogues	Fluorouracil (5-FU)	Squamous cell carcinoma of head and neck Conjunctival or corneal neoplasia Adenoid cystic carcinoma	Anorexia, nausea, stomatitis, diarrhea
		Tegafur	Squamous cell carcinoma of head and neck	Anorexia, nausea, stomatitis, diarrhea
Natural products	*Vinca* alkaloids	Vincristine	Lymphoma Sarcomas/Osteosarcoma	Neurological manifestations
		Vinblastine	Rosai–Dorfman	Neurological manifestations
	Epipodophyllotoxins	Etoposide	Lymphoma Sarcoma	Leukopenia, nausea, vomiting, stomatitis, diarrhea myelosuppression
	Antibiotics	Dactinomycin (actinomycin D)	Lymphoma	Anorexia, nausea, vomiting
		Doxorubicin (Adriamycin)	Osteosarcoma Sarcoma Adenoid cystic carcinoma Basal cell carcinoma Squamous cell carcinoma Lymphoma	Myelosuppression, cardiomyopathy, alopecia
		Bleomycin	Lymphoma Adenoid cystic carcinoma	Significant cutaneous toxicity, pulmonary toxicity, nausea, vomiting
		Mitomycin C	Conjunctival and corneal dysplasia and neoplasia Conjunctival melanoma Primary acquired melanosis with atypia	Ocular surface irritation, myelosuppression, nausea, vomiting, diarrhea, dermatitis, fever and malaise

(continued)

TABLE 35.1. Summary of Chemotherapeutic Agents Used in Orbital Disease. (*continued*)

Class	*Type of agent*	*Other names*	*Orbital disease*	*Clinical toxicity*
	Taxoids	Docetaxel	Squamous cell carcinoma of head and neck	Myelosuppression, asthenia, nausea, vomiting, hepatotoxicity, parasthesias, allergic reaction
		Paclitaxel	Squamous cell carcinoma of head and neck	Myelosuppression, asthenia, nausea, vomiting, hepatotoxicity, parasthesias, allergic reaction
	Biological response modifiers	Interferon alfa	Basal cell carcinoma Squamous cell carcinoma Malignant melanoma	Flulike symptoms
		Interleukin 2	Malignant melanoma	Flulike symptoms, cardiotoxicity, gastrointestinal disorders, dyspnea, metabolic disorders, rash, leukopenia
		GM-CSF	Malignant melanoma	Flulike symptoms, gastrointestinal disorders, metabolic disorders, rash
Miscellaneous agents	Platinum coordination complexes	Cisplatin	Adenoid cystic carcinoma Sarcomas/Osteosarcoma Basal cell carcinoma Squamous cell carcinoma of head and neck	Peripheral neuropathy, renal toxicity, ototoxicity, nausea, vomiting
		Carboplatin	Adenoid cystic carcinoma Sarcomas/Osteosarcoma Basal cell carcinoma Squamous cell carcinoma of head and neck	Myelosuppression
	Substituted Urea	Urea	Conjunctiva and corneal dysplasia and neoplasia	Hematopoietic depression
	Immunosuppressive agents	Cyclosporine	Thyroid eye disease Pseudotumor	Nephrotoxicity, hypertension, hepatotoxicity, neurotoxicity, nausea, vomiting, diarrhea
		Azathioprine	Thyroid eye disease	Gastrointestinal disorder, leukopenia, thrombocytopenia
	Immune modulation	Dinitrochlorobenzene (DNCB)	Conjunctival and corneal dysplasia and neoplasia	Myelosuppression
	Corticosteroids	Prednisone, prednisolone	Thyroid eye disease Pseudotumor Lymphoma Rosai–Dorfman	Fluid and electrolyte abnormalities, hypertension, hyperglycemia, osteoporosis, myopathy, behavioral disturbances, cataracts, growth arrest, striae, ecchymoses, hirsutism
	Monoclonal antibodies	Infliximab	Pseudotumor	Septicemia, latent tuberculosis reactivation, optic neuritis, dymelinating disease
		Rituximab	Lymphoma	Interstitial pneumonitis, Stevens–Johnson disease, tumor lysis syndrome
		Cetuximab	Squamous cell carcinoma of head and neck	Fever, asthenia, transaminase elevation nausea, skin toxicity

fluorouracil, and tegafur. The predominant side effects of these drugs include myelosuppression, nausea, vomiting, and mucositis.

Vincristine is a *Vinca* alkaloid and has associated neurological side effects, such as paresthesias, neuritic pain, muscle weakness, ptosis, and diplopia. Etoposide is an epipodophyllotoxin. Its most common side effects are myelosuppression, alopecia, and gastrointestinal disturbances. Secondary acute myelogenous leukemia has been reported following chemotherapy with etoposide. Dactinomycin, doxorubicin, bleomycin, and mitomycin C are antibiotics. In toxicity profile, they are similar to the alkylating agents already discussed. Doxorubicin may cause a cardiomyopathy. Ventricular ejection may be monitored during treatment to detect early cardiotoxicity. A reversible alopecia also occurs with doxorubicin. Bleomycin has been reported to cause pulmonary toxicity. Mitomycin C induces a severe myelosuppression and thus has limited utility for systemic administration. Topical mitomycin C is well tolerated when delivered onto an intact conjunctival and corneal epithelium. Reported side effects have been transient and resolved upon discontinuation of the drug. These include conjunctival injection, chemosis, epiphora, and punctate keratitis.[90–92,109,110] This is in contrast to earlier studies in which topical mitomycin C was applied to bare sclera, with a resultant scleral necrosis.[16,117] The taxoids docetaxel and paclitaxel are derivatives of the yew tree. Their principal toxicity is myelosuppression and a severe allergic reaction. The first dose of should be administered under close observation. Interferon-alfa, interleukin 2, and granulocyte colony-stimulating factor cause flulike symptoms that may be accompanied by a rash or metabolic abnormalities.

The platinum-coordinated complexes include cisplatin and carboplatin. Their most significant side effect is myelosuppression. Cisplatin, unlike carboplatin, is more likely to be associated with nephrotoxicity and ototocixity. Cyclosporine and azathioprine are immunosuppressive agents. Cyclosporine can cause nephrotocixity, neurotoxicity, and hepatoxicity, while azathioprine's most significant side effects are leukopenia and gastrointestinal distress.

Numerous side effects have been associated with prolonged use of corticosteroids. Most notably these include avascular necrosis of the hip, cataracts, cushingoid features, diabetes, glaucoma, hypertension, increased appetite, mood disturbances, osteoporosis, and gastric ulcers. Corticosteroid use should be limited to a few months. Agents that protect against osteoporosis and gastric irritation should be considered.

The monoclonal antibodies represent a new approach to chemotherapy, targeting specific cell surface markers in an attempt to maximize therapeutics and minimize toxicity. Infliximab, an inhibitor of tumor necrosis factor-α, has been associated with severe septicemia and reactivation of latent tuberculosis.[32,33,118,119] Rare cases of optic neuritis and exacerbation of demyelinating diseases have been reported in patients receiving infliximab.[120,121] Rituximab, an anti-CD20 monoclonal antibody, has been associated with hypersensitivity reactions resulting in interstitial pneumonitis and Stevens–Johnson syndrome.[122,123] Rapid cell death following administration may result in tumor lysis syndrome and acute renal failure.[124] Phase I to III trials with cetuximab, an antiepidermal growth factor receptor antibody, have reported fever, asthenia, transaminase elevation, nausea, and skin toxicities as the most adverse reactions.[87–89]

References

1. Wilson MW, Grossniklaus HE. Orbital disease in North America. *Ophthalmol Clin North Am* 1996;9:539–547.
2. Wilson MW, Buggage RR, Grossniklaus HE. Orbital lesions in the southeastern United States. *Orbit* 1996;24:17–24.
3. Henderson J. *Orbital Tumors*. 3rd ed. New York: BC Decker; 1994:43–51.
4. Kennedy RE. An evaluation of 829 orbital cases. *Trans Am Ophthalmol Soc* 1984;82:134–155.
5. Rootman J. *Diseases of the Orbit*. Philadelphia: JB Lippincott; 1988:119–139.
6. Shields JA, Bakewell B, Augsburger JJ, et al. Classification and incidence of space-occupying lesions of the orbit: a survey of 645 biopsies. *Arch Ophthalmol* 1984;102:1606–1611.
7. Gayre GS. Medical management of thyroid eye disease. In: Dutton JJ, Haik BG, eds. *Thyroid Eye Disease: Diagnosis and Treatment*. New York: Dekker; 2002:335–346.
8. Coday MP, Dallow RL. Managing Graves' orbitopathy. *Int Ophthalmol Clin* 1998;38:103–115.
9. Bartalena L, Marcocci C, Bogazzi F, et al. Glucocorticoid therapy of Graves' ophthalmopathy. *Exp Clin Endocrinol* 1991; 97:320–328.
10. Day RM, Carroll FD. Corticosteroids in the treatment of optic nerve involvement associated with thyroid dysfunction. *Trans Am Ophthalmol Soc* 1967;65:41–51.
11. Panzo GJ, Tomsak RL. A retrospective review of 26 cases of dysthyroid optic nerve neuropathy. *Am J Ophthalmol* 1988; 197:75–84.
12. Borel JF, Ryffel B. The mechanism of action of cyclosporin: continuing puzzle. In: Schindler R, ed. *Cyclosporin in Autoimmune Disease*. Berlin: Springer-Verlag; 1985:25–32.
13. Editorial. Cyclosporine in autoimmune disease. *Lancet* 1985; 1:909–911.
14. Weetman AP, Ludgate M, Mills PVB, et al. Cyclosporine improves Graves' ophthalmopathy. *Lancet* 1983;3:486–489.
15. Kahaly G, Schrezenmeir J, Krause U, et al. Cyclosporin and prednisone v. prednisone in the treatment of Graves' ophthalmology: a controlled, randomized and prospective study. *Eur J Clin Invest* 1986;16:415–422.
16. Prummel MF, Mourtis MP, Berghout A, et al. Prednisone and cyclosporine in the treatment of severe Graves' ophthalmopathy. *N Engl J Med* 1989;321:1353–1359.
17. Kahaly G. Nonsteroid immunosuppressants in endocrine orbitopathy. *Exp Clin Endocrinol* 1991;97:316–319.
18. Petros P, Weightman DR, Crobie AL, Kendall-Taylor P. Azathioprine in the treatment of thyroid associated ophthalmopathy. *Acta Endocrinol* 1990;122:8–12.
19. Mombaerts I, Schlingeman RO, Goldschmeding R, Koornneff L. Are corticosteroids useful in the management of orbital pseudotumor? *Ophthalmology* 1996;103:521–528.

20. Jakobiec FA. Orbital inflammation and lymphoid tumors. In: *Proceedings of the New Orleans Academy of Ophthalmology*. St Louis: CV Mosby; 1982:52–85.
21. Jakobiec FA, Jones IS. Orbital Inflammations. In: Jones IS, Jakobiec FA, eds. *Diseases of the Orbit*. Hagerstown, MD: Harper & Row; 1979:187–262.
22. Kennerdell JS, Dresner SC. The nonspecific orbital inflammatory syndromes. *Surv Ophthalmol* 1984;29:93–103.
23. Lanciano R, Fowble B, Sergott RC, et al. The results of radiotherapy for orbital pseudotumor. *Int J Radiat Oncol Biol Phys* 1990;18:407–411.
24. Donald SS, McDougall IR, Egbert PR, et al. Treatment of orbital pseudotumor (idiopathic orbital inflammation) by radiation therapy. *Int J Radiat Oncol Biol Phys* 1980;6:79–86.
25. Paris GL, Waltuch GF, Egbert PR. Treatment of refractory orbital pseudotumor with pulsed chemotherapy. *Ophthalmic Plast Reconstr Surg* 1990;6:96–101.
26. Eagle K, King A, Fisher C, Souhami R. Cyclophosphamide induced remission in relapsed, progressive idiopathic orbital inflammation ('pseudotumor'). *Clin Oncol R (R Coll Radiol)* 1995;7:402–404.
27. Garrity JA, Kennerdell JS, Johnson BL, Ellis LD. Cyclophosphamide in the treatment of orbital vasculitis. *Am J Ophthalmol* 1986;102:97–103.
28. Bielory L, Frohman LP. Low dose cyclosporine therapy of granulomatous optic neuropathy and orbitopathy. *Ophthalmology* 1991;98:1732–1736.
29. Diaz-Llopis M, Menezo JL. Idiopathic inflammatory orbital pseudotumor and low-dose cyclosporine. *Am J Ophthalmol* 1989;15:547–548.
30. Shah SS, Lowder CY, Schmitt MA, et al. Low-dose methotrexate therapy for ocular inflammatory disease. *Ophthalmology* 1992;99:1419–1423.
31. Smith JR, Levinson RD, Holland GN, et al. Differential efficacy of tumor necrosis factor inhibition in the management of inflammatory eye disease and associated rheumatic disease. *Arthritis Rheum* 2001;45:252–257.
32. Joseph A, Raj D, Dua HS, et al. Infliximab in the treatment of refractory posterior uveitis. *Ophthalmology* 2003;110: 1449–1453.
33. Jakobiec FA, Bilyk JR, Font RL. Orbit. In: Spencer WH, ed. *Ophthalmic Pathology: An Atlas and Textbook*. 4th ed. Philadelphia, WB Saunders; 1996:2686–2736.
34. McCormick SA, Milite JP. Lymphoproliferative disease of the orbit: a practical histopathologic approach to recognition, classification and therapy. *Ophthalmol Clin North Am* 693–704.
35. Gospodarowicz M, Tsang R. Mucosa-associated lymphoid tissue lymphomas. *Curr Oncol Rep* 2000;2:192–198.
36. Bairey O, Kremer I, Radowsky E, et al. Orbital and adnexal lymphoma in systemic non-Hodgkin's lymphoma. *Cancer* 1994;73:2395–2399.
37. Tranfa F, Di Matteo G, Strianese D, et al. Primary orbital lymphoma. *Orbit* 2001;20:119–124.
38. Antle CM, White VA, Horsman DE, Rootman J. Large cell lymphoma in patients with acquired immune deficiency syndrome. Case report and review. *Ophthalmology* 1990;97: 1494–1498.
39. Reifler DM, Warzynski MJ, Blount WR, et al. Orbital lymphoma associated with acquired immune deficiency syndrome (AIDS). *Surv Ophthalmol* 1994;38:371–380.
40. Leff SR, Shields JA, Augsburger JJ, et al. Unilateral eyelid, conjunctival, and choroids tumors as initial presentation of diffuse large-cell lymphomas. *Br J Ophthalmol* 1985;69:861–864.
41. Esmaeli B, Murray JL, Ahmadi MA, et al. Immunotherapy for low-grade non-Hodgkin secondary lymphoma of the orbit. *Arch Ophthalmol* 2002;120:1225–1227.
42. Cohen Y, Amir G, Rachmilewitz EA, Polliack A. Sustained complete remission following a combination of very low intensity chemotherapy with rituximab in an elderly patient with Burkitt's lymphoma. *Haemotologica* 2002;87:(01)ELT04.
43. Foucar E, Rosai J, Dorfman R. Sinus histiocytosis with massive lymphadenopathy (Rosai–Dorfman disease): review of the entity. *Semin Diagn Pathol* 1990;7:19–73.
44. Pulsoni A, Anghel G, Falcucci P, et al. Treatment of sinus histiocytosis with massive lymphadenopathy (Rosai–Dorfman disease): report of a case and literature review. *Am J Hematol* 2002;69:67–71.
45. Horneff G, Jürgens H, Hort W, et al. Sinus histiocytosis with massive lymphadenopathy (Rosai–Dorfman disease): response to methotrexate and mercaptopurine. *Med Pediatr Oncol* 1996;27:187–192.
46. Childs HA, Yim RY. Radiation response of Rosai–Dorfman disease presenting with involvement of the orbits. *Am J Clin Oncol* 1999;22:526–528.
47. Carbone A, Passannante A, Gloghini A, et al. Review of sinus histiocytosis with massive lymphadenopathy (Rosai–Dorfman disease) of head and neck. *Ann Otol Rhinol Laryngol* 1999;108:1095–1104.
48. Jakobiec FA, Bilyk JR, Font RL. Orbit. In: Spencer WH, ed. *Ophthalmic Pathology: An Atlas and Textbook*. 4th ed. Philadelphia: WB Saunders; 1996:2494–2509.
49. Font RL, Gamel JW. Adenoid cystic carcinoma of the lacrimal gland: a clinicopathologic study of 79 cases. In: Nicholson DH, ed. *Ocular Pathology Update*. New York: Masson; 1980:277–283.
50. Gamel JW, Font RL. Adenoid cystic carcinoma of the lacrimal gland: the clinical significance of a basaloid histologic pattern. *Hum Pathol* 1982;13:219–225.
51. Bartley GB, Harris GJ. Adenoid cystic carcinoma of the lacrimal gland: is there a cure . . . yet? *Ophthalmic Plast Reconstr Surg* 2002;18:315–318.
52. Meldrum ML, Tse DT, Benedetto P. Neoadjuvant intracarotid chemotherapy for treatment of advanced adenocystic carcinoma of the lacrimal gland. *Arch Ophthalmol* 1998;116: 315–321.
53. de Haan LD, de Mulder PH, Vermorken JB, et al. Cisplatin-based chemotherapy in advanced adenoid cystic carcinoma of the head and neck. *Head Neck* 1992;14:273–277.
54. Ikegawa A, Sida T, Obayashi H, et al. Cisplatin combination chemotherapy in squamous cell carcinoma and adenoid cystic carcinoma of the skin. *J Dermatol* 1989;16:227–230.
55. Petursson SR. Adenoid cystic carcinoma of the esophagus. Complete response to combination chemotherapy. *Cancer* 1986;57:1464–1467.
56. Budd GT, Groppe CW. Adenoid cystic carcinoma of the salivary gland. Sustained complete response to chemotherapy. *Cancer* 1983;51:589–590.
57. Skibba JL, Hurley JD, Ravelo HV. Complete response of a metastatic adenoid cystic carcinoma of the parotid gland to chemotherapy. *Cancer* 1981;47:2543–2548.
58. Antman KH, Eilber FR, Shiu MH. Soft tissue sarcomas: current trends in diagnosis and management. *Curr Probl Cancer* 1989;13:337–367.
59. Wall N, Starkhammar H. Chemotherapy of soft tissue sarcoma—a clinical evaluation of treatment over ten years. *Acta Oncol* 2003;42:55–61.
60. Hirano N, Sasaki A, Watanabe T, et al. Malignant fibrous histiocytoma of the lateral wall of the orbit. *Neurol Med Chir (Tokyo)* 1996;36:246–250.
61. Papai Z, Bodoky G, Szanto J, et al. The efficacy of a combination of etoposide, ifosfamide, and cisplatin in the treatment of patients with soft tissue sarcoma. *Cancer* 2000;89:177–180.
62. Dorfman HD, Czerniak B. *Osteosarcoma. Bone Tumors*. St Louis: CV Mosby; 1998:128–252.
63. Gurney JG, Severson RK, Davis S, Robison LL. Incidence of

cancer in children in the United States. *Cancer* 1995; 75:2186–2195.

64. Daw NC, Mahmoud HH, Meyer WH, et al. Bone sarcomas of the head and neck in children: the St. Jude Children's Research Hospital experience. *Cancer* 2000;88:2172–2180.
65. Newton WA, Meadows AT, Shimada H, et al. Bone sarcomas as second malignant neoplasms following childhood cancer. *Cancer* 1991;67:193–201.
66. Wong FL, Boice JD, Abramson DH, et al. Cancer incidence after retinoblastoma. Radiation dose and sarcoma risk. *JAMA* 1997;278:1262–1267.
67. Mohney, BG, Robertson, DM, Schomberg, PJ, Hodge, DO. Second nonocular tumors in survivors of heritable retinoblastoma and prior radiation therapy. *Am J Ophthalmol* 1998; 126:269–277.
68. Jaffe N, Frei E, Traggis D, Bishop Y. Adjuvant methotrexate and citrovorum-factor treatment of osteogenic sarcoma. *N Engl J Med* 1974;291:994–997.
69. Cortes EP, Holland JF, Wang JJ, et al. Amputation and Adriamycin in primary osteosarcoma. *N Engl J Med* 1974;291: 998–1000.
70. Meyers PA, Gorlick R, Heller G, et al. Intensification of preoperative chemotherapy for osteogenic sarcoma: results of the Memorial Sloan-Kettering (T12) protocol. *J Clin Oncol* 1998; 16:2452–2458.
71. Meyer WH, Pratt CB, Poquette CA, et al. Carboplatin/ifosfamide window therapy for osteosarcoma: results of the St Jude Children's Research Hospital OS-91 trial. *J Clin Oncol* 2001;19:171–182.
72. Guthrie TH Jr, Porubsky ES. Successful systemic chemotherapy of advanced squamous and basal cell carcinoma of the skin with *cis*-diamminedichloroplatinumIII and doxorubicin. *Laryngoscope* 1982;92:1298–1299.
73. Guthrie TH Jr, McElveen LJ, Porubsky ES, Harmon JD. Cisplatin and doxorubicin. An effective chemotherapy combination in the treatment of advanced basal cell and squamous cell carcinoma of the skin. *Cancer* 1985;55:1629–1632.
74. Guthrie TH Jr, Porubsky ES, Luxenberg MN, et al. Cisplatin-based chemotherapy in advanced basal and squamous cell carcinomas of the skin: results in 28 patients including 13 patients receiving multimodality therapy. *J Clin Oncol* 1990; 8:342–346.
75. Luxenberg MN, Guthrie TH Jr. Chemotherapy of basal cell and squamous cell carcinoma of the eyelids and periorbital tissues. *Ophthalmology* 1986;93:504–510.
76. Greenway HT, Cornell RC, Tanner DJ, et al. Treatment of basal cell carcinoma with intralesional interferon. *J Am Acad Dermatol* 1986;15:437–443.
77. Lamont EB, Vokes EE. Chemotherapy in the management of squamous-cell carcinoma of the head and neck. *Lancet Oncol* 2001:2;261–269.
78. Regine WF, Valentino J, Arnold SM, et al. A phase II study of concomitant hyperfractionated radiation therapy and double dose intra-arterial cisplatin for squamous cell carcinoma of the head and neck. *Technol Cancer Res Treat* 2002;1:133–140.
79. Marcu L, van Doorn T, Olver I. Cisplatin and radiotherapy in the treatment of locally advanced head and neck cancer—a review of their cooperation. *Acta Oncol* 2003;42:315–325.
80. Argiris A, Smith SM, Stenson K, et al. Concurrent chemotherapy for N2 or N3 squamous cell carcinoma of the head and neck from an occult primary. *Ann Oncol* 2003;14:1306–1311.
81. Haddad R, Colevas AD, Tishler R, et al. Docetaxel, cisplatin and 5-fluorouracil-based induction chemotherapy in patients with locally advanced squamous cell carcinoma of the head and neck: the Dana-Farber Cancer Institute experience. *Cancer* 2003;97:412–418.
82. Haddad R, Tishler RB, Norris CM, et al. Docetaxel, cisplatin, 5-fluorouracil (TPF)-based induction chemotherapy for head and neck cancer and the case for sequential, combined-modality treatment. *Oncologist* 2003;8:35–44.
83. Tishler RB, Norris CM, Colevas AD, et al. A phase I/II trial of concurrent docetaxel and radiation after induction of chemotherapy in patients with poor prognosis squamous cell carcinoma of the head and neck. *Cancer* 2002;95: 1472–1481.
84. Glisson BS, Murphy BA, Frentte G, et al. Phase II trial of docetaxel and cisplatin in patients with squamous cell carcinoma of the head and neck. *J Clin Oncol* 2002;20:1593–1599.
85. Hitt R, Paz-Ares L, Brandariz A, et al. Induction chemotherapy with paclitaxel, cisplatin, and 5-fluorouracil for squamous cell carcinoma of the head and neck: long-term results of a phase II trial. *Ann Oncol* 2002;13:1665–1673.
86. Wang HM, Wang CS, Chen JS, et al. Cisplatin, tegafur, leucovorin: a moderately effective and minimally toxic outpatient neoadjuvant chemotherapy for locally advanced squamous cell carcinoma of the head and neck. *Cancer* 2002;94: 2989–2995.
87. Robert F, Ezekiel MP, Spencer SA, et al. Phase I study of anti-epidermal growth factor receptor antibody cetuximab in combination with radiation therapy in patients with advanced head and neck cancer. *J Clin Oncol* 2001;19:3234–3243.
88. Kies MS, Harari PM. Cetuximab (Imclone/Merck/ Bristol-Myers Squibb). *Curr Opin Invest Drugs* 2002;3:1092–1100.
89. Baselga J. The EGFR as a target for anticancer therapy—focus on cetuximab. *Eur J Cancer* 2001;37(suppl 4):S16–S22.
90. Frucht-Pery J, Rozenman Y. Mitomycin C therapy for corneal intraepithelial neoplasia. *Am J Ophthalmol* 1994;117:164–168.
91. Heigle TJ, Stulting RD, Palay DA. Treatment of recurrent conjunctival epithelial neoplasia with topical mitomycin C. *Am J Ophthalmol* 1997;124:397–399.
92. Wilson MW, Hungerford JL, George SM, Madreperla SA. Topical mitomycin C for the treatment of conjunctival and corneal epithelial dysplasia and neoplasia. *Am J Ophthalmol* 1997;124:303–311.
93. Yeatts RP, Ford JG, Stanton CA, Reed JW. Topical 5-fluorouracil in treating epithelial neoplasia of the conjunctiva and cornea. *Ophthalmology* 1995;102:1338–1344.
94. de Keizer RJ, de Wolff-Rouendaal D, van Delft JL. Topical application of 5-fluorouracil in premalignant lesions of cornea, conjunctiva and eyelid. *Doc Ophthalmol* 1986;64:31–42.
95. Danopoulos ED, Danopoulou IE, Lairikos SB, Merkuris KM. Effects of urea treatment on malignancies of the conjunctiva and cornea. *Ophthalmologica* 1979;178:198–203.
96. Ferry AP, Meltzen MA, Taub RN. Immunotherapy with dinitrochlorobenzene (DCNB) for recurrent squamous cell carcinoma of conjunctiva. *Trans Am Ophthalmol Soc* 1976;74: 154–171.
97. Font RL. Eyelids and lacrimal drainage system. In: Spencer WH, ed. *Ophthalmic Pathology: An Atlas and Textbook*. 4th ed. Philadelphia: WB Saunders; 1996:2270–2278.
98. Wilson MW, Fleming JC, Fleming RM, Haik BG. Sentinel node biopsy for orbital and adnexal tumors. *Ophthalmic Plast Reconstr Surg* 2001;17:338–345.
99. Esmaeli B. Sentinel lymph node mapping for patients with cutaneous and conjunctival malignant melanoma. *Ophthalmic Plast Reconstr Surg* 2000;16:170–172.
100. Ridolfi R, Tanganelli L, Scelzi E, et al. (Italian Melanoma Intergroup). Chemotherapy and bio-chemotherapy in patients with advanced melanoma: combination therapy with nitrosourea. *J Chemother* 2003;15:198–202.
101. Keilholz U, Gore ME. Biochemotherapy for advanced melanoma. *Semin Oncol* 2002;29:456–461.
102. Flaherty LE, Atkins M, Sosman J, et al. Outpatient biochemotherapy with interleukin-2 and interferon alpha-2b in

patients with metastatic melanoma: results in two phase II cytokine working group trials. *J Clin Oncol* 2001;19:3194–3202.

103. Hakansson A, Hakansson L, Gustafsson B, et al. On the effect of biochemotherapy in metastatic malignant melanoma: an immunopathological evaluation. *Melanoma Res* 2003;13: 401–407.
104. Agarwala SS, Kirkwood JM. Update on adjuvant interferon therapy for high-risk melanoma. *Oncology (Huntington)* 2002;16: 1177–1187.
105. Dillman RO, Wiemann M, Nayak SK, et al. Interferon-gamma and granulocyte-macrophage colony stimulating factor administered as adjuvants with a vaccine of autologous tumors cells from short-term cell line culture: a randomized phase 2 trial of the cancer biotherapy research group. *J Immunother* 2003;26:367–373.
106. Dranoff G. GM-CSF secreting melanoma vaccines. *Oncogene* 2003;22:3188–3192.
107. Baroody M, Hartstein ME, Holds JB. Immunotherapy for melanoma metastatic to the orbit. *Ophthal Plast Reconstr Surg* 2003;19:270–274.
108. Folberg R. Melanocytic lesions of the conjunctiva. In: Spencer WH, ed. *Ophthalmic Pathology: An Atlas and Textbook*. 4th ed. Philadelphia: WB Saunders; 1996:125–147.
109. Finger PT, Czechnoska G, Liarikos S. Topical mitomycin C chemotherapy for conjunctival melanoma and PAM with atypia. *Br J Ophthalmol* 1998;82:476–479.
110. Frucht-Pery J, Peer J. Use of mitomycin C in the treatment of conjunctival primary acquired melanosis with atypia. *Arch Ophthalmol* 1996;114:1261–1264.
111. Gündüz K, Shields CL, Shields JA, et al. Plaque radiotherapy for management of ciliary body and choroidal melanoma with extraocular extension. *Am J Ophthalmol* 2000;130:97–102.
112. Savier E, Azoulay D, Huguet E, et al. Percutaneous isolated hepatic perfusion for chemotherapy: a phase I study. *Arch Surg* 2003;138:325–332.
113. Rothbarth J, Woutersen RA, Sparidans RW, et al. Melphalan antitumor efficacy and hepatotoxicity: the effect of variable infusion duration in the hepatic artery. *J Pharmacol Exp Ther* 2003;305:1098–1103.
114. Christoforidis D, Martinet O, Lejeune FJ, Mosimann F. Isolated liver perfusion for non-resectable liver tumours: a review. *Eur J Surg Oncol* 2002;28:875–890.
115. Chabner BA, Allegra CJ, Curt GA, Calabresi P. Chemotherapy of antineoplastic agents. In: Hardman JG, Limbard LE, eds. *The Pharmacologic Basis of Therapeutics*. 9th ed. New York: McGraw-Hill; 1996:1233–1287.
116. Fukamichi Y, Hikita N. Ocular complications following pterygium operation and installation of mitomycin C. *Folia Ophthalmol Jpn* 1981;32:197–201.
117. Yamanouchi U, Takaku I, Tsuda N. Scleromalacia presumably due to mitomycin C instillation after pterygium excision. *Jpn J Clin Ophthalmol* 1979;33:139–144.
118. Long R, Gardam M. Tumor necrosis factor-alpha inhibitors and the reactivation of latent tuberculosis infection. *Can Med Assoc J* 2003;168:1153–1156.
119. Natea MG, Radastake T, Joosten LA, et al. Salmonella septicemia in rheumatoid arthritis patients receiving anti-tumor necrosis factor: association with decreased interferon-gamma production and *Toll*-like receptor 4 expression. *Arthritis Rheum* 2003;48:1853–1855.
120. Foroozan R, Buono LM, Sergott RC, Savino PJ. Retrobulbar optic neuritis associated with infliximab. *Arch Ophthalmol* 2002;120:985–987.
121. Mohan N, Edwards ET, Cupps TR, et al. Demyelination occurring during anti-tumor necrosis factor alpha therapy for inflammatory arthritides. *Arthritis Rheum* 2001;44:2862–2869.
122. Burton C, Kaczmarski R, Jan-Mohamed R. Interstitial pneumonitis related to rituximab therapy. *N Engl J Med* 2003;348: 2690–2691.
123. Lowndes S, Darby A, Mead G, Lister A. Stevens–Johnson syndrome after treatment with rituximab. *Ann Oncol* 2002;13: 1948–1950.
124. Yang H, Rosove MH, Figlin RA. Tumor lysis syndrome occurring after the administration of rituximab in lymphoproliferative disorders: high-grade non-Hodgkin's lymphoma and chronic lymphocytic leukemia. *Am J Hematol* 1999;62:247–250.

Index